# Nursing

# HERBAL MEDICINE HANDBOOK

# Nursing

# HERBAL MEDICINE HANDBOOK

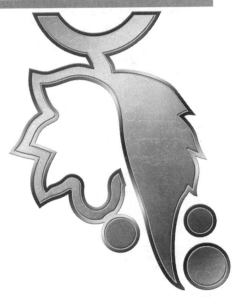

Springhouse Corporation
Springhouse, Pennsylvania

# Staff

**Senior Publisher**
Donna O. Carpenter

**Editorial Director**
William J. Kelly

**Clinical Director**
Marguerite S. Ambrose, RN, MSN, CS

**Creative Director**
Jake Smith

**Art Director**
Elaine Kasmer Ezrow

**Drug Information Editor**
Tracy Roux, RPh, PharmD

**Senior Associate Editor**
Ann E. Houska

**Clinical Project Editor**
Eileen Cassin Gallen, RN, BSN

**Editors**
Rita M. Doyle, Catherine Harold,
Peter Johnson

**Clinical Editors**
Heather Rischel Burcher, RN; Margaret
Friant Cramer, RN, MSN; Christine M.
Damico, RN, MSN, CPNP; Nancy Laplante,
RN, BSN; Lori Musolf Neri, RN, MSN,
CCRN, CRNP; Kimberly A. Zalewski, RN,
MSN, CEN

**Copy Editor**
Leslie Dworkin

**Designers**
Arlene Putterman (associate design
director), Joseph John Clark, David
Beverage, Susan Hopkins Rodzewich

**Typographers**
Diane Paluba (manager), Joy Rossi Biletz

**Manufacturing**
Patricia K. Dorshaw (manager), Otto
Mezei (book production manager)

**Editorial Assistants**
Carol A. Caputo, Arlene Claffee, Beth
Janae Orr

**Indexer**
Deborah K. Tourtlotte

Visit our website at NDHnow.com

ISBN 1-58255-100-6
NHMH-D    N O S A J J M A M F J
03 02 01  04 10 9 8 7 6 5 4 3 2 1

**Library of Congress Cataloging-in-Publication Data**

Nursing herbal medicine handbook.
    p.;cm.
    Includes bibliographical references and index.
    1. Herbs – Therapeutic use – Handbooks, manuals, etc. 2. Nursing – Handbooks, manuals, etc.
I. Lippincott Williams & Wilkins. Springhouse Division.
    [DNLM: 1. Medicine, Herbal – Handbooks.
WB 39 N9747 2001]
RM666.H33 N87 2001
615'.321 – dc21               00-066120
ISBN 1-58255-100-6 (casebound)

# Contents

# Clinical contributors and consultants

*At the time of publication, the contributors and consultants held the following positions.*

**Aimee F. Ansari, PharmD**
Assistant Professor of Clinical
  Pharmacy
St. John's University College of
  Pharmacy and Allied Health
  Professions
Jamaica, N.Y.

**Denise L. Balog, PharmD**
Assistant Professor of Clinical
  Pharmacy
St. John's University College of
  Pharmacy and Allied Health
  Professions
Jamaica, N.Y.

**Julie F. Barnes, RPh, PharmD**
Clinical Specialist, Nephrology
Clinical Assistant Professor
Medical University of South
  Carolina
Charleston, S.C.

**L. Ronald Batcheller, RPh, MBA**
Pharmacist Consultant
RBS Consulting
Minneapolis

**Maryam Behta, RPh, PharmD**
Clinical Coordinator, Infectious
  Diseases
New York Presbyterian Hospital
New York

**Dawna Benanchietti, RN, MSN**
Clinical Office Manager
MCP Hahnemann
  University-Partnership
Philadelphia

**Charles R. Bonapace, PharmD**
Pharmacotherapy Fellow,
  Infectious Diseases
Medical University of South
  Carolina
Charleston, S.C.

**Michael Briggs, RPh, PharmD**
Pharmacist, Co-owner
Lionville Natural Pharmacy
Exton, Pa.

**Yoon Ju Cha, RPh, PharmD**
Clinical Pharmacist
Johns Hopkins Hospital,
  Medicine/Surgery Pharmacy
Baltimore

**Dina M. Cheiman, PharmD**
Biomedical Writer, Assistant
  Professor
University of Michigan, College
  of Medicine and Surgery
Walled Lake, Mich.

**Barbara S. Chong, PharmD, BCPS**
Assistant Professor and Clinical
  Pharmacist
Medical University of South
  Carolina
Charleston, S.C.

**Linda M. Eugenio Clark, PharmD**
Assistant Professor of Clinical
  Pharmacy
Massachusetts College of
  Pharmacy and Health Sciences
Boston

**Wendell L. Combest, PhD**
Associate Professor,
  Biopharmaceutical Sciences
Shenandoah University School of
  Pharmacy
Winchester, Va.

**Jason C. Cooper, PharmD**
Assistant Professor
Medical University of South
  Carolina
Charleston, S.C.

**Ami Dansby, RPh**
Registered Pharmacist, Natural
  Medicine Consultant
Natural Alternatives
Greensboro, N.C.

**Teresa Dunsworth, PharmD,
BCPS**
Associate Professor of Clinical
  Pharmacy
West Virginia University School
  of Pharmacy
Morgantown, W.Va.

**Lana Dvorkin, RPh, PharmD**
Assistant Professor of Clinical
  Pharmacy
Massachusetts College of
  Pharmacy and Health Sciences
Boston

**Jerold H. Fleishman, MD, LAc**
Director of Clinical
  Neurophysiology; Section
  Chief, Department of
  Neurology
Franklin Square Hospital
Baltimore

**Nicole T. Galenas, PharmD**
Pediatric Clinical Pharmacist
Charleston Area Medical Center,
  Women and Children's Division
Charleston, W.Va.

**Tatyana Gurvich, PharmD**
Clinical Pharmacologist
Glendale Adventist Family
  Practice Residency Program
Glendale, Calif.

**Sheryl J. Herner, PharmD**
Assistant Professor of Pharmacy
  Practice
University of Wyoming
  School of Pharmacy
Laramie, Wyo.

**AnhThu Hoang, PharmD**
Clinical Coordinator,
  Infectious Diseases
New York Presbyterian Hospital
New York

**Scott Hodges, PharmD**
Clinical Pharmacist
Clark Memorial Hospital
Jeffersonville, Ind.

**Jennifer H. Justice, PharmD**
Clinical Assistant Professor of
  Pharmacy Practice
West Virginia University
Charleston, W.Va.

**Tina J. Kanmaz, PharmD**
Assistant Clinical Professor
St. John's University College of
  Pharmacy and Allied Health
  Professions
Jamaica, N.Y.

**Nishaminy Kasbekar, PharmD**
Clinical Specialist,
  Infectious Diseases
Presbyterian Medical Center
University of Pennsylvania
  Health System
Philadelphia

**Mary Kate Kelly, PharmD**
Manager, Ambulatory Care;
  Retail Pharmacist
Suburban Apothecary
Norristown, Pa.

**Julia N. Kleckner, RPh, PharmD**
Pharmacist
Mercy Community Hospital,
  Lionville Natural Pharmacy
Exton, Pa.

**Michelle Kosich, PharmD**
Mercy Community Hospital
Havertown, Pa.

**Gary L. Kracoff, RPh, BS**
Pharmacist, Owner
Bailey's Pharmacy
Allston, Mass.

**Susan A. Krikorian, RPh, MS**
Associate Professor of Clinical
  Pharmacy
Massachusetts College of
  Pharmacy and Health Sciences
Boston

**Robert J. Krueger, PhD**
Professor of Pharmacognosy
College of Pharmacy,
  Ferris State University
Big Rapids, Mich.

**Lisa M. Kutney, RPh, BS,
PharmD**
Medical Writer
Robbinsville, N.J.

**Mabel Lam, BS, PharmD**
Medical Information Specialist
Lyons Lavey Nickel Swift, Inc.
New York

**Kristi L. Lenz, PharmD**
Oncology Clinical Pharmacy
  Specialist and Assistant
  Professor
Medical University of South
  Carolina
Charleston, S.C.

**Heidi L. Liston, PharmD**
Clinical Research Fellow
  Pharmacokinetics/Pharmaco-
  dynamics of Psychoactive
  Agents
Medical University of South
  Carolina, Department of
  Psychiatry and Behavioral
  Sciences
Charleston, S.C.

**Yun Lu, PharmD**
Clinical Specialist
Hennepin County Medical
  Center
Minneapolis

**Kristy H. Lucas, PharmD**
Clinical Assistant Professor
West Virginia University,
  Schools of Pharmacy
  and Medicine
Charleston, S.C.

**Susan Luck, RN, BS, MA, HNC, CCN**
Holistic Nurse Consultant,
  Certified Clinical Nutritionist
Biodoron Immunology Center
Hollywood, Fla.

**Bonnie Mackey, MSN, ARNP, MTC, HNC**
Holistic Nurse Practitioner
Clinical Master Herbalogist and
  Herbalist
Mackey Health Institute, Inc. and
  Stoney Field Herbs
West Palm Beach, Fla.

**John S. Markowitz, PharmD, BCPP**
Assistant Professor, Department
  of Pharmaceutical Sciences
Medical University of South
  Carolina
Charleston, S.C.

**June H. McDermott, RPh, MSPharm, MBA, FASHP**
Clinical Assistant Professor,
  School of Pharmacy
University of North Carolina at
  Chapel Hill
Chapel Hill, N.C.

**Maryam R. Mohassel, PharmD**
Assistant Professor, Department
  of Pharmacy Practice
Long Island University
Arnold and Marie Schwartz
  College of Pharmacy and
  Health Sciences
Brooklyn, N.Y.

**Jane L. Murray, MD**
Medical Director
Sastun Center of Integrative
  Health Care
Mission, Kans.

**Jolynne Myers, RNCS, MSN, MSEd, ARNP**
Adult Nurse Practitioner
Independence Primary Care
Independence, Mo.

**George Nemecz, PhD**
Assistant Professor
Campbell University School of
  Pharmacy
Buies Creek, N.C.

**Steven G. Ottariano, RPh**
Clinical Herbal Pharmacist
V.A. Medical Center
Manchester, N.H.

**Robert Lee Page II, PharmD**
Assistant Professor, University of
  Colorado Health Sciences
  Center, School of Pharmacy
Denver

**June Riedlinger, RPh, PharmD**
Assistant Professor
Director, Center for Integrative
  Therapies in Pharmaceutical Care
Massachusetts College of
  Pharmacy and Health Sciences
Boston

**Sophie Robert, PharmD**
Practice Resident, Psychiatric
  Pharmacy
Medical University of South
  Carolina
Charleston, S.C.

**Ruthie Robinson, RN, MSN, CCRN, CEN**
Adjunct Instructor, Nursing
Lamar University
Beaumont, Tex.

**Michael S. Rocco, RPh**
Senior Medical Information
Specialist
Medical Information Source
New York

**Cynthia A. Ruiz, PharmD**
Assistant Professor of Pharmacy
Practice
St. Louis College of Pharmacy
St. Louis, Mo.

**Brian T. Sanderoff, PD**
Co-Director
Riverhill Wellness Center
Clarksville, Md.

**Cynthia A. Sanoski, PharmD**
Assistant Clinical Professor
St. John's University College of
Pharmacy and Allied Health
Professions
Jamaica, N.Y.

**Amy Sayner-Flusche, BSPharm, PharmD**
Geriatric Specialty Pharmacy
Resident
St. Louis College of Pharmacy
St. Louis, Mo.

**Sharon See, PharmD**
Assistant Clinical Professor
St. John's University,
College of Pharmacy
Jamaica, N.Y.

**Alexandra L. Stirling, PharmD**
Assistant Clinical Professor
St. John's University,
College of Pharmacy
Jamaica, N.Y.

**Maria A. Summa, BCPS, PharmD**
Assistant Professor of Clinical
Pharmacy
Massachusetts College of
Pharmacy and Health Sciences
Boston

**Dorota Szarlej, PharmD**
Clinical Pharmacist, Drug Use
Policy and Clinical Services
Thomas Jefferson University
Hospital
Philadelphia

**Nannette M. Turcasso, RPh, BCPS, PharmD**
Assistant Professor, Department
of Pharmacy Practice
Director, Drug Information
Medical University of South
Carolina, College of Pharmacy
Charleston, S.C.

**Amy M. VandenBerg, RPh, PharmD**
Pharmacy Practice Resident
Medical University of South
Carolina
Charleston, S.C.

**Laurie Willhite, RPh, PharmD**
Clinical Pharmacy Specialist,
Clinical Instructor
University of Minnesota College
of Pharmacy
Fairview University Medical
Center
Minneapolis

**Cindy J. Wordell, BS, PharmD**
Assistant Director of Pharmacy
  for Drug Use Policy and
  Clinical Services
Thomas Jefferson University
  Hospital
Philadelphia

**Lai Ha Yee, PharmD**
Distribution Coordinator
Carney Hospital, Inc.
Boston

# Preface

Disillusioned with traditional medicines, their costs, and their adverse effects, many people take treatment into their own hands and turn to herbal medicine. About 80% of the world's population use herbs and other dietary supplements for a variety of ailments. And nearly three-quarters of these people never inform their health care professionals that they use herbs.

Such unmonitored herb use can cause several problems. Whenever a patient adds a prescription medicine to the herbal chemical mixture he's already taking, the potential exists for the herbal base to raise or lower the levels of the prescribed drug significantly. Herbal medicines contain many pharmacologically active chemicals, which can conflict with the therapeutic goals of conventional drug regimens. Enhanced adverse effects can result if the herb and drug contain similar compounds. These facts raise many questions. For example, should a patient with diabetes or heart disease avoid a certain herb? Could there be an interaction between an herb and the conventional drug regimen the patient is following?

As a nurse, your first challenge is to elicit a detailed history from your patient, including his use of alternative medicines. Your second challenge is to find a reliable nursing reference that will give you information about the herb the patient is using and practical patient-teaching advice that you can give your patient.

Now, *Nursing Herbal Medicine Handbook,* which covers nearly 300 herbs, helps you meet these needs. The logical A-to-Z format lists herbs by their popular names, and the consistent layout of each monograph helps you locate the specific information you need right away. You'll find the information you need to teach your patient about the actions, common uses and dosages, adverse reactions, and interactions of the herb he's using. Facts about herb-drug, herb-herb, herb-food, and herb-lifestyle reactions are at your fingertips. You'll find out which herbs and which foods or medicines your patient should avoid if he's taking a certain herb because of the unpredictable, and potentially harmful, ways these substances can interact. In some cases, an entire herb is toxic, and only very small doses of it or certain parts of it can be tolerated.

This handbook is intended to give you information about herbs your patients may be using. But because these herbs and dietary supplements haven't been approved by the FDA and have no xiv

standard indications or dosages, this book neither recommends nor endorses their use.

If you keep this book handy during patient assessment, and remember to ask about your patient's herb intake early on, you'll be able to quickly spot potential dangers hidden in the use of these natural remedies.

# How to use this book

The *Nursing Herbal Medicine Handbook* provides comprehensive information on almost every herb used today, arranged alphabetically by popular name for easy access. This information was written and reviewed by pharmacists and nurses to provide a much-needed practical nursing handbook on herbs. The uses for each herb are listed, to give nurses a solid background on everything from basic pharmacology to management of toxicity and overdose.

In each self-inclusive entry, the herb's popular name is followed by a list of alternative popular names, which precedes an alphabetical list of common trade names.

Next, *How supplied* describes the forms in which each herb is available and provides information on the parts of the herb that are used to manufacture the product. The preparations available for each herb are listed (for example, tablets, capsules, elixirs, teas, and extracts) with known dosage forms and strengths.

*Actions & components* details how each herb works, including its actions on body systems. An herb's anesthetic or stimulating effects, if any, can be found in this section. An asterisk following a liquid herbal formulation (such as tincture) indicates that the liquid may contain alcohol, an important fact when your patient is a child, a recovering alcoholic, or someone with other alcohol-related problems.

*Uses* lists the therapeutic claims for each herb. This section may help you determine why your patient is using the herb.

*Dosage & administration* includes information on the various forms of the herbs and the amounts reported to achieve the desired effects. Keep in mind that dosages may vary widely, depending on the indication, herbal form used, and literature cited.

*Adverse reactions* lists the undesirable effects that may result from use of the herb. These effects are arranged by body system (CNS, CV, EENT, GI, GU, Hematologic, Hepatic, Metabolic, Musculoskeletal, Respiratory, Skin, and Other). Adverse reactions not specific to a single body system (for example, the effects of hypersensitivity) are listed under Other. Life-threatening reactions are presented in ***bold italic*** type.

The *Interactions* section provides cautions against potentially significant additive, synergistic, or antagonistic effects that may result from combined use of the herb with other elements. Interactions are broken down into four categories: herb-drug, herb-herb, herb-food, and herb-lifestyle. The interacting agent is italicized.

*Cautions* lists situations in which the patient shouldn't use the herb. These include hypersensitivity, pregnancy, breast-feeding, and certain diseases, as well as the presence of other drugs or herbs.

*Nursing considerations* offers practical information regarding herb use. An "Alert" logo signals cautionary tips and warnings on the toxic effects of certain herbs, life-threatening results of taking an herb in high doses, and herbs that have poisonous components.

*Patient teaching* contains points for the patient who is taking a particular herb, such as the signs of toxicity and the importance of alerting his pharmacist to any herbal medicine he's taking before having a new prescription filled.

To earn continuing education contact hours based on the information in this book, visit NDHnow.com, the web site of the Nursing Drug Handbook series.

| | | | | |
|---|---|---|---|---|
| AIDS | acquired immuno-deficiency syndrome | | GGT | gamma glutamyl-transferase |
| ALT | alanine aminotrans-ferase | | G6PD | glucose-6-phosphate dehydrogenase |
| AST | aspartate aminotrans-ferase | | GI | gastrointestinal |
| | | | gtt | drops |
| ATP | adenosine triphosphate | | GU | genitourinary |
| AV | atrioventricular | | HIV | human immuno-deficiency virus |
| AZT | zidovudine | | | |
| b.i.d. | twice a day | | h.s. | at bedtime |
| BPH | benign prostatic hyper-plasia | | I.D. | intradermal |
| | | | I.M. | intramuscular |
| BUN | blood urea nitrogen | | INR | international normal-ized ratio |
| cAMP | cyclic 3',5' adenosine monophosphate | | | |
| | | | IU | international unit |
| CBC | complete blood count | | I.V. | intravenous |
| CK | creatine kinase | | kg | kilogram |
| CNS | central nervous system | | L | liter |
| COPD | chronic obstructive pulmonary disease | | LD | lactate dehydrogenase |
| | | | $m^2$ | square meter |
| CPR | cardiopulmonary resuscitation | | MAO | monoamine oxidase |
| | | | mcg | microgram |
| CSF | cerebrospinal fluid | | mEq | milliequivalent |
| CV | cardiovascular | | mg | milligram |
| CVA | cerebrovascular accident | | MI | myocardial infarction |
| | | | ml | milliliter |
| CVP | central venous pressure | | $mm^3$ | cubic millimeter |
| DIC | disseminated intravas-cular coagulation | | ng | nanogram (millimicro-gram) |
| DNA | deoxyribonucleic acid | | NG | nasogastric |
| ECG | electrocardiogram | | NSAID | nonsteroidal anti-inflammatory drug |
| EEG | electroencephalogram | | | |
| FDA | Food and Drug Administration | | OTC | over-the-counter |
| | | | P.O. | by mouth |
| g | gram | | P.R. | per rectum |
| G | gauge | | p.r.n. | as needed |
| GFR | glomerular filtration rate | | PT | prothrombin time |
| | | | PTT | partial thromboplastin time |

| | |
|---|---|
| PVC | premature ventricular contraction |
| q | every |
| q.d. | every day |
| q.i.d. | four times a day |
| RBC | red blood cell |
| RNA | ribonucleic acid |
| SA | sinoatrial |
| S.C. | subcutaneous |
| SIADH | syndrome of inappropriate antidiuretic hormone |
| S.L. | sublingually |
| SSRI | selective serotonin reuptake inhibitor |
| $T_3$ | triiodothyronine |
| $T_4$ | thyroxine |
| t.i.d. | three times a day |
| UTI | urinary tract infection |
| WBC | white blood cell |

# Overview of Herbal Medicine

For thousands of years, cultures around the world have used herbs and plants to treat illness and maintain health. What's more, archaeological evidence shows that prehistoric man had a basic healing flora from which he selected remedies.

Many drugs prescribed today are derived from plants that cultures used for medicinal purposes. (The word *drug* comes from the Old Dutch word *drogge* meaning "to dry" because pharmacists, doctors, and ancient healers commonly dried plants for use as medicines.) In fact, about one-fourth of all conventional drugs—including about 120 of the most commonly prescribed modern drugs—contain at least one active ingredient derived from plants. The rest are chemically synthesized. (See *Common plant-based drugs*.)

Herbs and plants are valuable not only for their active ingredients but also for their minerals, vitamins, volatile oils, glycosides, alkaloids, acids, alcohols, and esters. And these components come from all parts of the plant—including the leaves, flowers, stems, berries, seeds, fruit, bark, and roots.

The World Health Organization estimates that 80% of the world's population uses some herbal remedy. Still, health care providers in the United States are largely unaware of which herbal remedies are successful, and many patients are reluctant to reveal their use of such remedies to their health care providers.

Today, however, renewed interest in all forms of alternative medicine is encouraging patients, health care providers, and drug

## Common plant-based drugs

Many drugs commonly used today have botanical origins.

| Drug | Therapeutic class | Botanical origin |
|---|---|---|
| aspirin | Analgesic | White willow bark and acid meadowsweet plant |
| atropine | Antiarrhythmic | Belladonna leaves |
| codeine, morphine | Potent narcotics | Opium poppy |
| colchicine | Antigout drug | Autumn crocus |
| digoxin | Antiarrhythmic | Foxglove, a poisonous plant |
| ephedrine | Bronchodilator | Ephedra |
| paclitaxel | Antineoplastic | Yew tree |
| quinine | Antimalarial | Cinchona bark |
| vinblastine, vincristine | Anticarcinogens | Periwinkle |

researchers to reexamine the value of herbal remedies. One of the most newsworthy plants being studied is St. John's wort. This perennial herb, commonly used in Europe as a tonic for anxiety and depression, contains xanthones and flavonoids that act as MAO inhibitors.

Because of the staggering number of stories touting herbal remedies in the media, you're likely to encounter patients who have read claims about certain herbs and who want your opinion about them. This chapter provides a general overview of the subject.

## History of herbal medicine

Also known as *phytotherapy* or *phytomedicine* (especially in Europe), herbal medicine has been practiced since the beginning of recorded history, with specific remedies being handed down from generation to generation. In ancient times, medicinal plants were chosen because of their color or the shape of their leaves. For example, heart-shaped leaves were used for heart problems, and plants with red flowers were used to treat bleeding disorders. This approach is known as the *Doctrine of Signatures.* The best use for each plant was determined by trial and error.

The formal study of herbs, known as *herbology,* goes back to the ancient cultures of the Middle East, Greece, China, and India. These cultures revered the power of nature and developed herbal remedies based on the plants that were found in their home environ-

ments. Written evidence of the medicinal use of herbs has been found on Mesopotamian clay tablets and ancient Egyptian papyrus.

The first known compilation of herbal remedies was ordered by the king of Sumeria around 2000 B.C. and included 250 medicinal substances, including garlic. Ancient Greece and Rome produced their own compilations, including the *De Materia Medica,* written in the 1st century A.D. Of the 950 medicinal products described in this work, 600 are derived from plants and the rest from animal or mineral sources. The Arab world added its own discoveries to the Greco-Roman texts, resulting in a compilation of more than 2,000 substances that was eventually reintroduced to Europe by Christian doctors traveling with the Crusaders.

Herbal therapy is also a major component of India's Ayurvedic medicine, traditional Chinese medicine, Native American medicine, homeopathy, and naturopathy.

In the United States, herbal remedies handed down from European settlers and learned from Native Americans were a mainstay of medical care until the early 1900s. The rise of technology and the biomedical approach to health care eventually led to the decline of herbal medicine. However, interest in herbal preparations has been revived in the United States for various reasons, including general disillusionment with modern medicine, the high cost and adverse effects of prescription drugs, the widespread availability of herbal drugs, and increased interest in self-care.

## Regulation

In 19th century America, many bogus remedies were sold to gullible, desperate people. The federal government finally took action against disreputable purveyors of phony remedies with the Food and Drug Act of 1906. This law addressed problems of mislabeling and adulteration of plant remedies but didn't address safety and effectiveness.

Today, regulatory bodies are reviewing herbal remedies on a regular basis, and laws are providing guidelines for their labeling. The FDA regulates herbal remedies as dietary supplements, not drugs. This means the FDA can challenge any herbal product that has proven to be harmful. The Dietary Supplement Health and Education Act of 1994 (DSHEA) requires that the contents of herbal remedies be indicated on the label. It also permits manufacturers and marketers of dietary supplements to make limited claims regarding their health benefits. For herbs and other supplements that don't provide nutritional support in a conventional nutritional manner, the law allows the manufacturer to make claims about how the product affects the body's structure or function. However, labels can't claim that the herbal remedy can treat, mitigate, prevent, or cure a disease or condition, nor can they mention a specific pathologic condition.

So, when it comes to buying herbal remedies in the United States, the message is "Buyer beware." Consumers should be well informed about the herbal products they plan to use and should seek advice from a trained practitioner before trying a product, especially for a serious condition. (See *Herbal remedies: Patient precautions,* pages 4 and 5.)

In Europe, millions of people use herbal and homeopathic remedies. Government bodies and the scientific community are much more open to natural remedies, especially those that have a long history of use. In Great Britain and France, traditional medicines that have been used for years with no serious adverse effects are approved for use under the "doctrine of reasonable certainty" when scientific evidence is lacking.

Also, the European Economic Community has established guidelines that standardize the quality, dosage, and production of herbal remedies. These guidelines are based on the World Health Organization's 1991 publication *Guidelines for the Assessment of Herbal Medicines,* which addresses concerns about the safety and efficacy of herbal medicines and establishes guidelines for pharmacopoeia monographs. (See *World Health Organization guidelines*, page 6.)

## Therapeutic uses

Herbal remedies are used primarily to treat minor health problems, such as nausea, colds and flu, coughs, headaches, aches and pains, GI disorders such as consti-

## Herbal remedies: Patient precautions

Many patients take for granted the safety of the foods and drugs they purchase. However, if your patient is taking or is considering taking any herbal remedies, he should be aware that no government agency reviews these products for quality, dosage, safety, or efficacy. Also, advise him of the general precautions and specific warnings listed below.

### General precautions

● Advise your patient to consult with his health care provider before using any herbal product, especially if he's also taking a prescription drug. Also, tell him to inform his herbalist of any prescription drugs he's taking. Many herbal remedies contain chemical substances that can interact with other drugs.

● Caution the patient that the FDA regulates herbal products only as food supplements, not as drugs. Labels on the products should contain information about product ingredients and use; however, ultimately, he and his health care provider are responsible for keeping informed and monitoring the risks, adverse effects, and possible harmful interactions with other substances.

● Tell your patient that herbal products may contain ingredients other than those indicated on the label. For example, one brand of Siberian ginseng capsules was found to contain a weed full of male hormone-like chemicals. Regulatory agencies continue to monitor product contents and labeling.

● Remind the patient that each person metabolizes and absorbs botanical and synthetic drugs differently, so there's no way to know whether the herb is in a form that his body can absorb or whether the recommended dosage on the label is right for him.

● Inform your patient that most botanical products sold in the United States haven't been scientifically tested. Their claimed benefits are largely based on observation through systematic testing of substances on patients for the purpose of learning more about the action of the herb.

● Tell your patient that commercially grown herbs are subject to contamination from pesticides, polluted water, and automobile exhaust fumes.

● Inform your patient that the quantity of the active ingredient varies from brand to brand—and possibly from bottle to bottle—within a particular brand.

● Caution the patient that products promising to cure specific health problems earn a red flag. Labeling laws prohibit claims of treating, mitigating, preventing, or curing a disease or condition.

● Advise your patient not to take herbal products for serious or potentially serious medical conditions, such as heart disease or bleeding disorders, unless they're used under the care of a well-trained health care provider.

● Advise the patient to seek guidance from a knowledgeable and experienced health care provider before using herbal preparations before, during, or after pregnancy or breast-feeding because many of the effects of the herbs on the fetus are unknown. Listings of the herbs indicated and contraindicated in each of the three trimesters of pregnancy, as well as for breast-feeding, are available.

● Caution the patient that many herbal remedies containing two or more herbs, also known as compounded herbal remedies, haven't been adequately researched.

● Advise the patient to be informed of reputable herbal companies and cautious about products sold through magazines, brochures, the broadcast media, or the Internet.

● Tell the patient to talk to a health care provider who's well-trained in herbology when in doubt about using herbal remedies—and to remember that the clerk at the health food store is a salesperson, not a trained practitioner.

## Warnings about specific products

● *Bloodroot*—which is promoted as an expectorant, purgative, stimulant, diaphoretic, plaque and cavity preventer, and treatment for rheumatism—is used in such a range of doses that it can be dangerous, and fatal if used as an emetic.

● *Chaparral tea*, which is promoted as an antioxidant and a pain reliever, may cause liver failure.

● *Coltsfoot*, which is used for respiratory problems, may cause liver problems and cancer.

● *Comfrey*, which is used for arthritis, may cause liver problems and cancer.

● *Indian herbal tonics* may cause lead poisoning.

● *Jin bu huan*, an ancient Chinese sedative and analgesic, contains morphinelike substances and may contribute to hepatitis.

● *Kombucha tea*, which is made from mushroom cultures and used as a cure-all, can cause death from acidosis.

● *Lobelia*, which is used to treat respiratory congestion, may contribute to respiratory paralysis and death.

● *Ma huang*, or *ephedra*, an ingredient in many diet pills, is a potentially dangerous drug because it can raise blood pressure and produce an irregular heartbeat. Also sold under such names as Herbal Ecstasy, Cloud 9, and Ultimate Xphoria to induce a high, it can cause heart attacks, seizures, psychotic behavior, and even death.

● *Mistletoe* has been falsely touted as a cure for cancer.

● *Pau d'Arco tea* has been falsely touted as a cure for cancer and AIDS.

● *Pennyroyal*, which is used to treat coughs and upset stomach, may have toxic effects on the liver, inhibiting blood clotting. Use of its essential oil has been fatal.

● *Sassafras*—which is a tonic used for fever reduction, skin disorders, and rheumatism—has been banned in the United States for causing liver damage and has been implicated in narcotic poisoning and accidental abortion.

● *Yohimbe bark*, which is used as an aphrodisiac, can severely lower blood pressure and may contribute to psychotic behavior.

## World Health Organization guidelines

In 1991, the World Health Organization (WHO) published Guidelines for the Assessment of Herbal Medicines, which establishes standards for determining the safety, quality, and efficacy of herbal preparations and the development of pharmacopoeia monographs. A summary of these guidelines appears below.

### Guidelines regarding safety
● If the product traditionally has been used without demonstrated harm, no specific restrictive action should be taken unless new evidence demands a revised risk-benefit assessment.
● Prolonged and apparently uneventful use of a substance is considered testimony to its safety.

### Guidelines regarding efficacy
● For treatment of minor disorders and for nonspecific indications, some relaxation is justified in the requirements for proof of efficacy, taking into account the extent of traditional use.
● The same considerations can apply to prophylactic use.

### Guidelines regarding pharmacopoeia monographs
● If a pharmacopoeia monograph exists, it should be sufficient to make reference to this monograph.
● If a monograph doesn't exist, one must be supplied and should be prepared in the same way as in an official pharmacopoeia.

### World Health Organization monographs
The WHO also published the WHO Monographs on Selected Medicinal Plants. This publication is used to validate the growing use of herbs, phytomedicines, and medicinal plant preparations as official medicines. An international team of scientific experts that the WHO assembled extensively reviewed the monographs. These monographs contain most of the elements needed to determine baseline standards for identity and quality and to assess the relative safety and efficacy of each medicinal plant. Monographs also have a therapeutics section that includes levels of medicinal uses—that is, those supported by clinical data, those described in pharmacopoeias and traditional systems of medicines, and those described in folk medicine but not supported by experimental or clinical data.

pation and diarrhea, menstrual cramps, insomnia, skin disorders, and dandruff. These therapeutic uses also serve as a way to categorize herbal remedies. (See *Herbal classifications,* page 8.)

Some herbalists have also reported success in treating certain chronic conditions—such as peptic ulcers, colitis, rheumatoid arthritis, hypertension, and respiratory problems, such as bronchitis and asthma—and illnesses usually treated only with prescription drugs, such as heart failure, hepatitis, and cirrhosis. However, advise any patient with a serious disorder who expresses an interest in herbal remedies not to discontinue ongoing medical treatment and to consult his health care provider about possible interactions between prescribed drugs and herbal remedies.

Numerous studies have been done on herbal remedies in Europe and Asia, where phytomedicine has a long history. European studies have shown that such herbs as ginkgo, bilberry, and milk thistle are beneficial in treating various chronic disorders. Chinese researchers have done extensive studies on many herbs, such as ginseng, ginger, foxglove, licorice, and wild chrysanthemum. Indian researchers using modern scientific methods recently studied various Ayurvedic herbs, including Indian gooseberry and turmeric. European researchers have broadly researched and published a comprehensive herbal guidebook, *The Complete German Commission E Monographs: Therapeutic Guide to Herbal Medicines.* Many health care providers, pharmaceutical companies, schools, and universities in the United States have adopted the English translation of it as an official herbal guidebook.

The United States lags behind other countries in herbal medicine research for a number of reasons:

● Until the establishment of the National Institutes of Health's Office of Alternative Medicine (OAM) in 1992, there was no federal support for research on natural remedies.

● Pharmaceutical companies have little financial incentive to develop herb-based drugs because botanical products can't be patented; therefore, the companies could never recoup their research investment.

● According to Western pharmaceutical standards, an inherent difficulty in studying herbs exists. These standards favor isolating a single active ingredient; however, herbs may contain several active ingredients that work together to produce a specific effect.

Despite the large gaps in research, many herbal medicine clinical trials are underway in the United States. The OAM has more than 110 research centers throughout the United States, established for the purpose of using credible scientific methods in research related to complementary medicine and health care. Collaborative research efforts among the OAM, National Institutes of Health, Office of Dietary Supplements, and many other organizations continue.

## Forms of herbal preparations

Herbs are available in various forms, depending on their medicinal purpose and the body system involved. They may be bought individually or in mixtures formulated for specific conditions. Herbs may be prepared as tinctures, extracts, capsules, tablets, lozenges, teas, juices, vapor treatments, and bath products. Some herbs are applied topically with a poultice or compress; others are rubbed into

## Herbal classifications

Herbs are commonly classified by their effects on patients, as follows:

- *Adaptogenic herbs* work on the adrenal gland to increase the body's resistance to illness.
- *Anthelminthic herbs* work to eliminate intestinal worms from the body.
- *Anti-inflammatory herbs* reduce the tissues' inflammatory response.
- *Antimicrobial herbs* boost the immune system by destroying disease-causing organisms or helping the body resist them.
- *Antispasmodic herbs* ease skeletal and smooth muscle cramps and tension.
- *Astringent herbs*, applied externally, work on the mucous membranes, skin, and other tissues to reduce inflammation, irritation, and the risk of infection.
- *Bitter herbs* work on the CNS, playing a major role in preventive medicine. Bitter herbs are recommended to increase the secretion of digestive juices, stimulate the appetite, and promote liver detoxification.
- *Carminative herbs* (aromatic oils) stimulate proper function of the digestive system, soothe the lining of the GI tract, and reduce gas, inflammation, and pain.
- *Delmucent herbs,* rich in mucilage, soothe and protect irritated or inflamed tissue and mucous membranes.
- *Diuretic herbs* increase the production and elimination of urine.
- *Emmenagogic herbs* stimulate menstrual flow.
- *Expectorant herbs* work to eliminate mucus from the lungs.
- *Hepatic herbs* work to increase the strength and tone of the liver, increase the flow of bile, and increase the production of hepatocytes.
- *Hypotensive herbs* work to decrease abnormally high blood pressure.
- *Laxative herbs* relieve constipation and promote digestion.
- *Nervine herbs* are divided into three groups based on their role in helping the nervous system: those that strengthen and restore, those that ease anxiety and tension, and those that stimulate nerve activity.
- *Stimulating herbs* stimulate the body's physiologic and metabolic activities.
- *Tonic herbs*, the foundation of traditional Chinese medicine and Ayurvedic (Indian) medicine, enliven and invigorate by promoting the "vital force," the key to health and longevity.

the skin as an oil, ointment, or salve.

### Tinctures and extracts

An herb placed in alcohol or liquid glycerin and reduced over time is known as a tincture or an extract. (Tinctures contain more alcohol than extracts.) The alcohol draws out the active chemical properties of the herb, concentrates it, and helps preserve it. The body easily absorbs alcohol. The full taste of the herb comes through in the alcohol and can be strong or unpleasant. Alcohol-based tinctures and extracts have a shelf life of 3 to 5 years.

Liquid glycerin extracts called *glycerites* are an alternative to alcohol extracts and are better suited to some patients. Glycerites are generally sweet and feel warm on the tongue. Glycerin is processed in the body as a fat, not a sugar, which is important to patients, such as diabetics, who must limit sugar intake. Patients should be aware that taking more than 1 oz (30 ml) of glycerin can have a laxative effect. In general, glycerin isn't an efficient solvent for most herbs, especially those that contain resins and gums. These herbs require alcohol for extraction.

Glycerin-based extracts should contain at least 60% glycerin with 40% water to ensure preservation. The shelf life of these extracts is shorter than that of alcohol-based extracts. An extract that contains citric acid can last for more than 2 years if stored properly.

Tinctures or extracts may be taken as drops in a tea, diluted in spring water, used in a compress, or applied during body massage. If the alcohol content of a tincture is a concern—for example, when administering the remedy to a child—a few drops may be placed in ¼ cup of very hot water and left to stand for 5 minutes. As the tincture stands, most of the alcohol evaporates and the mixture becomes cool enough to drink.

An herbal tincture is made by filling a glass bottle or jar with carefully calculated and weighed plant parts (cut fresh herbs or crumbled dry herbs); adding the appropriate amount of natural ethanol, such as vodka; sealing the container; and placing it in a warm area (70° to 80° F [21° to 27° C]) for 3 to 4 weeks. The mixture should be shaken daily. After 3 to 4 weeks, the herbs are strained, leaving the residue that contains the chemical constituents of the herb.

Extracts are also made with alcohol, water, or both to bring out the herb's essence. The product label should indicate which base was used. Extracts have about the same advantages and disadvantages as tinctures, except they're more concentrated and usually require less of a dose to be effective. Because of their strong herbal taste, they're usually diluted in juice or water.

## Capsules and tablets

Capsules and tablets contain the ground or powdered form of the raw herb and are much less potent than tinctures; however, they're easier to transport and generally tasteless. The capsule or tablet should be made within 24 hours of milling the herb because herbs degrade very quickly. The best products use fresh herbs, which should be indicated on the label. Capsules can be a hard or soft gel made of animal or vegetable gelatin. Most patients find capsules easier to swallow than tablets.

The patient should be aware that both capsules and tablets may contain a large amount of filler, such as soy or millet powder. Filler makes the herb difficult to identify in the powdered form, and a poorer quality herb may be substituted without the patient's knowledge. Tablets may also contain a binder, such as magnesium stearate or dicalcium phosphate, which may contain lead. Binders are used to help the herb absorb water and break down more readily for easy absorption by the body.

Capsules or tablets can be swallowed whole, as indicated, or they may be mixed with a spoonful of cream-style cereal or applesauce. They may also be dissolved in sweet fruit juice.

## Lozenges

Herbal lozenges are nutrient-rich, naturally sweetened preparations that dissolve in the mouth. They're available in various formulations, such as cough suppressant, decongestant, or cold fighting. Most lozenges have added vitamin C. One type that has become popular is the horehound lozenge, used to relieve coughs and minor throat irritation.

Lozenges should be taken as directed by a knowledgeable practitioner or as indicated on the package.

## Teas

Herbal teas, which can be made from most herbs, are used for various purposes, with formulations aimed at specific conditions or desired effects. These teas are generally prepared by infusion or decoction. An *infusion* is prepared by allowing a dried herb to steep in hot water for 3 to 5 minutes. A *decoction* is made by setting the herb into a gentle rolling boil of water

for 15 to 20 minutes, a method preferable for denser plant materials, such as roots or bark. Teas may be steeped in a muslin or conventional tea bag or tea ball or used in loose form for their fragrant, aromatic flavor.

Some teas, such as barberry, taste bitter because they contain alkaloids or, like oak bark, highly astringent tannins. In some cases, the bitterness promotes the digestive reflex, thereby stimulating the production of gastrin and cholecystokinin. The digestive reflex is commonly altered in people with liver, colon, or other digestive problems. Tasting the bitterness of the tea, then, becomes an important part of the treatment. For other patients, teas may be sweetened with the herbal sweetener Stevial or with honey. However, caution is needed when using honey in young children because of the risk of infant botulism.

For infants, the tea may be mixed with breast milk or formula, then put into a bottle, an eyedropper, or an empty syringe without a needle and gently squirted into the infant's mouth. If a breast-feeding mother takes an adult dose of an herbal remedy, the effect will be transmitted to her child through her breast milk.

The Chinese teach that the heat of the water and the taste of the herb enhance its effectiveness. Steeping an herb in hot water draws out its therapeutic essence. Generally, 1 to 2 heaping tablespoons of dried herb are used for each cup of tea, unless the product label says otherwise. The herbs should be placed in a china or glass teapot or cup, because plastic and metal containers are considered unsuitable for steeping; immersed in 8 oz of freshly boiled water for each cup; and covered.

Leaf or flower herbs are generally steeped for 5 to 10 minutes. Roots or bark are simmered or boiled for 10 minutes, then steeped for an additional 5 minutes. After steeping, the tea is strained and allowed to cool to a comfortable temperature before serving. If a tincture or extract is being placed in the tea, the cup of hot water should sit for 5 minutes to allow the alcohol to evaporate. Teas may be served hot, cold, or iced, depending on the purpose and according to instructions.

Five parts of a fresh herb generally equal one part of a dry herb. Bark, root, seeds, and resins must be powdered to break down the cell walls before they're added to water. Seeds should be slightly bruised to release the volatile oils from the cells. An aromatic herb may be infused in a pot with a tight lid to decrease the loss of volatile oil through evaporation. Because roots, wood, bark, nuts, and certain seeds are tough and their cell walls strong, they should be gently boiled in water to release their properties.

### Juices

Juices are made by washing fresh herbs under cold running water, cutting them into smaller-sized pieces with scissors, and then running them through a juice extractor until they turn into a liquid.

Juices are usually administered by placing a few drops in tea or spring water. They also may be applied externally by dabbing them on the affected part of the body. Ideally, fresh juices should be taken immediately after extraction; however, they may be stored in a small glass bottle, corked tightly, and refrigerated for several days without appreciable oxidation and loss of vital properties.

### Vapor and inhalation treatments

Used primarily for respiratory and sinus conditions, vapor and inhalation treatments open congested sinuses and lung passages, help discharge mucus, and ease breathing. One inhalation method requires a sink and an herbal oil. The sink is filled with very hot water and 2 to 5 gtt of the herbal oil are added. Hot water should be allowed to trickle into the sink to keep the water steaming. As the mixture becomes diluted, a few more drops of the herbal oil may be needed. The patient should deeply inhale the steam for 5 minutes and repeat three or four times a day.

Another method involves heating a large, wide pot of water, adding a handful of dried or fresh herbs, and bringing the pot to a low boil. After the herbs have simmered for 5 minutes, the pot is removed from the heat and placed on a trivet to cool slightly. If an aromatic oil is being used, the water is first heated to just short of boiling and then removed from the heat. With the pot on a trivet, the patient adds 4 or 5 gtt of the oil, then drapes a towel over his head to form a tent and leans over the pot, inhaling the steam for 5 minutes. If the vapor is too hot, it can burn the nasal passages.

## Herbal baths

If the herb is in a soluble medium, such as baking soda or aloe gel, it may be dissolved in hot bath water. If the herb is an oatmeal-type preparation, it may be finely milled or whirled into a powder in a blender. Fresh or dried herbs also can be bagged in a square of cheesecloth or placed in a washcloth and tied securely. The goal is maximum release of the herbal essence without having parts of the herb floating in the bath water. Full baths require about 6 oz of dried or fresh herbs.

As the tub fills with water, the bagged herbs are placed under a forceful stream of comfortably hot water, then dragged through the bath water to better distribute the herbal essence. Squeezing the bag releases a rich stream of essence that may be directed to the affected body part. The bag may also be gently rubbed over itching skin. Herbs with pointy or rough edges may be too irritating to use in this manner.

An herbal infusion can also be added to bath water. To make the infusion, soak 6 tbs of dried or fresh herbs overnight in 3 cups of boiled water. The cup is usually covered with a saucer. The next morning, the strained infusion can be poured directly into the bath water.

## Poultices and compresses

A *poultice* is a moist paste made from crushed herbs that is either applied directly to the affected area or wrapped in cloth to keep it in place and then applied. Poultices are especially useful in treating bruises, wounds, and abscesses. A *compress* is made by soaking a soft cloth in a strong herbal tea, a tincture or glycerite, an oil, or aromatic water and then wringing it out and applying it to the affected area. Compresses are very effective for bleeding, bruises, muscle cramps, and headaches.

Only fresh herbs should be used for poultices. One preparation method involves wrapping the herbs in a clean white cloth, such as gauze, linen, cotton, or muslin; folding the cloth several times; and then crushing the herbs to a pulp with a rolling pin. Pulping the herb directly onto the poultice cloth helps to retain its juices and improves the effectiveness of the poultice. The pulp is then exposed and applied to the affected area. Wrapping the entire area with a woolen cloth or towel will trap the herbal juices and hold them in place. This type of poultice can remain in place overnight.

The herbs also may be prepared by placing them in a steamer, colander, strainer, or sieve over a pot of rapidly boiling water and allowing the steam to penetrate and wilt the herbs. After 5 minutes, the softened, warmed herbs are spread on a clean white cloth, such as loosely woven cheesecloth, and the cloth is applied to the affected area. Wrapping the poultice with a woolen cloth or towel helps retain the heat. This type of poultice can be left on for 20 minutes or overnight if the patient finds the wrap comforting and soothing.

Making a compress usually involves soaking a linen or muslin cloth in an herbal infusion, then wringing the cloth, folding it, and applying it to the affected area. A bandage or plastic wrap may be used to hold the compress, which may be hot or cold, in place.

### Oils, ointments, salves, and rubs

Herbal oils are usually expressed from the peels of lemons, oranges, or other citrus fruits. Because they may irritate the skin, they're commonly diluted in fatty oils or water before being applied topically. Essential oils are used in massage and aromatherapy; diluted oils can be used to prevent skin irritation.

To make an oil, the fresh herbs are first washed and left to dry overnight. The herbs are then sliced or, if using dry herbs, crumbled; placed in a glass bottle or jar; and covered by about 1" of light virgin olive oil, almond oil, or sesame oil. The container is covered tightly and allowed to stand in a very warm area, such as on a stove or in the sunshine, for 2 weeks. The oil should be strained before use.

Herbal ointments, salves, and rubs are applied topically for various conditions. Some examples are calendula ointment for broken skin and wounds; goldenseal for infections, rashes, and skin irritations; aloe vera gel for minor burns; and heat-producing herbs for muscle aches and strains.

Ointments can be made in a ceramic or glass double-boiler by heating 2 oz of vegetable lanolin or beeswax until it liquefies. When the lanolin or wax has melted, 80 to 120 gtt of tincture are added and the compound is mixed together. The formula should then be poured into a glass container and refrigerated until it hardens.

### Visiting an herbalist

A visit to an herbalist begins with an evaluation that includes the patient's history. The herbalist may check the patient's pulse and tongue to assist in diagnosis and may perform a physical assessment. Some herbalists also assess the iris, a technique known as iridology, to aid in diagnosis; this procedure involves correlating minute markings on the iris with specific parts of the body.

Most herbalists also ask which drugs and herbs the patient is already taking, to help guard against interactions. For example, the herb St. John's wort, which is used as an antidepressant, shouldn't be taken with prescription antidepressants.

Like conventional health care providers, the herbalist asks whether the patient is pregnant or breast-feeding because certain herbs can induce miscarriage or be passed to the infant in breast milk, causing adverse reactions.

After the evaluation, the herbalist suggests individual herbs or combinations of herbs for the treatment of a particular condition.

Medicinal plants may be combined to increase their therapeutic effect, alter the individual actions of each herb, or minimize or negate toxic effects of stronger herbs. As with traditional drug combinations, herbal compounds have a synergy that allows the remedy to function more effectively. The art of herbal compounding has been practiced for more than 5,000 years and is the basis of today's herbal practice.

## Determining dosages

Dosages for herbal remedies have been established over the years, but these guidelines for quantity and frequency must be adjusted for each individual, based on factors such as age, weight, and use of other herbs or drugs. (See *Understanding herbal dosages*.)

Herbal remedies take time to work. The length of time a particular herb is used depends on whether it's being used as a therapy to relieve symptoms, a tonic to build strength, or both. An herb that's being used therapeutically may only be taken for a brief period—typically, 1 to 4 weeks. As with other drugs, herbs should be taken at certain times of the day. Some herbs are more effective when taken in the morning; others, in the evening.

An herbal remedy that's being used as a tonic generally requires a longer period of use—usually 4 to 6 months or longer. For example, hawthorn berry, a CV tonic, is most effective when used for 6 to 12 consecutive months.

Some herbs work best if used with a resting cycle. For example,

the patient might use an herb for 6 days, followed by 1 day off, 6 weeks on and 1 week off, 6 months on and 1 month off, or some similar pattern. The theory behind a resting cycle is that each period of rest from the herb treatment allows its effect to become integrated into the patient's physiology. If the desired effect doesn't appear in the specified time, or if adverse effects develop, the dosage or herb may be changed.

## Nursing perspective

Although the overall risk of herbal remedies to public health appears to be low, some traditional remedies have been associated with potentially serious adverse effects. For example, ma huang, an ingredient in numerous diet pills, contains the same active ingredient that's in the bronchodilator ephedrine and can cause irregular heartbeats, seizures, and even death.

If your patient is taking or considering taking an herbal remedy, make sure he understands the potential risks involved in treating himself. These include misdiagnosing his ailment, taking the wrong herb, worsening his condition by delaying conventional treatment, having the herbal drug counteract or interact with prescribed medical treatment, and aggravating other disorders.

Make sure your patient is aware of the actions and adverse effects of the herb he'll be taking *before* he begins taking it. Possible signs and symptoms of sensitivity or an adverse reaction include headache,

## Understanding herbal dosages

### Age and weight dosing

The *age-dosing guideline,* useful for treating infants and younger children, is based on organ maturity—the organ's ability to metabolize, use, and eliminate herbs. The *weight-to-dose guidelines* are based on the principle that the herb is distributed to different parts of the body. This method is used for patients who fall outside the normal weight range, requiring either an increased or decreased dose; however, it may not be reliable for very young children. It's similar to Clark's rule, which is used to verify pediatric dosages.

### Homeopathic prescribing

*Homeopathic prescribing* is based on the homeopathic principle of "like cures like." For example, cantharis or apis causes burning urination and kidney damage in high doses, but is given in low doses to treat UTIs and kidney disease.

### Pharmacologic prescribing

Most herbal dosages are set by a method called *pharmacologic prescribing,* in which the amount of a botanical preparation is sufficient to induce definite, visible, strong, sustained changes in the patient. The oldest dosage method and best represented by the British herbal tradition, pharmacologic prescribing can mask symptoms if the dose is improper or used too long.

### Physiologic prescribing

In *physiologic prescribing,* the herbalist recommends the minimum dosage of an herb required to induce a physiologic change. For example, he'd give a laxative only until a change in bowel action occurs.

### Prescribing herbal extracts

The standard dose of herbal extracts for the average adult is 6 g per day. However, this dose is only a guideline and may be modified for patients who aren't average sized.

### Wise woman prescribing

Based on ancient wisdom, *wise woman prescribing* is also known as folk herbalism. Herbs are taken in large doses like foods. The herbalist avoids strong, toxic, and rare plants, choosing those that grow freely and are close at hand.

upset stomach, and rash. Also, some patients are predisposed to react to particular herbs. For example, a patient with depressive symptoms shouldn't take certain herbs that treat insomnia—hops, for example—because they can heighten symptoms of depression. This warning may appear on the herbal remedy package, but there's no guarantee that all remedies will carry adequate warnings.

Advise your patient to discontinue using an herb if he develops an adverse reaction—such as headache, upset stomach, or rash—and to notify his health care provider.

Inform your patient that if his responses to an herb are favorable but too intense, he should decrease the dose or stop taking the herb altogether. For example, if the laxative he's taking for constipation causes diarrhea, he should stop taking the laxative.

If the patient is experiencing adverse effects, find out if he's using the correct herb, if he has been taking it too often, or if he has been using it for too long. Sometimes symptoms are related to incorrect dosage. For example, chamomile taken orally daily over an extended period may cause an allergy to ragweed. Also, taking black licorice in moderate to large quantities daily can lead to high blood pressure or intraocular pressure.

Many patients today are disillusioned with conventional medicine, and many have turned to self-treatment using herbal remedies. As a nurse, you're in a position to learn about drug interactions and adverse reactions caused by herbal therapy and to educate and caution patients about potential dangers.

# acacia gum

*Acacia senegal*

**Common trade names**
*Acacia Vera, Cape Gum, Egyptian
Thorn, Gum Acacia, Gum Arabic,
Gum Senegal, Gummae Mimosae,
Gummi Africanum, Kher, Somali
Gum, Sudan Gum Arabic, Yellow
Thorn*

## HOW SUPPLIED
Available as flakes, granules, powder, and spray-dried formulations.

As a component in a drug preparation, amount varies with the preparation. For periodontal use, concentrations range from 0.5% to 1%.

## ACTIONS & COMPONENTS
Derived from the sap of the acacia tree, *A. senegal*. Naturally appears as odorless, white or yellow-white to pale amber brittle tears. The main component of the gum is arabin, which is the calcium salt of arabic acid. It's almost completely soluble in water, but it doesn't dissolve in alcohol and is hydrolyzed to form arabinose, galactose, and arabinosic.

## USES
The dry powder form is commonly used as a stabilizer in drug emulsions and as an additive in various oral combinations.

Acacia gum is dissolved in water to make a mucilage. Although acacia gum is commonly used to reduce cholesterol levels, it may actually elevate these levels in serum and tissue.

Acacia is used to soothe throat and stomach irritation, to treat diarrhea, and to impede absorption of certain substances. It's used in cough drops.

Chewing acacia-based gum may limit development of periodontal disease and may also prevent plaque deposit. Whole gum mixtures of 0.5% to 1% may prevent growth of periodontal bacteria, and mixtures of 0.5% may inhibit bacterial protease enzyme.

Acacia also masks acrid substances such as capsicum and is used as a treatment for catarrh, as a mild stimulant, as a food stabilizer, and a film-forming agent in peel-off skin masks. It's also used in some wound-healing preparations.

## DOSAGE & ADMINISTRATION
*Mucilage:* Usual dose is 1 to 4 tsp P.O.

## ADVERSE REACTIONS
**Respiratory:** *severe bronchospasm.*
**Skin:** skin lesions.

## INTERACTIONS
**Herb-drug.** *Alkaloids:* When mixed, acacia gum may partially degrade certain alkaloids. Monitor patient closely.
*Ethyl alcohol:* Acacia is insoluble in substances containing ethyl alcohol concentrations of more

*Liquid contains alcohol.

than 50%. Advise patient not to mix the two together.

*Iron:* Ferric iron salt solutions may gelatinize acacia. Monitor patient closely.

*Oral drugs:* The fiber component of acacia may impair absorption of oral drugs. Monitor patient for loss of therapeutic effect.

## CAUTIONS
Those with allergy or hypersensitivity to acacia dust should avoid use. Pregnant and breast-feeding patients should avoid use because the effects of the herb are unknown.

## NURSING CONSIDERATIONS
• Find out why patient is using the herb.

• Acacia gum, which is essentially nontoxic, has no significant systemic effects when taken orally.

• Monitor patient for allergic reactions to acacia dust, including severe bronchospasm and skin lesions.

⚠ALERT: Don't confuse acacia gum with sweet acacia (*A. farnesiana*) or products from trees of the genus *Albizia*. These products may not be substituted for one another.

• Dry powder, flake, and granule formulations should be stored in tightly closed containers.

### Patient teaching
• Advise patient to consult with his health care provider before using an herbal preparation because a treatment with proven efficacy may be available.

• Tell patient to remind pharmacist of any herbal or dietary supple-

ment that he's taking, when filling a new prescription.

• Inform patient that if he delays seeking diagnosis and treatment from a health care provider, conditions such as hyperlipidemia, periodontal infection, and GI and throat irritation could worsen.

• Advise patient allergic to acacia dust not to use acacia gum because severe reactions may occur.

• Inform patient that acacia gum may affect the absorption of other oral drugs and that he should notify his health care provider before using the herb.

• Advise patient to store dry powder, granule, or flake formulations in tightly closed containers.

## acidophilus

*Lactobacillus acidophilus*

**Common trade names**
*Acidophilus, Bacid, Kala, Lactinex, More-Dophilus, Pro-Bionate, Probiotics, Superdophilus*

## HOW SUPPLIED
Available as capsules, granules, milk, powders, tablets, and yogurt.

## ACTIONS & COMPONENTS
*L. acidophilus* grows naturally in the human GI tract along with *Bacteroides, Escherichia coli, Streptococcus faecalis,* and other microorganisms. Each bacterial strain prevents the others from overgrowth in the intestine. Acidophilus produces hydrogen peroxide and lactic acid to suppress pathogenic bacteria.

---

## USES
Used for lactose intolerance, digestive disorders, or antibiotic-induced diarrhea because it helps replace intestinal flora. Also used to ease the pain of a sore mouth caused by oral candidiasis, and to treat fever blisters, canker sores, hives, and acne.

Lactobacillus products have also been used to treat vaginal yeast or bacterial infections and uncomplicated lower UTIs. They're administered intravaginally to treat bacterial vaginosis in pregnant women in the first trimester, thus restoring normal vaginal flora and acidity.

When antibiotics are given, growth of susceptible bacteria may decline, allowing for overgrowth of other bacteria; acidophilus is taken to restore intestinal flora and, thus, homeostasis.

Some herbal practitioners claim acidophilus may also retard the growth of tumors and reduce cholesterol levels; however, no data support this.

Although sometimes used to treat irritable bowel syndrome or inflammatory bowel disease, acidophilus probably isn't effective for these conditions.

## DOSAGE & ADMINISTRATION
*Bacid:* 2 capsules P.O. b.i.d. to q.i.d.
*Lactinex:* 1 packet added to or taken P.O. with food, milk, juice, or water b.i.d. or q.i.d.
*More-Dophilus:* 1 tsp P.O. q.d. with liquid.
*Pro-Bionate capsules:* 1 capsule P.O. q.d. to t.i.d.

*Pro-Bionate powder:* ¼ to 1 tsp P.O. q.d. to t.i.d.
*Superdophilus:* ¼ to 1 tsp P.O. q.d. to t.i.d.
*To decrease recurrence of vaginal candidiasis:* 1 cup of yogurt containing *L. acidophilus* P.O.

## ADVERSE REACTIONS
**GI:** flatulence.

## INTERACTIONS
None reported.

## CAUTIONS
Patients with sensitivity to dairy and children younger than age 3 should avoid using acidophilus.

Those with high fevers should use caution when using acidophilus.

## NURSING CONSIDERATIONS
● Find out why patient is using the herb.
● *L. acidophilus* is found in some dairy products such as milk and yogurt. Some products may contain other strains of *Lactobacillus,* such as *L. bulgaricus.*
● Some products labeled to contain *L. acidophilus* contain little to no active ingredient, whereas others contain contaminants such as *Clostridium sporogenes, Enterococcus faecium,* and *Pseudomonas.*
● Products may be administered orally or intravaginally, depending on intended use.
● The strength of an acidophilus product is commonly quantified by the number of living organisms per capsule. This number typically ranges from 1 to 10 billion viable organisms in three to four divided doses every day.

*Liquid may contain alcohol.

- Flatulence is prevalent with initial dosing but decreases with continued use.
- Acidophilus shouldn't be used for longer than 2 days.
- Refrigeration is recommended to maintain potency.

**Patient teaching**
- Advise patient to consult with his health care provider before using an herbal preparation because a treatment with proven efficacy may be available.
- Tell patient to remind pharmacist of any herbal or dietary supplement that he's taking, when filling a new prescription.
- Inform patient that if he delays seeking medical diagnosis and treatment, conditions such as inflammatory bowel disease, vaginal infections, UTIs, thrush, hyperlipidemia, antibiotic-associated diarrhea, and developing tumors could worsen.
- Advise patient not to use acidophilus for longer than 2 days or while he has a high fever, unless his health care provider has instructed him to do so.
- Advise patient with sensitivity to dairy to avoid oral use of *L. acidophilus*.
- Inform patient that flatulence may occur initially but usually decreases with continued use.
- Advise patient to store acidophilus in the refrigerator.

## aconite

*Aconitum napellus,* aconite, friar's cap, helmet flower, monkshood, soldier's cap, wolfsbane

**Common trade names**
*Aconiti, Aconiti Tuber, Blue Rocket, Mousebane*

**HOW SUPPLIED**
Available as the dried tuberous root of *A. napellus.*

**ACTIONS & COMPONENTS**
Root contains many alkaloids, with aconite being the most pharmacologically active; other alkaloids include hypaconitin and mesaconitin.

Aconitin increases membrane permeability for sodium ions and slows repolarization. Initially, aconitin is stimulating, but then it causes paralysis in the CNS and other nerve endings. In small doses, aconitin causes bradycardia and hypotension; in higher doses, it has an initial positive inotropic effect, then causes tachycardia, cardiac arrhythmias, and cardiac arrest.

The other alkaloids have comparable effects, with hypaconitin being the strongest.

**USES**
Liniments made from aconite are used for neuralgia, sciatica, and rheumatism.

Aconite is used as a cardiac depressant and as a component in some cough mixtures.

---

*Bold italic type* indicates that reaction may be life-threatening.

In traditional Chinese medicine, aconite is used to treat everything from sciatica to nephritis. In homeopathic preparations, aconite is used as an analgesic, antipyretic, and hypotensive.

## DOSAGE & ADMINISTRATION
*External use:* Average dose of Aconiti tinctura is 0.1 to 0.2 g, applied topically with a brush. Maximum daily dose is 0.6 g.

## ADVERSE REACTIONS
**CV:** *heart failure, arrhythmias, paralysis of cardiac muscle.* **Respiratory:** *paralysis of respiratory center.*

## INTERACTIONS
None reported.

## CAUTIONS
Oral use of aconite isn't recommended.

Liniments absorbed through the skin may produce serious poisoning. Liniments containing aconite should never be applied to wounds or abrasions because of the potential for enhanced absorption, which could cause systemic toxicity.

## NURSING CONSIDERATIONS
• Find out why patient is using the herb.
⚡ALERT: Because of aconite's toxic effects, it's rarely used in the United States. These effects may be partially decreased by some manufacturing processes; however, inability to predict toxic effects among available products should discourage use.

• Several fatal poisonings and numerous nonfatal toxic effects have been reported, perhaps because aconite's therapeutic index is narrow and its potency varies. Even as little as 1 tsp of the root may cause paralysis of the respiratory center and cardiac muscle, leading to death.
• The onset of aconite poisoning is almost immediate, with the delay of symptom onset being as long as 1 hour. Death from aconite poisoning may occur from minutes to days after ingestion, depending on the dose.
⚡ALERT: Immediate symptoms of toxic reaction include burning sensation of lips, tongue, mouth, and throat. Numbness of the throat and inability to speak may follow. Numbness of fingers and toes and, eventually, the entire body may progress to a furry sensation. Body temperature may significantly decline. Excessive salivation, nausea, vomiting, urination, hypotension, and blurred vision with yellow-green visual disturbance may also follow initial symptoms.
• Treatment of aconite poisoning is symptomatic. Atropine has been used to treat aconite-induced cardiotoxicity in severe cases. Arrhythmias may not respond to procainamide and may worsen with verapamil. Gastric lavage may need to be performed or vomiting induced.

### Patient teaching
• Advise patient to consult with his health care provider before using an herbal preparation because a

---

*Liquid may contain alcohol.

treatment with proven efficacy may be available.

● Tell patient to remind pharmacist of any herbal or dietary supplement that he's taking, when filling a new prescription.

● Warn patient that use of this herb isn't recommended because it may have toxic effects and cause death.

## agar

*Gelidium amansii,* agar-agar, Chinese gelatin, colle du Japon, E406, gelose, Japanese gelatin, Japanese isinglass, layor carang, vegetable gelatin

**Common trade names**
*Gelatin, Gelosa, and various multiple-ingredient preparations including Agarbil, Agarol, Demosvelte N, Diet Fibre Complex 1500, Emulsione, Falqui, Gelogastrine, Lexat, Paragar, Pseudophage*

### HOW SUPPLIED
Available as a dry powder and as thin, odorless, and colorless to pale yellow, orange, or gray translucent strips, flakes, and granules.

### ACTIONS & COMPONENTS
Made up of two major polysaccharides: neutral agarose and charged agaropectin. These polysaccharides are extracted from various species of *Rhodophyceae algae.*

Agarose is the gelling component of agar. Agar aids peristalsis by increasing bulk in the intestines and by swelling the intestines, thus stimulating the intestinal muscles.

### USES
Used as an oral bulk laxative to treat chronic constipation. It's also used to make dental impressions and added to other drugs in compounding emulsions, suspensions, gels, and hydrophilic suppositories.

### DOSAGE & ADMINISTRATION
*Laxative:* 1 to 2 tsp of powder P.O. with liquid, fruit, or jam before meals, q.d. to t.i.d.
*Oral use:* 4 to 16 g q.d. or b.i.d. with at least 8½ oz of water.

### ADVERSE REACTIONS
**GI:** esophageal or bowel obstruction.
**Metabolic:** hypercholesterolemia.

### INTERACTIONS
**Herb-drug.** *Oral drugs:* The fiber in agar may impair absorption of oral drugs. Encourage patient to separate administration times.

### CAUTIONS
Patients with bowel obstruction or difficulty swallowing shouldn't use agar.

### NURSING CONSIDERATIONS
● Find out why patient is using the herb.
● Dry powder is soluble in boiling water and produces a clear liquid that gels when cooled.
● Agar strips, flakes, and granules are tough when damp but become brittle when dried.
● Monitor patient for chest pain, vomiting, and difficulty swallowing or breathing.

---

*Bold italic type* indicates that reaction may be life-threatening.

**Patient teaching**

• Advise patient to consult with his health care provider before using an herbal preparation because a treatment with proven efficacy may be available.

• Tell patient to remind pharmacist of any herbal or dietary supplement that he's taking, when filling a new prescription.

• Advise any patient who has difficulty swallowing not to use agar.

• Inform patient that agar may alter the effectiveness of oral drugs, and encourage him to notify his health care provider if he's taking it.

• Advise patient who is using agar to take it with plenty of fluid (at least 8 oz) to prevent blockage of the throat or esophagus, which could cause choking.

• Advise patient to seek immediate medical attention if he experiences chest pain, vomiting, or difficulty swallowing or breathing.

## agrimony

*Agrimonia eupatoria, A. procera,* church steeples, cocklebur, common agrimony, liverwort, philanthropos, sticklewort, stickwort

**Common trade names**
*Fragrant Agrimony, Herba eupatoriae. Multiple-ingredient preparations include Gall & Liver Tablets, NeoGallonorm–Dragees, Potter's Piletabs, and Rhoival*

**HOW SUPPLIED**
Available as pulverized or powdered herb and as other preparations used to make compresses, gargles, poultices, teas, and various bath preparations.

**ACTIONS & COMPONENTS**
The dried above-ground parts of the plant are harvested during flowering season.

Contains flavonoids and 4% to 10% condensed tannins, which give the herb astringent properties. The ethanolic extracts of agrimony are thought to have antiviral properties.

**USES**
Probably safe and effective as a mild topical antiseptic or astringent. May be effective for mild, nonspecific acute diarrhea and gastroenteritis.

Specifically used for sore throat, inflammation of mouth and pharynx, inflammation of the skin, and diabetes. Also used as an antitumorigenic, cardiotonic, antihistamine, antasthmatic, diuretic, sedative, dye or flavoring agent, and coagulant for skin rashes or cuts.

Historically, agrimony was used for gallbladder disorders (in "liver and bile" teas), tuberculosis, corns and warts, and catarrh (mucous membrane inflammation with discharge).

**DOSAGE & ADMINISTRATION**
*External use:* Topical poultices using 10% water extract can be made by boiling agrimony at low heat for 10 to 20 minutes. Poultice may be applied several times daily. *Oral use:* Average daily dose is 3 g P.O.

**ADVERSE REACTIONS**
**CV:** hypotension.
**GI:** GI upset, constipation.
**Metabolic:** hypoglycemia.
**Skin:** photodermatitis.

**INTERACTIONS**
**Herb-drug.** *Anticoagulants:* High doses of agrimony may influence anticoagulant effects. Monitor patient closely.
*Antihypertensives:* High doses of agrimony may cause added hypotensive effects. Monitor blood pressure.
*Insulin, oral antidiabetics:* Increased risk of hypoglycemia. Monitor blood glucose levels.
**Herb-lifestyle.** *Sun-exposure:* Increased risk of photosensitivity reactions. Advise patient to wear protective clothing and sunscreen and to limit his exposure to direct sunlight.

**CAUTIONS**
Oral use of agrimony may be un-`safe in pregnant women. Because of the tannin content, agrimony use may be unsafe in high topical or oral doses.

**NURSING CONSIDERATIONS**
• Find out why patient is using the herb.
• Short-term use of agrimony in appropriate doses is considered safe.
• Monitor patient taking high doses for nausea and vomiting.
• Monitor diabetic patients for hypoglycemia.
• Monitor blood pressure in patients taking high doses.

**Patient teaching**
• Advise patient to consult with his health care provider before using an herbal preparation because a treatment with proven efficacy may be available.
• Tell patient to remind pharmacist of any herbal or dietary supplement that he's taking, when filling a new prescription.
• Caution patient that if he delays seeking medical diagnosis and treatment, his condition could worsen.
• Inform diabetic patient that agrimony may cause hypoglycemia, so if he's taking a conventional antidiabetic, the dosage of that drug may need to be adjusted.
• Inform patient that agrimony may affect the menstrual cycle.
• Advise patient that high doses of this herb may cause nausea and vomiting.
• Caution patient not to exceed recommended doses because high doses may cause hypotension.
• Advise patient that long-term use isn't recommended because of the risk of adverse reactions.
• Warn patient of potential adverse effects, particularly if he's also taking a drug for blood pressure, an antidiabetic, or an anticoagulant.

## allspice

clove pepper, Jamaica pepper, pimenta, pimento

**Common trade names**
*Allspice*

## HOW SUPPLIED
Available as aqueous extract, oil, and powder, which consists of ground dried fruit.

## ACTIONS & COMPONENTS
Allspice berries and leaves contain a volatile oil that's 60% to 80% eugenol. The leaves contain more eugenol than the berries (up to 96%). The oil also contains caryophyllene, cineole, levophellandrene, and palmitic acid.

Eugenol is responsible for the herb's effects on the GI system and its analgesic properties. It works by depressing the CNS and inhibiting prostaglandin activity in the colon mucosa. It also increases the activity of some digestive enzymes like trypsin.

Eugenol has antioxidant properties and in vitro activity against yeast and fungi. Eugenol inhibits platelet activity.

## USES
Allspice is commonly used to enhance the taste of food and toothpaste and the smell of cosmetics. In herbal medicine, it's used for GI problems such as indigestion, stomachache, and flatulence; it's also used as a purgative. Topically, it's used as an analgesic for muscle pain or toothache and as an antiseptic for teeth and gums.

## DOSAGE & ADMINISTRATION
*Antiflatulent:* 0.05 to 0.2 ml allspice oil P.O.

## ADVERSE REACTIONS
**CNS:** CNS depression, *seizures (with high doses).*

**EENT:** mucous membrane irritation (with topical use).
**GI:** nausea, vomiting.

## INTERACTIONS
**Herb-drug.** *Anticoagulants, antiplatelet drugs:* Enhanced effect. Monitor patient for bleeding.

## CAUTIONS
Patients with intestinal disorders should avoid use because allspice and its extracts stimulate the GI tract and may irritate mucous membranes.

## NURSING CONSIDERATIONS
• Find out why patient is using the herb.
• Allspice is safe when used topically or when consumed in amounts typically found in foods.
⚡ALERT: Ingestion of large quantities may cause toxic reaction. Ingestion of more than 5 ml of allspice oil can cause nausea, vomiting, CNS depression, and seizures.

## Patient teaching
• Advise patient to consult with his health care provider before using an herbal preparation because a treatment with proven efficacy may be available.
• Tell patient to remind pharmacist of any herbal or dietary supplement that he's taking, when filling a new prescription.
• Advise patient not to ingest large quantities of allspice.
• Advise patient not to delay treatment for an illness that doesn't resolve after taking allspice.

*Liquid may contain alcohol.

## aloe

*Aloe barbadensis, A. capensis, A. vera,* Barbados aloes, burn plant, curacao, elephant's gall, first-aid plant, Hsiang-dan, lily of the desert, lu-hui, socotrine, Zanzibar

**Common trade names**
*Aloe Gel, Aloe Latex, Aloe Vera, Cape*

### HOW SUPPLIED
Available as dried latex for internal use, extract capsules, juice (99.7% of whole leaf aloe vera juice), tincture* (1:10, 50% alcohol), and topical gel.
*Extract capsules:* 75 mg, 100 mg, 200 mg
*Topical gel:* 98%, 99.5%, 99.6%, and 100% purity strengths

### ACTIONS & COMPONENTS
A solid residue is obtained by evaporating aloe latex. It contains aloinosides, which irritate the large intestine, increasing peristalsis, thereby producing a laxative effect. Water and electrolyte reabsorption is inhibited. Aloe can cause potassium loss.

Aloe gel is a clear, thin, viscous material obtained by crushing the mucilaginous cells found in the leaf. The gel contains a polysaccharide similar to guar gum.

Aloe gel's wound healing ability comes from its moisturizing effect, which prevents air from drying the wound. Mucopolysaccharides and sulfur and nitrogen compounds also stimulate healing.

Aloe gel may work as an antibacterial against *Staphylococcus aureus, Escherichia coli,* and *Mycobacterium tuberculosis,* but information is conflicting.

Aloe also contains bradykinase, which is a protease inhibitor that relieves pain and decreases swelling and redness. The antipruritic effect of aloe may be related to the antihistamine properties of magnesium lactate.

### USES
Used orally, aloe latex is a potent cathartic. It's used to treat constipation; to provide evacuation relief for patients with anal fissures, hemorrhoids, or recent anorectal surgery; and to prepare a patient for diagnostic testing of the GI tract.

Aloe gel is used to treat minor burns and skin irritation and to aid in wound healing. It may also be effective as an antibacterial.

### DOSAGE & ADMINISTRATION
*Laxative:* 100 to 200 mg of aloe capsules, 50 mg of aloe extract, or 1 to 8 oz of juice h.s. Or, 30 ml of aloe gel or 15 to 60 gtt of aloe tincture (1:10, 50% alcohol), p.r.n.
*Topical use:* Apply gel liberally three to five times daily, p.r.n.

### ADVERSE REACTIONS
**CV:** *arrhythmias,* edema.
**GI:** cramps, diarrhea.
**GU:** albuminuria, hematuria, nephropathy.
**Metabolic:** electrolyte abnormalities, weight loss.
**Musculoskeletal:** muscle weakness, accelerated bone deterioration.

---

*Bold italic type* indicates that reaction may be life-threatening.

**Skin:** nummular eczematous, papular dermatitis.

## INTERACTIONS
**Herb-drug.** *Antiarrhythmics, cardiac glycosides such as digoxin:* Oral administration with aloe may lead to toxic reaction. Monitor patient closely.
*Corticosteroids, diuretics:* Concomitant use can enhance potassium loss. Monitor potassium level.
*Disulfiram:* Any herbal preparation that contains alcohol can precipitate a disulfiram-like reaction. Advise patient not to use together.
**Herb-herb.** *Licorice:* Increased risk of potassium deficiency. Advise patient not to use together.

## CAUTIONS
Those with intestinal obstruction; those with Crohn's disease, ulcerative colitis, appendicitis, or abdominal pain of unknown origin; those who are pregnant; and children younger than age 12 should avoid taking aloe orally.

Products derived from the latex of aloe's outer skin should be used cautiously.

## NURSING CONSIDERATIONS
• Find out why patient is using the herb.
• Aloe's laxative effects are apparent within 10 hours of taking aloe.
• Monitor patient for signs of dehydration. Geriatric patients are particularly at risk.
• Monitor electrolyte levels, especially potassium, after long-term use.
• If patient is using aloe topically, monitor wound for healing.

## Patient teaching
• Advise patient to consult with his health care provider before using an herbal preparation because a treatment with proven efficacy may be available.
• Tell patient to remind pharmacist of any herbal or dietary supplement that he's taking, when filling a new prescription.
• Caution patient that if he delays seeking medical diagnosis and treatment, his condition could worsen.
• If patient is taking digoxin or another drug to control his heart rate, a diuretic, or a corticosteroid, warn him not to take aloe without consulting his health care provider.
• Advise patient to reduce dose if cramping occurs after a single dose and not to take aloe for longer than 1 to 2 weeks at a time without consulting his health care provider.
• Advise patient to notify his health care provider immediately if he experiences feelings of dehydration, weakness, or confusion, especially if he has been using aloe for a prolonged period.

*Liquid may contain alcohol.

## American cranesbill

*Geranium maculatum,* alum
bloom, alumroot, American
kino, chocolate flower, crow-
foot, dove's-foot, old maid's
nightcap, shameface, spotted
cranesbill, stinking cranesbill,
storkbill, wild cranesbill, wild
geranium

Common trade names
*None known*

### HOW SUPPLIED
Available as dried herb, essential
oil, liquid extract*, mouthwash,
and tincture.

### ACTIONS & COMPONENTS
High in tannins, which likely accounts for its antidiarrheal activity.
May have some antiviral and antibacterial properties. A preparation
with extract and 80% ethanol may
inhibit the growth of some gram-
negative bacteria.

### USES
Used for diarrhea, dysentery,
Crohn's disease, inflammation of
the mouth, liver and gallbladder
disease, calculosis, and inflammation of the mouth, kidney, and
bladder.
    Used as a gargle or mouthwash.
Fresh leaves are commonly
chewed.

### DOSAGE & ADMINISTRATION
*Liquid extract:* 1 to 2 ml P.O. t.i.d.
*Tea:* 1 to 2 g P.O. Prepared by
adding 1 tsp of herb to ½ qt of
cold water, bringing that to a boil,
and leaving it to draw. Daily dose
is 2 to 3 cups between meals.
*Tincture:* 3 ml P.O. t.i.d.

### ADVERSE REACTIONS
**GI:** upset stomach.

### INTERACTIONS
**Herb-drug.** *Disulfiram:* Any herbal preparation that contains alcohol can precipitate a disulfiram-
like reaction. Advise patient not to
use together.

### CAUTIONS
Those with digestive disorders
should avoid use because of the
herb's high tannin content.

### NURSING CONSIDERATIONS
• Find out why patient is using the
herb.
• Relatively little information is
available on this herb.

**Patient teaching**
• Advise patient to consult with his
health care provider before using
an herbal preparation because a
treatment with proven efficacy
may be available.
• Tell patient to remind pharmacist
of any herbal or dietary supplement that he's taking, when filling
a new prescription.
• Caution patient not to delay seeking medical evaluation for symptoms that may indicate a serious
medical condition.
• Inform patient with a sensitive
stomach that herb could cause
nausea or vomiting.
• Tell patient not to take a higher
dose than is recommended.

---

*Bold italic type* indicates that reaction may be life-threatening.

• Advise patient not to take cranesbill for longer than 1 to 2 weeks at a time without consulting his health care provider.

## angelica

*Angelica archangelica,* angelica root, angelique, dong quai, engelwurzel, European angelica, garden angelica, heiligenwurzel, root of the Holy Ghost, tang-kuei, wild angelica

**Common trade names**
*Nature's Answer Angelica Root Liquid*

### HOW SUPPLIED
Available as liquid extract, tincture, and essential oil.

### ACTIONS & COMPONENTS
The root and fruit seeds of angelica are used to extract the medicinally active part of the plant. Angelica contains alpha-angelica lactone, which augments calcium binding and calcium turnover. Its action may involve increasing the contraction-dependent calcium pool to be released upon systolic depolarization. The coumarins and furanocoumarins may induce photosensitivity and may be photocarcinogenic and mutagenic.

### USES
Angelica seed is used as a diuretic and diaphoretic. It's also used to treat conditions of the kidneys and the urinary, GI, and respiratory tracts as well as rheumatic and neuralgic symptoms.

Angelica root is used orally for loss of appetite, GI spasm, and flatulence. It has been used topically to treat neuralgia. Other uses include treatment for coughs and bronchitis, anorexia, dyspepsia with intestinal cramping, and menstrual, liver, and gallbladder complaints.

Angelica seed has also been used as a flavoring in gin, some regional wines, candied leaves, and cake and pastry decorations.

### DOSAGE & ADMINISTRATION
*Crude root:* 4.5 g P.O. q.d.
*Essential oil:* 10 to 20 gtt P.O. q.d.
*Liquid extract (1:1):* 0.5 to 3 g P.O. q.d.
*Tincture (1:5):* 1.5 g P.O. q.d.

### ADVERSE REACTIONS
**Skin:** photodermatosis.

### INTERACTIONS
**Herb-drug.** *Antacids, $H_2$ blockers, proton pump inhibitors, sucralfate:* Angelica may increase acid production in the stomach and so may interfere with absorption of these drugs. Advise patient to separate administration times.
*Anticoagulants:* Potentiated effects with excessive doses of angelica. Monitor patient for bleeding.
**Herb-lifestyle.** *Sun exposure:* Increased risk of photosensitivity reactions. Advise patient to wear protective clothing and sunscreen and to limit direct exposure to sunlight.

### CAUTIONS
Pregnant and breast-feeding patients should avoid use because

---

*Liquid may contain alcohol.

angelica appears to stimulate menstruation and the uterus.

## NURSING CONSIDERATIONS
- Find out why patient is using the herb.
- Monitor patient for persistent diarrhea, which may be a sign of something more serious.
- Monitor patient for dermatologic reactions.
- Photodermatosis is possible after contact with the plant juice or plant extract.

### Patient teaching
- Advise patient to consult with his health care provider before using an herbal preparation because a treatment with proven efficacy may be available.
- Tell patient to remind pharmacist of any herbal or dietary supplement that he's taking, when filling a new prescription.
- Caution patient not to delay seeking medical treatment for symptoms that may be related to a serious medical condition.
- Advise patient not to take angelica if pregnant or if taking a gastric acid blocker or anticoagulant.
- Advise patient to notify his health care provider if he develops a skin rash.

## anise

*Pimpinella anisum,* aniseed, anise oil, semen anisi, sweet cumin

**Common trade names**
*None known*

## HOW SUPPLIED
Available as dried fruit, essential oil, and tea.

## ACTIONS & COMPONENTS
Anise oil is obtained from fruits of the herb. The highest quality oil comes from anise seeds. The major component of the oil is transanethole, which is responsible for the taste, smell, and medicinal properties of anise.

Structurally, anise is comparable to catecholamines (such as dopamine, epinephrine, and norepinephrine) and the hallucinogenic compound myristicin.

Bergapten, another component of anise, may cause photosensitivity reactions and may be carcinogenic.

## USES
Anise is used to treat coughs and colds and to decrease bloating and gas. In higher doses, anise is used as an antispasmodic and antiseptic for cough, asthma, and bronchitis.

Anise also has weak antibacterial effects against gram-positive and gram-negative organisms. The oil has been used for lice, scabies, and psoriasis.

Anise has also been used as flavoring in alcohols, various foods, perfumes, and soaps.

## DOSAGE & ADMINISTRATION
*Antiflatulent:* For adults, 1 tbs of tea several times q.d.; for breast-feeding babies, 1 tsp of tea P.O. p.r.n.
*Dried fruit:* 0.5 to 1 g P.O. Maximum daily dose is 3 g.
*Essential oil:* 50 to 200 ml P.O. q.d.

---

*Expectorant:* 1 cup of tea P.O. in the morning or the evening.
*Tea:* Prepared by steeping 1 to 2 tsp of crushed seed in water for 10 to 15 minutes and then straining. Tea may be taken t.i.d.

**ADVERSE REACTIONS**
**CNS:** *seizures.*
**GI:** nausea, vomiting, stomatitis.
**Respiratory:** pulmonary edema.
**Skin:** erythema, scaling, vesiculation, photosensitivity reactions.

**INTERACTIONS**
**Herb-drug.** *Anticoagulants, MAO inhibitors, oral contraceptives:* High doses of anise can interfere with these drugs. Monitor patient closely.
**Herb-lifestyle.** *Sun exposure:* Increased risk of photosensitivity reactions. Advise patient to wear protective clothing and sunscreen and to limit exposure to direct sunlight.

**CAUTIONS**
Those allergic to anise or anethole should avoid use. Pregnant patients should avoid using anise because it may cause abortion; those with dermatitis or inflammatory or allergic skin reactions should avoid using anise because it may cause photosensitivity.
   Those with coagulation problems should use anise cautiously.

**NURSING CONSIDERATIONS**
• Find out why patient is using the herb.
• Preparations containing 5% to 10% essential oil can be used externally.

⚡**ALERT:** Don't confuse anise with Chinese star anise.
• If overdose occurs, monitor patient for neurologic changes and provide supportive measures for nausea and vomiting.

**Patient teaching**
• Advise patient to consult with his health care provider before using an herbal preparation because a treatment with proven efficacy may be available.
• Tell patient to remind pharmacist of any herbal or dietary supplement that he's taking, when filling a new prescription.
• If patient is pregnant, instruct her not to use anise.
• If patient is taking an anticoagulant or an antiplatelet drug, advise him not to take anise.
• Instruct patient not to exceed the daily recommended dose.
• Advise patient to report any skin changes to his health care provider.

## arnica

*Arnica montana,* arnica flowers, arnica root, common arnica, Leopard's bane, mountain snuff, mountain tobacco, sneezewort, wolfsbane

**Common trade names**
*Arnica Flowers Extract, Arnica Gel, Arnicalm, Arnica Ointment, Arnica-Si, Weleda Massage Balm*

**HOW SUPPLIED**
Available, for external use only, as ointment, semisolid cream, and tincture for poultice preparation.

Also available in tablets for home-opathic preparations.

## ACTIONS & COMPONENTS
Typically, the dried yellow to orange-yellow flower heads of the plant are used to extract the active compounds. Parts of the rhizome at the base of the plant may also be used.

The plant contains many chemical compounds, including oils and fatty acids. Its sesquiterpene lactones have mild analgesic and anti-inflammatory effects. Helenalin and dihydrohelenalin, additional sesquiterpenes, may also have antibacterial and additional anti-inflammatory effects. Some components may reduce bleeding times and inhibit platelet function. Arnica may also have antifungal effects.

Arnica, which has some immunostimulatory activity, contains a group of polysaccharides that can modify the immune response.

## USES
Poultices and ointments have been used topically to treat skin inflammation, acne, bruises, sprains, blunt injuries, and rheumatic muscle and joint problems.

Oral rinses have been used to treat inflammation of the mouth and pharynx; however, ingestion of arnica can cause severe toxic reaction, including death, so its use as an oral rinse should be avoided or carefully monitored.

Arnica has also been used to treat heart problems, improve circulation, stimulate the CNS, provide analgesia, and treat surgical or accidental trauma and postoperative thrombophlebitis and pulmonary emboli.

## DOSAGE & ADMINISTRATION
*Oral rinse:* Tincture diluted 10 times with water.
*Poultice preparation:* Tincture diluted 3 to 10 times with water.

## ADVERSE REACTIONS
**CNS:** *coma,* drowsiness.
**CV:** *cardiac arrest.*
**GI:** stomach pain, diarrhea, vomiting, gastroenteritis.
**Respiratory:** dyspnea.
**Skin:** contact dermatitis, irritation of mucous membranes, and eczema (with prolonged use of topical preparation).

## INTERACTIONS
**Herb-drug.** *Aspirin, heparin, warfarin:* Increased risk of bleeding. Monitor patient closely.
**Herb-herb.** *Angelica, anise, asafoetida, bogbean, boldo, capsicum, celery, chamomile, clove, danshen, fenugreek, feverfew, garlic, ginger, ginkgo, ginseng, horse chestnut, horseradish, licorice, meadowsweet, onion, papain, passion flower, poplar bark, prickly ash, quassia wood, red clover, turmeric, wild carrot, wild lettuce, willow:* Possible increased bleeding times or altered platelet function. Caution patient about concomitant use.

## CAUTIONS
Pregnant and breast-feeding patients and those allergic to arnica, tansy, sunflowers, or chrysanthemums should avoid use.

---

*Bold italic type* indicates that reaction may be life-threatening.

Any patient taking a drug that affects coagulation or platelet function should use arnica cautiously.

**NURSING CONSIDERATIONS**
• Find out why patient is using the herb.
🖉ALERT: Arnica should only be used externally because internal use may result in severe toxic reaction or death.
• The typical extract strength of the tincture is ⅛ oz of flower heads in 3½ oz of water.
• Arnica oil is usually made with 1 part herb extract to 5 parts vegetable-fixed oil.
• In tablet form, the active ingredient is extremely diluted.
• Frequent topical use of arnica increases the likelihood of contact dermatitis reactions. Eczema may also result from prolonged contact of arnica-containing external dressings.
• Signs and symptoms of overdose include vomiting, diarrhea, drowsiness, dyspnea, and cardiac arrest.
• If overdose occurs, perform gastric lavage or induce vomiting, and follow with supportive treatment.

**Patient teaching**
• Advise patient to consult with his health care provider before using an herbal preparation because a treatment with proven efficacy may be available.
• Tell patient to remind pharmacist of any herbal or dietary supplement that he's taking, when filling a new prescription.
• Warn patient that arnica should only be used externally.

• Advise patient with history of dermatologic reactions to perfumes, cosmetics, hair tonics, and antidandruff preparations to use arnica cautiously because many of these products contain arnica, and he may be allergic to it.
• If patient is taking an anticoagulant or using long-term aspirin therapy, instruct him to use arnica cautiously and to notify his health care provider of any unusual bleeding or bruising.
• Warn patient that only diluted tincture should be used as a dressing.
• Advise patient that prolonged or frequent use of arnica dressings can increase the risk of skin reactions.
• Advise patient to store ointment and undiluted tincture out of children's reach and away from pets.

## artichoke

*Cynara scolymus*, garden artichoke, globe artichoke

**Common trade names**
*Artichoke Extract, Artichoke Ha, Artichoke Power, Cynara-SI Artichoke*

**HOW SUPPLIED**
Available as fresh pressed juice or fresh or dried leaf, stem, root, and capsules.

**ACTIONS & COMPONENTS**
Although the active component of artichoke hasn't been identified, cynarin or a mono-caffeoylquinic acid may have some cholesterol-lowering effects. Cynarin may

---

*Liquid may contain alcohol.

also have some liver-protective qualities, and it increases bile production.

**USES**
Used to treat dyspepsia, abdominal and gallbladder problems, and nausea. Also used as an antidiabetic, antilipemic, diuretic, and liver protectant. However, it's unknown whether artichoke reduces cholesterol in patients with types IIa or IIb familial hypercholesterolemia.

Artichoke has also been used to prevent the return of gallstones.

**DOSAGE & ADMINISTRATION**
*Dried leaf, stem, or root:* 1 to 4 g P.O. q.d.
*Dry extract:* 500 mg P.O. q.d. in a single dose.

**ADVERSE REACTIONS**
**Skin:** contact dermatitis.

**INTERACTIONS**
**Herb-drug.** *Insulin, oral antidiabetics:* Increased risk of hypoglycemia because both the drugs and the herb have glucose-lowering effects. Advise patient not to use together.

**CAUTIONS**
Those allergic to artichokes, marigolds, daisies, or chrysanthemums and those with bile duct obstruction should avoid use.

Those with gallstones should use artichoke cautiously.

**NURSING CONSIDERATIONS**
• Find out why patient is using the herb.

• Bile duct obstruction should be ruled out before artichoke is used medicinally.
• Artichoke preparations should be stored in a tightly closed container, away from light.
• Monitor blood glucose level in those with diabetes.

**Patient teaching**
• Advise patient to consult with his health care provider before using an herbal preparation because a treatment with proven efficacy may be available.
• Tell patient to remind pharmacist of any herbal or dietary supplement that he's taking, when filling a new prescription.
• Advise patient to avoid medicinal use of artichoke if he's allergic to artichokes, marigolds, daisies, or chrysanthemums.
• If patient has gallstones, advise him to consult with his health care provider before using artichoke medicinally.
• Advise patient to store artichoke preparations in a tightly closed container away from light.
• Advise diabetic patient that artichoke may have a hypoglycemic effect. If he's taking an antidiabetic, inform him that his dosage may need to be adjusted.

## asparagus

*Asparagus officinalis,* garden asparagus, sparrow grass

**Common trade names**
*ClearLung (combination product), Hy-C (Bu Yin), Tian Men Dong, Ultimate Urinary Cleanse*

---

*Bold italic type* indicates that reaction may be life-threatening.

## HOW SUPPLIED
Available as cut rhizome or root, fresh stalks, root powder, and tea.

## ACTIONS & COMPONENTS
Rich in vitamin A. Also contains folic acid. It has saponin components that act as mucous membrane irritants. The shoots have several sulfur-containing acids that can cause urine to become strong smelling.

## USES
Used with large amounts of liquid as irrigation therapy. Used to treat UTIs and rheumatic joint pain and swelling, to prevent kidney or bladder stones, and to provide contraception.

The seeds and root extracts are used in the production of alcoholic beverages. The seeds are also used in coffee substitutes, diuretic preparations, laxatives, and remedies for neuritis and rheumatism. The seeds may relieve toothaches, stimulate hair growth, and treat cancer. Topical preparations may have drying effects on acne.

Despite these varied uses, irrigation therapy is the only use with clinical supporting evidence.

## DOSAGE & ADMINISTRATION
*Daily dose:* 45 to 80 g P.O. q.d.
*Root powder:* 10 to 50 g mixed with milk and sugar P.O. b.i.d.
*Tea:* 40 to 60 g of cut rhizome or root P.O. q.d. The tea is prepared by steeping the herb in 5 oz of boiling water for 5 to 10 minutes and then straining the mixture.

## ADVERSE REACTIONS
**GI:** mucous membrane irritation.
**GU:** malodorous urine.
**Skin:** contact dermatitis (with external use).

## INTERACTIONS
**Herb-drug.** *Diuretics:* Possible increased effects. Monitor patient closely.

## CAUTIONS
Those with inflammatory kidney diseases should avoid use. Those with edema caused by heart or kidney disorders shouldn't use asparagus as an irrigant. Pregnant patients should avoid medicinal use of asparagus because the effects on the developing fetus are unknown.

## NURSING CONSIDERATIONS
• Find out why patient is using the herb.
• Patients using asparagus as a urinary irrigant should ensure adequate fluid intake.
• Asparagus may also be applied topically; however, no guidelines for concentration or dosing exist.

## Patient teaching
• Advise patient to consult with his health care provider before using an herbal preparation because a treatment with proven efficacy may be available.
• Tell patient to remind pharmacist of any herbal or dietary supplement that he's taking, when filling a new prescription.
• Encourage patient to drink plenty of fluids while taking asparagus.

---

*Liquid may contain alcohol.

• Inform patient that asparagus may cause his urine to develop a strong odor and that the odor may be more pronounced after eating fresh asparagus as opposed to taking the rhizome or root as a tea.

• If patient is pregnant, advise her to avoid using asparagus medicinally, but assure her that consuming fresh asparagus should be safe.

## autumn crocus

*Colchicum autumnale*, crocus, fall crocus, meadow saffron, mysteria, naked ladies, vellorita, wonder bulb

**Common trade names**
*None known*

### HOW SUPPLIED
Available as pulverized herb, freshly pressed juice, and other preparations for oral use.

### ACTIONS & COMPONENTS
Contains colchicine and other alkaloids. These components act as antichemotactics, antiphlogistics, and antimitotics. Overall, the herb decreases inflammation and collagen synthesis and inhibits cell division.

### USES
The plant and extracts have been used to treat arthritis, rheumatism, prostate enlargement, and gonorrhea. Extracts have also been used to treat cancer.

The FDA has approved the use of colchicine, the active ingredient in autumn crocus, for the treatment of gout.

Colchicine has also been used to treat multiple sclerosis, familial Mediterranean fever, hepatic cirrhosis, primary biliary cirrhosis; and as an adjunct therapy in primary amyloidosis, Bencet's disease, pseudogout, skin manifestations of scleroderma, psoriasis, palmoplantar pustulosis, and dermatitis herpetiformis.

### DOSAGE & ADMINISTRATION
*For acute gout attack:* One dose equivalent to 1 mg of colchicine P.O., followed by 0.5 mg to 1.5 mg P.O. every 1 to 2 hours until the pain diminishes. Total daily dose shouldn't exceed 8 mg of colchicine equivalent.
*For Mediterranean fever:* 0.5 mg to 1.5 mg of colchicine equivalent P.O. as a single dose.

### ADVERSE REACTIONS
**CNS:** peripheral neuritis, numbness of fingertips.
**EENT:** irritation of the nose and throat.
**GI:** GI disturbances.
**Hematologic:** *agranulocytosis, aplastic anemia.*

### INTERACTIONS
**Herb-drug.** *Colchicine:* Possible additive adverse and toxic effects. Advise patient not to use together.

### CAUTIONS
Pregnant and breast-feeding patients should avoid use because of its potential teratogenic effects and antimitotic properties.

---

## NURSING CONSIDERATIONS

• Find out why patient is using the herb.

⚡ **ALERT:** Because of plant's toxicity, internal use isn't recommended. Patient should consult a knowledgeable practitioner before use.

• Because many autumn crocus preparations aren't evaluated for colchicine content the way prescription colchicine products are, overdose is a concern.

• If patient insists on taking autumn crocus, advise him to alert his health care provider first and then to obtain the product from a reputable source.

• Monitor patient for agranulocytosis, aplastic anemia, and peripheral neuritis with prolonged use.

• Any patient who experiences nausea, vomiting, intense thirst, burning in the mouth, abdominal pain, or diarrhea after taking autumn crocus should immediately contact the poison control center. Diarrhea may be persistent and may lead to hypovolemic shock, renal impairment, and oliguria. Treatment for toxic reaction includes fluid replacement, induction of vomiting, and gastric lavage.

• Postmenopausal women and those using adequate contraceptive measures are the only women who should use autumn crocus. Any patient who may be pregnant should perform a pregnancy test before beginning therapy.

• Slicing the fresh corm can irritate the nose and throat and cause numbness of the fingers holding the corm.

## Patient teaching

• Advise patient to consult with his health care provider before using an herbal preparation because a treatment with proven efficacy may be available.

• Tell patient to remind pharmacist of any herbal or dietary supplement that he's taking, when filling a new prescription.

• Advise any patient who's pregnant, breast-feeding, or not using birth control and could become pregnant not to use autumn crocus. Further, instruct her to immediately discontinue use and notify her health care provider if pregnancy occurs.

• Advise any patient taking colchicine to avoid using autumn crocus.

• Warn patient that the entire plant is toxic and that he shouldn't take it orally, unless his health care provider has instructed him to do so.

• Advise any patient using autumn crocus to obtain it from a reputable source that clearly identifies the amount of colchicine that each dose contains.

• Advise patient to call a poison control center immediately if he experiences nausea, vomiting, burning in the mouth, or abdominal pain after taking a dose.

## avens

Geum urbanum, avens root, bennet's root, blessed herb, city avens, colewort, European avens, geum, goldy star, herb bennet, star of the earth, way bennet, wild rye, yellow avens

**Common trade names**
*None known*

### HOW SUPPLIED
Available as aerial parts and root, dried and made into a tea for oral consumption, and liquid extract* containing alcohol for oral consumption.

### ACTIONS & COMPONENTS
Contains tannins and phenolic glycosides, including eugenol, which give avens roots a clovelike odor. Both components have astringent properties that cause tissues to contract.

### USES
Used to treat diarrhea, digestive complaints, ulcerative colitis, intermittent fevers, sore throats, gingivitis, and halitosis.

### DOSAGE & ADMINISTRATION
*Extract (contains 25% alcohol):* 1 to 4 ml P.O. t.i.d.
*Tea:* 1 to 4 g steeped in boiling water and strained, P.O. t.i.d.

### ADVERSE REACTIONS
None known.

### INTERACTIONS
None reported.

### CAUTIONS
Pregnant and breast-feeding patients should avoid use because of a possible effect on the menstrual cycle.

### NURSING CONSIDERATIONS
• Find out why patient is using the herb.
🗲 **ALERT:** Don't confuse avens with Water Avens (*Geum rivale,* Chocolate Root).
• Avens is rarely used in herbal medicine.

**Patient teaching**
• Advise patient to consult with his health care provider before using an herbal preparation because a treatment with proven efficacy may be available.
• Tell patient to remind pharmacist of any herbal or dietary supplement that he's taking, when filling a new prescription.
• If patient is pregnant, breast-feeding, or planning pregnancy, advise her not to use avens and to notify her health care provider if she becomes pregnant during therapy.
• If patient is using avens to treat diarrhea, advise him to contact his health care professional if the diarrhea persists.

---

*Bold italic type* indicates that reaction may be life-threatening.

## balsam of Peru

*Myroxylon balsamum,* balsam tree, Peruvian balsam, tolu balsam

Common trade names
*None known*

### HOW SUPPLIED
Available in shampoo, lotions, and syrups.

### ACTIONS & COMPONENTS
Contains 50% to 70% ester mixtures, the greatest quantity being benzyl ester of benzoic, cinnamein, and cinnamic acid.

### USES
Used externally to help heal infected and poorly healing wounds, burns, pressure ulcers, frostbite, sore nipples, leg ulcers, bruises from prostheses, and hemorrhoids. Used to stimulate the heart, increase blood pressure, and reduce mucous secretions. Used as an antiparasitic to treat scabies and for fevers, colds, cough, bronchitis, tendency to infection, and mouth and pharynx inflammation. Also used to treat pruritus and later stages of acute eczema.

### DOSAGE & ADMINISTRATION
*Daily topical dosage:* Preparations containing 5% to 20% Peruvian balsam may be used for up to 1 week.
*Extensive application:* Preparations containing not more than 10% Peruvian balsam may be used for up to 1 week.
*Tolu balsam for internal use:* The average dose is 0.5 g P.O. q.d.

### ADVERSE REACTIONS
**GI:** aphthoid oral ulcers.
**GU:** renal damage.
**Skin:** allergic skin reactions, urticaria, purpura, photodermatosis, phototoxicity.
**Other:** Quincke's disease.

### INTERACTIONS
**Herb-drug.** *Sulfur-containing products:* Additive effects. Advise patient to use cautiously.
**Herb-lifestyle.** *Sun exposure:* Increased risk of photosensitivity reactions. Advise patient to wear protective clothing and sunscreen and to limit exposure to direct sunlight.

### CAUTIONS
Contraindicated in those with a propensity for allergies.

Those with hypertension should use balsam of Peru cautiously because it may increase blood pressure if ingested.

### NURSING CONSIDERATIONS
• Find out why patient is using the herb.
• If skin reaction occurs, patient should discontinue use.

### Patient teaching
• Advise patient to consult with his health care provider before using an herbal preparation because a

---

*Liquid may contain alcohol.

treatment with proven efficacy may be available.

● Tell patient to remind pharmacist of any herbal or dietary supplement that he's taking, when filling a new prescription.

● Warn patient to seek appropriate medical evaluation before using balsam of Peru to treat wound infection or pressure ulcers, to avoid a delay in healing and a worsening of the condition.

● Advise patient not to use herb with products containing sulfur.

● Advise patient to discontinue use if skin reaction occurs.

● Instruct any patient using the herb externally to treat sore nipples to remove residue from her breasts before breast-feeding an infant.

● Advise patient to limit external application to 1 week or less.

## barberry

*Berberis vulgaris,* berberry, jaundice berry, mountain grape, Oregon grape, pepperidge bush, pipperidge, sour-spine, sow berry, trailing mahonia, wood sour

**Common trade names**
*Barberry-Berberis Vulgaris*

### HOW SUPPLIED
Available as liquid extract, tablets, and tea.
*Tablets:* 400 mg

### ACTIONS & COMPONENTS
Contains isoquinolone alkaloids in the root and bark, including the alkaloid berberine. Berberine is effective in managing bacterial-induced diarrhea. In small doses, it stimulates the respiratory system; in large doses, it may produce dyspnea and lethal respiratory system paralysis.

### USES
Used to dilate blood vessels and stimulate the circulatory system, to treat GI ailments, and to relieve or reduce fever. May be beneficial as a bactericidal and for cholera-induced diarrhea, may stimulate uterine contractions, and may have some laxative effects.

### DOSAGE & ADMINISTRATION
*Dried root:* 2 to 4 g P.O.
*Fluidextract (1:1):* 2 to 4 ml P.O.
*For cholera-induced diarrhea:* 100 mg of berberine P.O. q.i.d. or 400 mg P.O. q.d., alone or with tetracycline. Maximum daily dose, 500 mg.
*Solid (powdered dry) extract (4:1) or 8% to 12% alkaloid content:* 250 to 500 mg P.O.
*Tea:* Prepared by pouring 5 oz of hot water onto 1 to 2 tsp whole or squashed barberries and straining after 10 to 15 minutes. Dosage is 2 to 4 g P.O. or 2 g in 8½ oz.
*Tincture (1:5):* 6 to 12 ml P.O.
*Tincture (1:10):* 20 to 40 gtt P.O. q.d.

### ADVERSE REACTIONS
**CNS:** stupor, lethargy.
**CV:** hypotension.
**EENT:** epistaxis, eye irritation.
**GI:** diarrhea.
**GU:** nephritis.
**Respiratory:** dyspnea.
**Skin:** skin irritation.

---

*Bold italic type* indicates that reaction may be life-threatening.

## INTERACTIONS
**Herb-drug.** *Antihypertensives:*
Possible increased effects. Monitor
blood pressure closely.

## CAUTIONS
Pregnant women should avoid use
of barberry because it may stimulate uterine contractions.

Patients with heart failure and
those with respiratory diseases
should use barberry cautiously.

## NURSING CONSIDERATIONS
● Find out why patient is using the
herb.
● If patient is using barberry to
treat diarrhea, monitor him to ensure the therapy is working.
● Ingestion of berberine in doses
exceeding 500 mg can produce
lethargy, nosebleeds, dyspnea, and
skin and eye irritation.
⚠ALERT: Signs of toxic reaction
include stupor, diarrhea, and nephritis. If signs or symptoms of toxic
reaction occur, patient should stop
using barberry and notify his
health care provider.

**Patient teaching**
● Advise patient to consult with his
health care provider before using
an herbal preparation because a
treatment with proven efficacy
may be available.
● Tell patient to remind pharmacist
of any herbal or dietary supplement that he's taking, when filling
a new prescription.
● Advise patient to avoid use during pregnancy and to discontinue
use if she becomes pregnant during barberry therapy.

● If patient is taking an antihypertensive, advise him to contact his
health care provider before taking
barberry.
● Caution patient that herb may be
useful in treating bacteria-induced
diarrhea only, so he shouldn't
delay seeking appropriate medical
evaluation for persistent diarrhea
or diarrhea of unknown cause.
● Advise patient not to take more
than 500 mg daily because doing
so may increase the risk of adverse
reactions, such as lethargy, nosebleeds, difficulty breathing, and
skin and eye irritation.
● Inform patient of the signs and
symptoms of toxic reaction, and
advise him to stop using barberry
if he experiences any of them.

## basil

*Ocimum basilicum,* common
basil, holy basil, St. Josephwort,
sweet basil

**Common trade names**
*None known*

## HOW SUPPLIED
Available as an oil and a spice.

## ACTIONS & COMPONENTS
Contains estragole (70% to 85%
of essential oil) as a major component and smaller amounts of safrole. Estragole may possess mutagenic effects if taken internally in
massive quantities. It's safe to use
as a spice. In vitro, basil is antimicrobial.

*Liquid may contain alcohol.

## USES
Used as an antiseptic, antimicrobial, diuretic, insect repellant, and antihypertensive. Also used to stimulate digestion and to treat halitosis.

## DOSAGE & ADMINISTRATION
*Insect repellant:* Patient should rub oil on exposed areas before he goes outdoors.

## ADVERSE REACTIONS
**CNS:** dizziness, confusion, headache, trembling.
**CV:** palpitations.
**Hepatic:** *hepatocarcinoma.*
**Metabolic:** hypoglycemia.
**Skin:** diaphoresis.

## INTERACTIONS
**Herb-drug.** *Antihypertensives:* May cause added hypotension. Monitor blood pressure.
*Insulin, oral antidiabetics:* May cause added hypoglycemia. Monitor blood glucose level.

## CAUTIONS
Pregnant or breast-feeding women, infants, and young children should avoid use.

Those with diabetes and those taking an antihypertensive should use basil cautiously because it may increase the therapeutic effect of conventional drugs.

## NURSING CONSIDERATIONS
• Find out why patient is using the herb.
• Estragole and safrole are procarcinogens with weak carcinogenic effects in the liver. Although the risk of developing cancer from use of basil is minimal, long-term or high-dose therapy isn't recommended.
• If a patient is taking both an antihypertensive and basil and his blood pressure stabilizes, the dosage of the conventional antihypertensive may need to be adjusted once he stops taking the herb.
• Taking medicinal doses of basil may disrupt a previously stable antidiabetic regimen.
• Monitor patient for signs and symptoms of hypoglycemia, such as dizziness, weakness, sweating, tachycardia, headache, confusion, and trembling.

**Patient teaching**
• Advise patient to consult with his health care provider before using an herbal preparation because a treatment with proven efficacy may be available.
• Tell patient to remind pharmacist of any herbal or dietary supplement that he's taking, when filling a new prescription.
• Advise patient that herb isn't recommended for use in large quantities because it may cause cancer; however, the amounts used in cooking appear to be safe.
• Advise pregnant or breast-feeding patient to avoid medicinal use of basil.
• Advise patient to avoid use in infants and children.
• Advise diabetic patient to consult his health care provider before using basil because it can cause hypoglycemia.
• If patient is taking an antihypertensive, inform him that basil may also lower blood pressure, causing

an additive effect on the blood pressure.

## bay

*Laurus nobilis,* bay laurel, bay leaf, bay tree, daphne, Grecian laurel, Indian bay, laurel, noble laurel, Roman laurel, sweet bay, true laurel

**Common trade names**
*None known*

### HOW SUPPLIED
Available as berries, extracts, leaves, oils, ointments, and soaps.

### ACTIONS & COMPONENTS
Contains 1,8-cineol, which may be bactericidal, and parthenolides, which may help prevent migraine. Lowers the blood glucose level by helping the body use insulin more effectively.

### USES
Used as an antiseptic and a stimulant. Used to treat the common cold and to relieve muscle spasms. Also found in some toothpastes because it may help prevent tooth decay.

### DOSAGE & ADMINISTRATION
Not well documented.

### ADVERSE REACTIONS
**Metabolic:** hypoglycemia.
**Respiratory:** asthma.
**Other:** allergic reactions.

### INTERACTIONS
**Herb-drug.** *Antidiabetics, insulin:* Bay may exacerbate the intended therapeutic effects of conventional drugs. Monitor blood glucose level.

### CAUTIONS
Patient shouldn't use internally. Pregnant and breast-feeding patients should avoid use.

Patients with diabetes who are taking an antidiabetic should use bay cautiously because it may exacerbate hypoglycemia, disrupting a previously stable antidiabetic regimen.

### NURSING CONSIDERATIONS
• Find out why patient is using the herb.
• Internal use may result in allergic reactions, including asthma.
• Monitor patient for signs and symptoms of hypoglycemia, such as confusion, dizziness, sweating, and trembling.

**Patient teaching**
• Advise patient to consult with his health care provider before using an herbal preparation because a treatment with proven efficacy may be available.
• Tell patient to remind pharmacist of any herbal or dietary supplement that he's taking, when filling a new prescription.
• Advise patient that bay isn't recommended for internal use because it can cause allergic reactions, including asthma.
• If patient has diabetes, advise him to consult with his health care provider before using bay because it can cause hypoglycemia.
• Advise patient to avoid use if she's pregnant or breast-feeding

*Liquid may contain alcohol.

and to notify her health care provider if she becomes pregnant during bay therapy.

## bayberry

*Myrica cerifera, M. cortex,* bog myrtle, candleberry, dutch myrtle, sweet gale, tallow shrub, vegetable tallow, wachsgagle, waxberry, wax myrtle

**Common trade names**
*Bayberry Bark, Bayberry Root Bark*

### HOW SUPPLIED
Available as capsules, liquid extract*, powder, and tea.
*Capsules:* 450 mg, 475 mg

### ACTIONS & COMPONENTS
Contains tannins, triterpenes, myricadiol, taraxerol, taraxerone, and flavonoid glycoside myricitrin.
   Tannins give bayberry its astringent properties. Myricadiol may have mineralocorticoid activity, myricitrin may stimulate the flow of bile, and the dried root may be antipyretic.

### USES
Used as a tea to treat diarrhea and as a gargle to treat sore throats. Also used internally for coughs and colds and for its antipyretic and circulatory stimulant properties. Used topically for its astringent properties.

### DOSAGE & ADMINISTRATION
*Liquid extract (1:1) in 45% alcohol:* 0.6 to 2 ml or 10 to 90 gtt P.O. t.i.d.

*Powdered bark:* 600 mg to 2 g P.O. t.i.d. by infusion or decoction.

### ADVERSE REACTIONS
**EENT:** sneezing.
**GI:** stomach upset, vomiting.
**Respiratory:** cough.

### INTERACTIONS
**Herb-drug.** *Antihypertensives, corticosteroids:* Possible additive effects. Bayberry may interfere with the intended therapeutic effects of conventional drugs.
*Iron:* Decreased absorption of iron. Advise patient to separate administration times by 2 hours.

### CAUTIONS
Patient shouldn't use internally. Pregnant patients, breast-feeding patients, and patients allergic to bayberry should avoid use. Patients taking a corticosteroid and those with hypertension, peripheral edema, heart failure, and other conditions in which mineralocorticoid use isn't advised should also avoid use.

### NURSING CONSIDERATIONS
● Find out why patient is using the herb.
● Bayberry has a high tannin content and commonly causes gastric distress and liver damage after long-term use.
● Long-term use of bark extract may result in malignant tumors.
● Heat, moisture, and light may cause bayberry to break down, so it should be stored in a dry, dark, cool place.

---

*Bold italic type* indicates that reaction may be life-threatening.

• Large doses have mineralocorticoid effects such as sodium and water retention and hypertension.

**Patient teaching**
• Advise patient to consult with his health care provider before using an herbal preparation because a treatment with proven efficacy may be available.
• Tell patient to remind pharmacist of any herbal or dietary supplement that he's taking, when filling a new prescription.
• If patient has high blood pressure or heart disease, advise him to consult with his health care provider before using the herb.
• Caution patient to avoid use if she's pregnant or breast-feeding and to notify her health care provider if she becomes pregnant during bayberry therapy.
• Caution patient that internal use of bayberry isn't recommended and that such use can cause stomach upset and vomiting.
• Advise patient to avoid using bayberry for extended periods because it can cause tumors or mineralocorticoid adverse reactions.
• Advise patient to store bayberry in a dry, dark, cool place.

## bearberry

*Arctostaphylos uva-ursi,* arberry, bearsgrape, kinnikinnick, manzanita, mealberry, mountain box, mountain cranberry, redberry leaves, rockbeery, sagackhomi, sandberry, uvaursi

**Common trade names**
*Uva-Ursi, Uva-Ursi Leaf, Standardized Uva-Ursi Extract*

### HOW SUPPLIED
Available as capsules, dried leaves, liquid extract, and tea bags.
*Capsules:* 455 mg, 460 mg (with dandelion), 500 mg, 505 mg capsules that contain 335 mg of leaf extract and 150 mg of uva-ursi leaves and millet
*Liquid extract (prepared from dried leaves):* Cold processed biochelated extract made from freshly manufactured uva-ursi leaves, vegetable glycerin, and grain neutral spirits (12% to 14% by volume)
*Tea bags:* Caffeine free

### ACTIONS & COMPONENTS
Bearberry leaves contain the hydroquinone derivatives arbutin, and methyl arbutin, in levels ranging from 5% to 15%. Arbutin is hydrolyzed to hydroquinone when it comes in contact with gastric fluid, which acts as a mild astringent and antimicrobial in alkaline urine.

Large amounts of bearberry must be ingested to achieve a significant antiseptic effect. The herb is effective against *Esche-*

---

*Liquid may contain alcohol.

*richia coli, Proteus mirabilis, P. vulgaris, Pseudomonas aeruginosa, Staphylococcus aureus,* and 70 other urinary tract bacteria.

Bearberry also contains ursolic acid and isoquercetin, which contribute to the plant's mild diuretic effect.

Bearberry may help treat hepatitis; reduce polyphagia, polydipsia, and weight gain resulting from diabetes; inhibit melanin production; and have anti-inflammatory effects.

## USES
Used as a urinary antiseptic and a mild diuretic. Also used to treat contact dermatitis, allergic-type hypersensitivity reactions, and arthritis.

## DOSAGE & ADMINISTRATION
*Capsules:* Doses vary depending on the formulation. Capsules should be taken with a meal or a glass of water.
*Cold maceration:* 3 g in 5 oz of water P.O. up to q.i.d. or 400 to 840 mg of hydroquinone derivatives calculated as water-free arbutin.
*Concentrated infusion:* 2 to 4 ml P.O.
*Dried leaves infusion:* Prepared by pouring boiling water over 2.5 g of finely cut or coarse powdered herb or placing the herb in cold water and rapidly bringing the mixture to a boil. Tea is strained after 15 minutes. (1 tsp is equivalent to 2.5 g of drug.)
*Liquid extract:* 1.5 to 4 ml (1:1 in 25% alcohol) P.O. t.i.d. Typically, 5 to 10 gtt of extract are mixed in

a small amount of spring or purified water b.i.d. or t.i.d.
*Tea bag infusion:* 1.5 to 4 g by infusion t.i.d. Prepared by placing 1 tea bag into a cup, adding no more than 6 oz of boiling water, and steeping for 3 minutes. Tea bag is pressed before it's removed to enhance the flavor.

Cold water, instead of hot water, is poured over the leaves to minimize the tannin content of the infusion. The tea steeps for 12 to 24 hours before the patient drinks it.

## ADVERSE REACTIONS
**CNS:** *seizures.*
**EENT:** tinnitus.
**GI:** nausea, vomiting.
**GU:** inflammation and irritation of the bladder and urinary tract mucous membranes, green-brown urine.
**Hepatic:** *hepatotoxicity.*
**Other:** cyanosis, collapse.

## INTERACTIONS
**Herb-drug.** *Dexamethasone, prednisolone:* Arbutin increases the inhibitory action of prednisolone and dexamethasone on contact dermatitis, allergic-type hypersensitivity reactions, and arthritis. Advise patient not to use together.
*Disulfiram:* Herbal products prepared with alcohol may cause a disulfiram-like reaction. Advise patient not to use together.
*Diuretics:* Enhanced effect. Monitor patient closely.
*Drugs known to acidify urine such as ascorbic acid or methenamine or to increase uric acid levels such as diazoxide, diuretics, or pyrazinamide:* May inhibit bearberry's

---

effects because bearberry needs an alkali environment. Advise patient to avoid using together.

**Herb-food.** *Foods known to increase uric acid levels in the bladder, such as those rich in vitamin C:* May inhibit bearberry's effects because bearberry needs an alkali environment and the urinary acidifier may inhibit the conversion of herb's arbutin to the active hydroquinone component. Advise patient to avoid using together.

CAUTIONS

Pregnant patients should avoid use because of bearberry's oxytocic effects; patients with kidney disease, because tannin components are believed to be excreted in the urine. Breast-feeding patients and children younger than age 12 should also avoid use.

NURSING CONSIDERATIONS
- Find out why patient is using the herb.
- Bearberry shouldn't be used for longer than 10 days at a time or more than five times per year.
- Bearberry contains 15% to 20% tannin, which may produce nausea and vomiting.
- Bearberry 9 g is equivalent to 400 to 700 mg of arbutin q.d.
- Signs and symptoms of overdose include inflammation and irritation of the bladder and urinary tract mucous membranes. Ingestion of 1 g can cause nausea, vomiting, tinnitus, cyanosis, seizures, and collapse. Ingestion of 5 g of hydroquinone can result in death.

- Hepatotoxicity may occur with prolonged use, especially in children.

**Patient teaching**
- Advise patient to consult with his health care provider before using an herbal preparation because a treatment with proven efficacy may be available.
- Tell patient to remind pharmacist of any herbal or dietary supplement that he's taking, when filling a new prescription.
- If patient has kidney disease or is pregnant or breast-feeding, advise her not to use bearberry.
- Advise patient to take bearberry with a meal or a glass of water.
- Inform patient that urine pH must be alkaline for bearberry to be effective and that a diet high in milk, vegetables (especially tomatoes), fruit, fruit juice, and potatoes can help keep urine alkaline. Tell him that he may also take 6 to 8 g of sodium bicarbonate a day to help keep his urine alkaline.
- Inform patient that the hydroquinone in the herb may discolor his urine green-brown.
- Advise patient to consult his health care provider if symptoms persist for more than 7 days or if he experiences high fever, chills, nausea, vomiting, diarrhea, or severe back pain.
- Inform patient that pouring hot water over the leaves when preparing a bearberry beverage may increase the tannin content of the infusion and, thus, increase the risk of stomach discomfort. Advise him instead to pour cold water over the leaves and to allow the

mixture to steep for 12 to 24 hours before drinking it.
- Advise patient not to take bearberry for more than 10 days at a time or more than five times per year.

## bee pollen

buckwheat pollen, maize pollen

**Common trade names**
*Bee Pollen, Health Honey, Super Bee Pollen Complex*

### HOW SUPPLIED
Available as capsules, chewable tablets, cream (in combination with other moisturizers), jelly, liquid (manufactured bee pollen extract, vegetable glycerin, and grain-neutral spirits), powder, raw granules, soft gel caps, and tablets.
*Capsules:* 265 mg, 500 mg, 580 mg, 586 mg
*Chewable tablets:* 500 mg
*Granules:* 154 servings/container
*Jelly:* 3,000 mg in 10-oz jar of honey
*Powder:* 5 g/1 heaping tsp
*Soft gel cap:* 100 mg
*Tablets:* 378 mg, 500 mg, 1,000 mg

### ACTIONS & COMPONENTS
Contains about 30% protein, 55% carbohydrates, 1% to 2% fat, 3% minerals, and trace vitamins. Components vary depending on plant source, geographic region, harvest methods, and season of the year. May contain up to 100 vitamins, minerals, enzymes, amino acids, and other substances, but the physiologic benefit of many of these components is unclear. Some

bee pollen supplements also contain 3.6% to 5.9% vitamin C.

### USES
Used to enhance athletic performance, minimize fatigue, and improve energy.

May relieve or cure cerebral hemorrhage, brain damage, body weakness, anemia, enteritis, colitis, constipation, and indigestion. May be beneficial in treating chronic prostatism and relieving symptoms of radiation sickness in those being treated for cervical cancer. May also be an effective prenatal vitamin and aid in weight loss.

Although bee pollen is used to treat allergic disorders, such use isn't recommended because bee pollen commonly causes allergic reactions.

### DOSAGE & ADMINISTRATION
*Granules:* Directions vary depending on product. One manufacturer recommends ingesting 1 tsp or more P.O. q.d. or sprinkling on food or mixing in drinks. Another manufacturer recommends ingesting 1 granule at lunchtime, increasing by 1 granule with each meal until 1 tsp is being eaten each meal.
*Liquid:* 10 to 12 gtt of extract mixed in a little water, b.i.d. or t.i.d.
*Oral use:* 1 to 3 g q.d. Dosage varies depending on product and manufacturer.
*Powder:* 1 to 2 tsp P.O. q.d. May be consumed as sold or may be blended or mixed with other foods.
*Soft gel cap:* 1 cap or more P.O. q.d.

*Tablets:* Dosage varies depending on the formulation and manufacturer. Tablets may be swallowed or dissolved with warm water and honey.

**ADVERSE REACTIONS**
**Other:** *acute anaphylactic reactions,* including sneezing, *generalized angioedema,* itching, dyspnea, and light-headedness; chronic allergic symptoms, including hypereosinophilia; and neurologic and GI complaints.

**INTERACTIONS**
None reported.

**CAUTIONS**
Those with sensitivity or allergies to pollen should avoid use.

Those with allergies to apples, carrots, or celery should use cautiously because of the potential for adverse reaction.

**NURSING CONSIDERATIONS**
• Find out why patient is using the herb.
• Overall, bee pollen hasn't been found to have significant nutritional or therapeutic benefit over more easily and safely administered nutritional products.
• Some bee pollen products also contain bee propolis extract and numerous other ingredients and vitamins.
• Doses as low as 1 tbs can cause acute anaphylactic reactions, including sneezing, generalized angioedema, itching, dyspnea, and light-headedness. Ask patient how much herb he uses daily.

• Patients taking bee pollen for longer than 3 weeks may experience chronic allergic symptoms, such as hypereosinophilia and neurologic and GI complaints; however, such symptoms are likely to resolve after the patient stops taking the bee pollen.

**Patient teaching**
• Advise patient to consult with his health care provider before using an herbal preparation because a treatment with proven efficacy may be available.
• Tell patient to remind pharmacist of any herbal or dietary supplement that he's taking, when filling a new prescription.
• Inform patient that bee pollen should be taken between meals, with a full glass of water.

## benzoin

*Styrax benzoin, S. paralleloneurus,* Benjamin tree, gum Benjamin, gum benzoin, Siam benzoin, Sumatra benzoin

**Common trade names**
*Benzoin Spray, Tincture of Benzoin, and various multiple-ingredient preparations*

**HOW SUPPLIED**
Available as compound tincture of benzoin* and tincture of benzoin spray*.

**ACTIONS & COMPONENTS**
Siam benzoin contains benzoate, alcohol, benzoic acid, d-siaresinolic acid, and cinnamyl benzoate. Sumatra benzoin contains benzoic

acid and cinnamic esters of ben-
zoresorcinol and coniferyl alcohol, free benzoic acid, cinnamic
acids, and other ingredients. These
components give benzoin its skin
protectant, expectorant, and soothing properties. Benzoic acid also
has antifungal and antibacterial
properties.

## USES
Used topically as a skin protectant.
Mixed with glycerin and water and
applied to cutaneous ulcers, bedsores, cracked nipples, and fissures
of the lips or anus. Also combined
with zinc oxide in baby ointments.

Administered on sugar or added
to hot water and inhaled as a vapor
to treat throat and bronchial inflammation, acute laryngitis, or croup.

## DOSAGE & ADMINISTRATION
*Inhalant use:* 1% in very hot
water.

## ADVERSE REACTIONS
**Skin:** irritation, urticaria at application site.

## INTERACTIONS
None reported.

## CAUTIONS
Those with hypersensitivity to
benzoin should avoid use.

## NURSING CONSIDERATIONS
● Find out why patient is using the
herb.
● Mild irritation may occur at the
application site.
● Benzoin should be stored in a
cool, dry place, away from excessive heat.

## Patient teaching
● Advise patient to consult with his
health care provider before using
an herbal preparation, because a
treatment with proven efficacy
may be available.
● Tell patient to remind pharmacist
of any herbal or dietary supplement that he's taking, when filling
a new prescription.
● Inform patient that mild irritation
may occur at application site.
● Instruct patient to store benzoin
in a cool, dry place, away from
excessive heat.

## betel palm

*Areca catechu,* piper betle

**Common trade names**
*Areca Nut, Betel Nut, Pinang,
Pinlang*

## HOW SUPPLIED
Available as quids, made from
powdered or sliced areca nut, tobacco, and slaked lime (calcium
hydroxide), obtained from powdered snail shells, and wrapped in
the betel vine leaf.

## ACTIONS & COMPONENTS
Contains arecoline, arecaidine,
arecaine, arecolidine, guvacine,
isoguvacine, and guvacoline,
which cause CNS stimulation.

Chewing the nut increases sali-
vary flow and aids digestion.

## USES
Used as a mild CNS stimulant
and a digestive aid. Used to treat
coughs, stomach complaints,

diphtheria, middle ear inflammation, and worm infestation.

Some patients steam the leaves and apply them as a facial dressing, but such use isn't recommended because of adverse dermatologic reactions.

## DOSAGE & ADMINISTRATION
*Quid:* 4 to 15 quids chewed q.d., for 15 minutes each.

## ADVERSE REACTIONS
**CNS:** *tetanic seizures.*
**EENT:** tooth discoloration, gingivitis, oral lichen planuslike lesion, *oral cancer including leukoplakia and squamous cell carcinoma,* periodontitis, resorption of oral calcium.
**Musculoskeletal:** chronic osteomyelitis.
**Respiratory:** asthma exacerbation.
**Skin:** contact leukomelanosis characterized by immediate bleaching, hyperpigmentation, and confetti-like depigmentation.

## INTERACTIONS
**Herb-drug.** *Fluphenazine, procyclidine:* May cause tremor, stiffness, akathisia because of decreased effectiveness of the drugs in the presence of herb's cholinergic alkaloid, arecoline. Advise patient to avoid using together.
*Prednisone, salbutamol:* May exacerbate asthma. Advise patient to avoid using together.

## CAUTIONS
Those with a history of asthma should avoid use because of bronchoconstriction; those who are pregnant, because of possible teratogenic or fetotoxic effects.

## NURSING CONSIDERATIONS
- Find out why patient is using the herb.

⚠ALERT: Arecaine, a compound of the herb, is poisonous, affects respiration and heart rate, and may cause seizures. Seed doses of 8 g can be fatal.
- Chewing betel palm can cause severe oral mucosal changes, including cancerous lesions.
- Chewing the betel palm–slaked lime mixture may place patient at higher risk for oral lesions than chewing betel palm alone.
- Monitor patient for asthmalike symptoms.
- Betel palm leaf facial dressings can cause severe dermatologic reactions, such as contact leukomelanosis, which occurs in three stages—immediate bleaching, hyperpigmentation, and confetti-like depigmentation.

### Patient teaching
- Advise patient to consult with his health care provider before using an herbal preparation because a treatment with proven efficacy may be available.
- Tell patient to remind pharmacist of any herbal or dietary supplement that he's taking, when filling a new prescription.
- Warn patient that chewing betel palm may cause cancerous lesions in mouth and that he should consult his health care provider immediately if he develops lesions.
- Advise patient who chews betel nut to contact his health care pro-

vider if he develops asthmalike symptoms.

• Advise patient not to apply betel palm leaves as a facial dressing because doing so could cause adverse dermatologic reactions.

## bethroot

*Trillium erectum, T. pendulum*, birthroot, coughroot, ground lily, Indian balm, Indian shamrock, jew's-harp plant, lamb's quarters, milk ipecac, nightshade, pariswort, purple trillium, rattlesnake root, snakebite, stinking benjamin, three-leaved, wake-robin

**Common trade names**
*None known*

### HOW SUPPLIED
Available as ground drug and liquid extract.

### ACTIONS & COMPONENTS
Contains a fixed oil, a volatile oil, a saponin called trillarin, a glycoside, tannic acid, and starch. The saponin glycosides have antifungal activity.

### USES
Used internally to treat long, heavy menstrual periods; to relieve pain; to control postpartum bleeding; and to manage diarrhea. Also used as an expectorant.

Used externally for varicose veins and ulcers, hematomas, and hemorrhoids. Also used externally as an astringent to minimize topical bleeding and irritation.

### DOSAGE & ADMINISTRATION
Ground drug and liquid extract are used for infusions and poultices.

### ADVERSE REACTIONS
**GI:** nausea, vomiting.
**GU:** promotes menstruation, promotes labor in pregnancy.
**Skin:** irritation at the application site.

### INTERACTIONS
None reported.

### CAUTIONS
Pregnant patients should avoid use because it stimulates the uterus.

### NURSING CONSIDERATIONS
• Find out why patient is using the herb.
• Monitor application site for irritation.

#### Patient teaching
• Advise patient to consult with his health care provider before using an herbal preparation because a treatment with proven efficacy may be available.
• Tell patient to remind pharmacist of any herbal or dietary supplement that he's taking, when filling a new prescription.
• Advise patient to avoid use during pregnancy.
• Inform patient that high doses of bethroot can cause nausea.
• Advise patient to discontinue use if skin irritation develops.

---

*Bold italic type* indicates that reaction may be life-threatening.

## betony

*Betonica officinalis, Stachys officinalis,* bishopswort, wood betony

**Common trade names**
*Betony, Betony Tincture, Wood Betony Capsules*

### HOW SUPPLIED
Available as a tincture*, powder, or in 450-mg capsules.

### ACTIONS & COMPONENTS
The basal leaves—which contain betaine, caffeic acid derivatives, and flavonoids—are the medicinal part of the herb. They're collected and dried in shade at a maximum temperature of 40° F (4.4° C).

Betony contains 15% tannins, which give the herb its astringent effects. Mixtures of flavonoid glycosides have hypotensive and sedative effects. Stachydrine is a systolic depressant and acts to decrease rheumatic pain.

### USES
Used as an antidiarrheal, a sedative, and an expectorant for coughs, bronchitis, and asthma. Also used to treat catarrh, heartburn, gout, nervousness, kidney stones, and inflammation of the bladder.

Used with other herbs such as comfrey or linden as a sedative, a mild hypotensive for treating neuralgia and anxiety, and a decongestant for treating sinus headache and congestion.

### DOSAGE & ADMINISTRATION
*Oral use:* 1 to 2 g q.d. in three divided doses.
*Topical use:* Extract or infusion is applied to the skin as an astringent or as a treatment for wounds. Or, fresh leaves are boiled and cooled and the liquid applied to skin.

### ADVERSE REACTIONS
**CNS:** drowsiness.
**GI:** GI irritation.

### INTERACTIONS
**Herb-drug.** *Antihypertensives, sedatives:* Betony may increase the intended therapeutic effect of these drugs. Advise patient to use cautiously.
*CNS depressants:* Additive effects. Advise patient to use cautiously.
*Disulfiram, metronidazole:* Tincture contains up to 40% ethyl alcohol and may cause a disulfiram or disulfiram-like reaction. Advise patient not to use together.
**Herb-lifestyle.** *Alcohol:* Additive effects. Advise patient to use cautiously.

### CAUTIONS
Patients who are pregnant or breast-feeding should avoid use.

### NURSING CONSIDERATIONS
• Find out why patient is using the herb.
• Large oral dosage may cause GI irritation because of the tannin content.
• Don't confuse with *Stachys officinalis* with *Stachys alpina.*

---

*Liquid may contain alcohol.

**Patient teaching**

- Advise patient to consult with his health care provider before using an herbal preparation because a treatment with proven efficacy may be available.
- Tell patient to remind pharmacist of any herbal or dietary supplement that he's taking, when filling a new prescription.
- Warn patient not to exceed the recommended dosage.
- Caution patient that internal use of betony may cause drowsiness.
- If patient is taking betony to treat diarrhea, advise him to consult his health care provider if it continues for longer than 2 days.
- If patient is taking betony to treat headache and it doesn't improve, advise him to discontinue use and consult his health care provider.

## bilberry

*Vaccinium myrtillus,* airelle, black whortles, bleaberry, bog bilberries, burren myrtle, dwarf bilberry, dyeberry, European blueberry, huckleberry, hurtleberry, hurts, trackleberry whortleberry, wineberry

Common trade names
*Bilberry, Bilberry Fruit, Bilberry Power, Bilberry Tincture, Dried Bilberry*

## HOW SUPPLIED

Available as dried fruit, 10% decoction for topical use, dry extract (25% anthocyanosides) in an 80-mg capsule, and fluidextract 1:1.

## ACTIONS & COMPONENTS

The fruit of the bilberry contains 5% to 10% tannins, which act as an astringent; these tannins may help target the bowel and help treat diarrhea.

The anthocyanidins in bilberry help prevent angina episodes, reduce capillary fragility, and stabilize tissues that have collagen-like tendons and ligaments. They also inhibit platelet aggregation and thrombus formation by interacting with vascular prostaglandins.

The anthocyanidins also help regenerate rhodopsin, a light-sensitive pigment found on the rods of the retina, so bilberry may help treat degenerative retinal conditions, macular degeneration, poor night vision, glaucoma, and cataracts.

Bilberry may have vasoprotective, antiedemic, and hepatoprotective properties because of its antioxidant effects from anthocyanidins. The anthocyanidin pigment in the herb may increase the gastric mucosal release of prostaglandin $E_2$, accounting for the antiulcerative and gastroprotective effects.

## USES

Used to treat acute diarrhea and mild inflammation of the mucous membranes of the mouth and throat. Used to provide symptomatic relief from vascular disorders (including capillary weakness, venous insufficiency, and hemorrhoids) and to prevent macular degeneration. Also used for its potential hepatoprotective properties.

---

*Bold italic type* indicates that reaction may be life-threatening.

## DOSAGE & ADMINISTRATION
*Dried fruit:* 4 to 8 g P.O. with water several times q.d.
*Fluidextract:* 2 to 4 ml P.O. t.i.d.
*For eye disorders:* 80 to 160 mg dry extract (25% anthocyanosides) P.O. t.i.d.
*For inflammation:* 10% decoction. Prepared by boiling 5 to 10 g of crushed dried fruit in 5 oz of cold water for 10 minutes and then straining while hot. Applied topically as an astringent.
*For treatment of acute diarrhea:* 20 to 60 g of dried fruit P.O. q.d.

## ADVERSE REACTIONS
None known.

## INTERACTIONS
**Herb-drug.** *Warfarin:* Possible additive effects. Monitor patient for bleeding or loss of therapeutic anticoagulation.

## CAUTIONS
Because the herb may inhibit platelet aggregation, it may be unsuitable for those with a bleeding disorder.

## NURSING CONSIDERATIONS
• Find out why patient is using the herb.
• Because bilberry may reduce a diabetic patient's blood glucose level, dosage of his conventional antidiabetic may need to be adjusted.
• Consistent dosing of bilberry is needed when using the herb to treat vascular or ocular conditions.
• Bilberry should be safe for pregnant and breast-feeding patients to use.

• Bilberry may be taken without regard to food.

**Patient teaching**
• Advise patient to consult with his health care provider before using an herbal preparation because a treatment with proven efficacy may be available.
• Tell patient to remind pharmacist of any herbal or dietary supplement that he's taking, when filling a new prescription.
• Tell patient that bilberry may be taken without regard to food.
• Advise any patient using the dried fruit to take each dose with a full glass of water.
• If patient is using bilberry to treat diarrhea, advise him to consult his health care provider if it doesn't improve in 3 to 4 days.

## birch

*Betula*, betula lenta

**Common trade names**
*Birch, Birch Leaf, Birch Tea*

## HOW SUPPLIED
Available as dried leaves for tea, freshly pressed plant juices for internal use, and ointment and birch tar for topical use.

## ACTIONS & COMPONENTS
Birch leaves are collected in spring and dried at room temperature in the shade. They contain tannin and gaultherine oil which, when mixed with water, yields methyl salicylate. Other components of the leaves are triterpene alcohol, flavonoids (1.5%), proan-

---

*Liquid may contain alcohol.

thocyanidins, and caffeic acid derivatives. These substances have a diuretic effect.

**USES**
Used as a gentle stimulant and astringent. Warm water infusion is used to stimulate diaphoresis, to flush out kidney stones, and to treat diarrhea, dysentery, cholera infantum, and UTIs.

Applied topically, birch may temporarily relieve rheumatic pain because of its menthyl salicylate content. Infusion is used to treat dandruff. Birch tar oil, or pix betulina, is used to treat scabies and skin infections.

**DOSAGE & ADMINISTRATION**
*Dried herb:* Average daily dose is 2 to 3 g several times a day.
*Infusion:* Taken between meals t.i.d. or q.i.d.
*Tea:* Prepared from dry leaves or fresh plant juice and used internally as is or used to make an infusion and then used internally.

**ADVERSE REACTIONS**
**Skin:** irritation from topical use.

**INTERACTIONS**
None reported.

**CAUTIONS**
Those who are dehydrated or allergic to birch trees should avoid use. Those with compromised cardiac or renal function shouldn't use birch to treat edema.

**NURSING CONSIDERATIONS**
• Find out why patient is using the herb.

• Make sure any patient taking the herb orally drinks plenty of fluids because birch has a diaphoretic effect.
• Birch ointment and oil could be lethal if used internally.
• Birch tar is a toxic substance that kills scabies. It shouldn't be overused because of the risk of systemic absorption.

**Patient teaching**
• Advise patient to consult with his health care provider before using an herbal preparation because a treatment with proven efficacy may be available.
• Tell patient to remind pharmacist of any herbal or dietary supplement that he's taking, when filling a new prescription.
• Advise patient not to exceed the average daily dose without consulting his health care provider.
• Advise patient to drink plenty of fluids if he's taking birch orally.
• Advise patient to consult with his health care provider if his condition doesn't improve in a few days.
• Instruct patient to discontinue use if his skin becomes irritated.

## bistort

*Persicaria bistorta,* adderwort, dragonwort, Easter giant, Easter mangiant, oderwort, osterick, patience dock, sankeweed, sweet dock

**Common trade names**
*None known*

**HOW SUPPLIED**
Available as a powder, which is

---

used to make an extract, infusion, ointment, or tincture for external use.

## ACTIONS & COMPONENTS
The powder is made from the leaves and rhizome of older plants; the parts are harvested, cleaned, freed from green parts, cut up, and dried in the sun.

Bistort contains 13% to 36% tannins, which give the herb the astringent effects that are helpful in treating diarrhea and sore or dry throat.

## USES
Used to treat digestive disorders, particularly diarrhea. Used as a gargle for mouth and throat infections and as an ointment for minor wounds.

## DOSAGE & ADMINISTRATION
*Tincture:* 10 to 40 gtt diluted in a small amount of water and used as a gargle.
*To treat minor mouth and throat irritations or infections:* An infusion is made with cold water. Used as a gargle or a rinse.

## ADVERSE REACTIONS
None reported.

## INTERACTIONS
**Herb-drug.** *Disulfiram, metronidazole:* Tincture contains alcohol and may precipitate a disulfiram or disulfiram-like reaction, including flushing, dyspnea, vomiting, syncope, and confusion. Advise patient to avoid using together.

## CAUTIONS
Pregnant and breast-feeding patients should avoid use.

## NURSING CONSIDERATIONS
• Find out why patient is using the herb.
• Bistort is rarely used, and dosage information for internal use is lacking.
• Because of the tannin content, overuse may increase mucous formation and irritate the intestines.

### Patient teaching
• Advise patient to consult with his health care provider before using an herbal preparation because a treatment with proven efficacy may be available.
• Tell patient to remind pharmacist of any herbal or dietary supplement that he's taking, when filling a new prescription.
• If patient is pregnant or breast-feeding, advise her not to use bistort.
• Warn patient that herb is rarely used and that few dosage guidelines exist.
• Instruct patient to keep herb away from children and pets.

## bitter melon

*Momordica charantia*, art pumpkin, balsam apple, balsam pear, bitter cucumber, bitter melon, carilla cundeamor, cerasee

### Common trade names
*Bitter Melon, Bitter Melon Juice, Bitter Melon Power, Bitter Melon Tincture*

---

*Liquid may contain alcohol.

## HOW SUPPLIED
Available as juice or as an extract in gel caps.

## ACTIONS & COMPONENTS
The hypoglycemic effect of bitter melon is the result of the melon's charantin, polypeptide P, and vicine components. These substances reduce the blood glucose level and improve glucose tolerance. The seeds of the bitter melon contain alpha-momorcharin and beta-momorcharin, which are abortifacients.

Bitter melon may have antimicrobial effects and may inhibit viruses, including polio, herpes simplex 1, and HIV. It may also have anti-inflammatory effects and improve GI ailments such as flatus, ulcers, constipation, and hemorrhoids.

## USES
Used to treat diabetes symptoms. May help treat GI disorders.

## DOSAGE & ADMINISTRATION
*To lower the blood glucose level:* 2 oz of the fresh juice q.d. or the equivalent of 15 g of the aqueous extract in gel cap form.

## ADVERSE REACTIONS
**CNS:** headache, *coma.*
**GI:** abdominal pain.
**GU:** uterine bleeding, uterine contractions, *abortion.*
**Hepatic:** *hepatotoxicity.*
**Metabolic:** hypoglycemia.
**Other:** fever.

## INTERACTIONS
**Herb-drug.** *Insulin, oral antidiabetics:* Possible increased hypoglycemic effect and rapid drop in blood glucose level. Monitor patient for signs of hypoglycemia.

## CAUTIONS
Because the red arils around the seeds may cause toxic reaction in children, bitter melon shouldn't be used in these patients. Also, pregnant women should avoid using it because it may cause uterine bleeding or miscarriage.

## NURSING CONSIDERATIONS
• Find out why patient is using the herb.
• The juice of bitter melon has a bitter taste.
• Bitter melon should be taken only in small doses, for no longer than 4 weeks.
• The hypoglycemic effects of bitter melon are dose related, so dosage should be adjusted gradually.
⚡**ALERT:** Bitter melon seeds contain vicine, which may cause an acute condition characterized by headache, fever, abdominal pain, and coma.

## Patient teaching
• Advise patient to consult with his health care provider before using an herbal preparation because a treatment with proven efficacy may be available.
• Tell patient to remind pharmacist of any herbal or dietary supplement that he's taking, when filling a new prescription.

---

*Bold italic type* indicates that reaction may be life-threatening.

- If patient is pregnant or breast-feeding, advise her not to use bitter melon.
- Advise patient to keep doses low and not to take bitter melon for longer than 4 weeks.
- Inform diabetic patient that herb may cause hypoglycemia.

⚡ALERT: Advise patient to store herb out of reach of children and pets because it can have toxic effects, including death.

- Instruct patient to immediately report headache, fever, and abdominal pain.

## bitter orange

*Citrus aurantium,* bigarade orange, cortenza de naranja amarga, neroli, orange, pomeranzenschale, zhi shi

Common trade names
*Bitter Orange Extract, Bitter Orange Peel, Oil of Bitter Orange*

### HOW SUPPLIED
Available as a crude, dry orange peel for use in tea and traditional Chinese medicine, capsules and tablets in weight-loss preparations, essential oil, and extracts for topical use.

### ACTIONS & COMPONENTS
An aromatic bitter with a spicy aroma and taste. Consists of the dry outer peel of both ripe and unripe fruits of *C. aurantium,* minus the white, spongy parenchyma.

Contains the flavanone glycosides naringin and neohesperidin, which are responsible for the bitter flavor. The volatile oils limonene,

jasmone, linalyl acetate, geranyl acetate, and citronellyl acetate contribute to the aroma.

A bitter orange aqueous extract may have vasoactive effects. Topical bitter orange has antifungal effects and may be useful as an antiseptic.

The plant that bitter orange comes from contains synephrine and other sympathomimetics that cause CNS stimulation, insomnia, hypertension, and tachycardia. Bitter orange may also have these effects.

### USES
Used to stimulate appetite, aid digestion, and relieve bloating. Used as an antifungal and as a gargle for sore throat. May also aid in weight loss.

In traditional Chinese medicine, it's used to treat prolapsed uterus, prolapsed anus or rectum, dysentery, abdominal pain, and other GI conditions.

Also used to improve the taste and smell of herbal teas and is commonly added to sedative teas containing valerian or balm leaves.

### DOSAGE & ADMINISTRATION
*Herb:* 4 to 6 g P.O. q.d.
*Extract:* 1 to 2 g P.O. q.d.
*Tea:* Prepared by steeping peel in 5 oz of boiling water for 10 to 15 minutes and then straining.
*Tincture:* 2 to 3 g P.O. q.d.

### ADVERSE REACTIONS
**Skin:** photosensitivity, erythema, blisters, pustules, dermatoses leading to scab formation, pigment spots.

*Liquid may contain alcohol.

## INTERACTIONS
**Herb-drug.** *Antihypertensives, anxiolytics, sedatives:* Possible decreased effectiveness. Advise patient to avoid using together.
**Herb-lifestyle.** *Sun exposure:* Increased risk of photosensitivity reactions. Advise patient to wear protective clothing and sunscreen and to limit exposure to direct sunlight.

## CAUTIONS
Pregnant and breast-feeding patients should avoid use because the effects are unknown. Patients with stomach or intestinal ulcers should avoid use because of bitter orange's toxic effect on the GI tract.

Those with CV disease, anxiety, or insomnia should use bitter orange cautiously.

Bitter orange may be unsafe for use in children because large amounts can cause intestinal colic, seizures, and death.

## NURSING CONSIDERATIONS
● Find out why patient is using the herb.
● Frequent contact with the peel or oil, as through occupational exposure, can cause erythema, blisters, pustules, dermatoses leading to scab formation, and pigment spots.

**Patient teaching**
● Advise patient to consult with his health care provider before using an herbal preparation because a treatment with proven efficacy may be available.
● Tell patient to remind pharmacist of any herbal or dietary supplement that he's taking, when filling a new prescription.
● Warn patient not to delay seeking appropriate medical evaluation for indigestion, abdominal pain, or bloating because doing so may delay diagnosis of a potentially serious medical condition.
● If patient is pregnant or breast-feeding, or is planning pregnancy or suspects that she may be pregnant, advise her not to use bitter orange.
● Advise patient to wash hands after handling the dry peel and oil and to avoid touching eyes because frequent contact with the skin can cause blistering and irritation.
● Advise patient that use of bitter orange may be unsafe in children.

## black catechu

*Acacia catechu,* cutch, gambier, gambir

**Common trade names**
*Black Catechu, Cutch, Diarcalm, Elixir Bonjean, Enterodyne, Spanish Tummy Mixture*

## HOW SUPPLIED
Available as dry powder, extract, lozenge, and tincture*.

## ACTIONS & COMPONENTS
Comes from *A. catechu,* a tree native to Burma and India. Dried extract is prepared from the bark and sapwood of the tree, boiled in water; this decoction is evaporated in syrup, cooled in molds, then broken into pieces. Contains 20% to 35% of catechutannic acid, 2% to

10% of acacatechin, quercetin, and red catechu.

The therapeutic properties of black catechu come from its tannic acid content. Tannic acid is an astringent with antisecretory properties. It acts locally by precipitating proteins such as damaged or necrotic tissue.

## USES
Used to treat diarrhea and other GI disorders. As a gargle or lozenge, used for its astringent effects on mucous membranes and to treat sore throat.

Externally, it's incorporated into ointments for boils, ulcers, and cutaneous eruptions. At one time, tannic acid was widely used to treat burns, but cases of fatal hepatotoxicity from systemic absorption ended this practice.

## DOSAGE & ADMINISTRATION
*Tincture:* 0.3 to 2 g P.O. q.d., divided t.i.d. Single dose is 0.5 g. Or, 20 gtt in a glass of lukewarm water P.O. or applied undiluted with a brush.

## ADVERSE REACTIONS
**GI:** nausea, vomiting, abdominal pain.
**Hepatic:** *liver damage caused by tannin content.*

## INTERACTIONS
**Herb-drug.** *Cardiac glycosides:* Possible reduced effectiveness of digoxin. Monitor patient closely.
*Disulfiram, metronidazole:* Tincture contains alcohol. Advise patient to avoid using together.

*Iron:* May interfere with iron absorption. Encourage patient to separate administration times.

## CAUTIONS
Pregnant and breast-feeding patients should avoid use because the effects are unknown; patients with liver disease, because of black catechu's tannin content.

Those with liver disease and those with a history of alcoholism should use black catechu cautiously.

## NURSING CONSIDERATIONS
● Find out why patient is using the herb.
● Black catechu may exacerbate the intended therapeutic effects of conventional drugs.
🖉 **ALERT:** Ingestion of large amounts of tannic acid can cause nausea, vomiting, abdominal pain, and liver damage. Tannic acid barium enemas and tannic acid burn treatments may cause fatal hepatotoxicity from systemic absorption. It isn't known how much black catechu is needed to cause these reactions.
● Many tinctures contain between 15% and 90% alcohol and may be unsuitable for children, alcoholic patients, and patients with liver disease.

### Patient teaching
● Advise patient to consult with his health care provider before using an herbal preparation because a treatment with proven efficacy may be available.
● Tell patient to remind pharmacist of any herbal or dietary supple-

ment that he's taking, when filling a new prescription.

• Warn patient not to delay seeking appropriate medical evaluation for symptoms of GI disorders because doing so may delay diagnosis of a potentially serious medical condition.

• If patient is pregnant or breast-feeding or is planning pregnancy, advise her not to use black catechu.

• Advise patient that safe oral dosing information is unknown.

• Instruct patient with history of alcoholism or liver disease to check label of black catechu products carefully because they may contain alcohol.

• Advise patient not to apply black catechu to burned, damaged, or abraded skin.

## black cohosh

*Cimicifuga racemosa,* baneberry, black snake root, bugbane, bugwort, cimicifuga, rattle root, rattleweed, richweed, squaw root

**Common trade names**
*Black Cohosh Liquid Extract, Black Cohosh Root Powder, NuVeg Black Cohosh Root, Remifemin, Wild Countryside Black Cohosh*

### HOW SUPPLIED
Available as capsules, liquid extract*, powder, tablets, and tincture*.

### ACTIONS & COMPONENTS
Obtained from the fresh or dried rhizome with attached roots of *C. racemosa.* Triterpene glycosides—

including actein, cimicifugoside, and 27-deoxyactein—may produce the therapeutic effects. Black cohosh also contains salicylic acid.

May affect hormones such as estradiol, luteinizing hormone, follicle-stimulating hormone, and prolactin. However, the herb probably isn't estrogenic.

### USES
German Commission E has approved black cohosh for premenstrual discomfort, dysmenorrhea, and menopausal symptoms of the autonomic nervous system.

Black cohosh, specifically the Remifemin product, is effective for treating somatic and psychological symptoms of menopause, including hot flushes, sweating, sleep disturbance, and anxiety. It doesn't affect vaginal epithelium and may be ineffective for treating menopausal vaginal dryness.

May be safe for women with a history of breast cancer and other estrogen-sensitive cancers.

### DOSAGE & ADMINISTRATION
*Liquid extract (1:1 in 90% alcohol):* 0.3 to 2.0 ml P.O.
*Remifemin:* 20 mg P.O. b.i.d.
*Tincture (1:10 in 60% alcohol):* 2 to 4 ml P.O.

### ADVERSE REACTIONS
**GI:** GI discomfort.

### INTERACTIONS
**Herb-drug.** *Disulfiram, metronidazole:* Tinctures contain alcohol and may cause a disulfiram or disulfiram-like reaction. Advise patient to avoid using together.

---

*Bold italic type* indicates that reaction may be life-threatening.

## CAUTIONS

Pregnant patients should avoid use because large doses may cause miscarriage or premature birth. Breast-feeding patients should avoid use because the effects aren't known.

Those who are salicylate sensitive—including those with asthma, gout, peripheral vascular disease, diabetes, hemophilia, and kidney and liver disease—should use cautiously.

## NURSING CONSIDERATIONS

● Find out why patient is using the herb.
● Effective doses are equivalent to 40 mg per day of crude drug.
● The adverse reactions of and precautions for salicylates may apply to black cohosh.
🖉ALERT: Don't confuse black cohosh with blue or white cohosh.
● Black cohosh has no known benefits for osteoporosis or CV disease.
● Tincture may contain up to 90% alcohol and so may be unsuitable for children, alcoholic patients, and those with liver disease.
● Black cohosh isn't recommended for use for longer than 6 months.
● Signs and symptoms of overdose include nausea, vomiting, dizziness, nervous system and visual disturbances, reduced pulse rate, and increased perspiration.

### Patient teaching

● Advise patient to consult with her health care provider before using an herbal preparation because a treatment with proven efficacy may be available.

● Tell patient to remind pharmacist of any herbal or dietary supplement that he's taking, when filling a new prescription.
● If patient is pregnant or breast-feeding or is planning pregnancy, advise her not to use this herb.
● Encourage patient to have a proper medical evaluation before treating symptoms of menopause.
● Inform patient with history of alcoholism or liver disease that tincture contains alcohol.
● Inform patient that he shouldn't use black cohosh for longer than 6 months.
● Advise patient to keep black cohosh away from children and pets.

## black haw

*Viburnum prunifolium,* American sloe, cramp bark, dog rowan tree, European cranberry, guelder rose, high cranberry, King's crown, May rose, red elder, rose elder, silver bells, snowball tree, stagbush, viburnum, water elder, Whitsun bosses, Whitsun rose, wild guelder rose

Common trade names
*Black Haw Bark*

## HOW SUPPLIED

Available as dried black haw bark and tincture*.

## ACTIONS & COMPONENTS

Obtained from the root and stem bark of the plant, which contain scopoletin, tannins, oxalic acid, salicin, and salicylic acid. Scopoletin may be a uterine relaxant.

*Liquid may contain alcohol.

## USES
Used to relieve menstrual cramps. Used as an antidiarrheal, diuretic, antispasmodic, and antasthmatic. Also used to prevent miscarriage.

## DOSAGE & ADMINISTRATION
*Tea:* 2 tsp of dried bark boiled and simmered in 1 cup of water for 10 minutes, and then strained.
*Tincture:* 5 to 10 ml P.O. t.i.d.

## ADVERSE REACTIONS
None reported.

## INTERACTIONS
**Herb-drug.** *Anticoagulants such as heparin, and low-molecular-weight heparin and warfarin; antiplatelets such as aspirin, clopidogrel, dipyridamole, NSAIDs, and ticlopidine:* Enhanced effects of these drugs. Advise patient to use cautiously.
*Disulfiram, metronidazole:* Tincture contains alcohol and may cause a disulfiram or disulfiram-like reaction. Advise patient to avoid using together.
**Herb-herb.** *Feverfew, garlic, ginger, ginkgo, ginseng:* Black haw may have antiplatelet effects, which may interact with anticoagulant or antiplatelet herbs, and produce increased bleeding tendencies. Advise patient to use cautiously.

## CAUTIONS
Pregnant patients shouldn't use black haw without the consent of an obstetrician. Breast-feeding patients should avoid use because the effects aren't known.

Those with history of kidney stones should use cautiously because black haw contains oxalic acid.

## NURSING CONSIDERATIONS
- Find out why patient is using the herb.
- Tincture may contain up to 90% alcohol and so may be unsuitable for children, alcoholic patients, and those with liver disease.
- Black haw may have antiplatelet effects, which can increase a patient's tendency for bleeding. Monitor patient for bleeding.
- Black haw may increase the intended therapeutic effect of conventional drugs.

### Patient teaching
- Advise patient to consult with his health care provider before using an herbal preparation because a treatment with proven efficacy may be available.
- Tell patient to remind pharmacist of any herbal or dietary supplement that he's taking, when filling a new prescription.
- Warn patient not to delay seeking appropriate medical evaluation because doing so may delay diagnosis of a potentially serious medical condition.
- If patient has a history of kidney stones, advise him to consult with his health care provider before using black haw.
- If patient is pregnant or breast-feeding, advise her to avoid use of black haw unless she has her health care provider's approval.
- Inform patient with a history of liver disease or alcoholism that tincture contains alcohol.

---

*Bold italic type* indicates that reaction may be life-threatening.

• Tell patient to report unusual bleeding or bruising.
• Instruct patient to keep herb away from children and pets.

## black root

*Leptandra virginica,* beaumont root, Bowman's root, Culveris root, hini, oxadoddy, physic root, tall speedwell, tall veronica, whorlywort

**Common trade names**
*Black Root Tincture, Dried Black Root, Powdered Black Root Bark*

**HOW SUPPLIED**
Available as dried root, powdered root bark, and tincture*.

**ACTIONS & COMPONENTS**
Derived from the whole root or root bark, which contains tannic acid, volatile oils, gum, resin, a crystalline principle, a saccharine principle resembling mannite, and a glucoside-resembling senegin. Tannic acid has astringent and antisecretory properties.

**USES**
The fresh root is used as an emetic. The dried root has a gentler action and is used to treat constipation and liver and gallbladder disease, and to increase bile flow.

Historically, black root was used to treat bilious fever.

**DOSAGE & ADMINISTRATION**
*Powdered root bark:* 1 to 4 g P.O.
*Tea:* Prepared by steeping 1 tsp of black root in 1 cup boiling water for 30 minutes, and then straining.

Dosage is ⅓ cup before each meal, not to exceed 1 cup of tea per day.
*Tincture:* 2 to 4 gtt P.O. in water.

**ADVERSE REACTIONS**
**GI:** nausea, vomiting, abdominal cramps.
**Hepatic:** *hepatotoxicity.*

**INTERACTIONS**
**Herb-drug.** *Cardiac glycosides such as digoxin:* Possible reduced effectiveness of digoxin. Monitor patient closely.
*Iron:* Decreased absorption. Encourage patient to separate administration times.
*Laxatives:* May increase the cathartic effects of black root. Monitor patient for dehydration and hypokalemia. Hypokalemia also increases the risk of digoxin toxicity.
**Herb-herb.** *Herbs with laxative effects such as aloe, blue flag rhizome, butternut, cascara sagrada bark, castor oil, colocynth fruit, manna bark exudate, podophyllum root, rhubarb root, senna, wild cumber fruit, yellow dock root:* Increased cathartic effects of black root. Monitor patient for dehydration and hypokalemia.
*Herbs with potassium-wasting effects such as gossypol, horsetail, and licorice:* Additive effects. Monitor patient for hypokalemia.

**CAUTIONS**
Those with gallstones or bile duct obstruction should avoid using black root because it may worsen these diseases; pregnant patients, because the fresh root has abortifacient and teratogenic effects. Also, breast-feeding patients

*Liquid may contain alcohol.

should avoid use because the effects are unknown.

Those with a GI disease like colitis or irritable bowel syndrome that may be aggravated by the cathartic effects of black root should use black root cautiously.

**NURSING CONSIDERATIONS**
• Find out why patient is using the herb.
• A patient using black root should only use the dry root, not the fresh root.
⚡ALERT: Ingesting tannic acid in large amounts can cause nausea, vomiting, abdominal pain, and liver damage. Tannic acid barium enemas and tannic acid burn treatments can cause fatal hepatotoxicity after systemic absorption. It isn't known how much black root is required to cause these symptoms.
• Monitor patient for excessive diarrhea.

**Patient teaching**
• Advise patient to consult with his health care provider before using an herbal preparation because a treatment with proven efficacy may be available.
• Tell patient to remind pharmacist of any herbal or dietary supplement that he's taking, when filling a new prescription.
• Warn patient not to delay seeking appropriate medical evaluation because doing so may delay diagnosis of a potentially serious medical condition.
• If patient is pregnant or breastfeeding or planning pregnancy, advise her not to use this herb.

• Caution patient not to use fresh black root, only dried.
• Advise patient not to drink more than 1 cup of black root tea per day.
• Advise patient to use caution when combining black root with other herbal, OTC, or prescription laxatives.

## blackthorn

*Berry: Prunus spinosa fructus,* blackthorn fruit, sloe, sloe berry

*Flower: Prunus spinosa flos,* sloe flower, wild plum flower

Common trade names
*None known*

**HOW SUPPLIED**
Available as dried flowers and fresh or dried fruit of *P. spinosa,* juice, marmalade, syrup, tea, and wine.

**ACTIONS & COMPONENTS**
The tannins in blackthorn berry have astringent effects, which help reduce mucous membrane inflammation. Blackthorn flower contains cyanogenic glycosides.

**USES**
Blackthorn berry is added to mouth rinse and used to decrease mild inflammation of the oral and pharyngeal mucosa.

Blackthorn syrup and wine are used to purge the bowels and induce sweat, and blackthorn marmalade is used to relieve symptoms of dyspepsia.

Blackthorn flower is used orally to prevent gastric spasms and to treat common colds, respiratory

---

*Bold italic type* indicates that reaction may be life-threatening.

tract disorders, bloating, general exhaustion, dyspepsia, rashes, skin impurities, and kidney and bladder ailments. And, it's used for its laxative, diuretic, diaphoretic, and expectorant effects.

Blackthorn flower is also a component of blood-cleansing teas, which may help purify the blood.

## DOSAGE & ADMINISTRATION
*Oral berry:* Mouth rinse up to b.i.d. Daily dose is 2 to 4 g.
*Oral flower:* 1 to 2 cups of tea during the day or 2 cups in the evening.
*Tea:* Both berry and flower teas are prepared by steeping and stirring 1 to 2 g of blackthorn in 5 oz of water for 10 minutes, and then straining.

## ADVERSE REACTIONS
None reported.

## INTERACTIONS
None reported.

## CAUTIONS
Pregnant patients should avoid use because of its teratogenic cyanogenic compounds. Breast-feeding patients should also avoid use.

## NURSING CONSIDERATIONS
• Find out why patient is using the herb.
• Blackthorn isn't recommended for long-term use.
• Blackthorn flower could be toxic because it contains cyanogenic glycosides.
• Blackthorn may be stored for up to 1 year, away from light and moisture.

## Patient teaching
• Advise patient to consult with his health care provider before using an herbal preparation because a treatment with proven efficacy may be available.
• Tell patient to remind pharmacist of any herbal or dietary supplement that he's taking, when filling a new prescription.
• If patient is pregnant or breast-feeding, advise her not to use blackthorn.
• Warn patient that blackthorn is for short-term use only.
• Tell patient that although the safety and effectiveness of the herb are uncertain, use as a coloring agent for tea is regarded as safe.
• Inform patient that blackthorn may be stored for up to 1 year, away from light and moisture.

## blessed thistle

*Cnicus benedictus,* benediktenkraut, cardin, holy thistle, spotted thistle, St. Benedict thistle

Common trade names
*Blessed Thistle Combo, Blessed Thistle Herb*

## HOW SUPPLIED
Available as capsules, decoction, dried herb, fluidextract, infusion, oil, tea, and tincture. Extracts appear in "healing" skin lotions, creams, and salves.
*Capsules:* 325 mg, 340 mg
*Dried herb:* 1-oz packets
*Tincture:* 1-oz containers

---

*Liquid may contain alcohol.

**ACTIONS & COMPONENTS**
Contains the sesquiterpene lactones cnicin and salonitenolide.

Cnin, a glycoside, is responsible for the herb's bitterness, which stimulates the appetite and aids in digestion by encouraging the secretion of saliva and gastric juice. It may also act directly on the stomach and part of the small intestine.

Blessed thistle stimulates menstruation. It's characterized as a bitter tonic, astringent, diaphoretic, antibacterial, expectorant, antidiarrheal, antihemorrhagic, vulnerary, antipyretic, and galactagogue. The antibacterial properties come from the volatile oil and the cnicin component.

**USES**
Used orally to treat digestive problems such as liver and gallbladder diseases, loss of appetite, indigestion and heartburn, constipation, colic, diarrhea, dyspepsia, and flatulence. May also improve memory, relieve menstrual complaints, control amenorrhea, regulate the menstrual cycle, increase perspiration, lower fever, boost a mother's milk production, dissolve blood clots, control bleeding, and reduce rheumatic pain. And it's also used as an expectorant and antibiotic.

Topically, blessed thistle poultice is used for boils, wounds, ulcers, and hemorrhage.

Blessed thistle is added to alcoholic beverages during manufacturing as flavoring.

**DOSAGE & ADMINISTRATION**
*Capsules:* 2 capsules P.O. t.i.d.
*Decoction:* 1 cup P.O. 30 minutes before meals. Prepared using 1.5 to 2 g of finely chopped herb in a cup of water.
*Extract:* 10 to 20 gtt P.O. in water q.d.
*Mean daily dose:* 4 to 6 g of herb or equivalent preparations.
*Tea:* 3 cups P.O. q.d.—that is, 2 g of dried herb added to 1 cup of boiling water and steeped for 10 to 15 minutes.
*Tincture:* 1 to 2 ml P.O. t.i.d.

**ADVERSE REACTIONS**
**GI:** nausea, vomiting, diarrhea.
**Skin:** contact dermatitis.

**INTERACTIONS**
**Herb-drug.** *Antacids, $H_2$ antagonists, proton pump inhibitors, sucralfate:* Because the herb increases stomach acidity, it may interact with these drugs. Monitor patient closely.
*Insulin, oral antidiabetics:* Possible worsening of hypoglycemia. Monitor blood glucose level and adjust antidiabetic dosage as needed.
**Herb-herb.** *Echinacea:* May potentiate the antibiotic activity of echinacea. Monitor patient closely.
*Other herbs from the Compositae family such as mugwort and cornflower:* Possible cross-sensitivity. Advise patient to avoid using together.

**CAUTIONS**
Pregnant and breast-feeding patients should avoid using blessed thistle because it may promote menstruation; those with acute stomach inflammation, ulcers, or hyperacidity, because it stimulates gastric juices.

---

*Bold italic type* indicates that reaction may be life-threatening.

Those with a history of contact dermatitis, especially in relation to other members of the Compositae family—including ragweed, chrysanthemums, marigolds, and daisies—and those with diabetes, ulcers, acute stomach inflammation, and hyperacidity of the GI tract should used blessed thistle cautiously.

**NURSING CONSIDERATIONS**
• Find out why patient is using the herb.
• Infusions of more than 5 g per cup may cause vomiting and diarrhea.
• Blessed thistle may cross-react with mugwort and cornflower.
• If patient has diabetes, monitor his blood glucose level.
⚠ ALERT: Don't confuse blessed thistle with the closely named milk thistle *Silybum marianum*.

**Patient teaching**
• Advise patient to consult with his health care provider before using an herbal preparation because a treatment with proven efficacy may be available.
• Tell patient to remind pharmacist of any herbal or dietary supplement that he's taking, when filling a new prescription.
• Warn patient not to delay seeking appropriate medical evaluation for indigestion, anorexia, or heartburn because doing so may delay diagnosis of a potentially serious medical condition.
• If patient is pregnant or breastfeeding, advise her not to use blessed thistle.

• If patient is taking a drug for diabetes, ulcers, or heartburn, instruct him to contact his health care provider before taking blessed thistle because his drug dosage may need to be adjusted.
• If patient is collecting blessed thistle himself, advise him to wear protective clothes and glasses because the plant can cause inflammation of the skin, eyes, and mucous membranes.
• Advise patient not to add milk or cream to blessed thistle tea; doing so may mute the gastric acid secretion.
• If patient is diabetic, advise him to closely monitor his blood glucose level because blessed thistle may cause additive hypoglycemia.

## bloodroot

*Sanguinaria canadensis,* coon root, Indian Plant, Indian red plant, paucon, pauson, red Indian paint, red puccoon, red root, sanguinaria, snakebite, sweet slumber, tetterwort

**Common trade names**
*Lexat, Viadent (available in combination)*

**HOW SUPPLIED**
Available for external use as decoction, extract, ointment, powder, and tincture. Available for internal use as decoction and tincture. Extracts appear in commercial mouthwashes and toothpastes.

**ACTIONS & COMPONENTS**
Isoquinolone alkaloid components, primarily sanguinarine, have anti-

microbial, antiseptic, anti-inflammatory, antihistamine, expectorant, antispasmodic, emetic, cathartic, pectoral, and cardiotonic effects.

Sanguinarine converted to a negatively charged iminium ion helps to inhibit plaque from settling on tooth enamel. Antibacterial properties of bloodroot fight organisms responsible for bad breath.

Another alkaloid, cholerythrine, may have some anticarcinogenic effects.

## USES
Used as an emetic, cathartic, antispasmodic, decongestant, digestive stimulant, laxative, expectorant, dental analgesic, and general tonic. Also used to treat bronchitis, asthma, croup, laryngitis, pharyngitis, congestion, deficient capillary circulation, nasal polyps, rheumatism, warts, ear and nose cancer (Fell technique), fever, sore throat, skin burns, and fungal infection.

Topically, it's used as an irritant and debriding agent.

## DOSAGE & ADMINISTRATION
*Extract (1:1 in 60% alcohol):* 0.06 to 0.3 ml (1 to 2 ml for emetic dose) P.O. t.i.d.
*Rhizome:* 0.06 to 0.5 g (1 to 2 g for emetic dose) P.O. t.i.d.
*Tea:* 1 cup P.O. several times a day. Prepared by boiling 1 to 2 tbs of chopped rhizome in 17 oz of water for 15 minutes.
*Tincture:* 0.3 to 2 ml (2 to 8 ml for emetic dose) P.O. t.i.d.
*Wine:* Prepared by steeping chopped drug in brandy, and then filtering.

## ADVERSE REACTIONS
**CNS:** headache, CNS depression, ataxia, reduced activity, ***coma.***
**CV:** hypotension.
**EENT:** eye and mucous membrane irritation.
**GI:** nausea, vomiting.
**Other:** ***shock.***

## INTERACTIONS
**Herb-drug.** *Antihypertensives, dopamine, ganglionic or peripheral adrenergic blockers such as tubocurarine and norepinephrine:* May potentiate the action of these drugs. Advise patient to use cautiously.
*CNS depressants:* Possible additive effects. Advise patient to avoid using together.
*Corticotropin, corticosteroids:* May produce hypokalemia. Monitor potassium level.
**Herb-food.** *Sanguinarine products containing zinc:* Increased antimicrobial activity of sanguinarine. Advise patient to avoid using together.
**Herb-lifestyle.** *Alcohol:* Possible increased CNS effects. Advise patient to avoid using together.

## CAUTIONS
Pregnant and breast-feeding patients and those with infections or inflammatory GI conditions should avoid use.

Those with GI irritation should use bloodroot cautiously because it can irritate the GI tract; those with glaucoma, because it can affect glaucoma treatment.

---

*Bold italic type* indicates that reaction may be life-threatening.

**NURSING CONSIDERATIONS**
- Find out why patient is using the herb.
- In most countries, the drug isn't used orally.
- ⚡ALERT: Powdered rhizome or juice can destroy live tissue. Large doses of the internal formulations can be poisonous. The FDA has classified bloodroot as unsafe.
- Oral use can cause CNS depression and narcosis because of bloodroot's relaxant effect on smooth muscle.
- At higher doses, bloodroot produces interactions similar to diuretics and cathartics.
- If patient is taking an antihypertensive, monitor his blood pressure.
- Prolonged use of bloodroot may affect electrolyte levels, such as potassium, sodium, blood urea nitrogen, uric acid, and glucose.
- If overdose occurs or if patient ingests a large quantity of bloodroot, perform gastric lavage or induce vomiting and provide symptomatic treatment.

**Patient teaching**
- Advise patient to consult with his health care provider before using an herbal preparation because a treatment with proven efficacy may be available.
- Tell patient to remind pharmacist of any herbal or dietary supplement that he's taking, when filling a new prescription.
- Inform patient that bloodroot isn't recommended for oral use and that large doses can be poisonous.
- If patient is pregnant, advise her not to use bloodroot.

- Advise patient to avoid contact with the eyes and mucous membranes because of bloodroot's irritant properties. Also advise him to take protective measures so he doesn't inhale the herb during crude herb processing.
- Tell patient that toothpastes and mouthwashes containing bloodroot extracts are unlikely to cause harm if they aren't swallowed.
- Tell patient to avoid alcohol while using bloodroot because of the risk of enhanced CNS depression.
- Warn patient that a component of the herb may cause cataracts.

## blue cohosh

*Caulophyllum thalictroides,* beechdrops, blueberry, blueberry root, blue ginseng, papoose root, squawroot, yellow ginseng

**Common trade names**
*Blue Cohosh Root Liquid*

**HOW SUPPLIED**
Available as capsules, decoction, dried powder, liquid extract*, tablets, tea, and tincture.
*Capsules:* 500 mg
*Liquid extract:* 0.5 to 1 ml
*Tinctures:* 1-oz and 2-oz containers

**ACTIONS & COMPONENTS**
Made from the aerial parts of the plant, its roots, and its rhizomes. Pharmacologic effects are attributed to several glycosides and alkaloids, such as caulosaponin and methylcytisine.

*Liquid may contain alcohol.

Caulosaponin is responsible for the herb's oxytocic effects and its effects on coronary vasculature as well as its ability to stimulate intestinal contractions.

Methylcytisine produces nicotinic effects—for example, it elevates blood pressure and blood glucose level, stimulates respiration, and causes peristalsis.

## USES

Used to treat colic, sore throat, cramps, hiccups, epilepsy, hysterics, UTIs, inflammation of the uterus, asthma, memory problems, high blood pressure, muscle spasms, worm infestation, anxiety, restlessness and pain during pregnancy, and and labor pains. Used to stimulate uterine contractions and induce menstruation. Also used as an antispasmodic, antirheumatic, diaphoretic, expectorant, and laxative.

May also have some antimicrobial activity. Low doses of the extract may inhibit ovulation.

The roasted seeds of the herb are commonly used as a coffee substitute.

## DOSAGE & ADMINISTRATION

*Dried rhizome or root:* 0.3 to 1 g P.O. t.i.d.
*Tea:* Prepared by steeping the herb in 5 oz of boiling water, and then straining. Daily dose is t.i.d.
*Liquid extract (1:1 in 70% alcohol):* 0.5 to 1 ml P.O. t.i.d.

## ADVERSE REACTIONS

**CV:** chest pain, hypertension, vasoconstriction, hypotension.
**EENT:** mucous membrane irritation.
**GI:** GI irritation, severe diarrhea, cramping.
**Metabolic:** hypoglycemia.

## INTERACTIONS

**Herb-drug.** *Acetazolamide, corticosteroids, dextrothyroxine, epinephrine, glucagon, oral contraceptives, phenothiazines, rifampin, thiazide diuretics, thyroid-stimulating hormones:* Decreased antidiabetic action of blue cohosh. Monitor blood glucose level.
*Allopurinol, anabolic steroids, chloramphenicol, clofibrate, fenfluramine, guanethidine, MAO inhibitors, phenylbutazone, phenyramidol, probenecid, salicylates, sulfinpyrazone, sulfonamides, tetracyclines:* Increased antidiabetic action of blue cohosh. Monitor blood glucose level.
*Aminosalicylic acid, antihistamines, disulfiram, halothane, isoniazid, methylphenidate, phenothiazines, propoxyphene, sulfa drugs, troleandomycin:* Possible decreased metabolism of blue cohosh. Monitor patient closely.
*Antacids, mineral oil:* May reduce anthelminthic effect of blue cohosh. Monitor patient closely.
*Antianginals, nicotine replacement therapy:* Blue cohosh may interact with these drugs. Advise patient to avoid using together.
*Antihypertensives, peripheral adrenergic blockers:* Diuretic activity of blue cohosh may potentiate the action of these drugs. Monitor patient closely.
*Barbiturates, diazoxide, loxapine, and vitamin $B_6$:* Possible induced

---

*Bold italic type* indicates that reaction may be life-threatening.

metabolism of blue cohosh. Monitor patient closely.

*Clindamycin:* May enhance neuromuscular relaxing action of blue cohosh. Monitor patient closely.

*Corticosteroids, digoxin, fluroxene, methadone, metyrapone, oral contraceptives, phenytoin, tetracyclines:* Possible increased metabolism of these drugs. Monitor patient closely.

*Lithium:* May reduce renal clearance of lithium. Monitor patient for toxic reaction.

*Sparteine:* May produce synergistic oxytocic activity when used with blue cohosh. Monitor patient closely.

*Vasoconstrictors such as ephedrine, methoxamine, phenylephrine:* May cause severe hypertension. Advise patient to avoid using together.

**Herb-lifestyle.** *Alcohol:* May induce metabolism of blue cohosh, thus decreasing pharmacologic effects. Advise patient to avoid using together.

*Marijuana:* Decreased antidiabetic action of blue cohosh. Monitor blood glucose level.

## CAUTIONS
⚡ALERT: Blue cohosh shouldn't be used during labor. Several adverse effects have been reported to the FDA Special Nutritionals Adverse Event Monitoring System, including fetal toxicity, neonatal stroke and aplastic anemia after maternal use of herb during labor, and neonatal acute MI associated with heart failure and shock.

Pregnant patients should avoid use of blue cohosh because it may stimulate menstruation. Cardiac patients and those with GI conditions should also avoid use.

Those with hypertension or diabetes should use blue cohosh cautiously.

## NURSING CONSIDERATIONS
● Find out why patient is using the herb.
● Blue cohosh has held official drug status in the past, being listed in the USP and the National Formulary; however, because of serious safety concerns, its use isn't recommended.
● The root of this herb can be toxic, and the danger associated with its use seems to outweigh the reported medicinal benefits.
⚡ALERT: Raw blue cohosh berries are poisonous to children.
● Blue cohosh may increase the intended therapeutic effects of conventional drugs.
● Despite the common last name, blue cohosh isn't related to black cohosh.
● Monitor blood pressure and blood glucose, BUN, uric acid, and protein-bound iodine levels.
● Signs and symptoms of overdose resemble those of nicotine toxicity. Monitor patient for evidence of these signs and symptoms.
● If overdose occurs, perform gastric lavage or induce vomiting, if needed.

**Patient teaching**
● Advise patient to consult with his health care provider before using an herbal preparation—especially if patient has diabetes, hypertension, or hypoglycemia or is taking

other drugs—because a treatment with proven efficacy may be available.

• Tell patient to remind pharmacist of any herbal or dietary supplement that he's taking, when filling a new prescription.

• Warn patient to avoid using blue cohosh during pregnancy, labor, and breast-feeding.

## blue flag

Dagger flower, daggers, dragon flower, flaggon, flag lily, fleur-de-lis, fliggers, Florentine orris, flower-de-luce, gladyne, iris, Jacob's sword, liver lily, myrtle flower, orris root, poison flag, segg, sheggs, snake lily, water flag, white flag root, wild iris, yellow flag, yellow iris

Common trade names
*Irisin*

### HOW SUPPLIED
*Fluidextract:* 0.5 to 1 fluidram
*Powdered root:* 20 grains
*Solid extract:* 10 to 15 grains
*Tincture:* 1 to 3 fluidrams

### ACTIONS & COMPONENTS
Blue flag preparations are obtained from the rhizome portion of the plant. Primary components are iridin and oleoresin.

Blue flag may stimulate the flow of bile from the gallbladder to the duodenum. It's used as an anti-inflammatory, diuretic, laxative, and sialagogue, as well as a hepatic and dermatologic herb.

### USES
Used to purify blood and free it from toxins. Used to treat heartburn, belching, nausea, and headaches resulting from digestive disorders as well as disorders of the respiratory tract and thyroid gland. Used for its cathartic, emetic, and diuretic effects.

Applied externally on sores and bruises to decrease inflammation.

### DOSAGE & ADMINISTRATION
*Decoction:* 1 cup of preparation P.O. t.i.d. Prepared by placing ½ to 1 tsp of dried herb in 1 cup of boiling water and simmering for 10 to 15 minutes.
*Solid extracts, powdered root:* 10 to 20 grains P.O.
*Tincture:* 2 to 4 ml P.O. t.i.d.

### ADVERSE REACTIONS
**CNS:** headache.
**EENT:** lacrimation, eye inflammation, throat irritation.
**GI:** iridin poisoning in humans and animals, severe nausea and vomiting after consumption of fresh root.
**Other:** mucous membrane irritation from the furfural component.

### INTERACTIONS
**Herb-drug.** *Anticoagulants:* May potentiate these drugs by reducing absorption of vitamin K from the gut. Monitor patient for bleeding. *Antihypertensives, ganglionic, or peripheral adrenergics:* May potentiate the action of these drugs. Monitor patient closely.
*Beta blockers such as meprobamate, phenobarbital, propranolol, and other sedative hypnotics such*

---

*Bold italic type* indicates that reaction may be life-threatening.

*as chloral hydrate:* Blue flag's anti-inflammatory effects may be decreased. Monitor patient closely. *Corticosteroids, corticotropin:* May produce hypokalemia. Monitor blood glucose level and adjust antidiabetic dosage, as needed. *Lithium:* Possible reduced renal clearance. Monitor patient for toxic reaction and discourage concomitant use.

**Herb-herb.** *Stimulant laxative herbs such as aloe, buckthorn fruit and bark, butternut, cascara sagrada bark, castor oil, colocynth fruit pulp, gamboge bark exudate, podophyllum root, rhubarb root, senna leaves and pods, yellow dock root, potassium-wasting herbs such as horsetail plant and licorice rhizome, and wild cucumber fruit:* Blue flag may increase depletion of potassium when used with listed herbs. Monitor patient for hypokalemia.

**CAUTIONS**
Pregnant and breast-feeding patients and patients with infectious or inflammatory GI conditions should avoid use.

Those with infectious or inflammatory conditions of the GI tract should use blue flag cautiously because it can irritate the GI tract.

**NURSING CONSIDERATIONS**
• Find out why patient is using the herb.
◪ ALERT: The fresh root of blue flag is poisonous, so if patient chooses to use the herb, he should use only small doses of the dried root.

• If patient is also taking digoxin, monitor his blood digoxin levels.
• Monitor blood pressure and blood glucose, serum electrolyte, and uric acid levels.
• If patient is also taking an anticoagulant, monitor INR.

**Patient teaching**
• Advise patient to consult with his health care provider before using an herbal preparation because a treatment with proven efficacy may be available.
• Tell patient to remind pharmacist of any herbal or dietary supplement that he's taking, when filling a new prescription.
• Advise patient to avoid taking blue flag internally.
• If patient is pregnant or breast-feeding, advise her not to use blue flag.
• Caution patient that blue flag can cause severe irritation if it comes in direct contact with eyes, ears, nose, or mouth.

## bogbean

*Menyanthes trifoliata,* bean trefoil, bog hop, bog myrtle, bog nut, brook bean, buck bean, marsh clover, marsh trefoil, moon flower, trefoil, water shamrock, water trefoil

**Common trade names**
*Bogbean Extract, Bogbean Leaf, Bogbean Leaf Powder*

**HOW SUPPLIED**
Available as a fluidextract, tablet, powder, and whole leaf.

## ACTIONS & COMPONENTS

Obtained from the dried rhizome of *M. trifoliata*. Main components are a small quantity of volatile oil and the glucoside menyanthin.

Menyanthin is reported to stimulate saliva production and gastric secretion.

## USES

Used to treat loss of appetite, dyspepsia, gout, rheumatoid arthritis, osteoarthritis, rheumatism, and skin diseases. Used as a bitter to promote gastric secretion. In large doses, it's also used as an emetic.

## DOSAGE & ADMINISTRATION

*Infusion:* ½ cup P.O., unsweetened, before each meal.
*Tea:* Prepared by steeping 0.5 to 1 g of finely cut herb in boiling water—or in cold water that's rapidly heated—for 5 to 10 minutes, and then straining. (1 tsp equals 0.9 g of herb.) Average daily dose is 1.5 to 3 g P.O.
*Tincture:* 1 to 4 ml P.O. t.i.d.

## ADVERSE REACTIONS

None reported.

## INTERACTIONS

**Herb-drug.** *Antacids, histamine₂ antagonists, proton pump inhibitors, sucralfate:* May negate the effects of these drugs because herb promotes gastric secretion. Advise patient to avoid using together.
*Stimulant laxatives:* May potentiate effects. Advise patient to avoid using together.

## CAUTIONS

Not for use in persons with diarrhea, dysentery, and colitis. Contraindicated in pregnant patients because it may stimulate menstruation and act as a stimulant laxative.

## NURSING CONSIDERATIONS

- Find out why patient is using the herb.
- Bogbean may alter the intended therapeutic effect of conventional drugs.
- If overdose occurs, induce vomiting.

### Patient teaching

- Advise patient to consult with his health care provider before using an herbal preparation because a treatment with proven efficacy may be available.
- Tell patient to remind pharmacist of any herbal or dietary supplement that he's taking, when filling a new prescription.
- Warn patient not to treat symptoms of anorexia, dyspepsia, or pain with bogbean before seeking appropriate medical evaluation because doing so may delay diagnosis of a potentially serious medical condition.
- Educate patient on possible adverse effects that result from overdose, such as vomiting.
- Advise patient with diarrhea, dysentery, or colitis not to use the herb.
- Advise patient to avoid use during pregnancy or breast-feeding.

---

*Bold italic type* indicates that reaction may be life-threatening.

# boldo

*Peumus boldus*, boldea, boldoa, boldu, boldus

**Common trade names**
*Boldo Extract, Boldo Leaf, Boldo Leaf Powder, Tincture of Boldo*

## HOW SUPPLIED
Available as capsules, fluidextract, tablets, and tincture of varying potencies.
*Capsules:* 250 mg, 400 mg; also in combination with other vitamins and herbal preparations

## ACTIONS & COMPONENTS
Comes from the dried leaves of *P. boldus.* Contains boldine, an isoquinoline alkaloid of the aporphine type and a volatile oil that contains ascaridiole.

Boldine may be effective as an antispasmodic, choleretic, and diuretic; it may also increase gastric secretions. The pharmacologic effects of the volatile oil are similar to those of boldine. Ascaridiole is an anthelminthic.

## USES
Used to treat liver and gallbladder complaints, loss of appetite, dyspepsia, and mild spastic complaints.

Boldo leaves, which are included in herbal teas for their diuretic and laxative effects, can cause significant diuresis. The oil is used to treat GU inflammation, gout, and rheumatism.

## DOSAGE & ADMINISTRATION
*Boldo oil:* 5 gtt P.O.

*Fluidextract (1:1):* 0.1 to 0.3 ml P.O. t.i.d.
*Pulverized herb for infusions:* Average daily dose is 4.5 g P.O.
*Tincture (1:10):* 0.5 to 2 ml P.O. t.i.d.

## ADVERSE REACTIONS
**CNS:** exaggerated reflexes, disturbed coordination, *seizures,* paralysis of motor and sensory nerves and muscle fibers.
**Respiratory:** *respiratory depression.*

## INTERACTIONS
**Herb-drug.** *Diuretics:* Additive effects. Advise patient to avoid using together.

## CAUTIONS
Those with bile duct obstruction, those with severe liver diseases, and pregnant patients should avoid use.

## NURSING CONSIDERATIONS
• Find out why patient is using the herb.
⚠ ALERT: In large doses, boldo stimulates the CNS, causing exaggerated reflexes, disturbed coordination, and seizures. In large doses, it may also paralyze motor and sensory nerves and muscle fibers, eventually causing death as a result of respiratory depression.
• Ascaridiole is a known toxin, and preparations of the volatile oil or distillates of the leaf should be avoided.
• If patient has gallstones or bile duct obstruction, monitor him for symptoms.

*Liquid may contain alcohol.

- Overdose may lead to respiratory depression, and patient may require intubation and respiratory support.

**Patient teaching**
- Advise patient to consult with his health care provider before using an herbal preparation because a treatment with proven efficacy may be available.
- Tell patient to remind pharmacist of any herbal or dietary supplement that he's taking, when filling a new prescription.
- If patient is pregnant, advise her not to use boldo.
- If patient has gallstones, advise him to consult his health care provider before using boldo.
- Advise patient to avoid preparations with the volatile oil of boldo because of the toxic effects of ascaridiole.
- Inform patient that preparations with virtually no ascaridiole are available.
- Inform patient not to delay seeking appropriate medical intervention if symptoms persist after taking this herb.
- Caution patient that overdose may lead to neurologic symptoms and, if severe enough, death.

## boneset

*Eupatorium perfoliatum,* agueweed, crosswort, eupatorium, feverwort, Indian sage, sweating plant, teasal, thoroughwort, vegetable antimony, wood boneset

**Common trade names**
*Alvita Tea, Boneset Extract, Boneset Herb Organic Alcohol, Boneset Leaf, Boneset Tops*

**HOW SUPPLIED**
Available as capsules, dried leaf or powder, fluidextract, and tablets. *Capsules:* 430 mg

**ACTIONS & COMPONENTS**
Obtained from the complete aerial part of *E. perfoliatum.* Contains the following components: a glucoside (eupatorin), volatile oil, resin, inulin, wax, sterols, triterpenes, and flavonoids. Also contains pyrrolizidine alkaloids, which cause hepatic impairment if consumed over a prolonged period, and tremetol, an unsaturated alcohol that lowers the blood glucose level.

Boneset acts as a diaphoretic, an antiphlogistic, and a bitter, which stimulates the appetite, aids digestion, and stimulates the body's immune system. Small doses of boneset may have diuretic and laxative effects, whereas large doses may result in vomiting and catharsis.

**USES**
Used as a tonic to help restore systemic vitality and as a nutritional

tonic to rejuvenate the body after a debilitating condition. Also used to treat colds, catarrh, influenza, rheumatism, most fevers, and inflammation of the nose, throat, or tongue.

### DOSAGE & ADMINISTRATION
*Fluidextract:* 2 to 4 g of plant P.O.
*Infusion:* Prepared by steeping 2 tsp to 2 tbs of crushed dried leaves and flowering tops in 8 to 16 oz of boiling water. Infusion should be administered t.i.d.
*Tincture:* 2 to 3 ml P.O. t.i.d.

### ADVERSE REACTIONS
**GI:** GI hemorrhage.
**GU:** fatty degeneration of the kidneys.
**Hepatic:** fatty degeneration of the liver, hepatic dysfunction.
**Metabolic:** hypoglycemia.
**Skin:** contact dermatitis.

### INTERACTIONS
**Herb-drug.** *Insulin, oral antidiabetics:* Increased risk of hypoglycemia. Monitor blood glucose level.

### CAUTIONS
Long-term use of boneset should be avoided. Those with liver disease and those who are pregnant or breast-feeding should avoid use.

### NURSING CONSIDERATIONS
● Find out why patient is using the herb.
● The herb contains pyrrolizidine alkaloids, which are hepatotoxic and hepatocarcinogenic, and so may cause hepatic dysfunction.

● If patient is diabetic and is taking an oral antidiabetic, closely monitor his blood glucose level.
● Symptoms of overdose include weakness, nausea, lack of appetite, thirst, and constipation. Severe poisoning may result in muscle trembling and loss of motor control, progressing to paralysis and death. For a toxic effect to occur, the cytochrome P-450 system must activate one of the herb's toxic components.

### Patient teaching
● Advise patient to consult with his health care provider before using an herbal preparation because a treatment with proven efficacy may be available.
● Tell patient to remind pharmacist of any herbal or dietary supplement that he's taking, when filling a new prescription.
● Warn patient not to delay seeking appropriate medical evaluation because doing so may delay diagnosis of a potentially serious medical condition.
● If patient is pregnant, advise her not to use boneset.
● Advise any diabetic patient who's also taking an antidiabetic to monitor his blood glucose level closely because the tremetrol component of the herb may have a hypoglycemic effect.

---

*Liquid may contain alcohol.

## borage

*Borago officinalis*, beebread, bugloss, burage, burrage, oxtongue, starflower

**Common trade names**
*Borage Bio-EFA Capsules, Borage Extract, Borage Leaf, Borage Leaf Powder, Borage Oil, Borage Oil Softgels, Borage-Power, GLA-320 Borage Capsules, Ultra GLA Capsules*

### HOW SUPPLIED
Available as dried leaf or powder, fluidextract, oil, and tablets.
*Oil:* 90-mg, 240-mg, 300-mg, 500-mg, and 1,000-mg capsules and softgels, in liquid form, and in combination with other vitamins in capsule and powder forms

### ACTIONS & COMPONENTS
Oil comes from the fatty oil of the seeds and flower of *B. officinalis.* Borage oil may contain between 17% and 25% gamma-linolenic acid (GLA). GLA has anti-inflammatory effects because of increased production of 15-hydroxy fatty acid and prostaglandin $E_1$, both metabolites of GLA, and astringent and sequestering effects. GLA is an essential fatty acid.

Leaves are the dried leaves and flower clusters of *B. officinalis.* They're harvested during the flowering period and are artificially dried at 104º F (40º C). They contain pyrrolizidine alkaloids, which are hepatotoxic and hepatocarcinogenic, and so may cause hepatic dysfunction. They also contain tannins, mucilage, malic acid, and potassium nitrate. In small amounts, borage may cause constipation because of its tannin content.

Borage's mucilage component may contribute to its expectorant effect; the malic acid and potassium nitrate components, to its mild diuretic effect.

### USES
Used externally as an astringent, a poultice for inflammation, and a treatment for eczema. The oil is used as treatment for neurodermatitis and as a GLA supplement.

Used for its sequestering and mucilaginous effects in treating coughs and throat illnesses. Used as an anti-inflammatory for kidney and bladder disorders and for rheumatism. Used as an analgesic, cardiotonic, sedative, and diaphoretic. Also used to enhance performance and to treat phlebitis and menopausal complaints.

### DOSAGE & ADMINISTRATION
*Borage oil:* Usually administered in vitamin capsules.
*Dried borage leaves:* For internal use, 1 oz of leaves is infused in 16 oz of boiling water and is taken in wineglassful (60-ml) doses.
*Fluidextract:* 2 to 4 ml P.O.

### ADVERSE REACTIONS
None reported.

### INTERACTIONS
**Herb-drug.** *Anticonvulsants:* May lower the seizure threshold. Advise patient to avoid using together.

---

*Bold italic type* indicates that reaction may be life-threatening.

## CAUTIONS
Long-term use of borage should be avoided. Those with liver disease or seizure disorders and those who are pregnant or breast-feeding should avoid use.

## NURSING CONSIDERATIONS
• Find out why patient is using the herb.
• Borage oil doesn't contain the potentially toxic pyrrolizidine alkaloids.
• Liver function tests may be needed to help monitor patient for hepatotoxicity.
• If patient has a history of seizures and is taking an anticonvulsant, monitor him for seizure activity because borage may lower the seizure threshold.
• Borage leaves should be protected from light and moisture.

### Patient teaching
• Advise patient to consult with his health care provider before using an herbal preparation because a treatment with proven efficacy may be available.
• Tell patient to remind pharmacist of any herbal or dietary supplement that he's taking, when filling a new prescription.
• If patient is pregnant or breast-feeding, advise her not to use borage.
• Warn patient of the potential for hepatic dysfunction and carcinogenic effects of borage plant preparations.
• Advise patient that borage oil is usually safe and free from adverse effects when taken in therapeutic doses.

• Advise patient not to delay seeking appropriate medical treatment if symptoms persist after taking borage.
• Advise patient to store dried leaves away from light and moisture.

## broom

*Cytisus scoparius,* basam, besenginsterkraut, besom, bizzom, breeam, broom top, browme, brum, ginsterkraut, green broom, hogweed, Irish broom top, Irish tops, sarothamni herb, Scotch broom, Scotch broom top

**Common trade names**
*Broomtops, Scotch Broom*

### HOW SUPPLIED
Available as an aqueous essential oil extract, liquid extract*, and tincture.

### ACTIONS & COMPONENTS
Derived from the dried and stripped flowers, the dried aerial parts, and the freshly picked flowers of *C. scoparius.*

The main alkaloid in broom is sparteine, a transparent, oily liquid, colorless when fresh, turning brown on exposure, with an aniline-like odor and a very bitter taste. It's slightly soluble in water, but readily soluble in alcohol and ether. Sparteine is a powerful oxytocic once used for inducing uterine contractions. It also has antiarrhythmic and bradycardic effects.

Scoparin, the other principal component, is a glucoside that occurs in pale yellow crystals, is tasteless, and is soluble in alcohol and hot water. It's responsible for broom's diuretic effect.

Broom also contains flavonoids, biogenic amines, isoflavonoids, and other alkaloids.

## USES
Aqueous essential oil extracts are used internally. Broom is used to treat hypertension and CV and circulatory disorders, as well as to stabilize circulation and to elevate blood pressure. Used as a cathartic and diuretic and, in large doses, as an emetic.

Also used to treat pathologic edema, cardiac arrhythmia, nervous cardiac complaints, menorrhagia, hemorrhage after birth, uterine contraction stimulant, low blood pressure, bleeding gums, hemophilia, gout, rheumatism, sciatica, gall and kidney stones, splenomegaly, jaundice, snake bites, and bronchial conditions.

Prepared as a cigarette and smoked like marijuana to produce euphoria and relaxation.

## DOSAGE & ADMINISTRATION
*Infusion:* 1 cup fresh infusion P.O. t.i.d.
*Liquid extract (25% alcohol):* 1 to 2 ml P.O. q.d.
*Tincture:* 0.5 to 2 ml P.O.

## ADVERSE REACTIONS
None reported.

## INTERACTIONS
**Herb-drug.** *Antihypertensives:* Additive effects. Monitor blood pressure.

*Disulfiram:* Herbal products prepared with alcohol may cause a disulfiram-like reaction. Advise patient to avoid using together.
*MAO inhibitors:* May cause a hypertensive crisis. Advise patient to avoid using together.
*Quinidine:* Additive effects. Advise patient to avoid using together.
**Herb-lifestyle.** *Nicotine, smoking:* Additive effects. Advise patient to avoid using together.

## CAUTIONS
Those taking an MAO inhibitor, those with high blood pressure or AV block, and those who are pregnant should avoid use.

## NURSING CONSIDERATIONS
• Find out why patient is using the herb.
• Monitor blood pressure.
• Broom has the potential for abuse.
• Doses that contain more than 300 mg sparteine, or 30 g of drug, may cause dizziness, headache, palpitations, weakness, sweating, sleepiness, pupil dilation, and ocular palsy.
• If overdose occurs and patient doesn't vomit on his own, perform gastric lavage and administer activated charcoal. Treat spasms with chlorpromazine or diazepam. If patient becomes asphyxiated, intubation and oxygen respiration may be needed.

**Patient teaching**
• Advise patient to consult with his health care provider before using an herbal preparation because a

---

*Bold italic type* indicates that reaction may be life-threatening.

treatment with proven efficacy may be available.

• Tell patient to remind pharmacist of any herbal or dietary supplement that he's taking, when filling a new prescription.

• Warn patient not to delay seeking appropriate medical evaluation for edema and cardiac complaints because doing so may delay diagnosis of a potentially serious medical condition.

• If patient is taking an MAO inhibitor or is pregnant, advise her not to use broom.

• Advise patient that broom should be used only under a health care provider's supervision.

## buchu

*Barosma* (synonym *Agathosma*) *betulina, B. crenulata, B. serratifolia,* bookoo, bucco, bucku, buku, long buchu, round buchu, short buchu

**Common trade names**
*Buchu Leaf Bulk*

### HOW SUPPLIED
Available as capsules, extract*, herbal tea, tablets, and tincture*. Also found in commercial herbal blends used for diuresis.

### ACTIONS & COMPONENTS
Consists of the dried leaves of *B. betulina, B. crenulata,* and *B. serratifolia.* Contains flavonoids, resin, and mucilage. Also contains volatile oil that's made up of more than 100 identified compounds. The principal component in the distilled oil is diosphenol, which crystallizes at room temperature (buchu camphor). Other major components of the oil include pulegone, limonene, and menthone.

Buchu is reported to have urinary antiseptic, antibacterial, diuretic, anti-inflammatory, and carminative properties. Diosphenol is thought to exert an antibacterial effect, similar to that of bearberry leaves. Like bearberry, this phenol is excreted as a glucuronic acid conjugate, which may account for similar antibacterial properties. Volatile oil and flavonoid components may be responsible for the anti-inflammatory effects.

Weak diuretic activity similar to coffee or tea may come from the flavonoids, diosphenol and terpinen-4-ol present in buchu leaf. Terpinen-4-ol increases glomerular filtration rate and may irritate the kidneys.

Pulegone is a hepatotoxin and an abortifacient that stimulates uterine contractions and may cause increased menstrual flow.

### USES
Used since the 16th century in Europe. Used widely by advocates of herbs, particularly in South Africa. However, German Commission E lists buchu as an unapproved herb whose effectiveness isn't documented.

Used to treat mild inflammation and infection of the kidneys and urinary tract in those with cystitis, urethritis, prostatitis, and venereal disease. Used to treat bladder irritation, gout, stomachache, and constipation. Also used as a mild

*Liquid may contain alcohol.

diuretic, antiseptic, tonic, and stimulant.

A douche prepared from an infusion of the leaves is used to treat yeast infections and leukorrhea.

## DOSAGE & ADMINISTRATION
*Fluidextract:* 0.3 to 1.2 ml P.O. t.i.d.
*For diuresis:* Tea is prepared by steeping 1 g of herb in boiled water, covered, for 10 minutes, and then straining. Taken P.O. several times a day.
*Oral use:* Daily dosage is 1 to 2 g.
*Tincture:* 2 to 4 ml P.O., up to t.i.d.

## ADVERSE REACTIONS
**GI:** stomach or bowel irritation.
**GU:** kidney irritation, increased menstrual flow.

## INTERACTIONS
**Herb-drug.** *Anticoagulants:* May enhance the effects of anticoagulants. Monitor patient for bleeding.
*Disulfiram:* Herbal products prepared with alcohol may cause a disulfiram-like reaction. Advise patient to avoid using together.

## CAUTIONS
Pregnant patients and those planning pregnancy should avoid use because of buchu's abortifacient effects. Those with kidney inflammation should avoid use.

Those with liver disease should use buchu cautiously because it may cause liver toxicity.

## NURSING CONSIDERATIONS
• Find out why patient is using the herb.

• Ingesting large amounts of buchu or the oil can irritate the GI tract and kidneys.
• Buchu may alter the intended therapeutic effect of conventional drugs.
• If patient is taking an anticoagulant, consider monitoring INR, PT, PTT, liver function, and menstruation.

## Patient teaching
• Advise patient to consult with his health care provider before using an herbal preparation because a treatment with proven efficacy may be available.
• Tell patient to remind pharmacist of any herbal or dietary supplement that he's taking, when filling a new prescription.
• Warn patient not to delay seeking appropriate medical evaluation because doing so may delay diagnosis of a potentially serious medical condition.
• If patient is pregnant or is planning pregnancy, advise her not to use buchu.
• If patient is taking an anticoagulant such as warfarin, advise him to notify his health care provider that he's using buchu because the herb can enhance the effects of such drugs.
• Advise patient to alert her health care provider if after using buchu she experiences profuse menstrual flow or kidney, stomach, or bowel irritation.

---

*Bold italic type* indicates that reaction may be life-threatening.

# buckthorn

*Rhamnus catharticus,*
*R. frangula,* alder buckthorn,
alder dogwood, arrow wood,
black alder bark, black
dogwood, buckthorn bark,
dogwood, frangula, frangula
bark, glossy buckthorn,
hartshorn, highwaythorn,
purging buckthorn ramsthorn,
waythorn

**Common trade names**
*None known*

## HOW SUPPLIED
Available as capsules, fluidextract,
liquid formulations, and tablets.
It's also an ingredient in various
teas.

## ACTIONS & COMPONENTS
Dried bark comes from the stems
and branches of the *R. frangula*
tree, which is imported from the
former USSR, former Yugoslavia,
and Poland. Contains anthranoids
and 3% to 9% anthraquinone glycosides, which include glucofrangulin A and B and frangulin A and
B, which have a laxative effect.

The fresh bark contains the reduced forms of anthrones and an-
throne glycosides, which have an
emetic component. Use of the un-
treated fresh herb can irritate the
stomach mucosa, causing severe
vomiting, colic, and bloody diarrhea.

Buckthorn's stimulant and irritant laxative effect on the large intestine is similar to, yet milder
than, that of cascara sagrada. It has
weaker antiabsorptive and hydra-

gogic properties. The herb takes
effect 6 to 8 hours after it's administered. Unlike bulk-forming laxatives, stimulant laxatives act directly on the intestinal mucosa and
commonly result in gripping and
loose stools.

Anthraquinones stimulate active
chloride secretion and increase the
amount of water and electrolytes
discharged into the large intestine
and passed in stool. The motility
of the colon is increased, as sta-
tionary and stimulating propulsive
contractions are inhibited, which
results in faster bowel movements.

## USES
Used orally to treat cancer. Used
as a laxative to treat constipation
and to ease bowel evacuation in
those who have anal fissures or
hemorrhoids and in those who
have had rectal-anal surgery. Also
used as a tonic.

Extracts of buckthorn bark are
used topically in sunscreen products.

## DOSAGE & ADMINISTRATION
*Daily doses:* The daily dose of
buckthorn bark is based on the
quantity of its key component anthranoid, not on the quantity of dry
herb.

The average daily dose based on
its hydroxyanthracine content is 20
to 180 mg; however, some sources
list the daily dose as 20 to 30 mg
of hydroxyanthracine derivative,
calculated as glucofrangulin A.
*Tea, infusion:* Prepared by pouring
boiling water over 2 g of finely
ground herb and straining after 10
to 15 minutes. A cold infusion can

---

*Liquid may contain alcohol.

be prepared by letting the herb steep for 12 hours at room temperature. (1 tsp equals about 2.4 g; 1 scant tsp, 2 g.)

## ADVERSE REACTIONS
**GI:** GI cramping or gripping.
**GU:** dark yellow or red urine.

## INTERACTIONS
**Herb-drug.** *Antiarrhythmics:* Overuse or abuse may interfere with the effects of antiarrhythmics because of potassium loss. With extended use of both, monitor serum potassium level.
*Cardiac glycosides such as digoxin:* Overuse or abuse may potentiate the adverse effects of cardiac glycosides because of potassium loss. With extended use of both, monitor serum potassium level.
*Corticosteroids:* Increased risk of hypokalemia may cause arrhythmias. With extended use of both, monitor serum potassium level.
*Thiazide diuretics such as furosemide:* Increased risk of hypokalemia. With extended use of both, monitor serum potassium level.
**Herb-herb.** *Licorice:* May increase the risk of hypokalemia. With extended use of both, monitor serum potassium level.
*Potassium-wasting herbs such as horsetail herb, stimulant laxative herbs such as aloe, black root, blue flag rhizome, butternut bark, cascara sagrada bark, castor oil, colocynth fruit pulp, gamboge bark exudate, jalap root, manna bark exudate, podophyllum root, rhubarb root, senna leaves and pods, wild cumber fruit* (Ecballium

elaterium), and *yellow dock root:* May increase the risk of hypokalemia. With extended use of both, monitor serum potassium level.

## CAUTIONS
Those with intestinal obstruction, abdominal pain of unknown origin, or acute inflammatory intestinal disease including appendicitis, colitis, Crohn's disease, and irritable bowel syndrome should avoid use. Pregnant and breast-feeding patients and children younger than age 12 should also avoid use.

Those with fluid or electrolyte imbalances should use buckthorn cautiously because long-term use or abuse can cause hypokalemia and loss of fluid.

## NURSING CONSIDERATIONS
● Find out why patient is using the herb.
● The fluidextract was once official in the National Formulary and USP.
● If buckthorn is being used as a laxative, the dosage should be individualized to the smallest dose required to produce a soft stool.
● Buckthorn may alter the intended therapeutic effect of conventional drugs.
● Patient shouldn't exceed the recommended dose or use buckthorn for longer than 2 weeks.
● Because buckthorn takes effect 6 to 8 hours after it's administered, it isn't suitable for rapid emptying of the bowels.
● Patient can decrease the adverse GI effects of buckthorn by reducing the dosage.

---

**Bold italic type** indicates that reaction may be life-threatening.

• If patient experiences diarrhea or watery stools, he should stop using buckthorn.

• Long-term use of buckthorn can cause loss of fluid and electrolytes, especially potassium, and eventual hyperaldosteronism. Consequences of chronic hypokalemia include aggravated constipation, accelerated bone deterioration, nephropathies, albuminuria, hematuria, damage to the renal tubules, heart function disorders, and muscular weakness, especially when patient is also taking a cardiac glycoside or a diuretic.

• Buckthorn may cause pigment changes in the intestinal mucosa that may be precancerous.

• It's unknown if the anthranoid level in buckthorn is high enough to cause diarrhea in breast-feeding infants.

☑ALERT: Don't confuse buckthorn bark with buckthorn berry (*Rhamnus cathartica*), which is also an anthranoid laxative used for constipation.

• Signs and symptoms of overdose include vomiting and severe GI spasms.

**Patient teaching**
• Advise patient to consult with his health care provider before using an herbal preparation because a treatment with proven efficacy may be available.

• Tell patient to remind pharmacist of any herbal or dietary supplement that he's taking, when filling a new prescription.

• Warn patient not to delay seeking appropriate medical evaluation because doing so may delay diagnosis of a potentially serious medical condition.

• If patient is pregnant or breast-feeding, is planning pregnancy, or has abdominal pain or diarrhea, advise her not to use buckthorn.

• Advise patient not to use buckthorn for longer than 2 weeks without consulting his health care provider because overuse can lead to severe electrolyte imbalances and intestinal sluggishness.

• Suggest that the patient try lifestyle changes to restore normal bowel function—such as increasing dietary fiber and fluid intake and increasing exercise—or even a bulk laxative as opposed to using buckthorn.

• Tell patient to report planned or suspected pregnancy to her health care provider.

• Warn patient not to exceed the recommended dose and to discontinue use if he develops diarrhea or watery stools.

• Inform patient that many so-called dieter's teas contain buckthorn.

## bugleweed

*Lycopus europaeus, L. virginicus,* archangel, green ashangee, gypsy weed, gypsywort, Paul's betony, sweet bugle, water bugle, water hoarhound, water horehound, wolf's foot, wolfstrappkraut

**Common trade names**
*Bugleweed Herb Vcaps*

**HOW SUPPLIED**
Available as capsules, freshly pressed juice, powdered herb, tea,

---

*Liquid may contain alcohol.

water-ethanol extract, and other galenic preparations for internal use.

*Capsules:* 350 mg

## ACTIONS & COMPONENTS

Consists of the fresh or dried leaves and tops of *L. europaeus* or *L. virginicus.* Contains flavonoids and hydrocinnamic and caffeic acid derivatives, including rosmaric acid, lithospermic acid, and their oligomerics, created through oxidation.

Herb may have antithyrotropic activity—specifically, it may inhibit peripheral deiodination of $T_4$. Herb may also have hypoglycemic and antigonadotropic activity and may also decrease serum prolactin levels.

## USES

Used for mild hyperthyroidism with disturbances of the autonomic nervous system, nervousness, insomnia, premenstrual syndrome, and breast pain.

Tinctures and infusions were once used to decrease bleeding of menorrhagia and nosebleeds.

## DOSAGE & ADMINISTRATION

*Teas:* 1 to 2 g P.O. q.d.

*Water-ethanol extracts:* Equivalent of 20 mg of herb P.O. q.d.

## ADVERSE REACTIONS

**Other:** enlargement of the thyroid, increased prolactin secretion.

## INTERACTIONS

**Herb-drug.** *Insulin, oral antidiabetics:* May increase the risk of hypoglycemia. Monitor blood glucose level.

*Iodine:* May interfere with metabolism of iodine. Advise patient to avoid using together.

*Thyroid hormones:* Reduced effectiveness of thyroid hormones, blocking peripheral conversion of thyroxin to $T_3$. Advise patient to avoid using together.

**Herb-herb.** *Thyroid-suppressing herbs such as balm leaf and wild thyme plant:* May have additive effects. Advise patient to avoid using together.

## CAUTIONS

Those with hypothyroidism or thyroid enlargement without functional disturbance and those receiving other thyroid treatments should avoid use. Pregnant and breast-feeding patients should also avoid use.

## NURSING CONSIDERATIONS

- Find out why patient is using the herb.
- Because every patient's optimal level of thyroid hormone is different, the dosages provided are only rough estimates. Both age and weight should be considered when determining dose.
- Bugleweed may interfere with control of the blood glucose level and may cause hypoglycemia. Monitor blood glucose level if patient has hypoglycemia or diabetes.
- Bugleweed therapy shouldn't be stopped abruptly because sudden withdrawal can lead to increased prolactin secretion or exacerbation of the disorder being treated.

---

*Bold italic type* indicates that reaction may be life-threatening.

• Bugleweed may interfere with diagnostic procedures using radio-isotopes.

**Patient teaching**
• Advise patient to consult with his health care provider before using an herbal preparation because a treatment with proven efficacy may be available.
• Tell patient to remind pharmacist of any herbal or dietary supplement that he's taking, when filling a new prescription.
• Advise patient with hyperthyroidism to consult a health care provider for treatment of condition.
• If patient is using other thyroid treatments, advise him not to use bugleweed.
• If patient is pregnant or breastfeeding or is planning pregnancy, advise her not to use bugleweed, unless a health care provider who's an expert in the appropriate use of this herb has directed otherwise.
• If patient is diabetic or hypoglycemic, advise him to alert his health care provider about taking this herb. Bugleweed may lower blood glucose level.
• Advise patient not to stop taking bugleweed abruptly. It should be discontinued gradually unless a health care provider has directed otherwise.

## burdock

*Arctium lappa*, bardana, bardane root, beggar's buttons, burr seed, clot-bur, cocklebur, cockle buttons, edible burdock, fox's clote, great burr, happy major, hardock, hareburr, lappa, lappa root, love leaves, personata, philanthropium, thorny burr

**Common trade names**
*Burdock root is a component in the following preparations: Arth Plus Capsules, Burdock Liquid Extract, Catarrh Mixture (oral liquid), Potter's G.B. Tablets and Gerard House Blue Flag Root Compound Tablets, Seven Seas Rheumatic Pain Tablets, Skin Eruptions Mixture (oral liquid), Tabritis Tablets*

**HOW SUPPLIED**
Available as capsules, liquid extract*, fresh root, tinctures*, and various topical formulations for cosmetic and toiletry-type products.
*Capsules:* 460 mg, 475 mg, 500 mg, 625 mg

**ACTIONS & COMPONENTS**
Consists of the fresh or dried, first-year root of great burdock, *A. lappa;* common burdock, *A. minus;* or woolly burdock, *A. tomentosum.* The leaves and fruits may also be used.
    Contains volatile oil, fatty oil, sucrose, resin, tannin, and large amounts of carbohydrate, specifically inulin. Active constituents include podophyllin-type lignan derivatives and guanidinobutyric acid.

---

*Liquid may contain alcohol.

The fresh root and root extracts may have mild bacteriostatic and fungistatic activity and may also stimulate the flow of bile from the gallbladder to the duodenum.

Polyacetylenes, specifically, arctiopiricin, may be responsible for the gram-positive and gram-negative antimicrobial properties.

Burdock may have antimutagenic, antitumorigenic, hypoglycemic, and uterine stimulant activity, and it may increase carbohydrate tolerance. The hypoglycemic and antimutagenic component may be a polyanionic, lignan-like compound. It's speculated that guanidinobutyric acid, a substance found in fruit extracts derived from burdock, may be responsible for the hypoglycemic activity.

Burdock may also have antipyretic, diuretic, and diaphoretic properties. It may inhibit HIV-1 infection, antagonize platelet activating factor, prevent tumors, and affect the digestion of dietary fiber.

## USES
Used orally to treat cancers, renal or urinary calculi, GI tract disorders, constipation, catarrh, fever, infection, gout, arthritis, and fluid retention. Also used as a blood purifier, aphrodisiac, and diaphoretic.

Used topically to promote healing and to treat various skin conditions, including hair loss, dandruff, eczema, scaly skin, psoriasis, acne, dry skin, and impure skin.

In traditional Chinese medicine, the fruits are commonly combined with other herbs to treat coughs, sore throat, tonsillitis, colds, sores, and abscesses. In Asia, the root is considered nutritious and is part of the diet.

German Commission E doesn't recommend burdock's use because of a lack of data and lists burdock as an unapproved herb.

## DOSAGE & ADMINISTRATION
*Liquid extract (1:1 in 25% alcohol):* 2 to 8 ml P.O. t.i.d.
*Oral:* 2 to 6 g of dried root P.O. t.i.d.
*Tea:* Prepared by placing 1 to 2.5 g of finely chopped or coarsely powdered herb into 5 oz of boiling water for 10 to 15 minutes, and then straining. 1 tsp equals 2 g of herb. Tea is consumed t.i.d.
*Tincture (1:10 in 45% alcohol):* 8 to 12 ml P.O. t.i.d.

## ADVERSE REACTIONS
**CNS:** headache, drowsiness, loss of coordination, slurred speech, incoherent speech, restlessness, hallucinations, hyperactivity, *seizures,* disorientation.
**CV:** flushing.
**EENT:** blurred vision, dryness of mouth and nose.
**Skin:** rash, lack of sweating, allergic dermatitis (topical).
**Other:** fever.

## INTERACTIONS
**Herb-drug.** *Disulfiram:* Herbal products prepared with alcohol may cause a disulfiram reaction. Advise patient to avoid using together.
*Insulin, oral antidiabetics:* May interfere with control of blood glu-

cose level. Monitor patient for hypoglycemia. Drug dosage may need to be adjusted.

**Herb-lifestyle.** *Alcohol:* Additive effects when used with alcohol-containing products. Advise patient to avoid using together.

## CAUTIONS

Pregnant patients should avoid use because it may cause uterine contractions; breast-feeding patients, because it isn't known whether herb appears in breast milk.

Patients allergic to ragweed, chrysanthemums, marigolds, and daisies should use burdock cautiously.

## NURSING CONSIDERATIONS

- Find out why patient is using the herb.
- Burdock is native to Europe but is now grown in the United States.
- In the past, burdock capsules, tinctures, and extracts appeared in the official monographs in the National Formulary and USP.
- None of the herb's properties have been proven to exist in the dried commercial product.
- Liquid extract and tincture contain alcohol and may be inappropriate for alcoholic patients or those with liver disease.
- Burdock should only be used when the fresh root or greens are collected by an expert with sufficient botanical knowledge.
- Burdock root closely resembles the toxic *Atropa belladonna,* commonly known as deadly nightshade root.
- Burdock may cause or exacerbate hypoglycemia. Monitor patient for

hypoglycemia and changes in the blood glucose level. Dosage of insulin or antidiabetic may need to be adjusted.

- Adverse reactions are related to atropine poisoning, which can occur if burdock is contaminated with the root of belladonna. Monitor patient for signs of belladonna toxicity.

### Patient teaching

- Advise patient to consult with his health care provider before using an herbal preparation because a treatment with proven efficacy may be available.
- Tell patient to remind pharmacist of any herbal or dietary supplement that he's taking, when filling a new prescription.
- Warn patient not to delay seeking appropriate medical evaluation because doing so may delay treatment of a potentially serious medical condition.
- If patient is pregnant or breast-feeding or is planning pregnancy, advise her not to use burdock.

⚡ALERT: Caution patient that burdock can cause poisoning if contaminated with belladonna (atropine) or deadly nightshade. Advise him to immediately report blurred vision, headache, drowsiness, slurred speech, loss of coordination, incoherent speech, restlessness, hallucinations, hyperactivity, seizures, disorientation, flushing, dry mouth and nose, rash, lack of sweating, and fever.

- Instruct patient to report any allergic symptoms to his health care provider.

- Inform patient with diabetes or hypoglycemia that burdock may lower his blood glucose level.
- Inform patient that some liquid formulations contain alcohol.

## butcher's broom

*Ruscus aculeatus,* Jew's myrtle, knee holly, kneeholm, pettigree, sweet broom

**Common trade names**
*None known*

### HOW SUPPLIED
Available as capsules, extracts, ointments, and suppositories.
*Capsules:* 75 mg, 100 mg, 370 mg, 470 mg, 475 mg, 675 mg

### ACTIONS & COMPONENTS
Consists of the dried rhizome and root of *R. aculeatus,* an evergreen shrub native to the Mediterranean. Contains the steroid saponins ruscin, ruscoside, aglycones, neuruscogenin, and ruscogenin. Also contains benzofuranes including euparone and ruscodibenzofurane.

Ruscogenin and neoruscogenin cause vasoconstriction by directly stimulating postjunctional alpha$_1$ and alpha$_2$ receptors of the smooth-muscle cells in the vascular wall. Two other steroid saponins may have cytostatic activity on a leukemic cell line.

Butcher's broom has diuretic, antipyretic, and anti-inflammatory properties. It may also be effective in treating venous disorders.

### USES
Used extensively in Europe to treat circulatory disorders and has gained popularity in the United States.

Used orally to treat conditions of venous insufficiency, such as pain, cramps, heaviness, and itching and swelling in the legs. Used to prevent atherosclerosis and to help mend broken bones. Also used as a laxative, a diuretic, and an anti-inflammatory.

Ointments and suppositories are used to relieve itching and burning from hemorrhoids.

In early cultures, the asparagus-like shoots of butcher's broom were eaten as food.

### DOSAGE & ADMINISTRATION
*Raw extract:* 7 to 11 mg P.O. q.d. based on the total ruscogenin content, determined as the sum of neoruscogenin and ruscogenin components.
*Root powder:* 100 to 3,000 mg P.O. q.d.

### ADVERSE REACTIONS
**GI:** GI discomfort, nausea.

### INTERACTIONS
None known.

### CAUTIONS
Pregnant and breast-feeding patients should avoid use.

### NURSING CONSIDERATIONS
- Find out why patient is using the herb.
- **⚡ALERT:** Don't confuse butcher's broom with the following herbs: Scotch broom, broom,

---

*Bold italic type* indicates that reaction may be life-threatening.

*Cytisus scoparius* L., or Spanish broom, *Spartium junceum* L.

**Patient teaching**
• Advise patient to consult with his health care provider before using an herbal preparation because a treatment with proven efficacy may be available.
• Tell patient to remind pharmacist of any herbal or dietary supplement that he's taking, when filling a new prescription.
• Warn patient not to delay seeking appropriate medical evaluation because doing so may delay treatment of a potentially serious medical condition.
• If patient is pregnant or breast-feeding, advise her to avoid use.
• Advise patient not to use with other treatments for circulatory disorders without consulting his health care provider.
• Inform patient that although products containing butcher's broom may claim to be effective for treating circulatory problems of the legs, these products aren't FDA approved and may be ineffective for these conditions.

## butterbur

*Petasites hybridus,* bladder-dock, bog rhubarb, bogshorns, butter-dock, butterfly dock, capdockin, flapperdock, langwort, petasites, umbrella leaves

**Common trade names**
*Butterbur Herb, Butterbur Root, Petadolex Standardized Extract*

**HOW SUPPLIED**
Available as capsules, dried herb, and dried root.
*Capsules:* 50 mg of butterbur root extract (Petadolex)

**ACTIONS & COMPONENTS**
Derived from the rhizome, or root-stock, and leaves of this perennial shrub. Contains sesquiterpene lactones including pestacins, angelicoyleneopetasol, fukinolide, and fukione. The antispasmodic and analgesic actions may result from the effects of pestacins on prostaglandin synthesis. The herb also contains volatile oils, pectin, mucilage, inulin flavonoids, and tannins.
Butterbur contains pyrrizolidine alkaloids, which are carcinogens and hepatotoxins.

**USES**
Used as an antispasmodic and analgesic. As an antispasmodic, it's used to treat urinary tract spasms, mild kidney stone disease, bile flow obstruction, dysmenorrhea, colic, bronchospasm, and cough.
As an analgesic, it's used for backache and migraine headache.

**DOSAGE & ADMINISTRATION**
*Capsules containing 50 mg of butterbur root extract—Petadolex:* 50 mg b.i.d. for migraine headache.
*GI disorders:* 5 to 7 g of dried herb q.d.

**ADVERSE REACTIONS**
**CNS:** sedation.
**Hepatic:** *hepatotoxicity.*
**Other:** *cancer.*

---

*Liquid may contain alcohol.

## INTERACTIONS
**Herb-drug.** *Antihistamines, atropine, phenothiazines, scopolamine, tricyclic antidepressants:* May have added anticholinergic adverse effects. Monitor patient closely.

## CAUTIONS
Pregnant patients should avoid use because of the herb's pyrrizolidine alkaloid content and antispasmodic effect; breast-feeding patients and those with liver disease, because of the herb's pyrrizolidine alkaloid content.

## NURSING CONSIDERATIONS
• Find out why patient is using the herb.
• German studies have shown a reduction in migraine severity and frequency after 4 weeks' treatment.
🖉 **ALERT:** Butterbur's pyrrizolidine alkaloids are known hepatotoxins and carcinogens.
• Because the pyrrizolidine alkaloids in butterbur are toxic, patient shouldn't use herb for longer than 4 to 6 weeks annually.
• Monitor liver function tests, as indicated.
• Butterbur may be unsafe for children.

### Patient teaching
• Advise patient to consult with his health care provider before using an herbal preparation because a treatment with proven efficacy may be available.
• Tell patient to remind pharmacist of any herbal or dietary supplement that he's taking, when filling a new prescription.
• If patient is pregnant or breast-feeding or is planning pregnancy, advise her not to use butterbur.
• Warn the patient not to delay treatment for an illness that doesn't resolve after taking butterbur.
• Instruct patient to stop using butterbur immediately if he experiences skin discoloration, abdominal pain, nausea, or vomiting.

---

*Bold italic type* indicates that reaction may be life-threatening.

# C

## cacao tree

*Theobroma cacao,* cocoa bean, theobroma; cocoa, chocolate, and cocoa butter are derived from this plant

**Common trade names**
*Cocoa Butter, Cocoa Powder, Cocoa Seed, Cocoa Seed Coat, Theobroma Oil*

### HOW SUPPLIED
Cacao seed is roasted, then pressed to express cocoa butter, also known as theobroma oil. The remaining cocoa cake is ground into cocoa powder.

### ACTIONS & COMPONENTS
Contains 0.5% to 2.7% theobromine and 0.25% caffeine; also contains other methylxanthine alkaloids. Unsweetened dark chocolate contains 47 mg of caffeine and 450 mg of theobromine per ounce. Milk chocolate contains about 6 mg caffeine and 45 mg of theobromine per ounce.

Theobromine has weaker stimulant effects than caffeine but is a more potent diuretic, CV stimulant, and coronary dilator. Cocoa contains the antioxidant catechin.

### USES
Cocoa powder and butter are widely used in food products; cocoa butter is used as a base for moisturizers, cosmetics, and suppositories.

Cocoa seed and seed coat are used to treat a wide variety of illnesses, such as intestinal conditions, diarrhea, liver, bladder and renal disease, and diabetes.

### DOSAGE & ADMINISTRATION
Dosage varies with the preparation.

### ADVERSE REACTIONS
**CNS:** CNS stimulation, tremor, insomnia.
**CV:** tachycardia.

### INTERACTIONS
**Herb-drug.** *Acetaminophen, aspirin:* Caffeine can increase the analgesic effects of these drugs. Monitor patient.
*Alendronate:* Coffee decreases alendronate bioavailability. Alendronate should be taken 2 hours before any food.
*Barbiturates:* Decreased caffeine effects because of increased metabolism and CNS depression. Monitor patient.
*Beta agonists such as albuterol, isoproterenol, terbutaline:* Increased CNS and CV stimulation. Monitor patient.
*Cimetidine, disulfiram, fluoroquinolones, such as ciprofloxacin, enoxacin, mexiletine, norfloxacin, oral contraceptives:* Increased caffeine effects resulting from decreased metabolism. Monitor patient closely.
*Clozapine:* Caffeine increases clozapine levels, increasing risk of adverse reactions. Monitor patient closely.

---

*Liquid may contain alcohol.

*Iron, zinc:* Decreased absorption of vitamins. Instruct patient to separate administration times by 2 hours.

*Lithium:* Increased lithium clearance. Monitor serum lithium levels closely.

*MAO inhibitors, such as isocarboxazid, phenelzine, tranylcypromine:* Large amounts of caffeine may result in hypertensive crisis. Discourage use of large doses of caffeine.

*Phenylpropanolamine:* Increased caffeine effect by additive sympathomimetic actions. Reports of manic psychosis with phenylpropanolamine and high caffeine doses. Monitor patient closely; discourage excessive caffeine use.

*Terbinafine:* Increased caffeine effects caused by decreased metabolism. Monitor patient.

*Theophylline:* Decreased theophylline levels with excessive caffeine intake. Monitor serum theophylline levels; discourage excess caffeine use.

*Verapamil:* Increased caffeine effects caused by decreased metabolism. Monitor closely.

**Herb-herb.** *Coffee, cola nut, ephedra, guarana, maté and tea, or ma huang:* The stimulant effects of cocoa products may be increased by these caffeine-containing herbs, and herbal sympathomimetics. Discourage using together.

## CAUTIONS
No studies or reports of women who consumed excessive doses of chocolate during pregnancy are known. Theobromine is teratogenic to animals when given in doses dozens to hundreds of times the equivalent of normal human consumption of chocolate. High doses of caffeine, that is more than 300 mg per day, have been associated with lower birth weight and higher risk of spontaneous abortion in some studies. Caffeine appears in small amounts in breast milk.

## NURSING CONSIDERATIONS
- Find out why patient is using the herb.
- Caffeine may interfere with phenobarbital and serum uric acid assay.
- Cocoa butter may be allergenic and comedogenic.
- Although no known chemical interactions have been reported in clinical studies, consideration must be given to the pharmacologic properties of the herbal product and their potential to exacerbate the intended therapeutic effect of conventional drugs.
- A link to migraine and tension headache is controversial.
- Herb use may worsen symptoms of irritable bowel syndrome.
- Chocolate contains relatively low amounts of caffeine compared with other food sources.

## Patient teaching
- Advise patient to consult with his health care provider before using an herbal preparation because a treatment with proven efficacy may be available.
- Tell patient to remind pharmacist of any herbal or dietary supplement that he's taking, when filling a new prescription.

---

*Bold italic type* indicates that reaction may be life-threatening.

- Advise pregnant or breast-feeding patient to avoid excessive chocolate consumption.
- Instruct patient to promptly report adverse effects.
- Inform the patient not to delay treatment for an illness that doesn't resolve after taking this herb.

## calumba

*Jateorhiza palmata,* colombo

**Common trade names**
*Calumba Dried Root*

### HOW SUPPLIED
Available as the dried root in pieces or powder.

### ACTIONS & COMPONENTS
The medicinal components of calumba aren't known.

### USES
Used as a bitter tonic to treat GI disorders such as diarrhea, dysentery, flatulence, colic, and GI upset.

### DOSAGE & ADMINISTRATION
Not well documented.

### ADVERSE REACTIONS
**CNS:** unconsciousness and paralysis (with very high doses).
**GI:** vomiting, epigastric pain.

### INTERACTIONS
None known.

### CAUTIONS
Pregnant patients should avoid use because the herb's effects on the fetus are unknown.

### NURSING CONSIDERATIONS
- Find out why patient is using the herb.
- Very little information is available on calumba.

**Patient teaching**
- Advise patient to consult with his health care provider before using an herbal preparation because a treatment with proven efficacy may be available.
- Tell patient to remind pharmacist of any herbal or dietary supplement that he's taking, when filling a new prescription.
- Warn patient not to treat symptoms of gastric distress with calumba before seeking appropriate medical evaluation because doing so may delay diagnosis of a potentially serious medical condition.
- Inform patient about other herbs and drugs, such as antidiarrheals or antiflatulents, that are more effective in treating GI disorders.
- Discuss dietary habits and fluid intake and their importance for proper bowel function.
- Advise pregnant or breast-feeding patient not to use calumba and to immediately report planned or suspected pregnancy to her health care provider.
- Tell patient the herb must be kept dry.

*Liquid may contain alcohol.

## capsicum

*Capsicum annuum, C. frutescens,* African chilies, bird pepper, capsaicin, cayenne, chilli pepper, goat's pod, grains of Paradise, Mexican chilies, red pepper, tabasco pepper, Zanzibar pepper

Common trade names
*Topical capsaicin products: Capsin (0.025% or 0.075% lotion), Capzasin-P (0.025% cream), Dolorac (0.025% cream in emollient base), No Pain-HP (0.075% roll-on), Pain Doctor (0.025% cream with methyl-salicylate and menthol), Pain-X (0.05% gel), R-Gel (0.025% gel), Zostrix (0.025% cream in emollient base), Zostrix-HP (0.075% cream in emollient base)*
*Oral capsaicin products: Cayenne Pepper Capsules and Alcoholic Extract*

### HOW SUPPLIED
Available as cayenne pepper capsules, alcoholic extract*, and topical preparation.

### ACTIONS & COMPONENTS
The active component of capsicum, capsaicin, is isolated from the membrane and seeds of the pepper.

Topically applied capsaicin depletes substance P from peripheral sensory neurons and blocks its synthesis and transport. Substance P is a neurotransmitter involved in transmitting pain and itch sensations from the periphery to the CNS and may have vasodilating effects. The effects may be similar to cutting or ligating a nerve.

Oral capsicum may inhibit gastric basal acid output and may inhibit platelet aggregation, but it doesn't alter PT or PTT. High-dose capsicum therapy may decrease coagulation (because of higher antithrombin III levels), lower plasma fibrinogen levels, and increase fibrinolytic activity.

Capsaicin also is highly irritating to mucous membranes and eyes.

### USES
The FDA has approved topical capsaicin for temporary relief of pain from rheumatoid arthritis, osteoarthritis, postherpetic neuralgia (shingles), and diabetic neuropathy. It's being tested for treatment of psoriasis, intractable pruritus, vitiligo, phantom limb pain, mastectomy pain, Guillain-Barré syndrome, neurogenic bladder, vulvar vestibulitis, apocrine chromhidrosis, and reflex sympathetic dystrophy. It's also used in personal defense sprays.

Oral capsicum is used for various GI complaints, including dyspepsia, flatulence, ulcers, and stomach cramps. It's used to treat hypertension and improve circulation. It's also used in some weight-loss and metabolic-enhancement products.

### DOSAGE & ADMINISTRATION
*Oral:* In some cultures, adults ingest up to 3 g P.O. q.d. of capsicum as a spice.
*Topical:* For adults and children ages 2 years and older, capsicum

---

***Bold italic type*** indicates that reaction may be life-threatening.

is applied topically to affected area, not more than t.i.d. or q.i.d. Hands should be washed immediately after capsicum is applied.

**ADVERSE REACTIONS**
**EENT:** eye irritation, corneal abrasion.
**GI:** oral burning, diarrhea, gingival irritation, bleeding gums.
**Respiratory:** cough, ***bronchospasm,*** respiratory irritation.
**Skin:** burning sensation, stinging sensation, erythema, contact dermatitis.

**INTERACTIONS**
**Herb-drug.** *ACE inhibitors:* Increased risk of cough when applied topically. Monitor patient closely.
*Anticoagulants:* May alter anticoagulant effects. Monitor PT and INR closely; advise patient to avoid using together.
*Antiplatelet drugs, heparin and low-molecular-weight heparin, warfarin:* Potential for interaction. Advise patient to avoid using together. If they must be used together, monitor patient for bleeding.
*Aspirin, salicylic acid compounds:* Reduced bioavailability of these drugs. Advise patient to avoid using together.
*Disulfiram:* Herbal products prepared with alcohol may cause a disulfiram-like reaction. Advise patient to avoid using together.
*Theophylline:* Absorption increased when administered with capsicum. Advise patient to avoid using together.

**Herb-herb.** *Feverfew, garlic, ginger, ginkgo, ginseng:* These anticoagulant or antiplatelet herbs may increase the anticoagulant effects of cayenne, thus increasing bleeding tendencies. Advise patient to avoid using together; if they must be used together, monitor patient closely for bleeding.

**CAUTIONS**
Pregnant patients should avoid use because the herb's effects on the fetus aren't known. Those with hypersensitivity to capsicum and those who are breast-feeding should also avoid use. Patients with irritable bowel syndrome should avoid use because of capsaicin's irritant and peristaltic effects.
⚡**ALERT:** Patients with asthma who use capsicum may experience bronchospasm.

**NURSING CONSIDERATIONS**
• Find out why patient is using the herb.
• Alcoholic extracts may be unsuitable for children, alcoholic patients, patients with liver disease, and those taking disulfiram or metronidazole.
• Topical product shouldn't be used on broken or irritated skin or covered with a tight bandage.
• Adverse skin reactions to topically applied capsaicin are treated by washing the area thoroughly with soap and water. Soaking the area in vegetable oil after washing provides a slower onset but longer duration of relief than cold water. Vinegar water irrigation is moder-

---

*Liquid may contain alcohol.

ately successful. Rubbing alcohol may also help.

●EMLA, an emulsion of lidocaine and prilocaine, provides pain relief in about 1 hour to skin that has been severely irritated by capsaicin.

🔏ALERT: Capsicum shouldn't be taken orally for longer than 2 days and then shouldn't be used again for 2 weeks.

**Patient teaching**
● Advise patient to consult with his health care provider before using an herbal preparation because a treatment with proven efficacy may be available.
● Tell patient to remind pharmacist of any herbal or dietary supplement that he's taking, when filling a new prescription.
● If patient is pregnant or breastfeeding or is planning pregnancy, advise her not to use this herb.
● If patient is applying capsicum topically, inform him that it may take 1 to 2 weeks for him to experience maximum pain control.
● If patient is using capsicum topically, instruct him to wash his hands before and immediately after applying it and to avoid contact with eyes. Advise contact lens wearer to wash his hands and to use gloves or an applicator if handling his lenses after applying capsicum.
● If patient is using capsicum topically, advise him not to use topical capsicum on broken or irritated skin and instruct him not to tightly bandage any area to which he has applied it.

● Inform patient not to delay treatment for an illness that doesn't resolve after taking capsicum. If he's applying it topically, advise him to promptly contact his health care provider if his condition worsens or if symptoms persist for 2 to 4 weeks.
● Tell patient to store capsicum in a tightly sealed container, away from light.

## caraway

*Carum carvi*

**Common trade names**
*Caraway Seed*

**HOW SUPPLIED**
Available as dried fruit and seed, alcoholic extract*, and tincture*.

**ACTIONS & COMPONENTS**
Caraway contains a volatile oil that produces its characteristic taste and smell. This oil contains carvole and d-limonene (carvene), which may be active against GI discomfort. Caraway may have weak antispasmodic activity.

**USES**
Most commonly used as a spice. Also used to treat GI upset, nausea, flatulence, bloating, menstrual discomfort, and incontinence; to promote lactation; and to stimulate appetite.
   Caraway oil is used to make liqueurs, such as aquavit, and herbal mouthwashes.

**DOSAGE & ADMINISTRATION**
*Dried fruit:* 1.5 to 6.0 g/day.

---

*Bold italic type* indicates that reaction may be life-threatening.

*Extract:* 3 or 4 gtt in liquid t.i.d. to q.i.d.
*Seeds:* Chew 1 tsp t.i.d. to q.i.d.
*Tea:* Prepared by steeping 1 to 2 tsp of freshly crushed fruit in 5 oz of boiling water for 5 to 10 minutes, and then straining. For adults, 1 cup of tea b.i.d. to q.i.d. between meals; for children, 1 tsp of tea.
*Tincture:* ½ to 1 tsp q.d. to t.i.d.

**ADVERSE REACTIONS**
**Skin:** contact dermatitis.

**INTERACTIONS**
**Herb-drug.** *Disulfiram:* Herbal products prepared with alcohol may cause a disulfiram-like reaction. Advise patient to avoid using together.

**CAUTIONS**
Pregnant and breast-feeding patients should avoid using caraway, even in food, because of its antispasmodic effects.

**NURSING CONSIDERATIONS**
• Find out why patient is using the herb.
• Many tinctures contain between 15% and 90% alcohol and may be unsuitable for children, alcoholic patients, patients with liver disease, and those taking disulfiram or metronidazole.
• Because the active component of caraway isn't water soluble, extracts and tinctures may be more effective than teas.

**Patient teaching**
• Advise patient to consult with his health care provider before using an herbal preparation because a treatment with proven efficacy may be available.
• Tell patient to remind pharmacist of any herbal or dietary supplement that he's taking, when filling a new prescription.
• If patient is pregnant, advise her not to use caraway.
• Inform patient not to delay treatment for an illness that doesn't resolve after taking caraway.
• Instruct patient to promptly report adverse reactions or new signs or symptoms.

## cardamom

*Elettaria cardamomum,* cardamom fruit, cardamom seeds

**Common trade names**
*Cardamom*

**HOW SUPPLIED**
Available as ground seeds and as a tincture*.

**ACTIONS & COMPONENTS**
Obtained from the dried, almost ripened fruit of *E. cardamomum.* Only the seeds of the fruit and the oils obtained from the seeds are used to prepare supplements.

The active ingredients of cardamom are believed to be the volatile oils contained within the seeds of the fruit. The volatile oils consist primarily of cineol, alphaterponyl acetate, and linalyl acetate.

Cardamom may have antiviral properties.

---

*Liquid may contain alcohol.

## USES
Used to soothe the stomach and treat dyspepsia. Used for its antispasmodic, antiflatulent, and motility-enhancing effects, making it potentially useful in other GI conditions.

## DOSAGE & ADMINISTRATION
*Ground seeds:* Average daily dose is 1.5 g.
*Tincture:* 1 to 2 g/day.

## ADVERSE REACTIONS
**Hepatic:** gallstone colic.

## INTERACTIONS
**Herb-drug.** *Disulfiram:* Herbal products prepared with alcohol may cause a disulfiram-like reaction. Advise patient to avoid using together.

## CAUTIONS
Patients with gallstones should avoid use. Pregnant and breast-feeding patients should avoid use.

## NURSING CONSIDERATIONS
• Find out why patient is using the herb.
• Tinctures may contain a significant amount of alcohol.

## Patient teaching
• Advise patient to consult with his health care provider before using an herbal preparation because a treatment with proven efficacy may be available.
• Tell patient to remind pharmacist of any herbal or dietary supplement that he's taking, when filling a new prescription.

• Warn patient not to treat symptoms of gastric distress with cardamom before seeking appropriate medical evaluation because doing so may delay diagnosis of a potentially serious medical condition.
• Instruct patient to promptly report adverse reactions and new signs or symptoms.

## carline thistle

*Carlina acaulis,* dwarf carline, ground thistle, southernwood root, stemless carlina root

**Common trade names**
*None known*

## HOW SUPPLIED
Obtained from the root of the *C. acaulis* plant. It's used both internally and externally. The dried root is used to prepare tea, wine, and tinctures*.

## ACTIONS & COMPONENTS
The medicinal portion of the plant is found in the root. The acetone extract and the essential oils found in the root of carline thistle are believed to possess antibacterial properties that seem to hinder the growth of *Staphylococcus aureus*.

## USES
Orally, carline thistle has been used to treat gallbladder disease, digestive problems, and alimentary tract spasms. It may also act as a mild diuretic and cause diaphoresis.

Externally, carline thistle has been used to treat dermatosis, rinse wounds and ulcers and, when used as a gargle, to alleviate symp-

---

*Bold italic type* indicates that reaction may be life-threatening.

toms associated with cancer of the tongue.

**DOSAGE & ADMINISTRATION**
*Tea:* Prepared by steeping 3 g of finely cut dried root in 5 oz of boiling water for 5 to 10 minutes, and then straining. Dosage is 3 cups q.d.
*Tincture:* Prepared by steeping 20 g of chopped root in 80 g of 60% ethanol for 10 days. Dosage is 40 to 50 gtt 4 to 5 times q.d.
*Topical preparation:* Prepared by steeping 30 g of dried root in 1 qt of boiling water for 5 to 10 minutes, and then straining.
*Wine:* Prepared by steeping 50 g of the dried root in 1 qt of white wine for a minimum of 12 days, and then straining. Dosage is one small glass before meals.

**ADVERSE REACTIONS**
**Other:** allergic reactions.

**INTERACTIONS**
**Herb-drug.** *Disulfiram:* Herbal products prepared with alcohol may cause a disulfiram-like reaction. Advise patient to avoid using together.

**CAUTIONS**
Pregnant and breast-feeding patients should avoid use.

**NURSING CONSIDERATIONS**
• Find out why patient is using the herb.
• Find out if patient has a history of seasonal allergies. He may be more likely to experience a hypersensitivity reaction.

• Wine and tincture preparations contain significant amounts of alcohol; therefore, these aren't suitable for children, alcoholic patients, and patients with liver disease.

**Patient teaching**
• Advise patient to consult with his health care provider before using an herbal preparation because a treatment with proven efficacy may be available.
• Tell patient to remind pharmacist of any herbal or dietary supplement that he's taking, when filling a new prescription.
• Encourage patient to consider other treatment options because little information about the safety and efficacy of carline thistle exists.
• Advise patient to seek medical attention immediately if he suspects he's having an allergic reaction to the herb.
• Instruct patient to promptly report adverse reactions or new signs and symptoms.

## carob

*Ceratonia siliqua,* locust bean, locust pods, St. John's bread, sugar pods

**Common trade names**
*None known*

**HOW SUPPLIED**
The fruit and seeds of the *C. siliqua* are used to prepare dry carob extracts.

---

*Liquid may contain alcohol.

## ACTIONS & COMPONENTS
Believed to act as a dietary binding drug and antidiarrheal; the exact mechanism of action is unknown.

May also have hypoglycemic and hypolipidemic effects, caused by an increase in the viscosity of GI contents.

## USES
Used orally to treat acute nutritional disorders, diarrhea, obesity, dyspepsia, enterocolitis, sprue, and celiac disease. It's also used for vomiting in infants and during pregnancy.

Carob can be found in health food products for weight loss and energy and as a chocolate substitute. Carob flour and extracts are used as flavoring agents in foods and beverages.

## DOSAGE & ADMINISTRATION
*For oral use:* 20 to 30 g of carob can be added to water, tea, or milk and can be consumed throughout the day.

## ADVERSE REACTIONS
None known.

## INTERACTIONS
None known.

## CAUTIONS
Pregnant and breast-feeding patients should consult their health care provider before use.

## NURSING CONSIDERATIONS
• Find out why patient is using the herb.

⚠ALERT: Don't confuse this product with Carob tree, Jacaranda procera, or Jacaranda caroba.

**Patient teaching**
• Advise patient to consult with his health care provider before using an herbal preparation because a treatment with proven efficacy may be available.
• Tell patient to remind pharmacist of any herbal or dietary supplement that he's taking, when filling a new prescription.
• Warn patient not to treat vomiting infant with carob before seeking appropriate medical evaluation because doing so may delay diagnosis of a potentially serious medical condition.
• Discuss with patient other options for treating diarrhea or GI complaints.
• Instruct patient to promptly report adverse reactions and new signs and symptoms.

## cascara sagrada

*Frangula purshiana, Rhamni purshianae cortex,* bitter bark, chittem bark, purshiana bark, sacred bark, yellow bark

**Common trade names**
*Aromatic cascara fluidextract, Cascara aromatci, Cascara sagrada, Cascara sagrada bark, Cascasa*

## HOW SUPPLIED
Available as cut bark, powder, and dry extracts.

---

*Bold italic type* indicates that reaction may be life-threatening.

## ACTIONS & COMPONENTS

Obtained from the dried bark of *R. purshianae;* the bark must be aged 1 year or heat treated before use. Anthraglycosides, or anthraquinones, which consist primarily of cascarosides A and B, are the active ingredients.

Cascara is referred to as a stimulant laxative. When ingested, the herb causes the secretion of water and electrolytes into the small intestine. In the large intestine, the absorption of these products is inhibited, allowing the contents of the bowel to grow in volume. This increased volume then stimulates peristalsis and advances the bowel contents quickly through the large intestine for evacuation.

Cascara may also have antileukemic properties.

## USES

Mainly used as a stimulant laxative to treat constipation; the FDA has approved the herb for this use. Used to make teas, decoctions, elixirs, or for cold maceration. Also used as sunscreens in cosmetic products.

## DOSAGE & ADMINISTRATION

*For constipation:* 20 to 70 mg q.d. P.O. of hydroxyanthracene derivatives, calculated as cascaroside A, from the cut bark, powder, or dry extract. Tea is prepared by steeping 2 g of finely cut bark in 5 oz of boiling water for 5 to 10 minutes and then straining it. The correct dose is the smallest necessary to maintain soft stools.

## ADVERSE REACTIONS

**CV:** *arrhythmias (with prolonged use).*
**GI:** abdominal cramping, abdominal discomfort, bloody diarrhea, colic (from intake of fresh rind).
**GU:** albuminuria, hematuria, kidney irritation (from intake of fresh rind).
**Metabolic:** potassium deficiency, weight loss.

## INTERACTIONS

**Herb-drug.** *Cardiac glycosides, digoxin:* Long-term use of cascara may lead to hypokalemia, which may enhance digoxin action. Monitor patient for signs of digoxin toxicity.
*Laxatives:* Concomitant use increases the likelihood of diarrhea and fluid or electrolyte disturbances. Advise patient to avoid using together.
*Potassium-sparing diuretics and corticosteroids:* Increased risk of potassium depletion. Advise patient to avoid using together.
**Herb-herb.** *Licorice root:* Increased risk of potassium depletion. Advise patient to avoid using together.

## CAUTIONS

Those with intestinal obstruction, ulcerative colitis, appendicitis, abdominal pain of unknown origin, diarrhea, or acute intestinal inflammation, such as Crohn's disease, should avoid use. Children younger than age 12 and pregnant or breast-feeding patients should also avoid use.

---

*Liquid may contain alcohol.

## NURSING CONSIDERATIONS
• Find out why patient is using the herb.
• Liquid and solid forms are for oral use only.
• Effects are generally seen within 6 to 8 hours.
• Long-term use may cause hypokalemia that can lead to cardiac problems and muscle weakness.
• Pseudomelanosis coli, a harmless pigmentation of the intestinal mucosa, may develop; it should reverse when patient stops taking the herb.
• Lazy bowel, an inability to move bowels without a laxative, may develop with long-term use of cascara.
• Herb may discolor urine, making diagnostic test interpretation more difficult.
• Fresh bark can cause severe vomiting or intestinal cramping.
• Overdose can cause diarrhea and fluid and electrolyte imbalance.

**Patient teaching**
• Advise patient to consult with his health care provider before using an herbal preparation because a treatment with proven efficacy may be available.
• Tell patient to remind pharmacist of any herbal or dietary supplement that he's taking, when filling a new prescription.
• Encourage patient to use milder methods of relieving constipation, including making dietary changes and using bulk-forming products, before using stimulant laxatives such as cascara.

• Tell patient not to begin using cascara if he's experiencing abdominal pain or diarrhea.
• Caution patient that children younger than age 12 and pregnant and breast-feeding patients shouldn't use cascara unless under the supervision of a health care provider.
• Advise patient not to use the fresh rind of the cascara plant because it can cause intestinal spasms, bloody diarrhea, or intestinal irritation.
• Advise patient that cascara isn't intended for long-term use and that he shouldn't use it for longer than 10 days without medical advice.
• Inform patient that if abdominal discomfort develops with cascara use, the discomfort may be resolved by lowering the dose. Patient should consult his health care provider.

## castor bean

*Ricinus communis,* African coffee tree, bofareira, castor, Mexico seed, Mexico weed, tangantangan oil plant, wonder tree

Common trade names
*Castor*

## HOW SUPPLIED
Available as a paste for external use.

## ACTIONS & COMPONENTS
Contains a constituent called ricin, a protoplasmic poison. Causes cell death after binding to normal cells

and disrupting DNA synthesis and protein metabolism. Ricin may have analgesic and antiviral properties.

## USES
Used externally as a paste to treat inflammatory skin conditions, boils, carbuncles, abscesses, inflammation of the middle ear, and migraines.

## DOSAGE & ADMINISTRATION
*Topical use:* A paste made from ground seeds can be applied externally to affected areas b.i.d. Treatment may take up to 15 days.

## ADVERSE REACTIONS
**Skin:** rash.
**Other:** *toxic reaction,* allergic reaction.

## INTERACTIONS
**Herb-drug.** *Digoxin:* Potassium depletion from herb use can increase body's sensitivity to drug. Advise patient to avoid using together.

## CAUTIONS
Pregnant and breast-feeding patients should avoid use.

## NURSING CONSIDERATIONS
• Find out why patient is using the herb.
• ALERT: Castor beans can be toxic when chewed and swallowed; 1 to 2 *chewed* seeds can be lethal for an adult. Leaves of the plants may also be poisonous.

• Signs and symptoms of overdose, or toxicity, include severe stomach pain, nausea, hemoptysis, bloody diarrhea, and burning of the mouth. Seizures, hepatic and renal failure, and death can occur.
• If overdose occurs, provide supportive therapy.
• Castor bean dust can be an inhalant allergen.

### Patient teaching
• Advise patient to consult with his health care provider before using an herbal preparation because a treatment with proven efficacy may be available.
• Tell patient to remind pharmacist of any herbal or dietary supplement that he's taking, when filling a new prescription.
• Advise patient not to use on broken or damaged skin.
• Advise patient to discontinue use if he develops a rash after using castor bean.
• Instruct patient to seek medical help immediately if he suspects he has taken an overdose.
• Warn patient to keep all herbal products away from children and pets.

## catnip

*Nepeta cataria,* catmint, catnep, catnip, catswort, field balm

### Common trade names
*Catnip Bulk Tea, Cat Nip, Catnip Herb, Leaves of Catnip*

### HOW SUPPLIED
Available as capsules, dried leaf, tea, and tincture*.

*Liquid may contain alcohol.

## ACTIONS & COMPONENTS
The volatile oil, nepetalactone, iridoids and tannins are the major active ingredients. The essential oil has sedative, carminative, and antispasmodic effects. It's a good source of iron, selenium, potassium, manganese, and chromium.

Catnip may also have diaphoretic and astringent effects. It may help relieve flatulence and colic.

## USES
Used to treat colds, cough, fever, migraines, and hives. Dry leaves are smoked to treat bronchitis and asthma. It's also used internally for menstrual cramps, dyspepsia, and colic because it helps relax smooth muscles.

This herb has been used for insomnia, diuresis, and diaphoresis and for children with diarrhea. Topical poultice is used to relieve swelling.

## DOSAGE & ADMINISTRATION
*Decoction:* 1 to 2 tsp of tea steeped in 6 to 8 oz of boiling water for 10 to 15 minutes. Or, 1 to 2 tsp of tea boiled in 6 to 8 oz of water, set to simmer at low heat for 3 to 5 minutes, and then strained.
*Infusion:* 2 tsp of dried herb infused in 8 oz of boiling water for 10 to 15 minutes. Dosage is 1 cup t.i.d.
*Tincture:* 2 to 4 ml t.i.d.

## ADVERSE REACTIONS
**CNS:** malaise, headache, sedation.
**GI:** abdominal discomfort, nausea, vomiting.

## INTERACTIONS
**Herb-drug.** *Benzodiazepines:* May cause additive CNS depression. Advise patient to avoid using together.
*Disulfiram:* Herbal products prepared with alcohol may cause a disulfiram-like reaction. Advise patient to avoid using together.

## CAUTIONS
Pregnant and breast-feeding patients should avoid use.

## NURSING CONSIDERATIONS
• Find out why patient is using the herb.
• The leaves and flowering tops and fennel of *N. cataria* are harvested between June and September and are used in the preparation of catnip products.
• Catnip was used for tea in Europe until Chinese tea was introduced.
• Children and geriatric patients start with weak preparations and increase the strength, as needed.
• Catnip abuse involves either smoking the dried leaves, similar to smoking marijuana, or making a volatile oil or extract of the herb, soaking the tobacco in the extract, and then smoking the tobacco. If abuse is suspected, watch patient for signs of mood elevation, such as giddiness.
• Monitor any patient using catnip for sedative effects.

## Patient teaching
• Advise patient to consult with his health care provider before using an herbal preparation because a

treatment with proven efficacy may be available.

- Tell patient to remind pharmacist of any herbal or dietary supplement that he's taking, when filling a new prescription.
- If patient is pregnant or is planning pregnancy, advise her not to use catnip.
- Caution patient about potential sedative effects and impairment of cognitive ability.
- Instruct patient to avoid activities that require mental alertness, such as driving, until CNS effects are known.
- Advise patient that extract may contain alcohol and may be unsuitable for children.
- Instruct patient that liquid form needs to be shaken well before each use.
- Warn patient to keep all herbal products and drugs away from children and pets.

## cat's claw

*Uncaria tomentosa*, life-giving vine of Peru, samento, una de gato

**Common trade names**
*Cat's Claw Bark, Cat's Claw Inner Bark Herbal Extract Alcohol Free, Cat's Claw-Power, Cat's Claw Standardized Extract, Cat's Claw Tea Bags, Cat's Claw (Una de Gato), Devil's Claw, Devil's Claw Root, Garbato, Paraguaya, Peruvian Cat's Claw Tincture Liquid, Premium Herb Cat's Claw, Secondary Root, Tambor Hausca, Toron*

**HOW SUPPLIED**
Available as capsules, dried inner stalk bark or root for decoction, extract*, powdered extract, and tea bags.
*Capsules:* 175 mg of standardized cat's claw bark extract delivering 7 mg of alkaloids, 3 mg total of oxindole alkaloids
*Extract:* 250 mg of cat's claw bark extract per milliliter, standardized to contain 3% of oxindole alkaloids; extract contains alcohol. An alcohol-free extract is available.
*Powdered extract:* Packed in 500-mg capsules

**ACTIONS & COMPONENTS**
Contains many alkaloids that are pharmacologically active dietary supplements and are produced from inner stalk bark, woody vine, or roots of *U. tomentosa*. It also inhibits urinary bladder contractions and has local anesthetic effects.

Most cat's claw alkaloids have immunostimulant properties, which may stimulate phagocytosis. The major alkaloids dilate peripheral blood vessels, inhibit the sympathetic nervous system, and relax smooth muscles.

Cat's claw may lower serum cholesterol levels and decrease heart rate.

**USES**
Used to treat GI problems—including Crohn's disease, colitis, inflammatory bowel disease, and hemorrhoids—and to enhance immunity. Also used in cancer patients for its antimutagenic effects. It's also used with AZT to stimu-

---

*Liquid may contain alcohol.

late the immune system in those with HIV infection.

Topically, it's used to relieve pain from minor injuries and to treat acne.

This herb has also been used to treat diverticulosis, ulcers, rheumatism, menstrual disorders, diabetes, prostate problems, gonorrhea, and cirrhosis and to prevent pregnancy.

**DOSAGE & ADMINISTRATION**
*Capsules:* 2 capsules (175 mg per capsule) P.O. q.d. or 3 capsules P.O. t.i.d.; dosage varies by manufacturer.
*Decoction:* 10 to 30 g inner stalk bark or root in 1 qt of water for 30 to 60 minutes. Dosage is 2 to 3 cups per day.
*Extract (alcohol free):* 7 to 10 gtt t.i.d.; may increase to 15 gtt five times a day.
*Liquid or alcohol extract:* 10 to 15 gtt b.i.d. to t.i.d., to 1 to 3 ml t.i.d.
*Powdered extract:* 1 to 3 capsules (500 mg per capsule) P.O. b.i.d. to q.i.d.

**ADVERSE REACTIONS**
**CV:** hypotension.

**INTERACTIONS**
**Herb-drug.** *Antihypertensives:* May potentiate hypotensive effects of conventional drugs. Advise patient to avoid using together.
*Immunosuppressants:* May counteract the therapeutic effects because herb has immunostimulant properties. Advise patient to avoid using together.

**Herb-food.** *Food:* Enhances absorption of herb. Advise patient to take herb with food.

**CAUTIONS**
Pregnant and breast-feeding patients, patients who've had transplant surgery, and patients who have autoimmune disease, multiple sclerosis, or tuberculosis should avoid use.

Those with a history of peptic ulcer disease or gallstones should use caution when taking this herb because it stimulates stomach acid secretion.

**NURSING CONSIDERATIONS**
• Find out why patient is using the herb.
• Some liquid extracts contain alcohol and may be unsuitable for children or patients with liver disease.
• This herb and its contents vary from manufacturer to manufacturer; the alkaloid concentration varies from season to season.

**Patient teaching**
• Advise patient to consult with his health care provider before using an herbal preparation because a treatment with proven efficacy may be available.
• Tell patient to remind pharmacist of any herbal or dietary supplement that he's taking, when filling a new prescription.
• This product and its contents may vary among manufacturers, and its alkaloid concentration varies from season to season. Advise patient to purchase cat's

---

*Bold italic type* indicates that reaction may be life-threatening.

claw from the same reputable source.
- Inform patient that herb should be used for no longer than 8 weeks without a 2- to 3-week rest period from the herb.
- Instruct patient to promptly report adverse reactions and new signs or symptoms.
- Warn patient to keep all herbal products away from children and pets.

## cat's foot

*Antennariae dioica,* cudweed, life everlasting, mountain everlasting

**Common trade names**
*Catsfoot, Cudweed*

### HOW SUPPLIED
Available as bulk dried herb.

### ACTIONS & COMPONENTS
Cat's foot flower consists of the fresh or dried flowers of *A. dioica.*

Cat's foot stimulates the flow of gastric and pancreatic secretions. It may raise blood pressure, and it may have spasmolytic, choleric, discutient, and astringent effects.

### USES
Used to stimulate the flow of bile from the gallbladder to the duodenum and to treat dysentery.

This herb has been used as a diuretic. In Europe, it's also used to cure quinsy and mumps and to treat bites of poisonous reptiles.

### DOSAGE & ADMINISTRATION
*Infusion:* Prepared by steeping 1 tsp fresh or dried flowering herb in ½ cup of boiling water for 10 minutes. Dosage is ½ to 1 cup P.O. q.d.

### ADVERSE REACTIONS
None known.

### INTERACTIONS
**Herb-drug.** *Antihypertensives:* Herb may interfere with the intended therapeutic effect of antihypertensives. Advise patient to use with caution.

### CAUTIONS
Pregnant and breast-feeding patients should avoid use.

### NURSING CONSIDERATIONS
- Find out why patient is using the herb.
- Therapeutic use of cat's foot isn't recommended.
- Monitor patient's blood pressure when therapy is initiated and regularly thereafter.

### Patient teaching
- Advise patient to consult with his health care provider before using an herbal preparation because a treatment with proven efficacy may be available.
- Tell patient to remind pharmacist of any herbal or dietary supplement that he's taking, when filling a new prescription.
- Instruct patient to promptly report adverse reactions and new signs or symptoms.

## celandine

*Chelidonii herba, Chelidonium majus,* celandine herb, greater celandine, jewel weed, pilewort, quick-in-the-hand, schöllkraut, slipperweed, tetterwort, touch-me-not

**Common trade names**
*Celandine, Swallow-Wort*

### HOW SUPPLIED
Available as dry plant, dry root, liquid extract\*, ointment, and tinctures\*. Also available in various multi-ingredient products.
*Liquid extract:* 1:1 in 25% alcohol
*Tinctures:* 1:10 in 45% alcohol

### ACTIONS & COMPONENTS
When used topically, celandine has analgesic, antiseptic, and caustic effects.

When taken orally, the herb may have cytostatic activity with non-specific immune stimulation and may facilitate bile flow in the GI system. It may also have antispasmodic and diuretic effects.

### USES
Used orally to treat nonobstructive cholecystitis, jaundice, cholelithiasis, hypercholesterolemia, angina pectoris, asthma, breast lumps, constipation, diffused latent liver complaints, stomach cancer, and gout. May also help manage blood pressure, but such use must be further investigated.

Used topically as an analgesic, antiseptic, and caustic agent for eczema, blister rashes, scabies, scrofulous diseases, and hemorrhoids.

### DOSAGE & ADMINISTRATION
*Herb decoction, infusion:* 2 to 4 g powdered herb, not root, in 1 cup of boiling water t.i.d.
*Liquid extract:* 1 to 2 ml P.O. t.i.d.
*Ointment:* Applied to affected area t.i.d. p.r.n., for insect bites or dermatitis.
*Root decoction, infusion:* Prepared by steeping 1 level tsp of rootstock in 1 cup of boiling water for 30 minutes. Dosage is ½ cup q.d., consumed when it's cold.
*Tincture:* 10 to 15 gtt S.L. t.i.d.
*Topical juice:* Mixed with vinegar and dabbed on no more than 2 or 3 warts at a time, b.i.d. to t.i.d.

### ADVERSE REACTIONS
**CNS:** stupor, *seizures,* drowsiness.
**GI:** burning in the mouth, abdominal discomfort, nausea, vomiting, bloody diarrhea, salivation.
**GU:** hematuria.
**Hepatic:** jaundice.
**Skin:** contact dermatitis.
**Other:** allergic response.

### INTERACTIONS
**Herb-drug.** *Disulfiram:* Products prepared with alcohol may cause a disulfiram-like reaction. Advise patient to avoid using together.

### CAUTIONS
Patients with latex or celandine allergy, pregnant patients, breast-feeding patients, and patients with painful gallstones, acute bilious colic, obstructive jaundice, or acute viral hepatitis should avoid use.

---

*Bold italic type* indicates that reaction may be life-threatening.

## NURSING CONSIDERATIONS
• Find out why patient is using the herb.
• Dried plant is less active than fresh.
• Patient should only use this herb under the supervision of a health care provider.
• A cross-sensitivity between latex allergy and celandine exists. A patient should carefully weigh the benefits against the risks before taking celandine orally.
• Overdose could be toxic and life-threatening.
⚡ALERT: Stem juice overdoses may cause paralysis and death.

### Patient teaching
• Advise patient to consult with his health care provider before using an herbal preparation because a treatment with proven efficacy may be available.
• Tell patient to remind pharmacist of any herbal or dietary supplement that he's taking, when filling a new prescription.
• Caution patient that he should only use celandine under a health care provider's supervision.
• If patient is pregnant or is planning pregnancy, advise her not to use celandine.
• Encourage patient to alert his health care provider if he's allergic to latex or herbs, before he starts celandine therapy.
• Warn patient not to exceed the recommended dosage.
• Advise patient to notify his health care provider if herb causes allergic reaction, yellowing of the skin, or sclera and to immediately

seek medical attention if any of these occur.
• Inform patient that herb isn't recommended for long-term use.

## celery, celery seed

*Apium graveolens,* celery fruit, celery herb, celery root, celery seed, celery seed oil, garden celery, smallage

### Common trade names
*Celery, Celery Fruit, Celery Seed*

### HOW SUPPLIED
Available as capsules, dried fruits, dried seeds, liquid extract*, tincture, and in multi-ingredient preparations for internal use.
*Capsules:* 450 mg of celery seed extract
*Liquid extract\*:* 1:1 in 50% alcohol

### ACTIONS & COMPONENTS
High in minerals, including sodium and chlorine, but is a poor source of vitamins. May have antirheumatic, anti-inflammatory, diuretic, sedative, anticonvulsive, fungicidal, and anticarcinogenic effects.
   The juice has antihypertensive effects, and the oil may cause hypoglycemia.

### USES
Celery is used to relieve GI gas and colic and to treat bladder and kidney disorders, rheumatic arthritis, gout, and calculosis. Dieters use celery because of its high fiber content.

Celery oil is used as a spasmolytic and sedative for nervousness and hysteria and as an antiflatulent. It's also used to manage hypertension and blood glucose level and to promote menses. Oil extract from the root is used to restore sexual potency impaired by illness.

Celery seeds are used to treat bronchitis and rheumatism.

**DOSAGE & ADMINISTRATION**
*Capsules:* 2 to 3 capsules P.O. b.i.d. to t.i.d.; dosage varies among products.
*Decoction:* Prepared by boiling ½ tsp of seeds in ½ cup of water briefly and straining. Taken t.i.d.
*Dried fruits:* 0.5 to 2 g or by prepared liquid substance 1:5 b.i.d. to t.i.d.
*Infusion:* Prepared by steeping 1 to 2 tsp of freshly crushed seeds in 1 cup of water for 10 to 15 minutes. Taken t.i.d.
*Juice:* 1 tbs b.i.d. to t.i.d. before meals.
*Liquid extract (1:1 in 50% alcohol):* 0.3 to 1.2 ml t.i.d.
*Oil:* 6 to 8 gtt in water b.i.d.
*Tincture:* 1 to 5 ml t.i.d.

**ADVERSE REACTIONS**
**CNS:** sedation.
**Respiratory:** respiratory difficulty.
**Skin:** dermatitis, urticaria, depigmentation, hyperpigmentation.
**Other:** *angioedema,* allergic reaction including ***anaphylactic shock.***

**INTERACTIONS**
**Herb-drug.** *Diuretics, antihypertensives:* Possible additive hypotensive effects. Advise patient to avoid using together.
*Insulin, oral antidiabetics:* Possible additive hypoglycemic effects. Advise patient to avoid using together.
**Herb-lifestyle.** *Sun exposure:* Increased risk of photosensitivity reactions. Advise patient to use sunscreen, wear protective clothing, and avoid prolonged exposure to the sun.

**CAUTIONS**
Pregnant patients shouldn't use celery seed and shouldn't use more than moderate amount of plant. Patients with renal infection or renal insufficiency should avoid use.

**NURSING CONSIDERATIONS**
• Find out why patient is using the herb.
• Ingestion of large amounts of celery oil may cause toxic reaction.
• If patient has diabetes, monitor blood glucose level because celery may cause hypoglycemia.
• If patient is also taking a diuretic or an antihypertensive, check his blood pressure regularly.

**Patient teaching**
• Advise patient to consult with his health care provider before using an herbal preparation because a treatment with proven efficacy may be available.
• Tell patient to remind pharmacist of any herbal or dietary supplement that he's taking, when filling a new prescription.

---

*Bold italic type* indicates that reaction may be life-threatening.

• Instruct patient to promptly report adverse reactions and new signs or symptoms.

• If patient has a kidney infection or kidney disease, advise him not to use celery medicinally because the volatile oils can irritate the renal system.

• If patient is pregnant or is planning pregnancy, advise her not to use celery seed and to be extremely cautious if using celery for its therapeutic effects.

• Tell patient that latent yeast infections may grow when the plant is stored, causing the furanocoumarin content to rise, which could lead to phototoxicosis.

# centaury

*Centaurii herba, Centaurium minus, Centaurium umbellatum, Erythraea centaurium,* centaury gentian, centory, Christ's ladder, feverwort, red centaury, tausendgüldenkraut

**Common trade names**
*Centaury*

## HOW SUPPLIED
Available as the dried flowering tops of common centaury and *E. centaurium,* liquid extract*, powder, tea, and tincture*.
*Tincture:* Essence of centaury, 27% alcohol content

## ACTIONS & COMPONENTS
Contains phenolic acids, alkaloids, monoterpenoids, triterpenoids, flavonoids, beta-coumaric, caffeic acids, xanthones, fatty acids, alkanes, and waxes. The major component, gentiopicroside, has antimalarial effects.

May have antipyretic and stomachic effects. The compounds erythro-centaurin and erytaurin may be responsible for centaury's bitter tonic effects. The phenolic acids may have antipyretic activity.

## USES
Mainly used to treat anorexia and dyspepsia.

## DOSAGE & ADMINISTRATION
*Liquid extract* (1:1 in 25% alcohol):* 2 to 4 ml P.O. up to t.i.d.
*Powder:* Sprinkle on a wafer with honey.
*Tea:* Prepared by steeping 2 to 3 g in 5 oz of boiling water for 15 minutes, and then straining.
*Tincture (27% alcohol)*:* 2 gtt in water or under tongue, p.r.n.

## ADVERSE REACTIONS
None reported.

## INTERACTIONS
**Herb-drug.** *Anticoagulants:* Possible antagonist effect of the anticoagulant. Advise patient to avoid using together.
*Disulfiram:* Herbal products prepared with alcohol may cause a disulfiram-like reaction. Advise patient to avoid using together.

## CAUTIONS
Those with hypersensitivity to centaury or any of its components and those with stomach or intestinal ulcers should avoid use. Pregnant and breast-feeding patients should also avoid use.

*Liquid may contain alcohol.

## NURSING CONSIDERATIONS
• Find out why patient is using the herb.
• Excessive use of centaury should be avoided because information about safety and toxicity is limited.
• Centaury may interfere with the intended therapeutic effect of conventional drugs.
• If patient is also taking an anticoagulant, monitor him for lack of therapeutic effect.

### Patient teaching
• Advise patient to consult with his health care provider before using an herbal preparation because a treatment with proven efficacy may be available.
• Tell patient to remind pharmacist of any herbal or dietary supplement that he's taking, when filling a new prescription.
• Encourage patient to promptly report adverse reactions and new signs and symptoms.
• Advise patient to avoid excessive use.
• If patient is taking disulfiram or metronidazole or if he has a history of alcoholism or cirrhosis, inform him that he should avoid centaury liquid extracts and tincture because of their alcohol content.

## chamomile

*Chamaemelum nobile* (English or Roman chamomile), *Chamomillae anthodium, Matricaria* (or *Chamomilla*) *recutita* (genuine, German, or Hungarian chamomile), anthemis nobilis, chamomilla, kamilenblüten, pin heads, wild chamomile

### Common trade names
*Azulon, Chamomile Flowers, Chamomile Tea, Kid Chamomile, Standardized Chamomile Extract, Wild Chamomile*

### HOW SUPPLIED
Available as capsules, fresh or dried flowerheads of *M. recutita* and *C. nobile,* liquid extract,* raw herb, tea, and topical cream.
*Capsules:* 350 to 400 mg/capsule (standardized to contain 1% apigenin and 0.5% essential oil)
*Liquid extracts*:* The strength of the liquid extracts available is usually 1:1 or 1:1.5. Some liquid extracts contain between 10% to 63% grain alcohol. Nature's Answer makes a liquid extract for children that contains glycerin, not alcohol.
*Raw herb:* Frontier offers whole German chamomile flowers to be used for making teas or massage oils.
*Teas:* Teas are made with the dried flowers of chamomile. Most chamomile teas are organic and caffeine free.

---

## ACTIONS & COMPONENTS

Contains a volatile oil that consists of up to 50% alpha-bisabolol. Bisabolol reduces inflammation and is an antipyretic. It also shortens the healing times of superficial burns and ulcers and inhibits development of ulcers. The essential oil also has antibacterial and slight antiviral effects.

Chamazulene, a minor component of the oil, has anti-inflammatory and antioxidant effects. The flavonoids apigenin and luteolin also contribute to the anti-inflammatory effect. Apigenin is primarily responsible for the anxiolytic and slight sedative effect through action on the CNS benzodiazepine receptors, unlike the benzodiazepines. Apigenin doesn't produce anticonvulsant effects.

Bisabolol, bisabolol oxides A and B, and the essential oil of chamomile are probably best known for their antispasmodic effects. Other compounds in chamomile that exert antispasmodic effects include apigenin, quercetin, luteolin, and the coumarins umbelliferone and herniarine.

## USES

Used orally to treat diarrhea, anxiety, restlessness, stomatitis, hemorrhagic cystitis, flatulence, and motion sickness.

Used topically to stimulate skin metabolism, reduce inflammation, encourage the healing of wounds, and treat cutaneous burns. Also used for its antibacterial and antiviral effects.

Teas are mainly used for sedation or relaxation.

## DOSAGE & ADMINISTRATION

*Liquid extracts\*:* For adults using 1:1 or 1:1.5 in 10% to 70% alcohol, 1 to 4 ml t.i.d.

**Children ages 2 and older:** Using a 1:4 strength alcohol-free extract.

**Children ages 2 to 4 years:** ⅛ to ¼ tsp directly or in water or juice b.i.d. to t.i.d.

**Children weighing 14 to 27 kg (31 to 60 lb):** ¼ to ½ tsp directly or in water or juice b.i.d. to t.i.d.

**Children weighing 27 to 41 kg (60 to 90 lb):** ½ to 1 tsp directly or in water or juice b.i.d. to t.i.d.

**Children weighing 41 to 54 kg (90 to 119 lb):** 1 to 2 tsp directly or in water or juice b.i.d. to t.i.d.

*Raw herb:* Used in massage oils, p.r.n.

*Teas*

For GI upset, tea is taken t.i.d. to q.i.d. between meals.

**Adults and children older than age 6:** Prepared by pouring boiling water over 1 tbs of chamomile or 1 chamomile tea bag, covering it for 5 to 10 minutes, and then passing it through a strainer (if using bulk herb). For inflammation of the mucous membranes in the mouth and throat, tea is used as a wash or gargle. For young children, tea should be diluted.

**Children ages 5 to 6:** 100 to 120 ml q.d. to q.i.d.

**Children ages 3 to 4:** 50 to 80 ml q.d. to q.i.d.

**Children ages 1 to 2:** 20 to 40 ml q.d. to q.i.d.

*Topical cream*

**Adults and children:** Apply q.i.d. to affected areas.

---

\*Liquid may contain alcohol.

**ADVERSE REACTIONS**
**EENT:** conjunctivitis, eyelid angioedema.
**GI:** nausea, vomiting.
**Skin:** eczema, contact dermatitis.
**Other:** *anaphylaxis.*

**INTERACTIONS**
**Herb-drug.** *Warfarin:* The coumarin content of chamomile may antagonize or potentiate the effect of an anticoagulant. Advise patient to avoid using together.

**CAUTIONS**
Patient with known or suspected allergy to chamomile or related members of the Compositae family should avoid use because of the potential for anaphylaxis. Pregnant patients should avoid use because of emmenagogue and abortifacient effects.

Chamomile shouldn't be used in teething babies or in children younger than age 2.

Safety in breast-feeding patients and those with liver or kidney disorders hasn't been established, so these patients should avoid use.

**NURSING CONSIDERATIONS**
• Find out why patient is using the herb.
🔊**ALERT:** People sensitive to ragweed and chrysanthemums or other Compositae family members (arnica, yarrow, feverfew, tansy, artemisia) may be more susceptible to contact allergies and anaphylaxis. Patients with hay fever or bronchial asthma caused by pollens are more susceptible to anaphylactic reactions.

• Signs and symptoms of anaphylaxis include shortness of breath, swelling of the tongue, skin rash, tachycardia, and hypotension.

**Patient teaching**
• Advise patient to consult with his health care provider before using an herbal preparation because a treatment with proven efficacy may be available.
• Tell patient to remind pharmacist of any herbal or dietary supplement that he's taking, when filling a new prescription.
• If patient is pregnant or is planning pregnancy, advise her not to use chamomile.
• If patient is taking an anticoagulant, advise him not to use chamomile because of possible enhanced anticoagulant effects.
• Advise patient that chamomile may enhance an allergic reaction or make existing symptoms worse in susceptible patients.
• Instruct parent not to give chamomile to any child before checking with a knowledgeable practitioner.

## chaparral

*Larrea tridentata,* chaparro, creosote bush, dwarf evergreen oak, el gobernadora, falsa alcaparra, greasewood, gumis, hediondilla, hideonodo, jarillo, shoegoi, Sonora covillea, tasago, ya-temp, zygophylacca

**Common trade names**
*Chaparral Capsules, Chaparral Leaf, Chaparral Liquid*

## HOW SUPPLIED
Available as bulk powder; capsules; the flowers, leaves, and twigs of the *L. tridentata;* liquid extract*; oil infusion; tablet; tea; and tincture*.
*Capsules:* 500 mg of chaparral leaf/capsule
*Liquid extracts:* 1:2.5 to 1:5 dry herb strength in 68% to 75% grain alcohol
*Tablets:* 500 mg of chaparral leaf/capsule combined with 100 mg of vitamin C, 65 mg of alfalfa, 10 mg of yucca, and 10 mg of zinc

## ACTIONS & COMPONENTS
Major constituent is the lignin nordihydroguaiaretic acid (NDGA), which makes up 1.84% of the plant's active compounds. NDGA has potent anti-inflammatory activity because of its ability to block the enzyme lipoxygenase. Lipoxygenase is a precursor to many inflammatory prostaglandins; therefore, by blocking this enzyme, chaparral may help treat certain inflammatory conditions.

Besides inhibiting platelet aggregation in those taking aspirin, NDGA also has some antioxidant effects. Other components of chaparral that add to its antioxidant activity include flavonoids, saponins, and lignins.

The lignins have amoebicidal, antiparasitic, and fungicidal activity. NDGA has also been reported to have antimicrobial activity against certain species of *Penicillium,* streptococci, *Staphylococcus aureus, Bacillus subtilis,* and *Pseudomonas aeruginosa.*

## USES
Used orally as supportive therapy for cancer, dyspepsia, venereal disease, tuberculosis, and parasitic infections. Used as an oral rinse to help prevent tooth decay, halitosis, and gum disease.

Used topically as supportive therapy for allergies, dysmenorrhea, intestinal cramping, rheumatoid arthritis, and wound healing.

## DOSAGE & ADMINISTRATION
*For antimicrobial use:* Swished with tea and spit out. Or, powder is applied directly to minor abrasions.
*To treat allergy symptoms:* Tea is prepared by steeping 1 tsp of leaves and flowers in 1 cup hot water for 10 to 15 minutes; 1 to 3 cups P.O. q.d. for several days. Or, 20 gtt of tincture of liquid extract P.O. q.d. to t.i.d. Alcohol content ranges between 68% and 75%.
*To treat arthralgia:* 1 to 3 cups of tea P.O. q.d. Or, 20 gtt of tincture or liquid extract q.d. to t.i.d. Treatment should be limited to a few days.
*To treat autoimmune disease:* 20 gtt of tincture P.O. q.d. to t.i.d.
*To treat dysmenorrhea or intestinal cramps:* Infused oil is applied topically to abdomen, p.r.n.
*To treat premenstrual syndrome:* 1 to 3 cups of tea P.O. q.d. Treatment should be limited to a few days. Or, 20 gtt of tincture P.O. q.d. to t.i.d.

## ADVERSE REACTIONS
**CNS:** fatigue.
**GI:** anorexia, abdominal pain, nausea, diarrhea, loose stools.

---

*Liquid may contain alcohol.

**GU:** dark urine, induction of cortical and medullary cysts in the kidney.

**Hepatic:** *hepatotoxicity, acute hepatitis,* jaundice, increased liver function test results, *cirrhosis, acute fulminant liver failure.*

**Metabolic:** weight loss.

**Skin:** pruritus, contact dermatitis.

**Other:** fever, tumor growth.

## INTERACTIONS

**Herb-drug.** *Anticoagulants, antiplatelet drugs:* NDGA, a component of chaparral, may interfere with platelet adhesion and aggregation in patients taking aspirin. Advise patient not to use the herb. *Disulfiram:* Herbal products prepared with alcohol may cause a disulfiram-like reaction. Advise patient to avoid using together. *MAO inhibitors including phenelzine, tranylcypromine:* Excessive doses of chaparral may interfere with MAO inhibitor activity. Advise patient to avoid using together.

## CAUTIONS

Those with a history of liver disease, alcohol abuse, hepatitis, renal insufficiency, preexisting renal disease, or chronic renal failure should avoid use. Neither pregnant nor breast-feeding patients should use the herb. Because pediatric dosing information isn't available, herb shouldn't be used in children.

## NURSING CONSIDERATIONS

• Find out why patient is using the herb.

• Dosages are for adults only.

• Most patients find chaparral teas' and tinctures' very strong taste disagreeable, which limits the amount they can tolerate before feeling nauseated.

• Monitor patient for signs or symptoms of hepatic failure. If patient experiences nausea, fever, fatigue, dark urine, or jaundice, he should stop using the herb.

⚡ALERT: Hepatotoxicity appears as toxic or drug-induced cholestatic hepatitis.

• Gastric lavage may be performed within 60 minutes of a potentially fatal ingestion.

• Activated charcoal may also be used when administered within 1 hour of a potentially fatal ingestion.

## Patient teaching

• Advise patient to consult with his health care provider before using an herbal preparation because a treatment with proven efficacy may be available.

• Tell patient to remind pharmacist of any herbal or dietary supplement that he's taking, when filling a new prescription.

• Warn patient not to delay seeking appropriate medical evaluation because doing so may delay diagnosis of a potentially serious medical condition.

• Instruct patient to stop taking chaparral if he develops nausea, fever, fatigue, dark urine, or jaundice.

---

*Bold italic type* indicates that reaction may be life-threatening.

## chaste tree

*Vitex agnus-castus,* chasteberry, Monk's pepper

### Common trade names
*Chasteberry Capsules, Chaste Tree Berry Liquid Herbal Extract, Chaste Tree Capsules, Chaste Tree Tincture, Vitex, Vitex Alfalfa Supreme, Vitex Extract, Vitex 40 Plus, Vitex 20 to 40 Vegicaps*

### HOW SUPPLIED
Available as capsules, elixir*, liquid extract, tablets, tea, and tinctures*. The herb is also contained in various women's multivitamin supplements and combination products used to alleviate menopausal symptoms.
*Capsules (Natrol, Nature's Way, Phytopharmica):* 150 to 325 mg/capsule (standardized to contain 0.5% agnuside)
*Elixir (Gaia):* Contains 85% alcohol
*Liquid extract (Gaia):* 1:1.5 double maceration strength. Contains 65% to 75% vegetable glycerine.
*Tablets (Rainbow Light):* 500 mg/capsule (standardized to contain 0.5% agnuside)
*Teas (Alvita):* Caffeine free
*Tinctures (Gaia):* Contain 40% grain alcohol

### ACTIONS & COMPONENTS
Derived from the dried, ripened fruit of *V. agnus-castus,* chaste tree is believed to act directly on the hypothalamic-pituitary axis.

Chaste tree contains the two iridoid glycosides agnuside and aucubin, flavonoids, essential oils,
and progestins. The berries exert a progesterogenic effect on women and an antiandrogenic effect on men. By increasing the release of luteinizing hormone, which in turn increases progesterone production in the ovaries, Vitex helps to regulate a woman's cycle. Progestin components include progesterone, testosterone, and androstenedione.

A component in chaste tree has been shown to bind to dopamine receptors, thereby inhibiting the release of prolactin. This is particularly useful in treating premenstrual breast pain associated with excess secretion of prolactin. May also act as a diuretic to reduce water retention before menstruation.

### USES
Chaste tree fruit is used to treat menstrual irregularities, such as amenorrhea or excessive menstrual bleeding, and premenstrual complaints, menopausal symptoms, and fibroids.

Chaste tree is also used to increase breast milk production and treat fibrocystic breast disease, infertility in women, and acne.

### DOSAGE & ADMINISTRATION
*Capsules, tablets:* 150 to 325 mg (standardized to contain 0.5% agnuside) P.O. q.d. or b.i.d.
*Tinctures, liquid extracts:* German Commission E recommends aqueous-alcoholic extracts with 30 to 40 mg of the active herb. Extracts from the crushed fruits, which contain between 50% and 70% alcohol, are taken as liquid or dry extract.

---

*Liquid may contain alcohol.

## ADVERSE REACTIONS
**CNS:** headaches.
**GI:** GI upset.
**GU:** increased menstrual flow.
**Skin:** itching, urticaria.

## INTERACTIONS
**Herb-drug.** *Antihypertensives:*
May have an antagonistic effect.
Advise patient to avoid using to-
gether.
*Beta blockers:* Possible risk of hy-
pertensive crisis. Advise patient to
avoid using together.

## CAUTIONS
Men, pregnant patients, breast-
feeding patients, adolescents,
those with hypersensitivity to
chaste tree or its components,
those with active urticaria, those
receiving hormone replacement
therapy, and those taking oral contraceptives should avoid use.

## NURSING CONSIDERATIONS
● Find out why patient is using the
herb.
● Oral use of chaste tree can cause
urticaria and itching. If these
symptoms occur, patient should
discontinue use.
● If patient is using chaste tree
orally, monitor him for signs or
symptoms of hypersensitivity,
including shortness of breath and
swelling of the tongue.
● Chaste tree can be used for 4 to 6
months to treat premenstrual syndrome or to regulate the menstrual
cycle.
● Women with amenorrhea or infertility can use chaste tree for 12
to 18 months.

## Patient teaching
● Advise patient to consult with his
health care provider before using
an herbal preparation because a
treatment with proven efficacy
may be available.
● Tell patient to remind pharmacist
of any herbal or dietary supplement that he's taking, when filling
a new prescription.
● If patient is pregnant or breast-
feeding, advise her not to use
chaste tree.
● If patient is taking an antihypertensive, especially a beta blocker,
advise him not to use chaste tree
because of the potential for hypertensive crisis.
● Caution men against using this
herb because of the antiandrogen
effects.
● Inform patient that chaste tree
may cause rash or itching and that
he should stop taking it if either
develops.
● Remind patient that the herb isn't
fast acting.
● Warn patient to keep all herbal
products away from children and
pets.

## chaulmoogra oil

*Hydnocarpus,* chaulmogra,
chaulmugra, hynocardia oil,
hydnocarpus oil, kalaw tree oil,
leprosy oil, taraktogenos kurzii

**Common trade names**
*Chaulmoogra, Oleum
Chaulmoograe*

## HOW SUPPLIED
Available as oil and ointment.

---

## ACTIONS & COMPONENTS

Topical chaulmoogra oil comes from the expressed oil of the seeds of the chaulmoogra tree. The active ingredient in the oil is chaulmoogric acid, also known as hydnocarpic acid. The oil may have antimicrobial activity, especially against *Mycobacterium leprae.*

Other compounds that have been isolated from the chaulmoogra tree include palmitic acid, glycerol, phytosterols, and a mixture of fatty acids.

## USES

Used to treat rheumatoid arthritis, eczema, psoriasis, and tuberculosis as well as sprains, bruises, and other inflammation of the skin. Applied directly to open wounds and sores.

In the past, chaulmoogra oil was used for its antimicrobial effects as supportive treatment for leprosy. It has since been replaced with newer, more effective drugs.

## DOSAGE & ADMINISTRATION

*Oil:* 5 to 60 minims applied topically to lesions, p.r.n.

## ADVERSE REACTIONS

**Skin:** irritation.

## INTERACTIONS

None known.

## CAUTIONS

Those with hypersensitivity to chaulmoogra oil or any of its components, pregnant patients, breastfeeding patients, and children should avoid use.

## NURSING CONSIDERATIONS

• Find out why patient is using the herb.

🖉 ALERT: Chaulmoogra oil should never be taken orally because the seeds are poisonous from their cyanogenic glycoside content. If accidental ingestion occurs, patient will likely require emergency cardiac and respiratory treatment.

• Oil may be painful to administer to open wounds because it's highly viscous.

• Patients with leprotic wounds show significant improvement when they use chaulmoogra oil, but few data exist regarding chaulmoogra oil's safety and efficacy.

### Patient teaching

• Advise patient to consult with his health care provider before using an herbal preparation because a treatment with proven efficacy may be available.

• Tell patient to remind pharmacist of any herbal or dietary supplement that he's taking, when filling a new prescription.

• If patient is pregnant or breastfeeding, advise her not to use chaulmoogra oil.

• Advise parents not to use the oil for their children.

• Encourage patient with leprotic wounds or ulcers to seek out professional medical treatment and to discuss with his health care provider the possibility of using chaulmoogra oil ointment as adjunct therapy.

*Liquid may contain alcohol.

## chickweed

adder's mouth, mouse ear, passerina, satin flower, starweed, starwort, *Stellaria media,* stitchwort, tongue-grass, winterweed

**Common trade names**
*None known*

**HOW SUPPLIED**
Available as dry herb, fluidextract*, ointment, tea, and tincture*.

**ACTIONS & COMPONENTS**
The leaves of chickweed contain potassium, phosphorus, and nitrate salts. Chickweed also contains 150 to 550 mg of vitamin C per 100 g of herb and the flavonoid rutin, which may explain its topical effects in the treatment of rheumatism; rutin is a counterirritant or rubefacient.

**USES**
Used to treat respiratory problems, such as bronchitis, asthma, cold, flu, cough, and tuberculosis. Also used to treat constipation and blood disorders.

In homeopathic medicine, used to treat rheumatism, gout, blood disorders, eczema, and psoriasis.

**DOSAGE & ADMINISTRATION**
*Dried herb:* 1 to 5 g t.i.d.
*Fluidextract (1:1 in 25% alcohol):* 1 to 5 ml t.i.d.
*Ointment (1:5 in a lard or paraffin base):* External use only for eczema and psoriasis.
*Tea:* Made from ½ to 1 tsp dried herb.

*Tincture (1:5 in 45% alcohol):* 2 to 10 ml t.i.d.

**ADVERSE REACTIONS**
**CNS:** paralysis (from large amounts).

**INTERACTIONS**
**Herb-drug.** *Disulfiram:* Herbal products prepared with alcohol may cause a disulfiram-like reaction. Advise patient to avoid using together.

**CAUTIONS**
Those with hypersensitivity to the herb or its components should avoid use. Because chickweed contains high amounts of potassium and phosphorus, patients with chronic renal failure shouldn't use it. Pregnant and breast-feeding women should avoid ingesting amounts larger than those found in food.

**NURSING CONSIDERATIONS**
• Find out why patient is using the herb.
• Consuming excessive amounts of chickweed may cause nitrate poisoning.
• Monitor patient for hypersensitivity reaction.
• If patient is also taking a cardiac drug, monitor his electrolyte levels.

**Patient teaching**
• Advise patient to consult with his health care provider before using herbal therapy because a treatment with proven efficacy may already be available.

---

***Bold italic type*** indicates that reaction may be life-threatening.

- Tell patient to remind pharmacist of any herbal or dietary supplement that he's taking, when filling a new prescription.
- Warn patient not to delay seeking appropriate medical evaluation because doing so may delay diagnosis of a potentially serious medical condition.
- Advise patient to promptly report adverse reactions and new signs or symptoms.
- Advise patient not to consume excessive amounts of chickweed because it may cause nitrate poisoning.

## chicory

*Cichorium intybus,* blue sailor's succory, hendibeh, succory, wild chicory, wild succory

**Common trade names**
*Chicory*

### HOW SUPPLIED
Available as fresh and dried leaves, stems, and roots as well as dry root stock.

### ACTIONS & COMPONENTS
Choriin, a 6,7 hydroxycoumarin derivative, is a pharmacologically active component. Lactucin, a bitter component, may be responsible for chicory's sedative effects and ability to counteract the effects of caffeine. Other bitter substances—such as intybin, fructose, and inulin—may be responsible for chicory's actions on the GI tract as a digestive tonic. Inulin also has quinidine-like effects.

### USES
Used as a sedative, mild diuretic, laxative, and digestive agent to manage indigestion or dyspepsia. Also used as a salad green.

Used in the past to treat cardiac arrhythmias.

### DOSAGE & ADMINISTRATION
*Comminuted drug:* 3 to 5 g.
*Decoction:* Prepared by adding 1 tsp rootstock to ½-cup cold water, boiling, and then straining. Dosage is 1 to 1½ cups P.O. q.d. (1 mouthful at a time).
*Infusion, tea:* Prepared by steeping 2 to 4 g of whole herb in 7 oz of boiling water for 10 minutes, and then straining.

### ADVERSE REACTIONS
**CNS:** sedation.
**CV:** lower heart rate.
**Skin:** contact dermatitis.
**Other:** allergic toxic reaction.

### INTERACTIONS
None reported; however, herb has cardioactive effects and may interact with drugs affecting heart rate, heart rhythm, or blood pressure.

### CAUTIONS
Those with hypersensitivity to chicory and those who are pregnant should avoid use.

Those with sensitivity to ragweed, chrysanthemums, marigolds, or daisies should use cautiously.

### NURSING CONSIDERATIONS
- Find out why patient is using the herb.
- ALERT: Some commercially prepared chicory products may

---

*Liquid may contain alcohol.

contain crushed cashew shells, which can cause an allergic reaction similar to poison ivy.

• Chicory is generally recognized as safe. Monitor blood pressure and heart rate in those using it for its therapeutic effects.

• If patient is also taking warfarin, monitor international normalized ratio.

• Handling chicory can cause contact dermatitis.

**Patient teaching**

• Advise patient to consult with his health care provider before using an herbal preparation because a treatment with proven efficacy may be available.

• Tell patient to remind pharmacist of any herbal or dietary supplement that he's taking, when filling a new prescription.

• Advise patient to immediately report any heart abnormalities to his health care provider.

• Advise patient to watch for adverse reactions, especially sedation and contact dermatitis.

• Warn patient not to perform activities that require mental alertness until CNS effects on him are known.

## Chinese cucumber

*Trichsanthies kirilowii*, alphatrichosanthin, Chinese snake gourd, compound Q, GLQ 223, gua-lau, gualoupi (fruit peel), gualouzi (seed), snakegourd fruit, tian-hua-fen (root)

**Common trade names**
*None known*

### HOW SUPPLIED
Available as dry ripe fruit, dry seeds, dry roots, fresh roots, dry fruit peel, and purified trichosanthin.

### ACTIONS & COMPONENTS
Chinese cucumber juice contains trichosanthin and karasurin, which are abortifacient proteins. The purified protein alphatrichosanthin from the root of Chinese cucumber is cytotoxic to some HIV-infected macrophage and monocytes and may increase $CD_4$ cell counts in AIDS patients. Trichosanthin may be useful in treating lymphomas and leukemias by helping to kill leukemia-lymphoma cells.

The herb may have antitumorigenic effects.

### USES
Used to treat invasive moles.

In traditional Chinese medicine, herb is used with other drugs to treat fever, dry and productive cough, mastitis, angina, constipation, lung abscess, and appendicitis.

---

*Bold italic type* indicates that reaction may be life-threatening.

## DOSAGE & ADMINISTRATION
*To treat fever, congestion, or constipation:* 9 to 15 g of dried fruit.

## ADVERSE REACTIONS
**CNS:** cerebral edema, *cerebral hemorrhage, seizures.*
**CV:** myocardial damage.
**GI:** nausea, vomiting.
**Hematologic:** blood cell damage.
**Respiratory:** acute pulmonary edema.
**Other:** *fatal anaphylactic reactions, prolonged anaphylactic reactions,* including fever, follicular atresia, ovulation changes, decreased hormone levels.

## INTERACTIONS
**Herb-drug.** *Antidiabetics:* Additive hypoglycemic effects. Advise diabetic patients to avoid use.

## CAUTIONS
Those with a hypersensitivity to Chinese cucumber should avoid use. Patients who are pregnant or who are planning pregnancy should also avoid use.

## NURSING CONSIDERATIONS
• Find out why patient is using the herb.
🖉 **ALERT:** This herb is used by some HIV-positive patients as adjunctive treatment. However, the extracts can be extremely toxic and should be used only under the direction of a knowledgeable practitioner.
• Monitor patient closely for hypersensitivity reactions and mental status changes. Effects may occur more than a decade after a trichosanthin injection.
• Monitor CBC closely at regular intervals.
• If patient is receiving an antidiabetic or another herb that could cause hypoglycemic additive effects, monitor blood glucose level.
• Chinese cucumber may interfere with the intended therapeutic effect of conventional drugs.
• The herb is also being studied as a possible treatment for AIDS infections.

## Patient teaching
• Advise patient to consult with his health care provider before using an herbal preparation because a treatment with proven efficacy may be available.
• Tell patient to remind pharmacist of any herbal or dietary supplement that he's taking, when filling a new prescription.
• If patient is pregnant, advise her to avoid all contact with Chinese cucumber.
• Warn patient that extracts of Chinese cucumber are extremely toxic.
• Advise patient never to ingest this product, unless under the supervision of a qualified health care provider.
• Instruct patient to immediately report to his health care provider any shortness of breath or severe headache.
• Advise patient that he should follow up regularly with his health care provider to evaluate the effectiveness of therapy.

*Liquid may contain alcohol.

## Chinese rhubarb

*Rheum officinale, R. palmatum,
R. tanguitcum,* Canton rhubarb,
China rhubarb, chong-gi-huang,
da-huang, daio, Himalayan
rhubarb, Indian rhubarb,
Japanese rhubarb, medicinal
rhubarb, racine de rhubarbee,
rhabarber, Rhubarb, Rhubarb
root, Russian rhubarb, Shenshi
rhubarb, tai huang, Turkey
rhubarb

**Common trade names**
*Phytoestrol N; Multiple ingredient
preparations include: Abdominolon,
Certobil, Cholaflux, Colax,
Compound Fix Elixir, Dragees
Laxatives, Enteroton, Fam-Lax,
Herbalax, Herbal Laxative, Neo-
Cleanse, New-Lax, Plantago
Complax, Tisana Arnaldi, Vegebyl*

### HOW SUPPLIED
Available as dry roots, stem parts,
bark, and powder.

### ACTIONS & COMPONENTS
Contains the anthraquinone rhein,
so higher doses have a stimulant
laxative effect similar to that of
cascara and senna. In contrast,
lower doses have antidiarrheal
effects because tannins in the herb
have astringent effects; Chinese
rhubarb contains between 5% and
10% tannins. Laxative effects generally occur 6 to 10 hours after
ingestion.

May also increase cardiac con-
tractility, with the polysaccharides
inhibiting calcium influx in the
myocardium, as well as slow the
progression of diabetic nephropathy and chronic renal failure. It
may lower proteinuria, heal GI
bleeding ulcers, and have antiviral,
antibacterial, antineoplastic, and
diuretic effects. The anthraquinones rhein and emodin may
inhibit growth of *Staphylococcus
aureus.*

### USES
Used to treat jaundice, kidney
stones, gout, headache, toothache,
and skin and mucous membrane
inflammation. Also used to heal
skin sores and scabs.

German Commission E has approved the herb as a treatment for
constipation; lower dosages are
used to treat diarrhea.

In traditional Chinese medicine,
used to treat delirium, edema,
amenorrhea, and abdominal pain.

### DOSAGE & ADMINISTRATION
*To treat constipation:* 20 to 30 mg
of rhein (1.2 g of whole roots and
stem of Chinese rhubarb) as a single daily dose for a maximum of
14 days. Or, 1 tsp of powdered
root boiled in 1 cup of water for
10 minutes, taken 1 tbs at a time,
up to 1 cup q.d. Or, ½ to 1 tsp of
tincture q.d.
*To treat diarrhea:* ¼ to ½ tsp of
powdered root boiled in 1 cup of
water for 10 minutes, taken 1 tbs
at a time, up to 1 cup q.d. Or, ¼
tsp of tincture q.d.
*To treat toothache:* Tincture is
applied by cotton swab directly to
the painful tooth.

## ADVERSE REACTIONS
**GI:** abdominal cramping, diarrhea, nausea, vomiting, reduced gastric motility.
**GU:** kidney stones, hematuria, discolored urine.
**Metabolic:** hypokalemia, electrolyte imbalance.
**Musculoskeletal:** weakness.
**Other:** dehydration, pigmentation of the intestinal mucosa.

## INTERACTIONS
**Herb-drug.** *Calcium:* The oxalate in Chinese rhubarb may form an insoluble compound with calcium, which may cause kidney stones. Advise patient to avoid using together.
*Corticosteroids, potassium-wasting diuretics:* Herb may increase the risk of hypokalemia when given with these drugs. Monitor patient and serum potassium levels closely.
*Digoxin, other antiarrhythmics:* Chinese rhubarb may increase the cardiac toxicity of these drugs as a result of potassium loss and effects on drug absorption. Advise patient to avoid using together.
*Laxatives:* Chinese rhubarb may potentiate the effects of these drugs. Advise patient to avoid using together.
*Vitamin K:* Rhubarb may potentiate the anticoagulant effect by reducing absorption of vitamin K. Advise patient to avoid using together.

## CAUTIONS
Those with hypersensitivity to the herb or its components, pregnant patients, breast-feeding patients, and children should avoid use.

Those with intestinal obstruction or ileus; appendicitis, chronic intestinal inflammation, such as gastric duodenal ulcer, Crohn's disease, or ulcerative colitis; abdominal pain of unknown origin; or a history of kidney stones should also avoid use.

## NURSING CONSIDERATIONS
• Find out why patient is using the herb.
• Oral ingestion of Chinese rhubarb may cause hypokalemia. Monitor levels of potassium and other electrolytes carefully.
• Lazy-bowel syndrome may develop with prolonged use.
• If patient is also taking digoxin or another antiarrhythmic, monitor ECG results for cardiac toxicity.
• If patient is also taking an anticoagulant, watch his INR closely.
• Patient may experience red or bright yellow discoloration of urine.
• Use of Chinese rhubarb may interfere with diagnostic urine tests.

## Patient teaching
• Advise patient to consult with his health care provider before using an herbal preparation because a treatment with proven efficacy may be available.
• Tell patient to remind pharmacist of any herbal or dietary supplement that he's taking, when filling a new prescription.
▨ ALERT: Caution patient against using the leaf of Chinese rhubarb because it's extremely toxic.
• If patient has a medical condition such as small bowel disease, a

stomach ulcer, or heart disease, advise him not to use Chinese rhubarb.

● If patient is taking digoxin, warfarin, a corticosteroid, or a diuretic, tell him to notify his health care provider before using Chinese rhubarb.

● Although Chinese rhubarb has been used to treat constipation, instruct patient not to take it without medical advice and even then to only use it when needed, to help reduce likelihood of hypokalemia.

● Advise patient to use only the smallest possible dose to achieve therapeutic effect.

● Instruct patient not to take Chinese rhubarb for longer than 10 days.

● Warn patient about laxative dependency.

## chondroitin

CDS, chondroitin sulfate, chondroitin sulfate A, chondroitin sulfate C, chondroitin sulfuric acid, chonsurid, CSA, galacosaminoglucuronoglycan sulfate, structum

**Common trade names**
*Oral in combination with glucosamine: ChondroFlex, Cosamin DS, OsteoBiflex*
*Topical: Humatrix*

## HOW SUPPLIED

Available as a capsule containing bovine or shark cartilage, as a gel, or as a synthetic preparation.

## ACTIONS & COMPONENTS

Natural, biologic, high-viscosity polymer found in the matrix between joints. It helps maintain water content and elasticity of the cartilage between joints, allowing for easy, painless movement. Proper supplement of chondroitin may enhance repair of degenerative injuries and inflammation. Chondroitin attracts fluid and nutrients into the synovial space and thus may help protect that area.

Chondroitin is a minor component in the low-molecular-weight heparin derivative, danaparoid.

Chondroitin may help improve symptoms of osteoarthritis when it's used with glucosamine and manganese ascorbate; however, the American College of Rheumatology doesn't recommend substituting the traditional treatment with chondroitin.

## USES

Used to decrease pain and inflammation after extravasation with ifosfamide, vindesine, doxorubicin, or vincristine.

## DOSAGE & ADMINISTRATION

*To treat osteoarthritis:* 200 to 400 mg P.O. b.i.d. to t.i.d.; 1,200 mg P.O. q.d.; 1 tablet of Cosamin DS (contains chondroitin sulfate, glucosamine hydrochloride, manganese ascorbate) P.O. t.i.d.

## ADVERSE REACTIONS

**GI:** epigastric pain, nausea.
**Other:** allergic reaction.

## INTERACTIONS

None reported.

---

*Bold italic type* indicates that reaction may be life-threatening.

## CAUTIONS
Those with hypersensitivity to chondroitin or its components should avoid use.

## NURSING CONSIDERATIONS
● Find out why patient is using chondroitin.
● Chondroitin may alter the effects of conventional drugs.
● Monitor patient for allergic reactions, such as shortness of breath or rash.

### Patient teaching
● Advise patient to consult with his health care provider before self-treating bothersome symptoms because a treatment with proven efficacy may be available.
● Tell patient to remind pharmacist of any herbal or dietary supplement that he's taking, when filling a new prescription.
● Instruct patient not to discontinue other arthritis treatment without discussing it with his health care provider.
● Little information exists about chondroitin's long-term effects.
● Instruct patient to notify his health care provider if he experiences any allergic reactions, such as shortness of breath or rash.

## cinnamon

*Cinnamomum verum*

**Common trade names**
*Ceylon Cinnamon, Cinnamomon, Cinnamon*

## HOW SUPPLIED
Available as tea and tincture*.

## ACTIONS & COMPONENTS
The medicinal source of the herb is the oil extracted from the bark, the bark of young trees, and the leaf. Cinnamaldehyde accounts for 65% to 80% of the herb. This essential oil possesses analgesic, antifungal, and antidiarrheal effects. Specifically, the essential oils from cinnamon bark are active against *Aspergillus* species and inhibit aflatoxin growth.

## USES
Used to treat loss of appetite, GI upset, bloating, flatulence, infections, fever, colds, and diarrhea.

## DOSAGE & ADMINISTRATION
*Tea:* Prepared by steeping 0.5 to 1 g of bark into 7 oz of boiling water for 5 to 10 minutes, and then straining. Dosage is 1 cup of tea P.O.; daily dosage of bark is 2 to 4 g.
*Tincture:* Prepared by moistening 200 parts cinnamon bark evenly with ethanol and percolate to produce 1,000 parts tincture. Daily dosage of tincture is 2 to 4 ml t.i.d.

## ADVERSE REACTIONS
**CNS:** sedation, sleepiness, depression.
**CV:** tachycardia.
**EENT:** oral lesions.
**GI:** increased intestinal movement.
**Respiratory:** tachypnea.
**Skin:** allergic reactions to skin and mucosa, skin irritation, pruritus, increased perspiration.

*Liquid may contain alcohol.

## INTERACTIONS
None reported.

## CAUTIONS
Those with an allergy to cinnamon or Peruvian balsam should avoid use. Those who are pregnant or are planning pregnancy and those who have GI conditions, including ulcers, should avoid using cinnamon for therapeutic purposes because it may irritate the GI tract.

## NURSING CONSIDERATIONS
● Find out why patient is using the herb.
● Cinnamon may cause an allergic skin reaction.
● The oil contains trace amounts of coumarin. If patient is also taking warfarin, monitor him for bleeding.

### Patient teaching
● Advise patient to consult with his health care provider before using an herbal preparation because a treatment with proven efficacy may be available.
● Tell patient to remind pharmacist of any herbal or dietary supplement that he's taking, when filling a new prescription.
● If patient is pregnant or is planning pregnancy, advise her not to use cinnamon medicinally.
● If patient is taking warfarin, advise him to check with his health care provider before using cinnamon medicinally.
● Advise patient to stop using cinnamon and to promptly contact his health care provider if he experiences stomach upset, diarrhea, or signs of bleeding.

● Instruct patient to promptly report adverse reactions and new signs or symptoms.

## clary

*Salvia sclarea*

**Common trade names**
*Clary Sage, Clear Eye, Essential Oil Clary Sage, Muscatel Sage, See Bright*

## HOW SUPPLIED
Available as oil distilled from the flowering tops and leaves of the plant.

## ACTIONS & COMPONENTS
Yields an essential oil that's made up largely of alcohols and up to 75% linalyl acetate, linlol, pinene, myrcene, and phellandrene. May have muscle relaxant, analgesic, anxiolytic, and some antiestrogenic effects.

## USES
Used to treat mental fatigue, depression, anxiety, tension, and migraine. Used as an astringent, anti-inflammatory, and antispasmodic. Also used to help restore hormonal balance and relieve symptoms of premenstrual syndrome or menopause.

The essential oil is used as a decoction, tincture, and topical agent; in aromatherapy it's also used for baths, sprays, diffusers, and massages.

---

*Bold italic type* indicates that reaction may be life-threatening.

## DOSAGE & ADMINISTRATION

*Atomizer:* 8 gtt of the essential oil added to 1 oz of water in an atomizer.

*Bath:* 8 gtt of the essential oil blended with 1 tbs of unscented bath oil or water and stirred well to disperse oil.

*Diffuser:* 6 to 10 gtt of the essential oil added to 2 tbs water in diffuser bowl.

## ADVERSE REACTIONS

None known.

## INTERACTIONS

**Herb-lifestyle.** *Alcohol use:* Use with this essential oil may result in enhanced sedation. Advise patient to avoid using together.

## CAUTIONS

Those who are pregnant or are planning pregnancy should avoid use. Those who have breast cysts, uterine fibroids, or other estrogen-related disorders should avoid long-term use.

## NURSING CONSIDERATIONS

- Find out why patient is using the herb.
- Clary is intended primarily for aromatherapy use.
- 🖉 ALERT: This essential oil is for external use only.

**Patient teaching**

- Advise patient to consult with his health care provider before using an herbal preparation because a treatment with proven efficacy may be available.
- Tell patient to remind pharmacist of any herbal or dietary supplement that he's taking, when filling a new prescription.
- Warn patient not to treat migraine, depression, or anxiety with clary before seeking appropriate medical evaluation because doing so may delay diagnosis of a potentially serious medical condition.
- If patient is pregnant or is planning pregnancy, advise her not to use the essential oil.
- If patient is taking estrogen, instruct her to inform her health care provider.
- Warn patient that the essential oil is for external use only.
- Tell patient not to apply undiluted essential oils to skin.

## clove oil

*Syzygium aromaticum*

**Common trade names**
*Clove Buds, Clove Oil*

## HOW SUPPLIED

Available for topical use or as a mouthwash.

## ACTIONS & COMPONENTS

Clove oil's medicinal action comes from dried, powdered flower buds. The chief components of clove are the volatile oils eugenol (85%), eugenyl acetate, and beta-caryophyllene (5% to 8%).

The eugenyl acetate component has antihistaminic and spasmolytic properties. Eugenol suppresses the pain pathways and may also inhibit prostaglandin and leukotriene biosynthesis by inhibiting cyclo-oxygenase and lipoxygenase.

*Liquid may contain alcohol.

Clove oil inhibits gram-positive and gram-negative bacteria and may also have fungistatic, anthelminthic, and larvicidal effects.

## USES

Used as a dental analgesic and antiseptic. Also used to inhibit platelet aggregation.

Clove oil is used to relieve signs and symptoms of the common cold and to treat coughs, bronchitis, inflammation of the mouth and pharynx, and infections.

## DOSAGE & ADMINISTRATION

*Mouthwashes:* Aqueous solutions equal to 1% to 5% essential oil may be used as a rinse.

*Toothaches:* Cotton is dipped into undiluted oil and then applied topically to area of tooth pain.

## ADVERSE REACTIONS

**CNS:** depression.
**GI:** hemoptysis.
**Hepatic:** *liver failure.*
**Metabolic:** altered electrolyte levels.
**Respiratory:** *pulmonary toxicity*, blood-tinged sputum.
**Skin:** irritation of skin and mucous membranes.
**Other:** toxic reaction, *DIC.*

## INTERACTIONS

**Herb-drug.** *Platelet aggregation inhibitors:* Herb may increase the effects of these drugs. Advise patient to avoid using together.

## CAUTIONS

Clove oil isn't for use in children.

## NURSING CONSIDERATIONS

● Find out why patient is using the herb.
● No adverse effects are known with the proper use and administration of clove oil.
● Allergic reactions to clove oil are rare.
● Inspect patient's gums and mucous membranes for signs of local irritation.

### Patient teaching

● Advise patient to consult with his health care provider before using an herbal preparation because a treatment with proven efficacy may be available.
● Tell patient to remind pharmacist of any herbal or dietary supplement that he's taking, when filling a new prescription.
● Warn patient of the risks associated with clove oil and of its potential for altering the therapeutic effect of conventional drugs.
● Instruct patient to stop using clove oil if adverse reactions or local irritation occurs.

## coenzyme Q10

ubiquinone

**Common trade names**
*Maxi Cardio Co-Q10, Maxi-Sorb Co Q10, Mega Co Q10, My Fav Coenzyme Q10*

## HOW SUPPLIED

Available as capsules, softgels, and tablets.

---

*Bold italic type* indicates that reaction may be life-threatening.

## ACTIONS & COMPONENTS
A lipid-soluble benzoquinone that's structurally related to vitamin K. It's found in every cell in the body; it acts as a free radical scavenger and membrane stabilizer and is an important cofactor in mitochondrial transport.

## USES
Used to treat ischemic heart disease, hypertension, and heart failure. It's used to guard against doxorubicin cardiotoxicity and to protect the myocardium during invasive cardiac surgery.

## DOSAGE & ADMINISTRATION
*Oral use:* 30 to 300 mg q.d., divided b.i.d. to t.i.d.; however, dosages above 100 mg/day should be given in two or three divided doses.

## ADVERSE REACTIONS
**GI:** epigastric discomfort, loss of appetite, nausea, and diarrhea.

## INTERACTIONS
**Herb-drug.** *Beta blockers:* May inhibit coenzyme Q10–dependent enzymes. Monitor patient closely. *HMG-Co-A reductase inhibitors, gemfibrozil:* May decrease levels of coenzyme Q10. Monitor patient closely.
*Insulin:* Coenzyme Q10 may decrease insulin requirements in those with type 1 diabetes mellitus. Monitor blood glucose levels closely; adjust insulin dosage, as needed.
*Warfarin:* International normalized ratio (INR) may be affected when used with coenzyme Q10. Monitor INR closely.

**Herb-food.** *Food:* Food will maximize absorption. Advise patient to take coenzyme Q10 with food.

## CAUTIONS
Those with a hypersensitivity to coenzyme Q10, pregnant patients, and breast-feeding patients should avoid use.

## NURSING CONSIDERATIONS
• Find out why patient is using coenzyme Q10.
• Monitor vital signs and ECG, as needed.
• If patient has diabetes, monitor blood glucose level regularly.
• Adverse reactions to coenzyme Q10 are rare.

### Patient teaching
• Advise patient to consult with his health care provider before self-treating worrisome symptoms because a treatment with proven efficacy may be available.
• Tell patient to remind pharmacist of any herbal or dietary supplement that he's taking, when filling a new prescription.
• Warn patient not to treat signs and symptoms of heart failure—such as increasing shortness of breath, edema, or chest pain—with coenzyme Q10 before seeking appropriate medical evaluation because doing so may delay diagnosis of a potentially serious medical condition.
**⚡ALERT:** Advise patient with heart failure that coenzyme Q10 shouldn't replace conventional drug therapy. Encourage him to discuss use of coenzyme Q10 with

---

*Liquid may contain alcohol.

his health care provider so treatment may be properly monitored.
● If patient is pregnant, advise her not to use coenzyme Q10.
● If patient is diabetic, alert him to the signs and symptoms of hypoglycemia and hyperglycemia, and instruct him to monitor his blood glucose level.
● Instruct patient to inform his health care provider if he's taking a cholesterol or heart drug, an anticoagulant, or insulin.

## coffee

*Coffea arabica*, Arabian coffee, caffea

**Common trade names**
*Chock Full O'Nuts, Folgers, Maxwell House*

**HOW SUPPLIED**
Available as dried, freeze-dried, or ground beans.

**ACTIONS & COMPONENTS**
Medicinal components of coffee come from the seeds, or beans. The coffee seeds contain 1% to 2% caffeine, 0.25% trigonelline, 3% to 5% tannins, 15% glucose and dextrin, 10% to 13% fatty oil (trioleoyl glycerol and tripalmitoyl glycerol), and 10% to 13% proteins.

Caffeine is the active component of coffee and acts as a CNS stimulant. Caffeine has positive inotropic and chronic effects on the heart, may increase gastric secretions, and may relax smooth muscles of the blood vessels and the bronchioles of the respiratory tract. Caffeine may also increase LDL and total cholesterol levels in those consuming more than 5 cups of coffee per day.

**USES**
Used most notably for its stimulant effects and for its ability to relieve malaise and weariness. Also used for its diuretic and anti-inflammatory effects.

Spray-dried crystals are used for instant coffee.

**DOSAGE & ADMINISTRATION**
*Oral use:* Maximum daily dose shouldn't exceed 1.5 g/day, although nonpregnant adults should limit caffeine intake to less than 250 mg/day. Many health care providers advise pregnant patients to limit coffee intake to 1 cup/day. (1 cup brewed coffee = 100 to 150 mg caffeine.)

**ADVERSE REACTIONS**
**CNS:** anxiety, insomnia, irritability, nervousness, dizziness, headache.
**CV:** hypertension, tachycardia, palpitations, irregular heart rate.
**GI:** ulcers, heartburn, vomiting, diarrhea, loss of appetite, abdominal spasms.
**Metabolic:** increased total cholesterol and LDL levels, hyperglycemia, increased excretion of calcium.
**Musculoskeletal:** stiffness, muscle spasms.
**Respiratory:** tachypnea.

---

*Bold italic type* indicates that reaction may be life-threatening.

## INTERACTIONS
**Herb-drug.** *Benzodiazepines:* Reduced sedative effects. Advise patient to avoid using together.
*Beta blockers (metoprolol, propranolol):* Slight increase in blood pressure. Advise patient to avoid using together.
*Oral drugs:* Coffee charcoal may interfere with the absorption of other drugs. Monitor patient for lack of therapeutic effect.
*Phenylpropanolamine:* Significant elevation in blood pressure and mania. Advise patient to avoid using together.
*Theophylline:* May potentiate the adverse effects of drug and increase jitteriness. Monitor patient closely, and advise him to avoid excessive use.

## CAUTIONS
Pregnant patients, breast-feeding patients, those planning pregnancy, those with ulcers or chronic digestive disorders, and those with hypertension should avoid use.

## NURSING CONSIDERATIONS
● Find out why patient is using the herb.
⚡ALERT: Although lethal overdose is unlikely, the first signs and symptoms of poisoning are vomiting and abdominal spasms.
● Caffeine is believed to increase the risk of late first- and second-trimester miscarriages.
● Caffeine consumed by a breast-feeding mother can cause sleep disorders in her infant.
● Sustained intake of coffee can lead to physical dependence.

● Withdrawal symptoms include headache and sleep disorders.

**Patient teaching**
● Advise patient to consult with his health care provider before using an herbal preparation because a treatment with proven efficacy may be available.
● Tell patient to remind pharmacist of any herbal or dietary supplement that he's taking, when filling a new prescription.
● Advise patient with risk factors for heart disease—that is, increased cholesterol level or hypertension—to discuss caffeine consumption with his health care provider.
● Advise patient that if he experiences difficulty sleeping or develops stomach upset or irritation to inform his health care provider.
● Advise patient who's pregnant, breast-feeding, or planning pregnancy to consider avoiding or limiting her caffeine intake.
● Discuss potential adverse effects with patient and instruct him to promptly report signs and symptoms.

## cola

bissy nut, cola nut, cola seeds, guru nut, kola tree

**Common trade names**
*None known*

## HOW SUPPLIED
Available as liquid extract*, cola nut, cola extract, tea, tincture, and wine.

*Liquid may contain alcohol.

## ACTIONS & COMPONENTS

Medicinal properties are found in the plant's seed. Contains theobromine, theophylline, and 0.6% to 3.7% caffeine—all of which are CNS stimulants.

Cola also has a diuretic effect, stimulates gastric acid production and gastric motility, and has mild chronotropic activity. Cola may contain potentially carcinogenic primary and secondary amines as well as tannins.

## USES

Used as a stimulant to counteract mental and physical fatigue. Cola seeds are chewed to suppress hunger, thirst, morning sickness, and migraines.

## DOSAGE & ADMINISTRATION

*Cola extract:* 0.25 to 0.75 g q.d.
*Cola nut:* 2 to 6 g q.d.
*Liquid extract:* 2.5 to 7.5 g q.d.
*Tea:* 1 to 2 g of cola nut can be taken t.i.d.
*Tincture:* 10 to 30 g q.d.
*Wine:* 60 to 180 g q.d.

## ADVERSE REACTIONS

**CNS:** insomnia, restlessness, nervousness, excitability.
**CV:** tachycardia, palpitations, elevated blood pressure.
**GI:** gastric irritation.

## INTERACTIONS

**Herb-drug.** *Beta agonists, such as albuterol, metaproterenol, salmeterol, and terbutaline:* Enhanced cardiac stimulation. Advise patient to avoid using together.
*CNS stimulants, such as phenylpropanolamine and pseudoephedrine; decongestants:* Enhanced cardiac and CNS stimulation. Advise patient to avoid using together.
*Diuretics:* Enhanced diuretic effect. Monitor fluid status to avoid potential dehydration.
*Lithium:* Abrupt caffeine withdrawal can increase the risk of lithium toxicity. Recommend consistent intake of caffeine-containing products during lithium therapy.
*MAO inhibitors:* Hypertensive crisis can be precipitated after excessive amounts of caffeine. Recommend avoiding caffeine-containing products during MAO inhibitor therapy.
*Quinolone antibiotics:* Can result in decreased caffeine clearance leading to increased potential adverse effects, such as increased blood pressure and heart rate, and excessive CNS stimulation. Recommend limiting intake of cola during treatment with a quinolone antibiotic.
*Theophylline:* Enhanced adverse effects. Monitor patient for signs of excessive CNS stimulation and advise him to avoid using together.
**Herb-food.** *Caffeine-containing products:* Enhanced adverse effects. Advise patient to limit daily sources of caffeine, particularly if he has a history of CV disease.
*Grapefruit juice:* Possible increased caffeine levels leading to increased risk of adverse effects. Recommend avoiding grapefruit juice altogether or maintaining a consistent intake.

---

***Bold italic type*** indicates that reaction may be life-threatening.

## CAUTIONS

Those with underlying cardiac disease or renal insufficiency, geriatric patients, and those with a history of gastric or duodenal ulcers should avoid use. Pregnant and breast-feeding patients should limit use.

Those with renal dysfunction should use cola cautiously.

## NURSING CONSIDERATIONS

● Find out why patient is using the herb.
● Monitor heart rate and blood pressure.
● The diuretic effect of excessive cola may result in dehydration.
● Observe for signs of excess CNS stimulation. Before using a drug to treat symptoms of excitability such as insomnia, check to see if the patient should simply decrease his intake of cola.
● Because some preparations contain significant amounts of alcohol, children, alcoholic patients, patients with liver disease, patients receiving metronidazole or disulfiram, and pregnant and breast-feeding patients should avoid them.
● Abrupt withdrawal can sometimes lead to physical withdrawal, including headaches, irritability, dizziness, and anxiety. Monitor patient for these signs and symptoms.
● Geriatric patients may be especially prone to adverse cardiac and CNS effects.

## Patient teaching

● Advise patient to consult with his health care provider before using an herbal preparation because a treatment with proven efficacy may be available.
● Tell patient to remind pharmacist of any herbal or dietary supplement that he's taking, when filling a new prescription.
● Advise patient to limit his sources of caffeine, to avoid excessive cardiac and CNS stimulation.
● If patient has hypertension or heart disease or is pregnant or breast-feeding, advise him to avoid cola preparations.
● Advise patient to consult his health care provider if he experiences palpitations or dyspepsia.
● Tell patient to inform all his health care providers about his use of cola.
● Instruct patient and family to avoid using alcohol preparations of cola in children, those with a history of alcohol abuse or liver disease, and those taking disulfiram or metronidazole.
● Advise patient that yellow staining of oral mucosa is associated with chewing cola nuts.

## coltsfoot

*Tussilago farfara,* Ass's foot, British tobacco, bullsfoot, butterbur, coughwort, Donnhove, fieldhove, flower velure, foal's-foot, foalswort, hallfoot, horse-foot, horsehoof

**Common trade names**
*Coltsfoot Leaf, Coltsfoot Tea*

## HOW SUPPLIED

Available as bulk leaf, capsules, leaf extract*, and tincture*.

*Liquid may contain alcohol.

*Capsules:* 50 to 100 mg of coltsfoot combined with other natural products
*Leaf extract:* (1:1) strength
*Tincture:* (1:5) strength

**ACTIONS & COMPONENTS**
Contains 5% to 10% mucilage, which is believed to produce a soothing effect by physically coating the irritated mucosa of the mouth and throat. The plant's polysaccharides, flavonoids, and phenolic components may have antiinflammatory and antibacterial activity. Also, the plant contains tussilagone, a sesquiterpene thought to have CV and respiratory stimulant properties, and a number of pyrrolizidine alkaloids, primarily senkirkine and senecionine, which are converted to toxic metabolites in the liver and have been associated with hepatotoxicity.

The dried leaf is the part most commonly used for medicinal purposes. Although the flower also contains medicinal components, it's reported to have higher levels of pyrrolizidine alkaloids.

**USES**
Used to soothe throat irritation and mild inflammations of the mouth and throat, to alleviate cough, and to treat symptoms of respiratory infections, acute and chronic bronchitis, laryngitis, asthma, colds, and emphysema. Also used as a smoking mixture.

**DOSAGE & ADMINISTRATION**
*Extract:* 0.6 to 2 ml t.i.d. Daily dose shouldn't exceed 1 mcg of pyrrolizidine alkaloids with a 1,2 necine structure.
*Tea:* Prepared by adding 1.5 to 2.5 g of cut leaf to boiling water. Taken P.O. several times a day. Dose shouldn't exceed 6 g/day, or 10 mcg of pyrrolizidine alkaloids with a 1,2 necine structure.
*Tincture:* 2 to 8 ml t.i.d.

**ADVERSE REACTIONS**
**CNS:** lethargy.
**GI:** anorexia, abdominal pain and swelling, nausea, vomiting, right upper quadrant pain.
**Hepatic:** *hepatotoxicity,* liver changes, reversible hepatic veno-occlusive disease, jaundice.
**Other:** allergic reaction, *cancer.*

**INTERACTIONS**
**Herb-drug.** *Antihypertensives, cardiac drugs:* Excessive consumption of coltsfoot may interfere with these drug therapies. Advise patient to avoid using together.
*Disulfiram, metronidazole:* Herbal products prepared with alcohol may cause a disulfiram-like reaction. Advise patient to avoid using together.

**CAUTIONS**
Pregnant and breast-feeding patients should avoid use because of the herb's reported abortifacient effects. Those with underlying liver disease should avoid use because of the herb's hepatotoxic effects. Those with a history of heart disease, circulatory problems, alcohol abuse, or liver disease and those allergic to ragweed or other mem-

---

*Bold italic type* indicates that reaction may be life-threatening.

bers of the Asteraceae family should also avoid use.

Patients taking an antihypertensive should use coltsfoot with caution.

## NURSING CONSIDERATIONS

• Find out why patient is using the herb.

• Consider recommending alternative therapies that haven't been associated with severe adverse effects—for example, OTC lozenges or sprays.

• Many countries have banned the internal use of other herbal products containing pyrrolizidine alkaloids because of the risk of liver toxicity.

• Some extracts may contain up to 45% alcohol, so children, alcoholic patients, those with liver disease, and those receiving metronidazole or disulfiram should avoid them.

• Some of coltsfoot's components may antagonize the effect of antihypertensives on blood pressure.

• Those with an allergy to plants in the Asteraceae family (such as ragweed, marigolds, daisies, and chrysanthemums) may experience hypersensitivity reactions to coltsfoot.

• The active ingredient, mucilage, is destroyed when burned.

• Monitor blood pressure and liver function test results, and watch for signs and symptoms of liver dysfunction, such as right upper quadrant pain, nausea, vomiting, abdominal distention, and jaundice.

• Regardless of the preparation used, therapy should last no longer than 4 to 6 weeks per year, to prevent exposure to large amounts of pyrrolizidine alkaloids.

**Patient teaching**

• Advise patient to consult with his health care provider before using an herbal preparation because a treatment with proven efficacy may be available.

• Tell patient to remind pharmacist of any herbal or dietary supplement that he's taking, when filling a new prescription.

• If patient is taking metronidazole or disulfiram, advise him to avoid using coltsfoot.

• If patient has cancer or is undergoing chemotherapy, advise him to avoid using this herb.

• If patient is pregnant or breastfeeding or is planning pregnancy, advise her not to use this herb.

• Discuss with patient other OTC products, such as lozenges, that may be safer to use.

• Caution patients that manufacturers don't report the pyrrolizidine alkaloid content of their products, making it very difficult to determine the exact dose being ingested.

• Inform patient that coltsfoot shouldn't be used for longer than 4 to 6 weeks per year.

• Warn patient that use in higher doses or for longer than recommended may increase the risk of liver toxicity and malignancy.

• Instruct patient to report any signs or symptoms of hepatotoxicity, such as nausea, vomiting, right upper quadrant pain, and jaundice.

## comfrey

*Symphytum officinale,* ass ear, black root, blackwort, boneset, bruisewort, consound, gum plant, healing herb, knitback, knitbone, salsify, slippery root, wallwort

**Common trade names**
*Comfree, Comfrey Root, alcohol and pyrrolizidine free, Comfrey Root*

### HOW SUPPLIED
Available as alcohol-free root extract, capsules, compounded oil, cream, leaf extract*, ointment, and root extract*.
*Capsules:* 50 mg, 100 mg, and 225 mg, along with other natural products
*Compounded oil:* Contains multiple herbal components along with comfrey
*Cream, ointment:* Contains 5% to 20% leaf or root extract, for external use

### ACTIONS & COMPONENTS
Medicinal products are derived from the fresh or dried root and leaves of *S. officinale.* Also used are the leaves and roots from Russian comfrey, which is a hybrid between *S. officinale* and *S. asperum,* also known as prickly comfrey.
The medicinal effect may result from the allantoin content of this herb, which promotes cell proliferation and enhances wound healing. The roots contain more allantoin (0.6% to 0.7%) than the leaves (0.3%). Other components include rosmarinic acid—also believed to have anti-inflammatory properties—mucilage, and numerous pyrrolizidine alkaloids. Pyrrolizidine alkaloids are converted in the liver to toxic metabolites that have been linked to hepatotoxicity. The root contains a higher amount of pyrrolizidine alkaloids than the leaves.
Also, Russian comfrey contains echimidine, which may be the most toxic pyrrolizidine alkaloid found in comfrey.

### USES
Used to treat bruises, sprains, joint inflammation, swelling, ulcers, gastritis, cancer, angina, and diarrhea. Also used to help heal wounds.

### DOSAGE & ADMINISTRATION
*External use:* Ointments and other external preparations containing 5% to 20% dried herb should be applied topically to intact skin with the daily dose not exceeding 100 mcg of pyrrolizidine alkaloids with 1,2 unsaturated necine structure.
*Internal use:* Dose should be limited to 1 mcg/day pyrrolizidine alkaloids with 1,2 unsaturated necine moiety.

### ADVERSE REACTIONS
**GI:** *pancreatic islet cell tumors.*
**GU:** *urinary bladder tumors.*
**Hepatic:** *hepatotoxicity,* liver damage, veno-occlusive disease.
**Other:** *cancer.*

---

*Bold italic type* indicates that reaction may be life-threatening.

## INTERACTIONS
**Herb-drug.** *Disulfiram:* Herbal products prepared with alcohol may cause a disulfiram-like reaction. Advise patient to avoid using together.

## CAUTIONS
Patients who are pregnant or breast-feeding or are planning pregnancy should avoid use. Patients with a history of alcohol abuse or liver disease should also avoid use.

## NURSING CONSIDERATIONS
• Find out why patient is using the herb.

⚡**ALERT:** Several agencies including United States Pharmacopeia's expert advisory panel and the American Herbal Products Association have identified comfrey preparations as potentially harmful because of reports of liver toxicity. Many countries have banned internal use of comfrey, so such use is highly discouraged.

• Also, some comfrey preparations may contain significant levels of alcohol, so children, alcoholic patients, those with liver disease, and those receiving metronidazole or disulfiram should avoid them.

• Infants may be more susceptible to hepatic veno-occlusive disease.

• Patients who ingest comfrey should be monitored for signs and symptoms of hepatotoxicity, including abdominal distention, nausea, and abdominal pain, and elevated liver function test results.

• If patient is using comfrey to promote wound healing, monitor the wound being treated. Evaluate the possibility of an infectious cause of cellulitis and inflammation.

• Use of comfrey should be limited to 4 to 6 weeks per year, to prevent exposure to large amounts of pyrrolizidine alkaloids.

**Patient teaching**
• Advise patient to consult with his health care provider before using an herbal preparation because a treatment with proven efficacy may be available.

• Tell patient to remind pharmacist of any herbal or dietary supplement that he's taking, when filling a new prescription.

• If patient is pregnant or breast-feeding or is planning pregnancy, advise her not to use comfrey.

• Advise patient that the internal use of comfrey isn't recommended and should be avoided.

• Inform patient that external preparations shouldn't be applied to broken or abraded skin.

⚡**ALERT:** Advise patient that many comfrey preparations don't indicate the amount of pyrrolizidine alkaloids they contain, making it impossible to determine the dose of toxic alkaloids being ingested. Also, products labeled as comfrey may contain prickly comfrey, reported to provide the most toxic pyrrolizidine compounds.

• Advise patient that if he experiences any adverse reactions (such as visual disturbances, tachycardia or bradycardia, dry skin and mouth), he should discontinue the product and consult his health care provider.

• Warn patient to obtain herbal products from reputable sources to help ensure the product isn't contaminated.
• Warn patient to keep all herbal products away from children.
• Inform patient that internal use of this product is highly discouraged.

## condurango

*Marsdenia condurango,* condurango bark, condurango blanco, condurango cortex, eagle vine

**Common trade names**
*Condurango can be found in many homeopathic preparations*

**HOW SUPPLIED**
Available as liquid extract*.

**ACTIONS & COMPONENTS**
Medicinal components of this plant are found in the bark of the branches and trunk of *M. condurango.* Includes numerous glycosides, including condurangin, which stimulates saliva and gastric juice secretion.

**USES**
Used to stimulate appetite, alleviate dyspepsia, promote diuresis, and treat stomach cancer. Also used to increase peripheral circulation.

Commonly used in South America as an alternative treatment for chronic syphilis.

**DOSAGE & ADMINISTRATION**
*Aqueous extract:* 0.2 to 0.5 g q.d.

*Bark:* 2 to 4 g q.d.
*Liqueur, tea:* Prepared by steeping 50 to 100 g of bark in 1 qt of wine for several days. A cup of the liqueur or tea can be taken 30 minutes before each meal.
*Liquid extract, tincture:* 2 to 5 g p.r.n. for alcohol content.

**ADVERSE REACTIONS**
**CNS:** vertigo, paralysis.
**EENT:** visual changes.
**Other:** *anaphylactic reaction.*

**INTERACTIONS**
**Herb-drug.** *Disulfiram, metronidazole:* Herbal products prepared with alcohol may cause a disulfiram-like reaction. Advise patient to avoid using together.

**CAUTIONS**
Pregnant and breast-feeding patients should avoid using condurango because it has an alkaloid component that resembles strychnine. Children and geriatric patients should also avoid use.

Those with severe allergy to natural rubber latex should use cautiously because of the potential for cross-sensitivity.

**NURSING CONSIDERATIONS**
• Find out why patient is using the herb.
🖉 ALERT: If patient has a severe allergy to natural rubber latex, monitor him for signs and symptoms of cutaneous reactions or respiratory compromise, such as shortness of breath, hypotension, or tachycardia.
• If patient is taking condurango to alleviate dyspepsia, find out how

---

*Bold italic type* indicates that reaction may be life-threatening.

serious his condition is and whether he has tried other therapies to treat it.

• If patient is taking condurango to stimulate his appetite, evaluate possible causes of his condition and whether patient has also experienced significant weight loss, because this may indicate a more serious condition.

• Patients who also report melena or hematemesis should be referred for further workup.

• Overdose may produce seizures, resulting in paralysis, vertigo, and visual changes. Monitor patient closely for these.

**Patient teaching**

• Advise patient to consult with his health care provider before using an herbal preparation because a treatment with proven efficacy may be available.

• Tell patient to remind pharmacist of any herbal or dietary supplement that he's taking, when filling a new prescription.

• If patient has a latex allergy or is pregnant or breast-feeding, advise her not to take condurango.

• If patient has a history of alcohol abuse or liver disease or is taking disulfiram or metronidazole, advise him to avoid taking preparations that contain alcohol.

• Inform patient that dosing varies according to the preparation used.

• Warn patient to avoid using condurango with other drugs because information regarding interactions with them are lacking.

• Advise patient to report continued weight loss, GI bleeding, or

worsening dyspepsia to his health care provider.

• Teach patient the signs and symptoms of overdose, such as visual disturbances, seizures, and dizziness; tell him to seek medical attention immediately if these occur.

## coriander

*Coriandrum sativum,* Chinese parsley, coriander fruit, coriander seed, koriander

**Common trade names**
*None known*

**HOW SUPPLIED**
Available as capsules, pure coriander seed, essential oil, powder, and tea. Also available in natural deodorant products and in curry powder.
*Capsules:* Contain 83.3 mg coriander, along with other vitamins and natural products

**ACTIONS & COMPONENTS**
This medicinal seed is used ripe and dried. It contains 0.5% to 1% essential oil. The volatile oil, which consists primarily of linalool, stimulates gastric acid secretion and has spasmolytic properties. It also provides vitamin C, calcium, magnesium, potassium, and iron.

Coriander may have hypoglycemic, hypolipidemic, and antiseptic effects.

**USES**
Used to enhance appetite and treat dyspepsia, flatulence, diarrhea,

and colic. Also used to treat coughs, chest pains, fever, bladder ailments, halitosis, postpartum complications, colic, measles, dysentery, hemorrhoids, and toothaches.

In aromatherapy, the essential oil is used for its soothing effects and to improve blood circulation.

Coriander is also used as a flavoring agent, culinary spice, and fragrance in bath and beauty products. It can also be used to disguise the unpleasant taste of medicine.

## DOSAGE & ADMINISTRATION
*Dried seed:* 3 g/day.
*Tea:* Prepared by pouring 7 oz of boiling water over 1 to 3 g of crushed coriander seed, steeping for 10 to 15 minutes, and then straining. It's then ingested between meals.
*Tincture:* 10 to 20 gtt q.d. after meals.

## ADVERSE REACTIONS
**Other:** *anaphylactic reaction.*

## INTERACTIONS
**Herb-lifestyle.** *Sun exposure:* Increased risk of photosensitivity reactions. Patient should avoid unprotected exposure to sunlight.

## CAUTIONS
Patients with hypersensitivity to coriander or any of its components, pregnant patients, breastfeeding patients, and children should avoid use.

## NURSING CONSIDERATIONS
● Find out why patient is using the herb.
● Breathing difficulty, airway tightness, and urticaria may occur in patients with severe allergy to coriander. Monitor patient for signs and symptoms of respiratory distress and vital signs closely.
● Some preparations may contain alcohol, so children, geriatric patients, those with a history of alcohol abuse or liver disease, and those taking disulfiram or metronidazole should avoid them.
● Assess patient's use of other therapies to manage GI complaints.
● Evaluate patient for complications such as melena, hematemesis, and significant unintended weight loss.

## Patient teaching
● Advise patient to consult with his health care provider before using an herbal preparation because a treatment with proven efficacy may be available.
● Tell patient to remind pharmacist of any herbal or dietary supplement that he's taking, when filling a new prescription.
● Instruct patient not to take coriander if he is allergic to it or any of its components.
● Advise patient to seek emergency medical help immediately if he experiences adverse reactions, such as shortness of breath, rapid heart rate, or dizziness.
● Advise patient to wear sunscreen and protective clothing and to avoid exposure to direct sunlight.

---

*Bold italic type* indicates that reaction may be life-threatening.

## corkwood

*Duboisia myoporoides,*
corkwood tree, pituri

**Common trade names**
*None known*

### HOW SUPPLIED
Available as extract, leaves, and
twigs.

### ACTIONS & COMPONENTS
Contains alkaloids, including hyoscyamine, hyoscine, scopolamine,
atropine, and butropine. These
components have potent anticholinergic properties and can be
fatal in large doses.

### USES
Used for its stimulant, euphoric,
and hallucinogenic effects. Some
patients chew the leaves and twigs.

In homeopathy, corkwood is
used to treat eye disorders.

Corkwood was used as a substitute for atropine and scopolamine
before commercial sources were
readily available.

### DOSAGE & ADMINISTRATION
Not well documented.

### ADVERSE REACTIONS
**CNS:** drowsiness, euphoria, exci-
tation, hallucinations, other CNS
disturbances.
**CV:** altered heart rate.
**EENT:** blurred vision, dry mu-
cous membranes, paralyzed eye
muscles.
**GI:** constipation.
**GU:** urine retention.
**Respiratory:** tachypnea.

### INTERACTIONS
**Herb-drug.** *Anticholinergics, such
as atropine and tricyclic antidepressants:* Corkwood potentiates
the anticholinergic effects of these
drugs. Counsel patients on the increased risk of blurred vision, dry
mouth, urine retention, disorientation, and drowsiness. Advise patient to discontinue use if he experiences these.
*Antiparkinsonians:* Corkwood may
interfere with the efficacy of these
drugs. Monitor patient, provide
supportive care, and advise him to
stop using corkwood, if needed.
*Beta blockers, digoxin:* Corkwood
can alter heart rate and cardiac
work. Monitor patient closely, and
advise him to avoid using together.

### CAUTIONS
Patients with a history of allergy
to corkwood or any of its components, atropine, or scopolamine
should avoid use. Patients who are
pregnant or breast-feeding and patients with glaucoma, intestinal
disease or obstruction, heart disease, or myasthenia gravis should
avoid use.

### NURSING CONSIDERATIONS
• Find out why patient is using the
herb.
• Corkwood contains scopolamine,
which is fatal in large doses.
• Monitor patient for anticholinergic adverse effects and drug interactions, including rapid heart rate,
decreased salivation, urine retention, psychosis, and constipation.
• Signs and symptoms of overdose
include anticholinergic responses,
such as tachycardia, tachypnea,

constipation, urine retention, dry mouth, and CNS disturbances.
- Coffee or lemon juice is an antidote of homeopathic tinctures.

**Patient teaching**
- Advise patient to consult with his health care provider before using an herbal preparation because a treatment with proven efficacy may be available.
- Tell patient to remind pharmacist of any herbal or dietary supplement that he's taking, when filling a new prescription.
- If patient is pregnant or breast-feeding, advise her not to use corkwood.
- Inform patient that corkwood isn't recommended for medicinal use and can be dangerous or fatal in high doses.

## cornflower

*Centaurea cyanus*, bluebottle, bluebow, blue cap, cyani flos, cyani-flowers, hurtsickle

**Common trade names**
*None known*

**HOW SUPPLIED**
Available as ray flowers, dried ray florets, and tubular florets of the cornflower plant.

**ACTIONS & COMPONENTS**
Several compounds—including anthocyans, flavonoids, and bitter principles—may be responsible for cornflower's activity. The flowers are generally considered to have tonic, stimulant effects and an ability to stimulate menstruation, with effects similar to blessed thistle.

**USES**
Used as a diuretic, an expectorant, a laxative, and as a stimulant for liver and gallbladder function. Used to treat cough, fever, menstrual disorders, vaginal candidiasis, and eczema of the scalp. Also used as an eye wash to treat eye inflammation and conjunctivitis.

**DOSAGE & ADMINISTRATION**
Not well documented.

**ADVERSE REACTIONS**
**Other:** allergic reaction.

**INTERACTIONS**
None reported.

**CAUTIONS**
Those with an allergy to cornflower or any of its components, geriatric patients, pregnant patients, breast-feeding patients, and children should avoid use.

**NURSING CONSIDERATIONS**
- Find out why patient is using the herb.
- This herb shouldn't be used to treat amenorrhea.

**Patient teaching**
- Advise patient to consult with his health care provider before using an herbal preparation because a treatment with proven efficacy may be available.
- Tell patient to remind pharmacist of any herbal or dietary supplement that he's taking, when filling a new prescription.

---

*Bold italic type* indicates that reaction may be life-threatening.

- Warn patient not to treat irregular menstrual periods with cornflower before seeking appropriate medical evaluation because doing so may delay diagnosis of an underlying medical condition.

## couch grass

*Agropyron repens, Elymus repens, Graminis rhizome,* cutch, dog-grass, durfa grass, quack grass, quickgrass, quitch grass, Scotch quelch, triticum, twitch grass, witch grass

**Common trade names**
*Aqua-Rid, Arcocaps, Diuplex*

### HOW SUPPLIED
Available as capsules, liquid extracts, tablets, and teas.
*Capsules:* 380 mg
*Tablets:* 60 mg

### ACTIONS & COMPONENTS
Contains the carbohydrate tricitin, mucilages, sugar alcohols, soluble silicic acid, and volatile oils.

The essential oil has an antimicrobial effect. Couch grass may also have a diuretic effect, probably a result of its sugar content. It increases urine volume and prevents kidney stone formation.

### USES
Used to prevent kidney stones and to treat arthritis, bronchitis, the common cold, constipation, cough, fever, inflammatory diseases of the urinary tract, and premenstrual syndrome. It's also used as a diuretic.

German Commission E has approved couch grass to help treat UTIs.

### DOSAGE & ADMINISTRATION
*Oral use:* 6 to 9 g q.d. Diuplex tablets have a recommended dose of 2 to 3 tablets P.O. q.d. to b.i.d.

### ADVERSE REACTIONS
**Metabolic:** electrolyte depletion.
**Skin:** rash.

### INTERACTIONS
**Herb-drug.** *Disulfiram, metronidazole:* Herbal products prepared with alcohol may cause a disulfiram-like reaction. Advise patient to avoid using together.

### CAUTIONS
Patients with edema from cardiac or renal insufficiency should avoid use. Pregnant and breast-feeding patients should also avoid use.

### NURSING CONSIDERATIONS
- Find out why patient is using the herb.
- Liquid extracts may contain between 12% to 14% alcohol.
- Dietary supplements of couch grass may use the rhizome, roots, and short stems of the plant.
- Patients using couch grass for urinary tract irrigation should drink plenty of fluids.
- Safety and efficacy of couch grass in geriatric patients and children is unknown.

### Patient teaching
- Advise patient to consult with his health care provider before using an herbal preparation because a

---

*Liquid may contain alcohol.

treatment with proven efficacy may be available.
- Tell patient to remind pharmacist of any herbal or dietary supplement that he's taking, when filling a new prescription.
- Warn patient not to delay seeking appropriate medical evaluation because doing so may delay diagnosis of a potentially serious medical condition.
- If patient is pregnant or breast-feeding, advise her to avoid the use of couch grass.
- Advise parent that use of couch grass in children hasn't been studied, the herb shouldn't be given to them.
- If patient has a history of alcohol abuse or liver disease or takes metronidazole or disulfiram, advise him to avoid using alcohol preparations of couch grass.
- If patient is using couch grass to irrigate the urinary tract, advise him to drink plenty of fluids.

## cowslip

*Primula veris, P. officinalis,* arthritica, buckles, butter rose, crewel, fairy caps, herb Peterpaigle, key flower, key of heaven, mayflower, our lady's keys, palsywort, password, peagles, peggle, petty mulleins, plumrocks

**Common trade names**
*None known*

### HOW SUPPLIED
Available as flowers and roots of the plant, liquid extract*, and tea.

### ACTIONS & COMPONENTS
Contains flavonoids, saponin glycosides, and volatile oil, which may be responsible for its ability to inhibit or dry secretions.

### USES
Used to treat asthma, cardiac insufficiency, dizziness, gout, headache, nervous diseases, neuralgia, tremors, and whooping cough and to inhibit or dry secretions. Used as an antispasmodic, diuretic, expectorant, hypnotic, and sedative.

### DOSAGE & ADMINISTRATION
Dosage varies with herb form.

### ADVERSE REACTIONS
**CV:** *heart dysfunction.*
**GI:** nausea, vomiting, diarrhea, irritation of the digestive tract.
**Hematologic:** destruction of RBCs.
**Hepatic:** liver damage.
**Other:** allergic reaction.

### INTERACTIONS
**Herb-drug.** *Antihypertensives:* Cowslip may potentiate the effects of antihypertensives. Advise patient to avoid using together.
*Diuretics:* Cowslip may potentiate electrolyte depletion. Monitor serum electrolyte levels closely, especially potassium levels.
*Sedatives:* Cowslip may potentiate the effects of sedatives. Advise patients to avoid using together.

### CAUTIONS
Patients with an allergy to cowslip or any other member of the primrose family—such as primrose,

*Anagallis arvensis,* yellow loose-strife, moneywort, water violet, and cyclamen—should avoid use. Pregnant and breast-feeding patients should also avoid use.

## NURSING CONSIDERATIONS
• Find out why patient is using the herb.
• Internal use isn't recommended because of the toxic effects of cowslip.
• If patient is also taking a diuretic, monitor serum electrolyte levels.
• If patient is using cowslip externally, monitor for irritation to the skin and mucous membranes.
• If overdose occurs, perform gastric lavage, and then administer activated charcoal. Provide symptomatic and supportive measures.

**Patient teaching**
• Advise patient to consult with his health care provider before using an herbal preparation because a treatment with proven efficacy may be available.
• Tell patient to remind pharmacist of any herbal or dietary supplement that he's taking, when filling a new prescription.
• Warn patient not to delay seeking appropriate medical evaluation because doing so may delay diagnosis of a potentially serious medical condition.
• If patient is pregnant or breast-feeding or is taking a blood pressure drug or a diuretic, advise her not to use cowslip.
• Instruct patient to promptly report adverse reactions and new signs or symptoms.

## cranberry

bog cranberry, marsh apple, mountain cranberry

**Common trade names**
*Cran-Actin, Cranberry-Plus, Emergen-C Cranberry, Ultra Cranberry*

## HOW SUPPLIED
Available as capsules and tablets of concentrated extract, concentrated liquids*, syrups, tinctures*, juices, and sweetened juices.
*Capsules:* 300- to 1,000-mg

## ACTIONS & COMPONENTS
Obtained from the juice of the ripe cranberry fruit. Contains substances called proanthocyanidins that appear to prevent *Escherichia coli,* a common pathogen in UTIs, from adhering to the epithelial cells lining the bladder wall.

## USES
Used to prevent UTIs, particularly in women prone to recurrent infection. Also used to prevent kidney stones and to treat asthma, fever, and active UTI.

## DOSAGE & ADMINISTRATION
*Capsules, tablets:* 300 to 500 mg P.O. b.i.d. to t.i.d.
*Cranberry juice, unsweetened:* 8 to 16 oz/day.
*Cranberry tincture:* 3 to 5 ml t.i.d.

## ADVERSE REACTIONS
**GI:** diarrhea, irritation.

## INTERACTIONS
**Herb-drug.** *Alkaline drugs such as sodium bicarbonate and methotrexate:* Cranberry acidifies the urine and may increase the rate of excretion of these drugs. Monitor patient for lack of therapeutic effect.

## CAUTIONS
None reported.

## NURSING CONSIDERATIONS
• Find out why patient is using the herb.
• Tinctures may contain up to 45% alcohol.
• Contrary to early investigations focusing on cranberry's ability to acidify the urine, its ability to prevent bacteria from adhering to the bladder wall seems to be more important in preventing UTIs.
• Only the unsweetened, unprocessed form of cranberry juice is effective in preventing bacteria from adhering to the bladder wall.
• Cranberry is safe for use in pregnant and breast-feeding patients.
• When consumed regularly, cranberry may be effective in reducing the frequency of bacteriuria with pyuria in women with recurrent UTIs.

**Patient teaching**
• Advise patient to consult with his health care provider before using an herbal preparation because a treatment with proven efficacy may be available.
• Tell patient to remind pharmacist of any herbal or dietary supplement that he's taking, when filling a new prescription.

• Advise patient that an appropriate antibiotic is usually needed to treat an active UTI.
• If patient is using cranberry to prevent a UTI, advise him to notify his health care provider if signs or symptoms of a UTI appear.
• If patient has diabetes, inform him that cranberry juice contains sugar but that sugar-free cranberry supplements and juices are available.

## creatine monohydrate

creatine

**Common trade names**
*Available from many manufacturers in numerous combination products*

## HOW SUPPLIED
Available as pills, liquid, and powder.

## ACTIONS & COMPONENTS
Naturally occurring substance. Can be obtained in red meat and other dietary sources.

Creatine may also have an anti-inflammatory effect and may reduce levels of triglycerides in the blood.

## USES
Used as a dietary supplement to increase strength and endurance, produce energy, enhance muscle size, improve stamina, and promote faster muscle recovery.

## DOSAGE & ADMINISTRATION
*Adults:* 20 g P.O. q.d. for 3 days, then 5 g P.O. q.d. for the next 8 weeks followed by 4 weeks with

---

no supplementation. Cycle is then repeated.

*Powder:* Mixed with 4 to 8 oz of orange or grape juice, up to q.i.d.

## ADVERSE REACTIONS
**GI:** abdominal pain, bloating, diarrhea.

**Metabolic:** dehydration, electrolyte imbalances, increased body weight.

**Musculoskeletal:** muscle cramps.

**Renal:** altered renal function.

## INTERACTIONS
**Herb-drug.** *Cimetidine, probenecid, trimethoprim:* May inhibit the tubular secretion of creatine, causing an increase in serum creatinine levels. Monitor serum creatinine levels closely.

*Glucose:* May increase creatine storage in muscle. Advise patient to avoid using together.

*NSAIDs:* May adversely affect renal function. Advise patient to use cautiously.

**Herb-food.** *Caffeine:* May reduce creatine's effects. Advise patient to avoid intake of caffeine-containing products.

## CAUTIONS
Those with a history of renal disease and pregnant and breast-feeding patients should avoid use.

## NURSING CONSIDERATIONS
- Find out why patient is using creatine monohydrate.
- If muscle cramping occurs, patient should stop taking creatine and contact health care provider. A smaller dose may be needed.
- Monitor serum electrolyte levels and renal function, as needed.
- Monitor youths involved in sports for overuse or abuse of creatine.

## Patient teaching
- Advise patient to consult with his health care provider before using an herbal preparation or dietary supplement because a treatment with proven efficacy may be available.
- Tell patient to remind pharmacist of any herbal or dietary supplement that he's taking, when filling a new prescription.
- If patient is a young athlete, discuss creatine's use and adverse effects with both the parents and the patient. Advise parents to monitor young athlete's use of creatine and to promptly report adverse effects to the health care provider.
- If patient is taking cimetidine, probenecid, or an NSAID, advise him to consult his health care provider before taking creatine.
- Advise patient to drink plenty of fluids while taking creatine.
- Advise patient to watch for adverse reactions, especially muscle cramps, and to promptly report such reactions to his health care provider.
- Caution patient that this product is useful only for intense exercise and short duration or when short bursts of strength are needed.

*Liquid may contain alcohol.

## cucumber

*Cucumis sativus,* cowcumber, wild cucumber

**Common trade names**
*Cucumber Cleansing Bar, Sea Cucumber Vegi*

### HOW SUPPLIED
Available as emollient ointments and lotions.

### ACTIONS & COMPONENTS
Cucurbitin and fatty oil, contained in the cucumber seeds, may have mild diuretic properties when ingested and a soothing effect when used topically.

Cucumber flower may be an effective diuretic and may be effective in treating pulmonary diseases and diseases of the GI and GU systems. Cucumbers are high in potassium.

### USES
Used to treat high and low blood pressure, to cool and soothe irritated skin in patients with sunburn, and to provide fragrance in perfumes. Also used as a cooling and beautifying agent.

### DOSAGE & ADMINISTRATION
*Lotion, cream:* Apply topically to affected areas, as needed.

### ADVERSE REACTIONS
**Metabolic:** fluid loss, electrolyte imbalances.

### INTERACTIONS
**Herb-drug.** *Diuretics:* Excessive use of cucumber may potentiate the diuretic effect, leading to fluid and electrolyte disturbances. Advise patient to avoid using together.

### CAUTIONS
Pregnant and breast-feeding patients should avoid medicinal use of cucumber.

### NURSING CONSIDERATIONS
• Find out why patient is using the herb.
• Monitor patient for serum electrolyte imbalances.
• Monitor fluid intake and output.

**Patient teaching**
• Advise patient to consult with his health care provider before using an herbal preparation because a treatment with proven efficacy may be available.
• Tell patient to remind pharmacist of any herbal or dietary supplement that he's taking, when filling a new prescription.
• Warn patient not to treat swelling or edema with cucumber before seeking appropriate medical evaluation because doing so may delay diagnosis of a potentially serious medical condition.
• If patient is pregnant or breast-feeding, advise her not to use cucumber medicinally.
• Advise patient to promptly report adverse reactions to his health care provider.

# D

## daffodil

*Narcissus pseudonarcissus*,
asphodel, daffy-down-dilly, fleur
de coucou, goose leek, Lent lily

**Common trade names**
*None known*

### HOW SUPPLIED
Available as powder and extract.

### ACTIONS & COMPONENTS
Contains alkaloids such as lycorine and galanthamine.

In small doses, lycorine may
cause salivation, vomiting, and
diarrhea; in high doses, paralysis
and collapse. Galanthamine is an
anticholinesterase that also exhibits analgesic activity.

In resting bulbs, daffodil exhibits pilocarpine-like activity; in
flowering bulbs, atropine-like activity.

### USES
Used as a topical astringent for
treating various wounds, burns,
stiff joints, and strained muscles.

### DOSAGE & ADMINISTRATION
*Extract:* 2 to 3 grains.
*Powder:* 20 grains to 2 drams.

### ADVERSE REACTIONS
**CNS:** CNS disorders, paralysis,
fainting episodes.
**CV:** *CV collapse.*
**EENT:** irritation and swelling of
the mouth, tongue and throat,
miosis.

**GI:** vomiting, salivation, diarrhea.
**Respiratory:** *respiratory collapse.*
**Skin:** dermatitis.
**Other:** chills, shivering.

### INTERACTIONS
None known.

### CAUTIONS
🖉 ALERT: Patient shouldn't ingest any part of this herb orally
because the flowers and bulbs are
poisonous and can lead to rapid
death.

### NURSING CONSIDERATIONS
● Find out why patient is using the
herb.
● If daffodil bulbs are mistaken for
onions, accidental poisoning could
result.
● Daffodils may affect the CNS,
causing paralysis and possibly
death.

### Patient teaching
● Advise patient to consult with his
health care provider before using
an herbal preparation because a
treatment with proven efficacy
may be available.
● Tell patient to remind pharmacist
of any herbal or dietary supplement that he's taking, when filling
a new prescription.
● Instruct patient not to ingest any
part of a daffodil, explaining to
him daffodil's potentially adverse
effects.
● Instruct patient to seek immediate emergency medical help if

CNS symptoms, such as numbness of extremities or paralysis, occur.
● Warn patient to keep all herbal products away from children and pets.

## daisy

Bairnwort, bruisewort, common daisy, Day's eye, field daisy, moon daisy

**Common trade names**
*None known*

### HOW SUPPLIED
Available as dried herb, fresh herb, and oil.

### ACTIONS & COMPONENTS
Medicinal part is derived from the dried flowering herb. May have anti-inflammatory and astringent properties.

### USES
Used to treat migraine, neuralgia, rheumatism, GI complaints such as bloating and anorexia, and liver inflammation. Used to curb fevers.

The oil is used internally for rheumatic complaints, joint pain, and dysmenorrhea; externally, for gout, bruises, sprains, and wounds.

Daisy has been used as an ointment or salve, applied directly to the inflammation site.

### DOSAGE & ADMINISTRATION
*Infusion:* 1 tsp of dried herb steeped in boiling water for 10 minutes and taken t.i.d.
*Tincture:* 2 to 4 ml t.i.d.

### ADVERSE REACTIONS
None reported.

### INTERACTIONS
None known.

### CAUTIONS
⚠ALERT: Components of the volatile oil can vary with the variety of daisy from which the oil is derived. Those that have a high thujone content are particularly toxic. Internal use should be avoided.

Pregnant and breast-feeding patients should avoid use.

### NURSING CONSIDERATIONS
● Find out why patient is using the herb.
● Monitor patient for adverse reactions and new signs and symptoms.
● Monitor inflammation site for improvement, change, or worsening of inflammation.

### Patient teaching
● Advise patient to consult with his health care provider before using an herbal preparation because a treatment with proven efficacy may be available.
● Tell patient to remind pharmacist of any herbal or dietary supplement that he's taking, when filling a new prescription.
● Advise patient that daisy has a bitter, pungent taste.
● Instruct patient to promptly report adverse reactions and new signs and symptoms to his health care provider.

---

*Bold italic type* indicates that reaction may be life-threatening.

●Discuss with patient other proven medical treatments for his condition.

## damiana

*Turnera diffusa,* damiana herb, damiana leaf, herba de la pastora, Mexican damiana, old woman's broom

**Common trade names**
*Damiana, Damiana Root*

### HOW SUPPLIED
Available as capsules, powder, tea, and tincture.

### ACTIONS & COMPONENTS
The leaf and the stem of the damiana plant are the most commonly used components. Ethanolic extracts have CNS depressant activity, and the quinone arbutin may be responsible for antibacterial activities.

### USES
Used mainly for its aphrodisiac effects, for prophylaxis, and for treating sexual disturbances. Damiana is used to control bedwetting, depression, constipation, and nervous dyspepsia; to strengthen and stimulate during exertion; and to boost and maintain mental and physical capacity. It's also boiled in water, and the steam is inhaled to relieve headaches. There have been some reports of recreational use, with euphoric and hallucinogenic effects.

### DOSAGE & ADMINISTRATION
*Extract:* 2 to 4 ml.

*Oral:* 2 to 4 g (capsules) P.O. of dried leaf t.i.d. or 1 cup of tea (2 to 4 g) in 5 oz boiling water, P.O. t.i.d.

### ADVERSE REACTIONS
**CNS:** insomnia, headache, hallucinations.
**GU:** urethral mucous membrane irritation.
**Hepatic:** liver injury.

### INTERACTIONS
**Herb-drug.** *Antidiabetics:* Damiana may interfere with the action of antidiabetics. Monitor blood glucose level closely.

### CAUTIONS
Pregnant and breast-feeding patients should not use this herb because the effects on them are unknown.

### NURSING CONSIDERATIONS
●Find out why patient is using the herb.
●When more than 7 oz of extract is consumed, patient may display tetanus-like convulsions, and paroxysms.
●Diabetic patient should discuss the use of damiana with his health care provider before taking it with his antidiabetic.
●Monitor blood glucose level closely in diabetic patient taking both damiana and an antidiabetic.
●Monitor liver function test results, as needed.
●If patient claims to have had damiana-induced hallucinations, evaluate him for drug use.

*Liquid may contain alcohol.

## Patient teaching

- Advise patient to consult with his health care provider before using an herbal preparation because a treatment with proven efficacy may be available.
- Tell patient to remind pharmacist of any herbal or dietary supplement that he's taking, when filling a new prescription.
- Advise pregnant and breast-feeding patients and patients of childbearing age to avoid using this herb because of a lack of sufficient information about its safety.
- Advise patient to avoid performing activities that require mental alertness until the herb's CNS effects on him are known.
- Tell diabetic patient that damiana may interact with his antidiabetic drug.
- Advise diabetic patient to check blood glucose level regularly and to report changes.
- Tell patient to promptly report adverse reactions or new signs and symptoms to his health care provider.

## dandelion

*Taraxacum officinale,* blowball, cankerwort, dandelion herb, dandelion root with herb, lion's tooth, priest's crown, swine snout, wild endive

**Common trade names**
*Dandelion Leaf, Dandelion Leaf Tea, Dandelion Root Capsules, Dandelion Root Extract*

## HOW SUPPLIED
Available as fresh greens, capsules, extract, tablets, tea, and tincture.

## ACTIONS & COMPONENTS
Contains sesquiterpenes, triterpenes, fatty acids, flavonoids, minerals (297 mg of potassium, 7.6 mEq/100 mg of leaves), phenolic acids, phytosterols, sugars, vitamins (up to 14,000 IU of vitamin A/100 g of leaves), inulin, and taxarin, which makes it bitter. The leaves also contain the coumarins cichorin and aesculin.

Dandelion has a diuretic effect, probably from the sesquiterpenes and the high potassium content. It may help prevent and treat kidney stones because of its disinfectant and solvent actions on urinary calculi.

The enzyme taraxalisin is present in dandelion roots. The inulin component, with its hypoglycemic effects, may affect the blood glucose level.

Dandelion may have some immune-modulating effects. It may also stimulate nitric oxide production, which is involved with immune regulation and defense, and may induce tumor-necrosis-factor-alpha secretion in peritoneal cells.

## USES
Used in salads and wines. The dried roots are used as a coffee substitute. Traditionally used to treat liver, gallbladder, and spleen ailments.

In Germany, the herb with the root is used as an appetite stimulant, diuretic, bile stimulator, and treatment for dyspepsia. The herb without the root is used for loss of appetite and dyspepsia involving flatulence and feelings of fullness. Also used as a mild laxative and antidiabetic.

## DOSAGE & ADMINISTRATION
**Herb.** *Fluidextract (1 g/ml of 25% ethanol):* 4 to 10 ml P.O. t.i.d.
*Fresh herb:* 4 to 10 g cut herb P.O t.i.d.
*Infusion:* 4 to 10 g in 5 to 9 oz water P.O. t.i.d.
*Succus:* 5 to 10 ml pressed sap from fresh plant P.O. b.i.d.
*Tincture (1 g/5 ml of 25% ethanol):* 2 to 5 ml P.O. t.i.d.
**Herb with root.** *Fluidextract (1 g/ml of 25% ethanol):* 3 to 4 ml P.O. t.i.d.
*Infusion:* 1 tbs cut roots and herb in 5 oz water.
*Tincture (1 g/5 ml of 25% ethanol):* 10 to 15 gtt P.O. t.i.d.

## ADVERSE REACTIONS
**GI:** GI discomfort, GI or biliary tract blockage, gallbladder inflammation, gallstones.
**Skin:** contact dermatitis.
**Other:** allergic reaction.

## INTERACTIONS
**Herb-drug.** *Anticoagulants; antiplatelet drugs, including aspirin, clopidrogrel, heparin, ticlopidine, warfarin; and NSAIDs:* Increased risk in bleeding. Advise patient to use with caution.
*Antidiabetics:* Possible potentiated effects, leading to hypoglycemia. Advise patient to avoid using together.

*Antihypertensives:* Additive effects are possible. Advise patient to avoid using together.
*Ciprofloxacin:* Decreased blood ciprofloxacin levels. Advise patient to avoid using together.
*Fluoroquinolone antibiotics:* Dandelions are rich in minerals, such as magnesium, which are known binders of these drugs. Advise patient to avoid using together.

## CAUTIONS
Those allergic to the herb, those with photosensitive dermatitis and allergies to other Compositae plants, and those with bile obstruction, empyema, or ileus should avoid use.

## NURSING CONSIDERATIONS
• Find out why patient is using the herb.
• All parts of the dandelion plant are edible. The stems, leaves, and flowers can be harvested alone, or the whole plant including the roots can be used.
• Tinctures may contain between 15% and 60% alcohol and may be unsuitable for children, alcoholic patients, those with liver disease, and those taking metronidazole or disulfiram.
• Sesquiterpine lactones are thought to be the allergenic components, but not all people with dandelion dermatitis react to sesquiterpine patch testing.
• Three reports of allergic reactions to ingested bee pollen that contained dandelion pollen have been reported. All three patients were sensitive to the pollens of dande-

---

*Liquid may contain alcohol.

lions and other plants in the Compositae family.
● The bitter substances contained in the leaves may cause gastric discomfort.
● If patient is also taking an antidiabetic, monitor blood glucose level closely.

**Patient teaching**
● Advise patient to consult with his health care provider before using an herbal preparation because a treatment with proven efficacy may be available.
● Tell patient to remind pharmacist of any herbal or dietary supplement that he's taking, when filling a new prescription.
● Warn patient against harvesting dandelions from grounds that may have been treated with weed killer or fertilizer.
● Warn patient not to substitute dandelion therapy for a prescribed diuretic.
● If patient is taking a fluoroquinolone antibiotic, advise him not to use dandelions because of a possible decrease in blood antibiotic level.
● If patient is taking an antidiabetic, advise him to monitor his blood glucose level closely and to report alterations to his health care provider.
● Advise patient to immediately report any rashes or signs of bleeding to his health care provider.
● Instruct patient to contact his health care provider if symptoms don't resolve or if new symptoms develop.

## dehydroepiandrosterone (DHEA)

**DHEA-S** (sulfate conjugate of DHEA)

**Common trade names**
*DHEA Fuel, DHEA Power Combination products: Andro-Stack 850, EAS Andro-6, Twinlab Growth Fuel, Twinlab 7-Ketofuel, Twinlab Tribulus Fuel Stack*

**HOW SUPPLIED**
Available as tablets, capsules, sustained-release tablets, micronized tablets, chewing gum, liquid, S.L. drops, herbal tea, and cream.

**ACTIONS & COMPONENTS**
DHEA is a precursor of both estrogen and testosterone; it's secreted mainly by the adrenal glands. Both DHEA and its sulfate conjugate DHEA-S are converted in the periphery to androgens. Related compounds include androstenedione, a metabolite of DHEA, and pregnenolone, a precursor to DHEA. Circulating levels of DHEA increase during childhood into early adulthood. These levels drop with age; by age 60, levels are only 5% to 15% of what they are at age 20. Those with autoimmune and CV disease also have lower DHEA levels.
  Responses to DHEA appear to be gender specific. In women, supplementation increases both serum DHEA and testosterone levels; in men, it may have no effect on serum testosterone or estrogen levels.

---

*Bold italic type* indicates that reaction may be life-threatening.

DHEA may be useful as treatment for depression and as an anti-aging supplement to restore neuroendocrine function, thus improving mood and increasing feelings of well-being.

It may also be useful in treating systemic lupus erythematosus (SLE) and adrenal insufficiency.

## USES
Used to treat osteoporosis, depression, Alzheimer's dementia, Tourette syndrome, chronic fatigue syndrome, AIDS, migraines, erectile dysfunction, seizure disorders, and cancer. Also used to increase feelings of well-being, slow or reverse the aging process, increase sex drive, increase lean body mass, and decrease fat mass.

## DOSAGE & ADMINISTRATION
*Oral use:* 25 to 200 mg P.O. q.d.
*Creams (10%):* 3 to 5 g applied topically to skin q.d.

## ADVERSE REACTIONS
**CNS:** severe manic episode.
**CV:** *cardiac arrhythmias.*
**Skin:** acne.
**Other:** androgenic or masculinizing effects, including hirsutism, in women; estrogenic effects, including gynecomastia, in men; male-pattern baldness.

## INTERACTIONS
None known.

## CAUTIONS
Those with cancers that are stimulated by estrogen or testosterone such as breast or prostate cancer and those at risk for heart disease should avoid taking DHEA. Pregnant patients should also avoid use because DHEA may have androgenic effects on female fetuses, may induce spontaneous abortion, or may inhibit fetal development.

## NURSING CONSIDERATIONS
- Find out why patient is using DHEA.
- DHEA isn't a natural supplement. It's a hormone, synthetically manufactured from soybeans or wild yams. Contrary to advertising claims, wild yams don't contain DHEA. They contain diosgenin, a precursor of DHEA, which may not be converted to DHEA in the body.
- DHEA isn't intended for any patient younger than age 40 unless circulating levels of DHEA are less than 130 mg/dl if patient is a woman, or less than 180 mg/dl if patient is a man.
- DHEA has orphan drug status for the treatment of corticosteroid-dependent SLE and for the treatment of severe burns in those who require skin grafting.
- The typical dosage range is 50 to 200 ml daily, depending on the intended use and the person's response.
- DHEA may increase levels of insulin-like growth factor, which may represent a risk for those with prostate cancer.
- Monitor patient for adverse hormonal effects.
- Long-term safety of DHEA supplementation is unknown.

**Patient teaching**

• Advise patient to consult with his health care provider before using an herbal preparation because a treatment with proven efficacy may be available.

• Tell patient to remind pharmacist of any herbal or dietary supplement that he's taking, when filling a new prescription.

• Discuss with patient his reasons for taking DHEA.

• Advise female patient to inform her health care provider if she becomes pregnant or plans to do so in the near future.

• Instruct female patient to report any weight gain, hair loss, growth of facial hair, or other masculinizing effects to her health care provider.

• Instruct male patient to report signs of breast growth and development.

## devil's claw

*Harpagophytum procumbens,* grapple plant, wood spider

**Common trade names**
*Devil's Claw, Devil's Claw Root, Devil's Claw Tincture, Devil's Claw Tuber Powder*

**HOW SUPPLIED**
Available as capsules, fresh herb, and tincture.

**ACTIONS & COMPONENTS**
The iridoid glycosides harpagoside, harpagide, and procumbide—the chemically active components in devil's claw—and various other glycosides are found in the prima-

ry roots and the secondary roots, called tubers. The secondary roots contain more of the active ingredients than the primary roots. Trace amounts of these glycosides are also found in the leaves.

Devil's claw may have anti-inflammatory, analgesic, hypotensive, and bradycardic effects and may interfere with calcium influx into smooth-muscle cells. However, stomach acid may inactivate the iridoid glycosides, thus decreasing the herb's effectiveness.

**USES**
Used for its anti-inflammatory and analgesic effects. Also used to treat allergies, atherosclerosis, GI disturbances and heartburn, menstrual difficulties, menopausal symptoms, nicotine poisoning, neuralgia, and liver, kidney, and bladder diseases.

In Germany, devil's claw is approved for use as an appetite stimulant and digestive aid.

**DOSAGE & ADMINISTRATION**
**Loss of appetite.** *Decoction:* 0.5 g in 150 ml water P.O. t.i.d.
*Fluidextract (1 g/ml):* 0.5 ml taken P.O. t.i.d.
*Fresh cut tuber:* 1.5 g P.O. q.d.
**Other conditions.** *Decoction:* 1.5 g in 150 ml water P.O. t.i.d.
*Dried tuber/root:* 6 g P.O. q.d.
*Fluidextract (1 g/ml):* 1.5 ml P.O. t.i.d.
*Infusion:* Prepared by steeping 4.5 g of herb in 10 oz boiling water for 8 hours. Dosage is 3 portions P.O. q.d.
*Standardized extracts:* 600 to 800 mg P.O. t.i.d.; standardized to 2%

---

to 3% iridoid glycosides or 1% to 2% harpagoside.

## ADVERSE REACTIONS
**CNS:** headache.
**EENT:** tinnitus.
**GI:** anorexia.
**Other:** allergic reaction.

## INTERACTIONS
**Herb-drug.** *Disulfiram:* Herbal products prepared with alcohol may cause a disulfiram-like reaction. Advise patient to avoid using together.

## CAUTIONS
Patients with gastric or duodenal ulcers should avoid use because devil's claw increases production of stomach acid.

Patients taking a beta blocker, calcium channel blocker, antihypertensive, or antiarrhythmic should use cautiously because herb may have hypotensive, bradycardic, and antiarrhythmic effects. Patients with heart failure should use cautiously because herb may have negative inotropic effects at high doses.

## NURSING CONSIDERATIONS
• Find out why patient is using the herb.
• Devil's claw may increase the intended therapeutic effect of conventional drugs.
• Tinctures may contain between 15% and 60% alcohol and may be unsuitable for children, alcoholic patients, those with liver disease, and those taking metronidazole or disulfiram.

**Patient teaching**
• Advise patient to consult with his health care provider before using an herbal preparation because a treatment with proven efficacy may be available.
• Tell patient to remind pharmacist of any herbal or dietary supplement that he's taking, when filling a new prescription.
• Warn patient to seek appropriate medical evaluation right away to avoid delaying diagnosis of a potentially serious medical condition.
• If patient is taking a heart drug or a blood pressure drug, advise him to promptly report any lightheadedness, dizziness, abnormal heartbeats, or swelling.
• Instruct patient to seek medical attention if symptoms don't resolve.

## dill

*Anethum graveolens*, dill herb, dill seed, dill weed

**Common trade names**
*Dill Seed, Dill Weed*

## HOW SUPPLIED
Available as fresh greens, dried greens, or dried seeds.

## ACTIONS & COMPONENTS
The dried seeds contain an essential oil, carvone, that may have an effect on smooth and skeletal muscle response.

## USES
The upper stem and seeds of the plant are used, either fresh or

dried, as a flavoring agent and a garnish.

Dill is used to prevent and treat diseases affecting the GI and urinary tracts and kidneys as well as to treat sleep disorders and spasms.

Dill seed is used as an antispasmodic and bacteriostatic. Also used to treat dyspepsia.

## DOSAGE & ADMINISTRATION

*Oil of dill:* 0.1 to 0.3 g, or 2 to 6 gtt.

*Tea:* Prepared by steeping 2 tsp of mashed seeds in 1 cup of boiling water for 10 minutes. Dosage is 3 cups P.O. q.d.

*Tincture:* ½ to 1 tsp, up to t.i.d.

## ADVERSE REACTIONS
**Other:** allergies.

## INTERACTIONS

**Herb-drug.** *Disulfiram:* Herbal products prepared with alcohol may cause a disulfiram reaction. Advise patient to avoid using together.

**Herb-lifestyle.** *Sun exposure:* Contact with the juice from the fresh dill plant may cause skin to react badly when exposed to sunlight. Take precautions to avoid this.

## CAUTIONS

Those allergic to dill should avoid use.

## NURSING CONSIDERATIONS

● Find out why patient is using the herb.

● Dill weed is high in sodium. Discourage excessive use in those with conditions that require sodium restriction, such as heart failure or renal failure.

● Tinctures may contain between 15% and 60% alcohol and may be unsuitable for children, alcoholic patients, those with liver disease, and those taking metronidazole or disulfiram.

● Monitor patient's response to therapy, including improvement of symptoms and adverse reactions.

## Patient teaching

● Advise patient to consult with his health care provider before using an herbal preparation because a treatment with proven efficacy may be available.

● Tell patient to remind pharmacist of any herbal or dietary supplement that he's taking, when filling a new prescription.

● Advise any patient with an allergy to dill to avoid use of these products.

● Warn patient to seek appropriate medical evaluation right away, to avoid delaying diagnosis of a potentially serious medical condition.

● Instruct patient to promptly report adverse reactions and new signs or symptoms.

---

*Bold italic type* indicates that reaction may be life-threatening.

## dong quai

*Angelica polymorpha,* Chinese
angelica, dang-gui, tang-kuei

**Common trade names**
*Dong Kwai, Dong Quai Capsules,
Dong Quai Fluidextract, Dong Quai
Root, Women's Ginseng
Combination products: Dong Quai
and Royal Jelly, Menopausal
Formula, Nature's Fingerprint,
PMS Formula, Rejuvex*

### HOW SUPPLIED
Available in capsules and extract.
*Capsules:* 200 mg, 250 mg, 500
mg
*Extract in vegetable glycerin:* 565
mg

### ACTIONS & COMPONENTS
Dong quai dietary supplements are
obtained from the roots of *A. polymorpha.*

Dong quai extracts contain at
least 6 coumarin derivatives—
including bergapten, osthol, oxy-
peucedanin, and psoralen—and
two furocoumadin derivatives,
sen-byak-angelicole and 7-
demethylsuberosin. Coumarin
derivatives have anticoagulant,
vasodilating, and antispasmodic
activity. Also, osthol may have
CNS stimulant activity.

Other components found in the
essential oil include *n*-butyl-
phthalide, cadinene, isosafrole,
and safrole. Safrole may be carcinogenic, so ingestion should be
avoided.

Root extracts may contain various lactones and vitamins A, E,
and $B_{12}$. Dong quai extracts may
have a modulatory effect on endogenous estrogens.

### USES
Used to treat anemia, hepatitis,
hypertension, migraines, neural-
gias, rhinitis, and gynecologic disorders including irregular menstruation, dysmenorrhea, premenstrual syndrome, and menopausal
symptoms.

### DOSAGE & ADMINISTRATION
*Capsules:* 500 mg P.O., or 1 to 2
capsules t.i.d.
*Liquid extract:* 1 to 2 gtt t.i.d.

### ADVERSE REACTIONS
**EENT:** bleeding gums.
**GI:** diarrhea, blood in stool.
**GU:** hematuria.
**Skin:** photodermatitis.
**Other:** bleeding, fever, *cancer.*

### INTERACTIONS
**Herb-drug.** *Warfarin:* Can potentiate anticoagulant effects. Similar
effects possible with other anticoagulants. Avoid using together.
**Herb-lifestyle.** *Sun exposure:* Increased risk of photosensitivity
reactions. Advise patient to wear
protective clothing and sunscreen
and to limit exposure to direct sunlight.

### CAUTIONS
Patients taking an anticoagulant
should avoid use. Because of potential effects on uterine contractions and unknown direct effects
on the developing fetus, pregnant
and breast-feeding patients should
not use dong quai.

---

*Liquid may contain alcohol.

## NURSING CONSIDERATIONS
● Find out why patient is using the herb.
● Monitor patient for signs of easy bruising or bleeding.
● If dong quai must be used with another anticoagulant, closely monitor PT and INR.
● Monitor patient for photosensitivity reactions.

### Patient teaching
● Advise patient to consult with his health care provider before using an herbal preparation because a treatment with proven efficacy may be available.
● Tell patient to remind pharmacist of any herbal or dietary supplement that he's taking, when filling a new prescription.
● If patient is pregnant or breast-feeding, advise her not to use dong quai.
● Instruct patient to avoid taking dong quai with an anticoagulant, unless otherwise instructed by his health care provider.
● Warn patient to keep all herbal products away from children and pets.

# E

## echinacea

*Echinacea angustifolia, E. pallida, E. purpurea*, American coneflower, black sampson, black susans, cockup hat, comb flower, hedgehog, Indian head, Missouri snakeroot, narrow-leaved purple coneflower, purple coneflower, purple Kansas coneflower, red sunflower, rudbeckia, scurvy root, snakeroot

**Common trade names**
*Coneflower Extract, EchinaCare Liquid, Echinacea, Echinacea Angustifolia Herb, Echinacea Extract, Echinacea Fresh Freeze Dried, Echinacea Glycerite, Echinacea Herbal Comfort, Echinacea Red Root Supreme, Echinacea Root Complex, Echinacea Root Extract, Echinacea Xtra, Echina Fresh, Echinagel, EchinaGuard Liquid, EchinaGuard Pro, Echinex, Enhanced Echinacea, Standardized Echinacea Extract*

---

### HOW SUPPLIED
Available as capsules, glycerite, expressed juice*, hydroalcoholic extract, lozenges, tablets, tea, tinctures (1:5, 15% to 90% alcohol)*, and whole dried root.
*Capsules:* 125 mg, 250 mg, 355 mg, and 500 mg
*Hydroalcoholic extracts (50%)**
*Tablets:* 335 mg

### ACTIONS & COMPONENTS
Obtained from the dried rhizomes and roots of *E. angustifolia* and *E. pallida* and the roots or above-ground parts of *E. purpurea*. Extracts of echinacea contain numerous components including alkylamides, caffeic acid derivatives, polysaccharides, essential oils, chicoric acids, flavonoids, and glycoproteins.

Echinacea may enhance immune system function, with the lipophilic fraction in the roots and leaves producing the most effective immunostimulation. When taken internally, echinacea may increase the number of circulating leukocytes, enhance phagocytosis, stimulate cytokine production, and trigger the alternate complement pathway. In vitro, some components are directly bacteriostatic and exhibit antiviral activity. Applied topically, echinacea can exert local anesthetic activity, antimicrobial activity, and anti-inflammatory activity, and it can stimulate fibroblasts

Also, echinacea's effects on cytokines may result in antitumorigenic activity.

### USES
Used to stimulate the immune system and treat acute and chronic upper respiratory tract infections and UTIs. Used also to heal wounds, including abscesses, burns, eczema, and skin ulcers. May be used as an adjunct to a conventional antineoplastic and

---

*Liquid may contain alcohol.

may provide prophylaxis against upper respiratory tract infections and the common cold.

**DOSAGE & ADMINISTRATION**
*Capsules containing powdered* E. pallida *root extract:* Equivalent to 300 mg P.O. t.i.d.
*Expressed juice of* E. purpurea *(2.5:1, 22% alcohol):* 6 to 9 ml P.O. q.d. When used externally, don't use for longer than 8 weeks.
*Hydroalcoholic tincture (15% to 90% alcohol):* 3 to 4 ml P.O. t.i.d.
*Tea*: Prepared by simmering ½ tsp of coarsely powdered herb in 1 cup of boiling water for 10 minutes. For colds, dosage is 1 cup of freshly made tea taken several times q.d.
*Whole dried root:* 1 to 2 g P.O. t.i.d.

**ADVERSE REACTIONS**
**EENT:** unpleasant taste.
**GI:** nausea, vomiting, minor GI symptoms.
**Other:** diuresis, allergic reaction, fever, tachyphylaxis.

**INTERACTIONS**
**Herb-drug.** *Disulfiram, metronidazole:* Herbal products that contain alcohol may precipitate a disulfiram-like reaction. Advise patient to avoid using together.
*Immunosuppressants such as cyclosporine:* Decreased effectiveness of these drugs. Advise patient to avoid using together.
**Herb-lifestyle.** *Alcohol:* Echinacea preparations containing alcohol may enhance CNS depression. Advise patient to avoid using together.

**CAUTIONS**
Patients with HIV infection, including AIDS, and patients with tuberculosis, collagen disease, multiple sclerosis, or other autoimmune disease should avoid use. Pregnant and breast-feeding patients should also avoid use.

**NURSING CONSIDERATIONS**
• Find out why patient is using the herb.
• Daily dose depends on the preparation and potency but shouldn't exceed 8 weeks. Consult specific manufacturer's instructions for parenteral administration, if applicable.
• Echinacea is considered supportive treatment for infection; it shouldn't be used in place of antibiotic therapy.
• Some active components may be water-insoluble.
• Echinacea is usually taken at the first sign of illness and continued for up to 14 days. Regular prophylactic use isn't recommended.
• Herbalists recommend using liquid preparations because it's believed that Echinacea functions in the mouth and should have direct contact with the lymph tissues at the back of the throat.
• Some tinctures contain between 15% and 90% alcohol, which may be unsuitable for children and adolescents, alcoholics, and patients with hepatic disease.

**Patient teaching**
• Advise patient to consult with his health care provider before using an herbal preparation because a

---

*Bold italic type* indicates that reaction may be life-threatening.

treatment with proven efficacy may be available.

• Tell patient to remind pharmacist of any herbal or dietary supplement that he's taking, when filling a new prescription.

• Advise patient not to delay seeking appropriate medical evaluation for a prolonged illness.

• Advise patient that prolonged use may result in overstimulation of the immune system and possible immune suppression. Echinacea shouldn't be used longer than 14 days for supportive treatment of infection.

• The herb should be stored away from direct light.

• Warn patients to keep all herbal products away from children and pets.

## elderberry

*Sambucus canadensis, S. ebulus, S. nigra,* black elder, black-berried alder, blood elder, blood hilder, boor tree, common elder, danewort, dwarf elder, elder, ellanwood, ellhorn, European alder

**Common trade names**
*Elderberry, Elderberry Flowers, Elderberry Powder*

### HOW SUPPLIED
Available as aqueous solution, berries, extract, flowers, oil, and wine*.

### ACTIONS & COMPONENTS
Extracts of the berries and flowers contain an essential oil, which is made up of free fatty acids such as palmitic acid, alkanes, triterpenes, ursolic acid, oleanic acid, betulin, and betulic acid. Other components found in leaves include the cyanogenic glucoside sambunigrin, flavonoids, and caffeic acids. Anthocyanin glucosides, a component of elderberry juice, may exhibit pro-oxidant activity. Elderberry extracts also inhibit the replication of certain strains of the human influenza virus and decrease inflammatory cytokines. The component sambuculin A may exhibit hepatoprotective effects.

### USES
Extracts are used to treat asthma, bronchitis, cough, epilepsy, fever, fungal infections, gout, headache, hepatic dysfunction, neuralgia, rheumatic diseases, and toothache. They're also used as diuretics, insect repellents, and laxatives.

### DOSAGE & ADMINISTRATION
*Infusion:* Prepared by adding 3 to 4 g of elderberry flowers to 5 oz of simmering water. The dose is 1 to 2 cups P.O., given several times q.d.

### ADVERSE REACTIONS
**GI:** diarrhea, nausea, vomiting.
**Other:** *cyanide-like poisoning.*

### INTERACTIONS
None known.

### CAUTIONS
Pregnant and breast-feeding patients should avoid use. All patients should avoid consumption of berries from the dwarf elder (*S. ebulus*) because it can contain an especially

---

*Liquid may contain alcohol.

high content of cyanide-like compounds.

**NURSING CONSIDERATIONS**
• Find out why patient is using the herb.
• Leaves and stems shouldn't be crushed when making elderberry juice because of potential for cyanide toxicity.
• Elderberry may interfere with the intended therapeutic effect of conventional drugs.
• Elderberry (especially *S. ebulus*) can cause cyanide-like poisoning—characterized by diarrhea, vomiting, vertigo, numbness, and stupor—particularly if uncooked portions are consumed. It can also cause toxic reaction in children if they use elderberry stems for peashooters.
• Uncooked elderberries are more likely to cause nausea.
• Monitor patients for nausea and vomiting.

**Patient teaching**
• Advise patient to consult with his health care provider before using an herbal preparation because a treatment with proven efficacy may be available.
• Tell patient to remind pharmacist of any herbal or dietary supplement that he's taking, when filling a new prescription.
• Warn patient not to treat symptoms of asthma, infection, or hepatic disease with elderberry before seeking appropriate medical evaluation because doing so may delay diagnosis of a potentially serious medical condition.

• Inform patient of the toxic potential of certain varieties of elderberry.
• Warn patients to keep all herbal products away from children and pets.

## elecampane

*Inula helenium,* elfdock, elfwort, horse-elder, horseheal, scabwort, velvet dock, wild sunflower

**Common trade names**
*None known*

**HOW SUPPLIED**
Available as fluidextract and in powdered root preparations.

**ACTIONS & COMPONENTS**
Obtained from the dried cut root and rhizomes of *I. helenium.* Extracts generally contain a volatile oil whose chief components are alantolactone; isoalantolactone; 11,13-dihydroisoalantolactone; 11,13-dihydroalanlantolactone; and other sesquiterpenlactones. These compounds may exhibit variable antiseptic, antibacterial, antifungal, diuretic, expectorant, and hypotensive activities.

**USES**
Used to treat diseases of the respiratory tract, such as bronchitis, asthma, and cough; diabetes; hypertension; diseases of the GI tract; and diseases of the kidney and lower urinary tract. Also used to stimulate appetite and bile production, to treat dyspepsia and

---

*Bold italic type* indicates that reaction may be life-threatening.

menstrual complaints, and to promote diuresis.

## DOSAGE & ADMINISTRATION
*Dried root:* 2 to 3 g P.O. t.i.d.
*Fresh root:* 1 to 2 tbs P.O. t.i.d.
*Tea:* Prepared by steeping 1 g of ground herb in boiling water for 10 to 15 minutes, and then straining. (1 tsp is equivalent to 4 g of drug.) Dosage is 1 cup t.i.d. to q.i.d. as an expectorant.

## ADVERSE REACTIONS
**CNS:** signs of paralysis with larger doses.
**EENT:** mucous membrane irritation.
**GI:** nausea, vomiting, diarrhea, and cramps with larger doses.
**Skin:** allergic contact dermatitis.

## INTERACTIONS
None reported.

## CAUTIONS
Those with a history of hypersensitivity or contact dermatitis should avoid use. Pregnant and breast-feeding patients should also avoid use.

## NURSING CONSIDERATIONS
• Find out why patient is using the herb.
• Elecampane may interfere with the intended therapeutic effect of conventional drugs.
• Monitor patient for signs of allergic reaction, especially dermatologic reactions.
• The alantolactone component can irritate mucous membranes.

• If overdose occurs, treat with gastric lavage, intestinal emptying, and activated charcoal.

## Patient teaching
• Advise patient to consult with his health care provider before using an herbal preparation because a treatment with proven efficacy may be available.
• Tell patient to remind pharmacist of any herbal or dietary supplement that he's taking, when filling a new prescription.
• Advise patient that little evidence exists supporting therapeutic use of elecampane and that the herb can cause an allergic reaction.
• Warn patients to keep all herbal products away from children and pets.
• Instruct patient not to store the herb in a plastic container.

## ephedra

*Ephedra sinica, E. shennungiana,* Brigham tea, cao ma huang (Chinese ephedra), desert herb, desert tea, eph-edrine, epitonin, joint fir, ma-huang, mahuuanggen (root), Mexican tea, Mormon tea, muzei mu huang (Mongolian ephedra), popotillo, sea grape, squaw tea, teamster's tea, yellow astringent, yellow horse, zhong ma huang

### Common trade names
*Available as combination products, including Chromemate, Escalation, Excel, Herbal Ecstasy, Herbal Fen-Phen, Herbalife, Metabolife, Power Trim, Up Your Gas*

---

*Liquid may contain alcohol.

## HOW SUPPLIED
Available as crude extracts of root and aerial parts of *E. sinica* and *E. shennungiana*; other forms include *E. nevadensis, E. trifurca, E. equisetina,* and *E. distachya.* Available also as capsules, tablets, teas, and tinctures*.

## ACTIONS & COMPONENTS
The primary active ingredient of ephedra extract is ephedrine, although extracts generally contain between 0.5% and 2.5% of alkaloids of the 2-aminophenylpropane type, including ephedrine, methylephedrine, pseudoephedrine, norephedrine, and norpseudoephedrine.

Similar to the structurally related drug amphetamine, ephedrine acts by directly stimulating the sympathomimetic system and the CNS (alpha and beta agonists), possibly increasing heart rate, myocardial contraction, peripheral vasoconstriction with associated elevations in blood pressure, bronchodilation, and mydriasis. Ephedrine is active when given orally, parenterally, or ophthalmically.

Other components in ephedra extracts include volatile oils, catechins, gallic acid, tannins, flavonoids, inulin, dextrin, starch, and pectin.

## USES
Used to treat respiratory tract diseases with mild bronchospasm. Allopathic practitioners have used it since the 1930s to treat asthma, but the herb has become less popular as more specific beta agonists have become available.

Also used as a CV stimulant. Pseudoephedrine remains a common ingredient in many OTC cough and cold preparations. Ephedrine is used to treat various other conditions, including chills, coughs, colds, flu, fever, headaches, edema, and nasal congestion; it's also used as an appetite suppressant. The alkaloid-free North American species is used to treat venereal disease.

## DOSAGE & ADMINISTRATION
*Extract:* 1 to 3 ml P.O. t.i.d.
*Oral use:* For adults, 15 to 30 mg total alkaloid, calculated as ephedrine, taken every 6 to 8 hours for a total maximum daily dose of 300 mg/day. In children older than age 6, 0.5 mg total alkaloid/kg. The recommended daily dose is 2 mg.
*Tea:* 1 to 4 g P.O. t.i.d.
*Tincture (1:1):* Medium single dose 5 g P.O.
*Tincture (1:4):* 6 to 8 ml P.O. t.i.d.

## ADVERSE REACTIONS
**CNS:** anxiety, confusion, dependency, dizziness, headache, insomnia, irritability, mania, motor restlessness, nervousness, psychosis, *seizure.*
**CV:** *arrhythmias, cardiac arrest,* hypertension, hypotension, *MI,* palpitations, tachycardia.
**GI:** nausea.
**GU:** uterine contractions, urinary disorders.
**Metabolic:** hyperglycemia, hypoglycemia.
**Skin:** dermatitis.

---

*Bold italic type* indicates that reaction may be life-threatening.

## INTERACTIONS
**Herb-drug.** *Beta blockers such as propranolol:* May enhance sympathomimetic effects on vasculature from unopposed alpha-agonist effects, thus increasing risk of hypertensive effects. Advise patient to avoid using together.
*Cardiac glycosides, halothane:* May disturb heart rhythm. Advise patient to avoid using together.
*CNS stimulants such as dextroamphetamine:* May pose risk of additive pharmacodynamic effects. Ad-vise patient to avoid using together.
*Guanethidine:* Increased sympathomimetic effect. Advise patient to avoid using together.
*MAO inhibitors:* May pose risk of hypertensive crisis. Advise patient to avoid using together.
*Oxytocin, secale alkaloid derivatives:* Increased blood pressure. Advise patient to avoid using together.
*Theophylline:* May increase risk of GI and CNS adverse effects. Advise patient to avoid using together.
**Herb-food.** *Caffeine:* Additive sympathomimetic and CNS stimulation. Advise patient to discontinue ephedra or reduce caffeine consumption.
**Herb-herb.** *Yohimbe:* Additive sympathomimetic and CNS stimulation. Advise patient to avoid using together.

## CAUTIONS
Pregnant patients should avoid use because of the risk of inducing uterine contractions and the unknown effects of the herb on the fetus. Those with glaucoma, pheochromocytoma, thyrotoxicosis, underlying CV disease, or a history of cerebrovascular disease should avoid use. Diabetic patients should avoid use because of potential hyperglycemic effects. Those with sleep, mood, anxiety, and psychotic disorders should use cautiously.

## NURSING CONSIDERATIONS
● Find out why patient is using the herb.
● Compounds containing ephedra have been linked to several deaths and more than 800 adverse effects, many of which appear to be dose related.
● Monitor patient's pulse and blood pressure.
● Ephedra shouldn't be used for more than 7 consecutive days because of the risk of tachyphylaxis and dependence.
● Patients with eating disorders may abuse this herb.
▨ALERT: Pills containing ephedra have been combined with other stimulants like caffeine and sold as "natural" stimulants in weight-loss products. Deaths from overstimulation have been reported.
▨ALERT: Dosages high enough to produce psychoactive or hallucinogenic effects are toxic to the heart and shouldn't be used.
● Signs and symptoms of toxic reaction include diaphoresis, dilated pupils, muscle spasms, fever, and cardiac and respiratory failure.
● If overdose occurs, perform gastric lavage and administer activated charcoal. Treat spasms with diazepam, replace electrolytes with

---

I.V. fluids, and prevent acidosis with sodium bicarbonate infusions.

**Patient teaching**
- Advise patient to consult with his health care provider before using an herbal preparation because a treatment with proven efficacy may be available.
- Tell patient to remind pharmacist of any herbal or dietary supplement that he's taking, when filling a new prescription.
- Advise patient not to use this herb in place of getting the proper medical evaluation of a prolonged illness.
- Advise patient with thyroid disease, hypertension, CV disease, or diabetes to avoid using ephedra.
- Recommend standard pharmaceutical formulations of ephedrine or pseudoephedrine for those with a valid need for these compounds because preparations may differ in ephedrine alkaloid content by 130%.
- Advise patient not to use ephedra-containing products for longer than 7 consecutive days.
- Advise patient not to use ephedra at dosages that are purported to produce psychoactive or hallucinogenic effects because such dosages are toxic to the heart.
- Advise patient to watch for adverse reactions, particularly chest pain, shortness of breath, palpitations, dizziness, and fainting.
- Instruct patient to store ephedra away from direct light.
- Warn patients to keep all herbal products away from children and pets.

## eucalyptus

*Eucalypti globulus,* blue gum tree, eucalyptol, fever tree, gum tree, red gum, stringy bark tree

**Common trade names**
*Eucalyptus Oil, Eucalyptus Rub*

**HOW SUPPLIED**
Available as dried herb, eucalyptus leaf, essential oil, and tea bags.

**ACTIONS & COMPONENTS**
The primary component of eucalyptus oil is the volatile substance 1,8-cineol (cineole). Oil preparations are standardized to contain 80% to 90% cineole.

The effectiveness of the herb as an expectorant is attributed to the local irritant action of the volatile oil.

**USES**
Used internally and externally as an expectorant. Used to treat infections and fevers. Also used topically to treat sore muscles and rheumatism.

**DOSAGE & ADMINISTRATION**
*Essential oil:* Use the oil in massage blends for sore, aching muscles, in foot baths or saunas, steam inhalations, chest rubs, room sprays, bath blends, and air diffusions. For external use only.
*Leaf:* Average dose is 4 to 16 g P.O. q.d. divided every 3 to 4 hours.
*Oil:* For internal use, average dose is 0.3 to 0.6 g P.O. q.d. For external use, oil with 5% to 20% con-

---

centration or a semisolid preparation with 5% to 10% concentration.
*Tea:* Prepared using one of two methods. For the infusion method, 6 oz of dried herb is steeped in boiling water for 2 to 3 minutes, and then strained. For the decoction method, 6 to 8 oz of dried herb is placed in boiling water, boiled for 3 to 5 minutes, and then strained.
*Tincture:* 3 to 4 g P.O. q.d.

### ADVERSE REACTIONS
**GI:** nausea, vomiting, diarrhea.
**Respiratory:** asthmalike attacks.

### INTERACTIONS
**Herb-drug.** *Antidiabetics:* Enhanced effects. Patient shouldn't use together unless under the direct supervision of a health care provider.
*Other drugs:* Eucalyptus oil induces detoxication enzyme systems in the liver; therefore, the oil may affect any drug that the liver metabolizes. Monitor patient for effect and toxic reaction.
**Herb-herb.** *Other herbs that cause hypoglycemia (basil, glucomannan, Queen Anne's lace):* Decreased blood glucose level. Monitor patient for effect.

### CAUTIONS
Patients who have had an allergic reaction to eucalyptus or its vapors should avoid use. Those who are pregnant or breast-feeding, have liver disease, or have intestinal tract inflammation should avoid use. Essential oil preparations shouldn't be applied to an infant's or child's face because of risk of severe bronchial spasm.

### NURSING CONSIDERATIONS
• Find out why patient is using the herb.
• Eucalyptus oil, also known as eucalyptol, is steam-distilled from the twigs and long leathery leaves of the eucalyptus tree. Eucalyptus folium contains the dried leaves of older eucalyptus globus trees. The leaves are collected after the tree has been cut down and allowed to dry in the shade.
• Monitor patient for allergic reaction.
• In susceptible patients, particularly infants and children, the application of eucalyptus preparations to the face or the inhalation of vapors can cause asthmalike attacks.
• Monitor blood glucose level in diabetic patient taking eucalyptus.
• Oral administration may cause nausea, vomiting, and diarrhea.
🖉 **ALERT:** The oil shouldn't be taken internally unless it has been diluted. As little as a few drops of oil for children and 4 to 5 ml of oil for adults can cause poisoning. Signs include hypotension, circulatory dysfunction, and cardiac and respiratory failure.
• If poisoning or overdose occurs, don't induce vomiting because of risk of aspiration. Administer activated charcoal and treat symptomatically.

### Patient teaching
• Advise patient to consult with his health care provider before using an herbal preparation because a

---

*Liquid may contain alcohol.

treatment with proven efficacy may be available.

- Tell patient to remind pharmacist of any herbal or dietary supplement that he's taking, when filling a new prescription.
- Advise the patient to stop taking eucalyptus immediately and to check with his health care provider if he has trouble breathing, hives, or skin rash.
- Inform patient of potential adverse effects.
- Instruct caregiver not to apply to the face of a child or infant, especially around the nose.
- Warn patients to keep all herbal products away from children and pets.

## evening primrose oil

*Oenothera biennis*, evening primrose, fever plant, king's cureall, night willow-herb, rock-rose, sand lily, scabish, sun-drop

### Common trade names
*Evening Primrose Oil Capsules, Mega Primrose Oil, Original Primrose for Women, Royal Brittany Evening Primrose Oil*

### HOW SUPPLIED
Available as capsules, liquid, oil, and tablets (evening primrose complex).
*Capsules:* 500 mg, 1,000 mg, and 1,300 mg
*Liquid, oil:* 2 oz, 4 oz

### ACTIONS & COMPONENTS
Contains the amino acid tryptophan and a high concentration of essential fatty acids, in particular *cis*-linoleic acid (CLA) and gamma-linoleic acid (GLA). The variety of evening primrose grown for commercial purposes produces oil with 72% CLA and 9% GLA. These fatty acids are prostaglandin precursors.

Conversion of the prostaglandin precursors into prostaglandins is the basis for using this oil to stimulate cervical ripening, prevent heart disease, and reduce symptoms of rheumatoid arthritis. Its efficacy in other clinical conditions may result from its supply of fatty acids.

### USES
Used by midwives to stimulate cervical ripening during pregnancy at or near term and to ease childbirth. Also used to manage cyclic mastitis, premenstrual syndrome, and neurodermatitis. Used as a dietary stimulant.

In Europe, used to treat eczema and diabetic neuropathy, although recent evidence doesn't support its use for these conditions. Also used to treat hypercholesterolemia, rheumatoid arthritis, inflammatory bowel disease, Raynaud's disease, Sjögren's syndrome, chronic fatigue syndrome, endometriosis, obesity, prostate disease, hyperactivity in children, and asthma.

### DOSAGE & ADMINISTRATION
*Cyclic mastitis:* 3 g P.O. q.d. in two or three divided doses.
*Diabetic neuropathy:* 4 to 6 g P.O. q.d.
*Eczema in children:* 2 to 4 g P.O. q.d.

---

*Bold italic type* indicates that reaction may be life-threatening.

*Oral use:* The usual dose is based on GLA content. Typical dose is 1 to 2 capsules (0.5 to 1 g) t.i.d. *Rheumatoid arthritis:* 5 to 10 g q.d.

**ADVERSE REACTIONS**
**CNS:** headache.
**GI:** nausea, diarrhea, bloating, vomiting, flatulence.
**Other:** allergic reactions.

**INTERACTIONS**
**Herb-drug.** *Drugs that lower the seizure threshold such as pheno-thiazines, tricyclic antidepres-sants,and other epileptogenic drugs:* Increased risk of seizures. Advise patient to avoid using to-gether.

**CAUTIONS**
Those with an allergy to evening primrose oil and pregnant and breast-feeding patients should avoid use. Those with a history of epilepsy and those taking a tri-cyclic antidepressant, phenothia-zine, or another drug that lowers the seizure threshold should avoid use.

**NURSING CONSIDERATIONS**
• Find out why patient is using the herb.
• Monitor patient for allergic reaction.
• The fatty oil, extracted from the seeds of the evening primrose plant by a cold extraction process, is available standardized for fatty acid content.
🖉**ALERT:** The oil may unmask previously undiagnosed epilepsy, especially when taken with a drug

that treats depression or schizo-phrenia.
• Drug effects may be delayed: cy-clic mastitis and premenstrual syn-drome, 4 to 6 weeks with maxi-mum benefit in 4 to 8 months; ec-zema, 3 to 4 months for decreased pruritus; diabetic neuropathy, 3 to 6 months.
• Vitamin E may be given with eve-ning primrose oil to prevent the formation of toxic metabolites.
• Drug should be taken with food to decrease adverse GI reactions.

**Patient teaching**
• Advise patient to consult with his health care provider before using an herbal preparation because a treatment with proven efficacy may be available.
• Tell patient to remind pharmacist of any herbal or dietary supple-ment that he's taking, when filling a new prescription.
• Tell patient to discontinue the herb if he has signs or symptoms of an allergic reaction, such as trouble breathing, hives, itchy or swollen skin, or rash.
• Advise patient to consult with her health care provider before using evening primrose oil during pregnancy or while breast-feeding.
• Advise patient to take herb with food to minimize adverse GI reac-tions.

## eyebright

*Euphrasia officinalis,* euphrasia

**Common trade names**
*Eyebright*

### HOW SUPPLIED
Available as capsules, dried herb, liquid extract*, tablets, and tincture*.
*Capsules, tablets:* 150 mg of eyebright combined with other herbs

### ACTIONS & COMPONENTS
Major components include a glycoside (aucuboside), a tannin (aucubin), caffeic and ferulic acids, sterols, choline, basic compounds, and a volatile oil. Also contains vitamins A and C.

### USES
Used topically in the form of lotions, poultices, and eye baths for ophthalmic disorders including treatment of blepharitis, conjunctivitis, styes, and eye fatigue. Also used internally for coughs, hoarseness, and respiratory infections.
   Many believe that eyebright has antibacterial and astringent properties, although none of the chemical components has been associated with a significant therapeutic effect. German Commission E recommends against the use of eyebright for therapeutic purposes.

### DOSAGE & ADMINISTRATION
*Capsules, tablets:* 1 to 2 capsules or tablets P.O. t.i.d.
*Liquid extract (alcohol free):* 1 to 2 ml (28 to 56 gtt) P.O. t.i.d.
*Liquid extract (25% alcohol):* 2 to 4 ml (40 to 80 gtt) P.O. t.i.d.
*Tea (prepared using one of two methods):* Infusion is prepared by steeping 1 to 2 tsp of finely cut herb in 6 oz of boiling water for 5 to 10 minutes, and then straining. Decoction is prepared by placing 1 to 2 tsp of finely cut herb in 6 to 8 oz boiling water, continuing to boil it for 3 to 5 minutes, and then straining. Although the 2% decoction may be used t.i.d. to q.i.d. for eye rinses, such use is strongly discouraged. Dosage is up to t.i.d. P.O.
*Tincture (45% alcohol):* 2 to 6 ml P.O. t.i.d.

### ADVERSE REACTIONS
**CNS:** confusion, cephalgia, insomnia, weakness.
**EENT:** intense pressure in the eyes with tearing, itching, redness, swelling, photophobia, changes in vision, sneezing, toothache, hoarseness.
**GI:** stomach upset.
**GU:** polyuria.
**Respiratory:** cough, dyspnea.
**Skin:** diaphoresis.
**Other:** yawning.

### INTERACTIONS
**Herb-drug.** *Disulfiram, metronidazole:* May precipitate a disulfiram-like reaction with preparations high in alcohol content. Advise patient to avoid using together.
**Herb-lifestyle.** *Alcohol:* Enhanced CNS effects if taken with preparations containing alcohol. Advise patient to avoid using together.

---

*Bold italic type* indicates that reaction may be life-threatening.

## CAUTIONS

Pregnant and breast-feeding patients and children should avoid use. Ophthalmic use is strongly discouraged. Patients with ophthalmic disease such as glaucoma should avoid use.

## NURSING CONSIDERATIONS

• Find out why patient is using the herb.

• Warn patient not to treat symptoms of ophthalmic disorders with eyebright before seeking appropriate medical evaluation because doing so may delay diagnosis of a potentially serious medical condition.

• Herbal products containing eyebright are prepared from the above-ground parts of the plant *E. officinalis.*

• Many tinctures contain between 25% and 45% alcohol and thus shouldn't be used by alcoholic patients, those with liver disease, or those taking disulfiram, metronidazole, a benzodiazepine, a barbiturate, or a cephalosporin.

• Topical ophthalmic use is a risk to the patient for hygienic reasons.

### Patient teaching

• Advise patient to consult with his health care provider before using an herbal preparation because a treatment with proven efficacy may be available.

• Tell patient to remind pharmacist of any herbal or dietary supplement that he's taking, when filling a new prescription.

• Caution patient not to apply eyebright directly to his eye because the sterility of the products can't be guaranteed.

• Tell patient that if he has trouble breathing or develops hives, or if his skin is itchy or swollen or breaks out in a rash, to stop taking this herb and contact his health care provider immediately.

• Warn patients to keep all herbal products away from children and pets.

*Liquid may contain alcohol.

# F

## false unicorn root

*Chamaelirium luteum,* blazing star, devil's bit, drooping starwort, fairy-wand, false unicorn, helonias root, rattlesnake

**Common trade names**
*False Unicorn*

### HOW SUPPLIED
Available as dried root or rhizome, liquid extract*, and tincture*.

### ACTIONS & COMPONENTS
The root, which is derived from *C. luteum,* contains the steroid saponin mixture chamaelirin. Other components that have been isolated from the root extract are oleic, linoleic, and stearic acids. Chamaelirin is believed to be responsible for the oxytocic, diuretic, and anthelmintic effects of the herb. Although the root probably has no effect on uterine tissue, it may exert its effect by increasing human chorionic gonadotropin release.

### USES
Used to treat dysmenorrhea, amenorrhea, and morning sickness and used as an appetite stimulant, anthelmintic, diuretic, emetic, and insecticide and as a uterine tonic during pregnancy to prevent miscarriage.

### DOSAGE & ADMINISTRATION
*Dried root or rhizome:* As a tea P.O. t.i.d.
*Liquid extract (45% alcohol):* 1 to 2 ml (20 to 40 gtt) P.O. t.i.d.
*Tincture (45% alcohol):* 2 to 5 ml P.O. t.i.d.

### ADVERSE REACTIONS
**GI:** gastric upset, vomiting.

### INTERACTIONS
**Herb-drug.** *Estrogen and progesterone:* False unicorn root may alter the action of hormones that affect the uterus. Monitor pregnant patient closely.

### CAUTIONS
Pregnant and breast-feeding patients should avoid use.

### NURSING CONSIDERATIONS
• Find out why patient is using the herb.
• Many tinctures contain between 25% and 45% alcohol and shouldn't be used by alcoholic patients, those with liver disease, or those taking a drug such as disulfiram, metronidazole, a barbiturate, a benzodiazepine, or a cephalosporin.
• High doses may cause stomach upset and vomiting.

#### Patient teaching
• Advise patient to consult with his health care provider before using an herbal preparation because a treatment with proven efficacy may be available.
• Tell patient to remind pharmacist of any herbal or dietary supple-

---

*Liquid may contain alcohol.

ment that he's taking, when filling a new prescription.

• Advise patient not to use false unicorn root without consulting her health care provider, especially if she's pregnant or breast-feeding.

• Warn patient not to delay seeking appropriate medical evaluation because doing so may delay diagnosis of a potentially serious medical condition.

• Tell patient that false unicorn root produces vomiting if used at high doses.

• Instruct patient to stop taking this herb and to contact health care provider immediately if he experiences difficulty breathing, hives, itchy or swollen skin, or a rash.

## fennel

*Foeniculum vulgare,* fenkel, large fennel, sweet or bitter fennel, wild fennel

### Common trade names
*Fennel, Fennel Herb Tea, Fennel Seed*

### HOW SUPPLIED
Available as essential oil, honey syrup, and seeds.

### ACTIONS & COMPONENTS
Fennel oil is obtained from the ripe or dried seeds of either sweet or bitter fennel. The composition of the oil varies slightly, depending on the source.

Fennel oil extracted from bitter fennel is made up primarily of 50% to 75% trans-anetholes, 12% to 33% fenchone, and 2% to 5% estragole. Fennel oil extracted

from sweet fennel is made up of 80% to 90% trans-anetholes, 1% to 10% fenchone, and 3% to 10% estragole. Additional components are present in smaller quantities. Fennel oil stimulates GI motility, and at high levels it has antispasmodic activity. The anethole and fenchone components have a secretolytic effect on the respiratory tract, probably a result of fennel's local irritant effects on the respiratory tract.

### USES
Used as an expectorant to manage cough and bronchitis. Also used to treat mild, spastic disorders of the GI tract, feelings of fullness, and flatulence. Fennel syrup has been used to treat upper respiratory tract infections in children.

### DOSAGE & ADMINISTRATION
*Essential oil:* 0.1 to 0.6 ml P.O. q.d. (equivalent to 0.1 to 0.6 g of fennel).
*Honey syrup with 0.5 g fennel oil/kg:* 10 to 20 g P.O. q.d.
*Seeds:* Crushed or ground; used for teas, tealike products, and internal use. Daily dose is 5 to 7 g.

### ADVERSE REACTIONS
**CNS:** *seizure (with use of oil),* hallucinations (with use of oil).
**GI:** nausea with oil, vomiting with oil.
**Respiratory:** *pulmonary edema (with use of oil).*
**Skin:** photodermatitis, contact dermatitis.
**Other:** allergic reaction.

---

*Bold italic type* indicates that reaction may be life-threatening.

## INTERACTIONS
**Herb-drug.** *Drugs that lower the seizure threshold, anticonvulsants:* Increased risk of seizure. Monitor patient very closely.

**Herb-lifestyle.** *Sun exposure:* Increased risk of photosensitivity reaction. Advise patient to wear protective clothing and sunscreen and to limit exposure to direct sunlight.

## CAUTIONS
Those with sensitivity to fennel, celery, or similar foods and herbs should avoid use. Pregnant patients, small children, and those with a history of seizures should also avoid use.

Diabetic patients should use the honey syrup cautiously because of the sugar content.

## NURSING CONSIDERATIONS
• Find out why patient is using the herb.
• Verify that the patient doesn't have an allergic response to celery, fennel, or similar spices and herbs.
🖉ALERT: Don't mistake poison hemlock for fennel. Hemlock can cause vomiting, paralysis, and death.

**Patient teaching**
• Advise patient to consult with his health care provider before using an herbal preparation because a treatment with proven efficacy may be available.
• Tell patient to remind pharmacist of any herbal or dietary supplement that he's taking, when filling a new prescription.

• If patient has diabetes, make sure that he's aware of the sugar content of the product.
🖉ALERT: Advise patient that the maximum length of use should be 2 weeks.
• Tell patient to stop taking this herb and contact health care provider immediately if he experiences difficulty breathing, hives, or a rash.

## fenugreek

*Foeniculum vulgare, Trigonella foenum-graecum,* bird's foot, bockshornsamen, fenugreek seed, foenugraeci semen, Greek hay seed

**Common trade names**
*Fenugreek, Fenugrene*

## HOW SUPPLIED
Available as capsules, paste, powder, ripe seeds, dried seeds, and as a spice.

## ACTIONS & COMPONENTS
Active components in fenugreek include mucilages, proteins, steroid saponins, flavonoids, and volatile oils. Trigonelline, an alkaloid found in fenugreek, is degraded to nicotinic acid (niacin), which may partially explain its ability to lower serum cholesterol levels. Steroid saponins may also lower blood glucose and plasma glucagon levels and enhance food consumption and appetite.

The seeds contain up to 50% mucilaginous fiber that, because of their ability to absorb and expand, are commonly used to treat diarrhea and constipation. The seeds also contain coumarin compounds.

## USES

Used to treat GI complaints and to relieve upper respiratory tract congestion and allergies. Used to lower cholesterol, blood glucose, insulin, and hemoglobin $A_{1C}$ levels and to improve glucose tolerance. Also used as an appetite stimulant.

Topically, it's applied to treat skin inflammation, muscle pain, and gout, and to aid in the healing of wounds or skin ulcers.

## DOSAGE & ADMINISTRATION

*External:* Poultice is prepared by mixing 50 g of powdered fenugreek with 1 qt of water. Applied topically to affected area, as needed.

*Internal:* Dosage is 6 g P.O., or a cup of tea taken several times a day. Infusion is prepared by steeping 0.5 g of fenugreek in cold water for 3 hours, and then straining. Honey may be used to sweeten the infusion.

## ADVERSE REACTIONS

**GU:** maple-syrup odor to urine.
**Hepatic:** *hepatotoxicity* including jaundice, nausea, vomiting, and increased bilirubin level.
**Metabolic:** hypoglycemia.
**Skin:** contact dermatitis (with external use), flushing.
**Other:** wheezing, watery eyes, numbness, rash, and *angioedema* (after inhalation, ingestion, or topical anesthesia).

## INTERACTIONS

**Herb-drug.** *Adrenergic blockers:* Additive vasodilating effect possibly leading to hypotension. Monitor blood pressure closely.
*Anticoagulants such as aspirin, heparin, low-molecular-weight heparins, NSAIDs, warfarin:* Increased PT and INR and potential risk of abnormal bleeding. Monitor PT and INR.
*Antidiabetics, including insulin:* Decreased blood glucose level. Monitor blood glucose level.
*Probenecid:* Decreased uricosuric effect. Monitor patient for therapeutic effect.
*Sulfinpyrazone:* Decreased uricosuric effect. Monitor patient for therapeutic effect.
*Other drugs:* Because of the fibrous content in fenugreek seeds and its binding potential, absorption of drugs may be altered. Advise patient to avoid using fenugreek within 2 hours of other drugs.

## CAUTIONS

Pregnant patients should avoid use because of the herb's potential abortifacient properties; alcohol and water extracts of the herb may stimulate uterine activity. Those with liver disease, peptic ulcers, or severe hypotension should avoid use because of the formation of nicotinic acid. Those who have had a previous allergic reaction to fenugreek or nicotinic acid and breast-feeding patients should also avoid use.

Those taking an anticoagulant—such as warfarin, heparin,

---

aspirin, or an NSAID—should use cautiously.

**NURSING CONSIDERATIONS**
• Find out why patient is using the herb.
• If patient is taking an anticoagulant, monitor INR, PTT, and PT. Also observe patient for abnormal bleeding.
• Appearance of rash or contact dermatitis may indicate sensitivity to fenugreek.
• Nausea, vomiting, jaundice, or elevated bilirubin level may indicate liver damage and hepatotoxicity from nicotinic acid. If patient develops these signs or symptoms, he should immediately stop using the herb.

**Patient teaching**
• Advise patient to consult with his health care provider before using an herbal preparation because a treatment with proven efficacy may be available.
• Tell patient to remind pharmacist of any herbal or dietary supplement that he's taking, when filling a new prescription.
• If patient is pregnant, planning to become pregnant, or breastfeeding, advise her not to use fenugreek.
• Caution patient that a rash or abnormal skin change may indicate an allergy to fenugreek and that nausea, vomiting, and skin color changes may indicate liver damage. Tell patient to discontinue use if such signs and symptoms appear.
• Remind patient not to take fenugreek at the same time as other

drugs and to separate administration times by 2 hours.

## feverfew

*Chrysanthemum parthenium, Tanacetum parthenium,* altamisa, bachelor's button, chamomile grande, featherfew, featherfoil, feather-fully, febrifuge plant, flirtroot, grande chamomile, midsummer daisy, mutterkraut, nose bleed, Santa Maria, tanacetum, vetter-voo, wild chamomile, wild quinine

**Common trade names**
*Feverfew, Feverfew Extract, Feverfew Extract Complex, Feverfew Leaf, Feverfew Leaf and Flower, Feverfew LF and FL-GBE, Feverfew Power, Fresh Freeze-Dried Feverfew, Migracare Feverfew Extract, Migracin, MigraSpray, MygraFew, Partenelle, Tanacet*

**HOW SUPPLIED**
Available as capsules, dried leaves, liquid, powder, seeds, and tablets.
*Capsules containing leaf extract:* 250 mg
*Capsules containing pure leaf:* 380 mg

**ACTIONS & COMPONENTS**
Has more than 35 chemical components. Of these, sesquiterpene lactones are the most well known and studied, and parthenolide, a germacranolide, is the most abundant of them. Monoterpenes, such as camphor; flavonoids, such as luteolin and apigenin; and volatile oils, including angelate, costic

acid, and pinene are also found in feverfew. Traces of melatonin appear in pure leaves and commercial preparations of the herb.

Parthenolide is thought to be the major component responsible for the pharmacologic effects of feverfew. It inhibits prostaglandin synthesis, platelet aggregation, serotonin release from platelets, release of granules from polymorphonuclear leukocytes, histamine release from mast cells, and phagocytosis. Parthenolide may have thrombolytic, cytotoxic, and antibacterial activity and may cause contraction and relaxation of vascular smooth muscle.

Monoterpenes, and possibly melatonin, may be responsible for feverfew's sedative and mild tranquilizing effects.

## USES
Used most commonly to prevent or treat migraine headaches and to treat rheumatoid arthritis. Used to treat asthma, psoriasis, menstrual cramps, digestion problems, and intestinal parasites; to debride wounds; and to promote menstrual flow. Also used as a mouthwash after tooth extraction, a tranquilizer, an abortifacient, and an external antiseptic and insecticide.

## DOSAGE & ADMINISTRATION
*Infusion:* Prepared by steeping 2 tsp of feverfew in a cup of water for 15 minutes. For stronger infusion, double the amount of feverfew and allow it to steep for 25 minutes. Infusion dose is 1 cup t.i.d.; stronger infusions are used for washes.

*Migraines:* 125 mg of dried leaf preparation q.d.; *T. parthenium* content should be standardized to contain at least 0.2% parthenolide, equivalent to 250 mcg of feverfew. *Powder:* Recommended daily dose is 50 mg to 1.2 g.

## ADVERSE REACTIONS
**CNS:** dizziness.
**CV:** tachycardia.
**EENT:** mouth ulcerations.
**GI:** GI upset.
**Skin:** contact dermatitis.

## INTERACTIONS
**Herb-drug.** *Anticoagulants, antiplatelet drugs including aspirin, and thrombolytics:* Feverfew inhibits prostaglandin synthesis and platelet aggregation. Monitor for increased bleeding tendency.

## CAUTIONS
Pregnant women should avoid use because of its potential abortifacient properties, and breast-feeding women should avoid use. Patients allergic to members of the daisy, or *Asteraceae*, family—including yarrow, southernwood, wormwood, chamomile, marigold, goldenrod, coltsfoot, and dandelion—and patients who have had previous reactions to feverfew shouldn't take it internally. Feverfew shouldn't be used in children younger than age 2.

Those taking an anticoagulant such as warfarin or heparin should use cautiously.

## NURSING CONSIDERATIONS
• Find out why patient is using the herb.

---

*Bold italic type* indicates that reaction may be life-threatening.

• If patient is taking an anticoagulant, monitor appropriate coagulation values—such as INR, PTT, and PT. Also, observe patient for abnormal bleeding.

• Rash or contact dermatitis may indicate sensitivity to feverfew. Patient should discontinue use immediately.

• Abruptly stopping the herb may cause "postfeverfew syndrome," involving tension headaches, insomnia, joint stiffness and pain, and lethargy.

**Patient teaching**

• Advise patient to consult with his health care provider before using an herbal preparation because a treatment with proven efficacy may be available.

• Tell patient to remind pharmacist of any herbal or dietary supplement that he's taking, when filling a new prescription.

• If patient is pregnant, planning to become pregnant, or breastfeeding, advise her not to use feverfew.

• Educate patient about the potential risk of abnormal bleeding when combining herb with an anticoagulant, such as warfarin or heparin, or an antiplatelet, such as aspirin or another NSAID.

• Caution patient that a rash or abnormal skin alteration may indicate an allergy to feverfew. Instruct patient to stop taking the herb if a rash appears.

## figwort

*Scrophularia nodosa,* carpenter's square, heal-all scrofula plant, kernelwort, rosenoble, throatwort

**Common trade names**
*None known*

### HOW SUPPLIED
Dried herb and root, liquid extract*, and tincture*.

### ACTIONS & COMPONENTS
Contains iridoids, flavonoids, tannins, and phenolic acids. Iridoid and phenylethanoid glycosides have also been isolated from the aerial parts of the plant. Two of these glycosides, harpagoside and harpagide, may have heart-strengthening and anti-inflammatory properties.

### USES
Used externally to treat skin conditions, such as eczema and psoriasis. May also help heal wounds, ulcers, burns, and hemorrhoids.

Used internally for its mild laxative effect and its mild diuretic and heart-strengthening properties.

In homeopathic medicine, used to treat decreased resistance, tonsillitis, and lymph edema.

### DOSAGE & ADMINISTRATION
*Liquid extract (1:1 preparation in 25% alcohol USP):* 2 to 8 ml P.O. t.i.d.
*Tea:* Prepared by steeping 2 to 8 g of dried leaves and stems in 5 oz of boiling water for 5 to 10 minutes. Dosage is t.i.d.

*Liquid may contain alcohol.

*Tincture (1:10 preparation in 45% alcohol USP):* 2 to 4 ml P.O. t.i.d.

**ADVERSE REACTIONS**
None reported.

**INTERACTIONS**
**Herb-drug.** *Antiarrhythmics, digoxin:* Figwort may contain cardiac glycosides; potential interactions may occur. Monitor patient for adverse reactions.
*Antidiabetics such as insulin, metformin, sulfonylureas:* Figwort may increase blood glucose level and therefore may decrease the effectiveness of these drugs. Monitor blood glucose level.
**Herb-herb.** *Other cardiac glycoside–containing herbs such as black hellebore, digitalis leaf, lily-of-the-valley, motherwort, oleander leaf, pheasant's eye, pleurisy root, uzara:* Increased cardiac effects. Advise patient to avoid using together.

**CAUTIONS**
Those with preexisting cardiac abnormalities including arrhythmias and conduction disturbances should avoid use. Pregnant and breast-feeding patients should also avoid use.

**NURSING CONSIDERATIONS**
● Find out why patient is using the herb.
● Figwort may interfere with the intended therapeutic effect of conventional drugs.
● Monitor patient for cardiac abnormalities.
● If patient has diabetes, monitor him for fluctuations in the blood

glucose level because herb may cause hyperglycemia.

**Patient teaching**
● Advise patient to consult with his health care provider before using an herbal preparation because a treatment with proven efficacy may be available.
● Tell patient to remind pharmacist of any herbal or dietary supplement that he's taking, when filling a new prescription.
● If patient is pregnant, planning to become pregnant, or breast-feeding, advise her not to use figwort.
● Inform patient about the potential for cardiac abnormalities. If patient experiences any cardiac disturbances while taking figwort, instruct him to discontinue the herb and to immediately report symptoms to his health care provider.
● Instruct diabetic patient to monitor blood glucose level frequently and to watch for abnormal fluctuations.
● Warn patient to keep all herbal products away from children and pets.

## flax

*Linum usitatissimum,* flaxseed, leinsamen, lini semen, linseed, lint bells, linum, winterlien

**Common trade names**
*Dakota Flax Gold, Flax Seed Oil, Flax Seed Whole*

**HOW SUPPLIED**
Available as capsules, flour, fresh flowering plant, oil, and whole

seeds. Also, many cereals, pancake and muffin mixes, and eggs contain flax.

*Capsules:* 1,000 mg, 1,300 mg

## ACTIONS & COMPONENTS

Contains mucilages, cyanogenic glycosides, 10% to 25% linoleic acid, oleic acid proteins (albumin), xylose, galactose, rhamnose, and galacturonic acid. Cyanogenic acids, with the activity of a certain enzyme, have the potential to release cyanide. Linolenic, linoleic, and oleic acids are classified as omega fatty acids.

The mucilaginous fiber absorbs and expands. The omega fatty acid component may decrease serum total cholesterol and low-density lipoprotein levels and may decrease platelet aggregation.

## USES

Used internally to treat diarrhea, constipation, diverticulitis, irritable bowel, colons damaged by laxative abuse, gastritis, enteritis, and bladder inflammation.

Used externally to remove foreign objects from the eye. Also used as a poultice for skin inflammation.

## DOSAGE & ADMINISTRATION

*For gastritis, enteritis:* 1 tbs of the whole or bruised seed, not ground, mixed with 5 oz of liquid and taken b.i.d. or t.i.d. Or, 5 to 10 g of whole seed soaked in cold water for 30 minutes; liquid is then discarded, the seeds are ground, and 2 to 4 tbs are used as linseed gruel. *Ophthalmic:* A single moistened flax seed is placed under the eyelid until the foreign object sticks to the mucous secretion from the seed. *Topical:* 30 to 50 g of the flour is used for a hot poultice or compress.

## ADVERSE REACTIONS

**GI:** intestinal blockage.

## INTERACTIONS

**Herb-drug.** *Oral drugs:* Because of its fibrous content and binding potential, drug absorption may be altered or prevented. Advise patient to avoid using flax within 2 hours of taking a drug.

## CAUTIONS

Those with an ileus, those with esophageal strictures, and those experiencing an acute inflammatory illness of the GI tract should avoid use. Pregnant and breastfeeding patients and those planning to become pregnant should also avoid use.

## NURSING CONSIDERATIONS

• Find out why patient is using the herb.
• When flax is used internally, it should be taken with more than 5 oz of liquid per tablespoon of flaxseed.
• Cyanogenic glycosides may release cyanide; however, the body only metabolizes these to a certain extent. At therapeutic doses, flax doesn't elevate cyanide ion level.
• Even though flax may decrease a patient's cholesterol level or increase bleeding time, it isn't necessary to monitor cholesterol level or platelet aggregation.

*Liquid may contain alcohol.

### Patient teaching
• Advise patient to consult with his health care provider before using an herbal preparation because a treatment with proven efficacy may be available.
• Tell patient to remind pharmacist of any herbal or dietary supplement that he's taking, when filling a new prescription.
• Warn patient not to treat chronic constipation or other GI disturbances or ophthalmic injury with flax before seeking appropriate medical evaluation because doing so may delay diagnosis of a potentially serious medical condition.
• If patient is pregnant, plans to become pregnant, or is breast-feeding, advise her not to use flax.
• Instruct patient to drink plenty of water when taking flaxseed.
• Instruct patient not to take any drug for at least 2 hours after taking flax.

## fumitory

*Fumaria officinalis,* beggary, common fumitory, earth smoke, fumitory wax dolls

### Common trade names
*None known*

### HOW SUPPLIED
Available as leaves, liquid extract*, powder, and tincture*.

### ACTIONS & COMPONENTS
The dried or fresh flowering plant—the above-ground parts—is used medicinally. Active components include isoquinoline alkaloids such as scoulerine, protopine, fumaricine, fumariline, fumaritine, flavonoids such as rutin, fumaric acid, and hydroxycinnamic acid derivatives.

Isoquinolone alkaloids may contribute to the herb's antispasmodic effects on the gallbladder, bile ducts, and GI tract. Cinnamic acid has a choleretic effect. Fumaric acid works as an antioxidant, a flavoring agent, and a chelating agent. Flavonoids and their derivatives may improve capillary function by decreasing abnormal leakage.

### USES
Used to relieve liver, gallbladder, and GI complaints and to treat cystitis, atherosclerosis, rheumatism, arthritis, hypoglycemia, and infections. Also used as a blood purifier.

Fumitory has been used to treat skin diseases such as chronic eczema and psoriasis.

### DOSAGE & ADMINISTRATION
*For gallbladder complaints:* Infusion is prepared by pouring boiling water over 2 to 3 g of fumitory, and then straining after 20 minutes. Dosage is 1 cup warmed and taken before meals.
*Internal use:* 6 g P.O. or 1 cup of tea several times a day.
*Liquid extract (1:1 preparation in 25% alcohol USP):* 2 to 4 ml P.O. t.i.d.
*Tincture (1:5 preparation in 45% alcohol USP):* 1 to 4 ml P.O. t.i.d.

### ADVERSE REACTIONS
**CV:** hypotension.
**EENT:** increased intraocular pressure.
**GU:** *acute renal failure.*

---

## INTERACTIONS

**Herb-drug.** *Antiglaucoma drugs:* Fumitory may increase intraocular pressure and reverse the effect of these drugs. Advise patient to use caution when using together.

*Antihypertensives:* Increased hypotension. Monitor blood pressure carefully.

*Disulfiram, metronidazole:* Tinctures and extracts contain significant levels of alcohol, increasing the risk for a disulfiram-like reaction. Advise patient to avoid using together.

*Oral drugs:* Fumaric acid is classified as a chelating agent; it may bind to other drugs and alter absorption. Advise patient to avoid using together.

**Herb-lifestyle.** *Alcohol use:* Increased CNS effects. Advise patient to avoid using together.

## CAUTIONS

Those with glaucoma and pregnant and breast-feeding women should avoid use. Because fumaric acid may cause renal failure, those with renal dysfunction should also avoid use.

Those taking an antihypertensive should use cautiously because of possible increased risk of hypotension.

## NURSING CONSIDERATIONS

● Find out why patient is using the herb.

● Monitor patient for renal dysfunction—serum creatinine and BUN levels—because fumaric acid may cause renal failure.

● Because tinctures and extracts contain significant levels of alcohol, they may be unsuitable for children, alcoholics, those with a previous history of alcohol abuse, those with preexisting liver disease, and those taking disulfiram or metronidazole.

## Patient teaching

● Advise patient to consult with his health care provider before using an herbal preparation because a treatment with proven efficacy may be available.

● Tell patient to remind pharmacist of any herbal or dietary supplement that he's taking, when filling a new prescription.

● If patient is pregnant or breast-feeding or is planning to become pregnant, advise her not to use fumitory.

● Inform patient of the potential for hypotension when using fumitory with an antihypertensive, and instruct him to report feelings of weakness, dizziness, or lightheadedness to his health care provider.

● Remind patient not to take fumitory with any drug; instruct him to separate administration times by 2 hours.

● Caution patient not to use fumitory with alcohol.

● Instruct patient to report feelings of increased eye pressure or pain and to stop taking the herb immediately if he experiences such symptoms.

*Liquid may contain alcohol.

# G

## galangal

*Alpinia officinarum,* catarrh root, China root, Chinese galangal, Chinese ginger, colic root, East India catarrh root, East India root, galanga, gargaut, greater galangal, India root, lesser galangal

**Common trade names**
*None known*

### HOW SUPPLIED
Available as dried powder, fluidextract*, oil, rhizome, and tea.

### ACTIONS & COMPONENTS
Dioxyflavanol whose rhizome contains a volatile oil, resin, galangal, kaempferid, galangin, and alpinin. The volatile oil may play a role in the herb's active medicinal properties such as calming the stomach.

### USES
Used to relieve flatulence, dyspepsia, nausea, vomiting, loss of appetite, and motion sickness. Used to treat fevers, colds, cough, sore throat, bronchitis, infection, rheumatism, and liver and gallbladder complaints. Used to inhibit prostaglandin synthesis. Used as an antibacterial and antispasmodic. Also used as a spice because of its pungent and spicy flavor and as a perfume.

Used in homeopathic medicine as a stimulant.

### DOSAGE & ADMINISTRATION
*Infusion:* Prepared by pouring boiling water over 0.5 to 1 g of galangal, and then straining after 10 minutes. Dosage is 1 cup 30 minutes before meals.
*Tincture or rhizome:* 2 to 4 g P.O. q.d.

### ADVERSE REACTIONS
**CNS:** hallucinations.

### INTERACTIONS
None known.

### CAUTIONS
Pregnant and breast-feeding patients should avoid use.

### NURSING CONSIDERATIONS
● Find out why patient is using the herb.
● Galangal isn't widely used in the United States and may be difficult to obtain. Patient should be careful when using products from unknown origins.
● This herb may interfere with the intended therapeutic effect of conventional drugs.

#### Patient teaching
● Advise patient to consult with his health care provider before using an herbal preparation because a treatment with proven efficacy may be available.
● Tell patient to remind pharmacist of any herbal or dietary supplement that he's taking, when filling a new prescription.

---

*Liquid may contain alcohol.

• Tell patient that galangal may be difficult to obtain in the United States, and advise him to obtain it only from a reputable, known source.

• Advise patient that dosing may be difficult if he's using galangal powder that's made for cooking. Tell him to consult with a health care provider with a background in natural medicine before use.

• Warn patient that this herb may cause hallucinations.

## galanthamine

*Galanthus nivalis, G. woronowii,* galanthamine hydrobromide

**Common trade names**
*Jilkon, Lycoremin, Nivalin*

### HOW SUPPLIED
Available as oral and I.V. solutions and tablets.

### ACTIONS & COMPONENTS
An alkaloid and a selective, long-acting acetylcholinesterase inhibitor from the plant *G. nivalis* or *G. woronowii.* Antagonizes muscle relaxation caused by nondepolarizing, curare-like muscle relaxants. May also modulate nicotinic cholinergic receptors and help improve daily functioning in patients with Alzheimer's disease.

### USES
Used to treat symptoms of Alzheimer's disease, neuromuscular disorders, and mania. Also used postoperatively to reverse the effects of neuromuscular blockers.

### DOSAGE & ADMINISTRATION
*Alzheimer's disease:* 20 to 50 mg P.O. q.d.
*Reversal of neuromuscular blockers:* 0.3 mg/kg I.V.

### ADVERSE REACTIONS
**CNS:** agitation, sleep disturbances, insomnia, light-headedness.
**CV:** *bradycardia.*
**GI:** nausea, vomiting, diarrhea, anorexia.

### INTERACTIONS
**Herb-drug.** *Other cholinergics (parasympathomimetics):* Potential to increase adverse effects including bradycardia, hypotension, and respiratory distress. Avoid using together.

### CAUTIONS
Those with a known allergy or hypersensitivity to galanthamine should avoid use. Patients with bradycardia, bronchial asthma, a siezure disorder, hyperkinesia, ileus, or ureter occlusion should avoid use. Pregnant and breast-feeding patients should also avoid use.

### NURSING CONSIDERATIONS
• Find out why patient is using the herb.

• Galanthamine is considered an investigational drug in the treatment of Alzheimer's disease. It may not be available for public use.

• Response to drug for Alzheimer's disease and mania may take 6 to 8 weeks.

• If patient is also taking an antiparkinsonian, monitor him closely

---

*Bold italic type* indicates that reaction may be life-threatening.

for symptom improvement or progression and adverse effects.
● Monitor patient for agitation, weight loss, and bradycardia.

**Patient teaching**
● Advise patient to consult with his health care provider before using an herbal preparation because a treatment with proven efficacy may be available.
● Tell patient to remind pharmacist of any herbal or dietary supplement that he's taking, when filling a new prescription.
● If patient is pregnant or breast-feeding, advise her not to use galanthamine.
● Tell patient to take with meals, if possible.

## garlic

*Allium sativum*, clove garlic, poor man's treacle, rustic treacle, stinking rose

**Common trade names**
*Garlicin, Garlic Powermax, Garlinase 4,000, GarliPure, Garlique, Garlitrin 4,000, Kwai, Kyolic Liquid, Wellness Garlicell*

**HOW SUPPLIED**
Available as aqueous extract (1:1), capsules, fermented garlic, fresh cloves, garlic oil maceration (1:1), powdered cloves, softgel capsules, solid garlic extract*, and tablets.

**ACTIONS & COMPONENTS**
Medicinal ingredients of garlic are obtained from the bulb of the *A. sativum* plant. The aroma, flavor, and medicinal properties of garlic

are primarily the result of sulfur compounds including alliin, ajoen, and allicin. Also found in garlic are vitamins, minerals, and the trace elements germanium and selenium.

Garlic inhibits lipid synthesis, thus decreasing cholesterol and triglyceride levels. Works as an anticoagulant by inhibiting platelet aggregation, which is probably the work of allicin and ajoen. Lowers blood pressure. Lowers the blood glucose level by increasing the body's circulating insulin and by increasing glycogen storage in the liver. Works as an antibacterial against both gram-positive and gram-negative organisms, including *Helicobacter pylori* (the causative organism in many peptic ulcers and in certain gastric cancers). May also have antifungal and antitumorigenic effects.

**USES**
Used most commonly to decrease total cholesterol and triglyceride levels and, increase HDL cholesterol level. Also used to help prevent atherosclerosis because of its effect on blood pressure and platelet aggregation. Used to decrease the risk of cancer, especially cancer of the GI tract. Used to decrease the risk of stroke and heart attack and to treat cough, colds, fevers, and sore throats.

Used orally and topically to fight infection through its antibacterial and antifungal effects.

**DOSAGE & ADMINISTRATION**
*To lower cholesterol:* 900 mg of dried power, 2 to 5 mg of allicin,

or 2 to 5 g of fresh clove. Average dose is 4 g of fresh garlic or 8 mg of essential oil q.d.

## ADVERSE REACTIONS
**CNS:** headache, insomnia, fatigue, vertigo.
**CV:** tachycardia, orthostasis.
**EENT:** halitosis.
**GI:** heartburn, flatulence, distress, nausea, vomiting, bloating, diarrhea.
**Respiratory:** asthma, shortness of breath.
**Skin:** contact dermatitis, burns.
**Other:** *hypersensitivity reactions,* facial flushing, body odor.

## INTERACTIONS
**Herb-drug.** *Acetaminophen and other drugs metabolized by the enzyme CYP 2E1, a member of the CYP 450 system:* Decreased metabolism of these drugs. Monitor for clinical effects and toxic reaction.
*Anticoagulants, NSAIDs, prostacyclin:* Combination may increase bleeding time. Advise patient to avoid using together.
*Antidiabetics:* Blood glucose level may be further decreased. Advise patient to use caution if using together and to monitor blood glucose level.
**Herb-herb.** *Other herbs that exert anticoagulation effects, such as feverfew and ginkgo:* Increased bleeding time. Advise patient to avoid using together.
*Other herbs that exert antihyperglycemic effects, like glucomannan:* Blood glucose level may be further decreased. Advise patient to use caution if using together, and monitor blood glucose level.

## CAUTIONS
Patients allergic to garlic should avoid use. Pregnant and breastfeeding patients should avoid use if consuming it in amounts greater than used in cooking.

Should be used cautiously in young children and in those with severe hepatic or renal disease.

## NURSING CONSIDERATIONS
- Find out why patient is using the herb.
- Garlic isn't recommended for patients with diabetes, insomnia, pemphigus, organ transplants, and rheumatoid arthritis, and in post-surgical patients.
- Consuming excessive amounts of raw garlic increases the risk of adverse reactions.
- Monitor patient for signs and symptoms of bleeding.
- Garlic may lower blood glucose level. If patient is taking an antihyperglycemic, watch for signs and symptoms of hypoglycemia and monitor his serum glucose level.

⚠ **ALERT:** Garlic oil shouldn't be used to treat inner ear infections in children.

### Patient teaching
- Advise patient to consult with his health care provider before using an herbal preparation because a treatment with proven efficacy may be available.
- Tell patient to remind pharmacist of any herbal or dietary supple-

---

*Bold italic type* indicates that reaction may be life-threatening.

ment that he's taking, when filling a new prescription.

• Advise patient not to delay seeking appropriate medical evaluation because doing so may delay diagnosis of a potentially serious medical condition.

• Advise patient to consume garlic in moderation, to minimize the risk of adverse reactions.

• Discourage heavy use of garlic before surgery.

• If patient is using garlic to lower his serum cholesterol levels, advise him to notify his health care provider and to have his serum cholesterol levels monitored.

• Advise patient that using garlic with anticoagulants may increase the risk of bleeding.

• If patient is using garlic as a topical antiseptic, avoid prolonged exposure to the skin because burns can occur.

## gentian

*Gentiana lutea,* bitterroot, bittersweet, pale gentian, stemless gentian, yellow gentian

**Common trade names**
*Gentian Root*

## HOW SUPPLIED
Available as bitter tonic*, dried powder, dried root, extract*, tincture*, and tea.

## ACTIONS & COMPONENTS
The medicinal components of gentian are derived from the roots and rhizome of the *G. lutea* species. Includes the following components: amarogentin, gentiopicrin,

gentiopicroside, swertiamarin, the alkaloids gentianine and gentialutine, xanthones, carbohydrates, pectin, tannins, triterpenes, and volatile oils.

Gentian may stimulate gastric secretions. Because it's usually administered with alcohol, it's difficult to determine whether the gentian or alcohol is having the gastric effects.

## USES
Used to stimulate appetite and to aid in digestion by stimulating gastric juices. May have some anti-inflammatory effects.

## DOSAGE & ADMINISTRATION
*Dried rhizome or root:* 2 to 4 g P.O. q.d.
*Liquid extract:* 2 to 4 g P.O. q.d.
*Tea:* Prepared by steeping 1 to 2 g of the herb in boiling water for 5 to 10 minutes.
*Tincture:* 1 to 4 ml P.O. t.i.d. The average dose is 1 to 3 g q.d.

## ADVERSE REACTIONS
**CNS:** headache.
**GI:** GI upset, nausea, vomiting.

## INTERACTIONS
**Herb-drug.** *Barbiturates, benzodiazepines:* Increased sedation because of the alcohol content in the liquid preparations. Advise patient to avoid using together.
*Cephalosporins, disulfiram, metronidazole:* Potential for disulfiram-like reactions because of the alcohol content in the liquid preparations. Advise patient to avoid using together.

---

*Liquid may contain alcohol.

## CAUTIONS
Patients with stomach or duodenal ulcers or excessive acid production should avoid use. Pregnant and breast-feeding patients should also avoid use.

Patients with GI disorders, such as peptic ulcer disease and Zollinger-Ellison syndrome, and patients with hypertension should use cautiously.

## NURSING CONSIDERATIONS
• Find out why patient is using the herb.

⚠ **ALERT:** Don't confuse gentian with gentian violet, also known as crystal violet; they have different uses.

### Patient teaching
• Advise patient to consult with his health care provider before using an herbal preparation because a treatment with proven efficacy may be available.
• Tell patient to remind pharmacist of any herbal or dietary supplement that he's taking, when filling a new prescription.
• Tell patient to discontinue use if stomach upset occurs.
• Advise patient that the tincture form contains alcohol.
• Advise patient to keep product out of direct light.

## ginger
*Zingiber officinale,* zingiber

**Common trade names**
*Alcohol-Free Ginger Root, Caffeine Free Ginger Root, Ginger Aid Tea, Ginger Kid, GingerMax, Ginger Powder, Ginger Root, Quanterra Stomach Comfort, Travellers, Travel Sickness, Zintona*

## HOW SUPPLIED
Available as candied ginger root, fresh root, oil, powdered spice, syrup, tablet, tea, and tincture.
*Capsules:* 250 mg, 410 mg, 550 mg

## ACTIONS & COMPONENTS
Rhizome or root of the plant *Z. officinale.* Its pungent properties also contribute to its pharmacologic activities. Ginger contains cardiotonic compounds known as gingerols, volatile oils, and other compounds such as (6)-, (8)-, and (10)-shogoal, (6)- and (10)-dehydrogingerdione, (6)- and (10)-gingerdione, zingerone, and zingibain.

The root has antiemetic effects, resulting from its carminative and absorbent properties and from its ability to enhance GI motility. The root can have positive inotropic effects on the CV system in large doses. Anti-inflammatory effects may result from ginger's ability to inhibit prostaglandin, thromboxane, and leukotriene biosynthesis; antimigraine effects, from ginger's ability to inhibit prostaglandins and thromboxane. Antithrombotic effects may result from ginger's ability to inhibit platelet aggregation. The volatile oil may have antimicrobial effects.

## USES
Used most commonly as an antiemetic in those with motion sickness, morning sickness, and generalized nausea. Used to treat colic, flatulence, and indigestion. Used to treat hypercholesterolemia, burns, ulcers, depression, impotence, and liver toxicity. Used as an antiinflammatory for those with arthritis and as an antispasmodic. Also used for its antitumorigenic activity in patients with cancer.

## DOSAGE & ADMINISTRATION
*As an antiemetic:* 2 g of fresh powder P.O. taken with some liquid. Total daily recommended dose is 2 to 4 g of dried rhizome powder.
*For arthritis:* 1 to 2 g q.d.
*For chemotherapy-associated nausea:* 1 g before chemotherapy.
*For migraine headache or arthritis:* Up to 2 g q.d.
*For motion sickness:* 1 g P.O. 30 minutes before travel, then 0.5 to 1 g q 4 hours. Also could begin 1 to 2 days before trip.
*Infusion:* To prepare, steep 0.5 to 1 g of herb in boiling water, and then strain after 5 minutes. (1 tsp = 3 g of drug.)

## ADVERSE REACTIONS
**CNS:** CNS depression with large doses.
**CV:** *cardiac arrhythmias (with large doses),* increased bleeding time (with large doses).
**GI:** heartburn.

## INTERACTIONS
**Herb-drug.** *Anticoagulants and other drugs that can increase bleeding time:* May further increase bleeding time. Advise patient to avoid using together.
**Herb-herb.** *Other herbs that may increase bleeding time:* May further increase bleeding time. Advise patient to avoid using together.

## CAUTIONS
Patients with gallstones or with an allergy to ginger should avoid use. Pregnant women and those with bleeding disorders should avoid using large amounts of ginger.
Patients taking a CNS depressant or an antiarrhythmic should use cautiously.

## NURSING CONSIDERATIONS
• Find out why patient is using the herb.
• Adverse reactions are uncommon.
• Monitor patient for signs and symptoms of bleeding. If patient is taking an anticoagulant, monitor PTT, PT, and INR carefully.
• Use in pregnant patients is questionable, although small amounts used in cooking are safe. It's unknown if ginger appears in breast milk.
• Ginger may interfere with the intended therapeutic effect of conventional drugs.
• If overdose occurs, monitor patient for arrhythmias and CNS depression.

## Patient teaching
• Advise patient to consult with his health care provider before using

---

*Liquid may contain alcohol.

an herbal preparation because a treatment with proven efficacy may be available.

• Tell patient to remind pharmacist of any herbal or dietary supplement that he's taking, when filling a new prescription.

• If patient is pregnant, advise her to consult with a knowledgeable practitioner before using ginger medicinally.

• Educate patients to look for signs and symptoms of bleeding, such as nosebleeds or excessive bruising.

• Tell patient to remind pharmacist of any herbal or dietary supplement that he's taking, when filling a new prescription.

• Warn patient to keep all herbal products away from children and pets.

## ginkgo

Ginkgo biloba, kew tree, maidenhair-tree, yinhsing

**Common trade names**
*Bioginkgo, Gincosan, Ginkgo Go!, Ginkgo Liquid Extract Herb, Ginkgo Nut, Ginkgo Power, Ginko Capsules, Ginkyo, Quanterra Mental Sharpness*

### HOW SUPPLIED
Available as tablets, capsules, and liquid preparations.

### ACTIONS & COMPONENTS
Medicinal parts include dried or fresh leaves and the seeds separated from the fleshy outer layer. The flavonoids and terpenoids of ginkgo extracts are considered antioxidants that serve as free-radical

scavengers. Other suggested mechanisms of action include arterial vasodilation, increased tissue perfusion, increased cerebral blood flow, decreased arterial spasm, decreased blood viscosity, and decreased platelet aggregation.

Ginkgo may be effective in the management of cerebral insufficiency, dementia, and circulatory disorders.

### USES
Primarily used to manage cerebral insufficiency, dementia, and circulatory disorders such as intermittent claudication. Also used to treat headaches, asthma, colitis, impotence, depression, altitude sickness, tinnitus, cochlear deafness, vertigo, premenstrual syndrome, macular degeneration, diabetic retinopathy, and allergies.

Used as an adjunctive treatment for pancreatic cancer and schizophrenia. Also used in addition to physical therapy for Fontaine stage IIb peripheral arterial disease to decrease pain during ambulation with a minimum of 6 weeks of treatment.

In Germany, standardized ginkgo extracts are required to contain 22% to 27% ginkgo flavonoids and 5% to 7% terpenoids.

### DOSAGE & ADMINISTRATION
*Tablets and capsules:* 40 to 80 mg P.O. t.i.d.
*Tincture (1:5 tincture of the crude ginkgo leaf):* 0.5 ml P.O. t.i.d.

### ADVERSE REACTIONS
**CNS:** headaches, dizziness, *subarachnoid hemorrhage.*

---

*Bold italic type* indicates that reaction may be life-threatening.

**CV:** palpitations, ***serious bleeding.***
**GI:** nausea, vomiting, flatulence, diarrhea.
**Other:** allergic reaction.

## INTERACTIONS
**Herb-drug.** *Anticoagulants, antiplatelets, and high-dose vitamin E:* May increase the risk of bleeding. Advise patient to avoid using together.
*MAO inhibitors:* Theoretically, ginkgo can potentiate the activity of these drugs. Advise patient to use together cautiously.
*Selective serotonin reuptake inhibitors:* Ginkgo extracts may reverse the sexual dysfunction associated with these drugs.
*Warfarin:* Possibly increased INR when taken together. Monitor INR.
**Herb-herb.** *Garlic and other herbs that increase bleeding time:* Potentiation of anticoagulant effects. Advise patient to use together cautiously.

## CAUTIONS
Patients with a history of an allergic reaction to ginkgo or any of its components should avoid use, as should patients with risk factors associated with intracranial hemorrhage (hypertension, diabetes). Patients receiving an antiplatelet or an anticoagulant should avoid use because of the increased risk of bleeding. Herb should be avoided in the perioperative period and before childbirth.

## NURSING CONSIDERATIONS
• Find out why patient is using the herb.

• Ginkgo extracts are considered standardized if they contain 24% ginkgo flavonoid glycosides and 6% terpene lactones.
• Treatment should continue for at least 6 to 8 weeks, but therapy beyond 3 months isn't recommended.
⚠️**ALERT:** Seizures have been reported in children after ingestion of more than 50 seeds.
• Patients must be monitored for possible adverse reactions such as GI problems, headaches, dizziness, allergic reactions, and serious bleeding.
• Toxicity may cause atonia and adynamia.

**Patient teaching**
• Advise patient to consult with his health care provider before using an herbal preparation because a treatment with proven efficacy may be available.
• Tell patient to remind pharmacist of any herbal or dietary supplement that he's taking, when filling a new prescription.
• If patient is taking the herb for motion sickness, advise him to begin taking it 1 to 2 days before taking the trip and to continue taking it for the duration of his trip.
• Inform patient that the therapeutic and toxic components of ginkgo can vary significantly from product to product. Advise him to obtain his ginkgo from a reliable source.
• Warn patient to keep all herbal products away from children and pets.
• Advise patient to discontinue use at least 2 weeks before surgery.

---

*Liquid may contain alcohol.

## ginseng, Asian

*Panax ginseng, P. quinquefolius,*
American ginseng, Chinese
ginseng, five-fingers, Korean
ginseng, Oriental ginseng

**Common trade names**
*American Ginseng, American
Ginseng Root, Centrum Ginseng,
Chikusetsu Ginseng, Chinese Red
Panax Ginseng, Concentrated
Ginseng Extract, Dwarf Ginseng,
Gin-Action, Ginsai, Ginsana,
Ginseng Concentrate, Ginseng
Manchurian, Ginseng Natural,
Ginseng Power Max 004X G-Sana,
Ginseng Up, Gin Zip, Herbal Sure
Chinese Red Ginseng, Herbal
Sure Korean Ginseng, Himalayan
Ginseng, Korean Ginseng, Korean
Ginseng Root, Korean White
Ginseng, Lynae Ginse-Cool, Man-
churian Ginseng, Natural Ginseng,
Power Herb Korean Ginseng,
Premium Blend Korean Ginseng
Extract, Sanchi Ginseng, The
Ginseng Solution, Time Release
Korean Ginseng Power, Zhuzishen*

**HOW SUPPLIED**
Available as powdered root, tablets, capsules, and tea.

**ACTIONS & COMPONENTS**
Ginseng's dried root is medicinal.
Contains triterpenoid saponins
called ginsenosides that appear to
be the active ingredients responsible for the plant's immunomodulatory effects. Ginsenosides seem to
increase natural-killer cell activity,
stimulate interferon production,
accelerate nuclear RNA synthesis,
and increase motor activity.

The ginsenosides have been
found to protect against stress
ulcers, to decrease blood glucose
level, to increase high-density
lipoprotein level, and to affect
CNS activity, which includes acting as a depressant, anticonvulsant, analgesic, and antipsychotic.

**USES**
Used to manage fatigue and lack
of concentration and to treat atherosclerosis, bleeding disorders, colitis, diabetes, depression, and cancer. Also used to help recover
health and strength after sickness
or weakness.

**DOSAGE & ADMINISTRATION**
*Powdered root:* For a healthy patient, 0.5 to 1.0 g of the root P.O.
q.d. in two divided doses for 15 to
20 days. The morning dose is usually taken 1 to 2 hours before
breakfast; the evening dose, 2
hours after dinner. If a second
course of therapy is desired, patient must wait at least 2 weeks
before starting ginseng again.
    For a geriatric or sick patient,
0.4 to 0.8 g of the root P.O. q.d.
taken continuously.
*Solid extracts in tablets and cap-
sules:* 100 to 300 mg P.O. t.i.d.
*Tea:* 1 cup q.d. to t.i.d. for 3 to 4
weeks. Prepared by steeping 3 g of
the herb in a cup of boiling water
for 5 to 10 minutes.

**ADVERSE REACTIONS**
**CNS:** headache, insomnia, dizzi-
ness, restlessness, nervousness.
**CV:** hypertension, hypotension.
**GI:** diarrhea, vomiting.

---

*Bold italic type* indicates that reaction may be life-threatening.

**GU:** estrogenic-like effects such as vaginal bleeding and mastalgia, in women.

**Other:** ginseng abuse syndrome including increased motor and cognitive activity combined with significant diarrhea, nervousness, insomnia, hypertension, edema, and skin eruptions.

### INTERACTIONS
**Herb-drug.** *Anticoagulants, antiplatelet drugs:* May decrease the effects of these drugs. Monitor PT and INR.

*Antidiabetics, insulin:* Increased hypoglycemic effects. Monitor serum glucose level.

*Drugs metabolized by CYP 3A4:* Ginseng may inhibit this enzyme system. Monitor for clinical effects and toxicity.

*Phenelzine, other MAO inhibitors:* Headache, irritability, and visual hallucinations. Other potential interactions may exist. Advise patient to avoid using together.

*Warfarin:* Possible decreased INR when taken together. Monitor INR.

### CAUTIONS
Patients with a history of an allergic reaction to the product or any of its components should avoid use, as should patients taking an MAO inhibitor.

Patients receiving an anticoagulant or an antiplatelet drug should use cautiously.

### NURSING CONSIDERATIONS
● Find out why patient is using the herb.

● The German Commission E doesn't recommend using ginseng for longer than 3 months.

● Ginseng is believed to strengthen the body and increase resistance to disease.

🖉**ALERT:** Reports have circulated of a severe reaction known as the ginseng abuse syndrome in patients taking large doses—more than 3 g per day for up to 2 years. Patients experiencing this syndrome report a feeling of increased motor and cognitive activity combined with significant diarrhea, nervousness, insomnia, hypertension, edema, and skin eruptions.

### Patient teaching
● Advise patient to consult with his health care provider before using an herbal preparation because a treatment with proven efficacy may be available.

● Tell patient to remind pharmacist of any herbal or dietary supplement that he's taking, when filling a new prescription.

● Inform patient that the therapeutic and toxic components of ginseng can vary significantly from product to product. Advise him to obtain his ginseng from a reliable source.

## ginseng, Siberian

*Acanthopanax senticosus,*
*Eleutherococcus senticosus*

### Common trade names
*Devil's Shrub, Eleuthero Ginseng,*
*Eleuthero Ginseng Root,*
*Pepperbush, Shigoka, Siberian*
*Ginseng Power Herb, Siberian*
*Ginseng Root, Spiny Ginseng,*
*Wild Pepper*

### HOW SUPPLIED
Available as tablets, capsules, liquid (ethanol extract)*, and tea.

### ACTIONS & COMPONENTS
The herb's dried root is medicinal.
Eleutheroside appears to be the active ingredient responsible for the plant's immunomodulatory effects. Eleutheroside may also affect the pituitary-adrenocortical system. Eleutheroside may also increase T-lymphocyte counts in healthy people. It's believed to strengthen the body and increase resistance to disease.

### USES
Used to manage fatigue and lack of concentration. Also used to treat hypotension, diabetes, cancer, and infertility.

### DOSAGE & ADMINISTRATION
*Capsules:* 1 g of powdered root in capsule P.O. q.d.
*Dry root:* 2 to 3 g P.O. q.d. for up to 1 month.
*Ethanol extract:* For a healthy patient, 2 to 16 ml P.O. q.d. to t.i.d. for up to 2 months. If a second course of therapy is desired, patient must wait 2 to 3 weeks before restarting Siberian ginseng.
For a sick patient, 0.5 to 6 ml P.O. q.d. to t.i.d. for 35 days. If a second course of therapy is desired, patient must wait 2 to 3 weeks before restarting Siberian ginseng.
*Root decoction:* 35 ml P.O. b.i.d.

### ADVERSE REACTIONS
**CNS:** drowsiness, anxiety, insomnia.
**CV:** tachycardia, hypertension, pericardial pain.
**Musculoskeletal:** muscle spasm.

### INTERACTIONS
**Herb-drug.** *Anticoagulants and antiplatelet drugs:* Decreased effectiveness of these drugs. Monitor PT and INR.
*Barbiturates:* Decreased metabolism of these drugs leading to additive adverse effects. Advise patient to use together cautiously.
*Digoxin:* Elevated serum digoxin levels. Other potential interactions may exist. Monitor serum digoxin level.
*Warfarin:* Possible decreased INR when taken together. Monitor INR.

### CAUTIONS
Patients with a history of allergic reactions to Siberian ginseng or its components should avoid use, as should patients with underlying hypertension.
Patients receiving an anticoagulant or an antiplatelet should use cautiously.

---

***Bold italic type*** indicates that reaction may be life-threatening.

## NURSING CONSIDERATIONS
- Find out why patient is using the herb.
- The German Commission E doesn't recommend using Siberian ginseng for longer than 3 months.
- ⚠ALERT: Adulterating ginseng with other herbs and caffeine is dangerous. Ginseng products, if contaminated with germanium, may cause nephrotoxicity.
- Monitor patient for adverse effects such as tachycardia, hypertension, pericardial pain, drowsiness, anxiety, muscle spasm, and insomnia.
- Siberian ginseng may increase serum alkaline phosphatase, gamma glutamyl transferase, BUN, and serum creatinine levels. It may also decrease serum glucose and serum triglyceride levels. Monitor these laboratory results, as needed.

### Patient teaching
- Advise patient to consult with his health care provider before using an herbal preparation because a treatment with proven efficacy may be available.
- Tell patient to remind pharmacist of any herbal or dietary supplement that he's taking, when filling a new prescription.
- Inform patient that the therapeutic and toxic components of Siberian ginseng can vary significantly from product to product. Advise him to obtain his ginseng from a reliable source.

## glucomannan
*Amorphophallus konjac,* koch, konjac, konjac mannan

**Common trade names**
*Glucomannan*

### HOW SUPPLIED
Available as tablets, capsules, liquid, powder, and hydrophilic gum.

### ACTIONS & COMPONENTS
Polysaccharide derived from the underground stems of *A. konjac.* Absorbs water. May increase the viscosity of the intestinal contents, decrease gastric emptying time, act as a barrier to diffusion, delay the absorption of glucose from the intestines, and decrease the need for antidiabetics in diabetic patients. May also inhibit the active transport of cholesterol in the jejunum and prevent the absorption of bile acids in the ileum.

### USES
Used to manage constipation, diabetes, obesity, hypercholesterolemia, and hyperlipidemia. Used to induce weight loss.

### DOSAGE & ADMINISTRATION
*For diabetes:* 3.6 to 7.2 g P.O. q.d.
*For hyperlipidemia:* 3.9 g P.O. q.d.
*For weight loss:* 1 g P.O. t.i.d. 2 hours before each meal.

### ADVERSE REACTIONS
**GI:** esophageal obstruction, flatulence, diarrhea.
**Metabolic:** hypoglycemia.

---

*Liquid may contain alcohol.

## INTERACTIONS
**Herb-drug.** *Oral antidiabetics or insulin:* May cause significant hypoglycemia. Use together cautiously and monitor serum glucose level. Antidiabetic dosage may need to be reduced.
*Oral drugs:* The fiber content of glucomannan may interfere with the absorption of various drugs. Advise patient to separate administration times by at least 2 hours.

## CAUTIONS
Patients with a history of an allergic reaction to glucomannan or any of its components should avoid use.

Patients with GI dysfunction, patients prone to hypoglycemia, and patients with underlying diabetes should use cautiously.

## NURSING CONSIDERATIONS
• Find out why patient is using the herb.
• Consuming glucomannan may result in a feeling of fullness, thereby decreasing the appetite.
• Monitor patient for adverse effects such as esophageal obstruction, lower GI obstruction, flatulence, diarrhea, and hypoglycemia.
• Monitor patient's weight and serum cholesterol and serum glucose levels.

**Patient teaching**
• Advise patient to consult with his health care provider before using an herbal preparation because a treatment with proven efficacy may be available.
• Tell patient to remind pharmacist of any herbal or dietary supplement that he's taking, when filling a new prescription.
• Advise patient to avoid using tablet form because it poses an increased risk of esophageal obstruction.
• Inform patient that the therapeutic and toxic components of glucomannan can vary significantly from product to product. Advise him to obtain his glucomannan from a reliable source.

## glucosamine sulfate
chitosamine

**Common trade names**
*Glucosamine*

## HOW SUPPLIED
Available as tablets.
*Tablets:* 500 mg

## ACTIONS & COMPONENTS
Glucosamine, an endogenous aminomonosaccharide, is a simple molecule found in mucopolysaccharides, mucoproteins, and chitin.

Stimulates the synthesis of glycosaminoglycans and proteoglycans, both of which are considered building blocks of the cartilage. Has weak anti-inflammatory effects. May inhibit degenerative enzymes responsible for destruction of the cartilage. Appears to be effective in reducing pain and improving range of motion in patients with osteoarthritis. May also slow the process of joint damage.

## USES
Used to treat osteoarthritis.

---

*Bold italic type* indicates that reaction may be life-threatening.

## DOSAGE & ADMINISTRATION
*Tablets:* 500 mg P.O. t.i.d.; duration of therapy has lasted anywhere from 2 weeks to 3 months. For obese patients, 20 mg/kg body weight P.O. q.d.

## ADVERSE REACTIONS
**CNS:** drowsiness, headache, insomnia.
**CV:** peripheral edema, tachycardia.
**GI:** nausea, vomiting, abdominal pain, diarrhea.
**Respiratory:** bronchopulmonary complications.
**Skin:** skin rash.

## INTERACTIONS
**Herb-drug.** *Antidiabetics, insulin:* Increased resistance to these drugs. Adjust dosage, as needed.
*Diuretics:* Decreased effectiveness of glucosamine. Dosage may need to be increased for full effect.

## CAUTIONS
Patients with a history of an allergic reaction to glucosamine or any of its components should avoid use.

Patients with diabetes mellitus should use cautiously.

## NURSING CONSIDERATIONS
• Find out why patient is using the herb.
• Glucosamine may increase the adverse effects of diabetes mellitus.
• Monitor patient for possible adverse effects such as peripheral edema, tachycardia, drowsiness, headache, insomnia, nausea, vom-
iting, abdominal pain, diarrhea, and skin rash.

## Patient teaching
• Advise patient to consult with his health care provider before using an herbal preparation because a treatment with proven efficacy may be available.
• Tell patient to remind pharmacist of any herbal or dietary supplement that he's taking, when filling a new prescription.
• Inform patient that the therapeutic and toxic components of glucosamine sulfate can vary significantly from product to product. Advise him to obtain his glucosamine sulfate from a reliable source.
• Advise patient that, although limited drug interactions have been reported with use of this product, more potential interactions may exist.
• Inform patient that it may take 4 to 6 weeks before maximum benefits are achieved.
• Warn patient to keep all herbal products away from children and pets.

## goat's rue

*Galega officinalis*, French honeysuckle, French lilac, Italian fitch

**Common trade names**
*Goat's rue*

## HOW SUPPLIED
Available as dried leaves.

---

*Liquid may contain alcohol.

## ACTIONS & COMPONENTS

Consists of the dried, above-ground parts of *G. officinalis*, which include the stalk, leaves, and flowers; the leaves are collected at the beginning of the flowering season. Contains lectins, flavonoids, and the alkaloids galegine and paragalegine. May have diuretic and hypoglycemic activity and may also promote weight loss. The effect on blood glucose level has been attributed to the galegine alkaloid constituent.

## USES

Used as a diuretic and lactogenic in breast-feeding patients. Also used to reduce hyperglycemia and treat plague, fever, and snakebites.

## DOSAGE & ADMINISTRATION

*Extract:* Prepared by steeping 1 tsp of dried leaves in 1 cup of boiling water for 10 to 15 minutes. The fluidextract is taken P.O. b.i.d.

## ADVERSE REACTIONS

**CNS:** headache, weakness, nervousness.

## INTERACTIONS

None reported.

## CAUTIONS

Children, pregnant patients, and breast-feeding patients should avoid use.

## NURSING CONSIDERATIONS

• Find out why patient is using the herb.
• Diabetic patients should be evaluated by their health care provider before using goat's rue.

• Goat's rue may affect the intended therapeutic effect of conventional medications.
• Fatal poisoning has occurred in animals grazing on the herb. Signs and symptoms of toxicity include salivation, labored breathing, spasms, and paralysis as well as asphyxiation leading to death.

### Patient teaching

• Advise patient to consult with his health care provider before using an herbal preparation because a treatment with proven efficacy may be available.
• Tell patient to remind pharmacist of any herbal or dietary supplement that he's taking, when filling a new prescription.
• If patient has diabetes, inform him that goat's rue isn't recommended for the management of this condition and that he should consult his health care provider for proper diabetes care.
• If patient is pregnant or breast-feeding, advise her not to use this herb.
• Warn patient to keep all herbal products away from children and pets.

## goldenrod

*Solidago virgaurea,* Aaron's rod, blue mountain tea, European goldenrod, sweet goldenrod

**Common trade names**
*None known*

## HOW SUPPLIED

Available as ethanolic and aqueous extracts*.

---

*Bold italic type* indicates that reaction may be life-threatening.

## ACTIONS & COMPONENTS
Consists of the above-ground parts of *S. virgaurea,* gathered during the flowering season. The active medicinal ingredients identified include flavonoids, saponins, tannins, diterpenes, and carotenoids. The herb also contains phenol glucosides and caffeic acid derivatives.

Flavonoids and saponins exert a diuretic action on the kidneys. Astringent properties are derived from tannins. The herb also has anti-inflammatory activity.

## USES
Used to treat and prevent the formation of kidney stones and to treat inflammatory diseases of the urinary tract.

German Commission E has approved goldenrod for use as a diuretic, an anti-inflammatory, and a mild antispasmodic.

## DOSAGE & ADMINISTRATION
*Daily dose:* 6 to 12 g of herb, as recommended by the German Commission E.
*Infusion:* Prepared by steeping 1 to 2 tbs of dried herb in 5 to 9 oz of boiling water, and then straining after 15 minutes. Dosage is b.i.d. to q.i.d. between meals.
*Liquid extract (1:1 in 25% ethanol):* 0.5 to 2 ml P.O. b.i.d. to t.i.d.
*Tincture (1:5 in 45% ethanol):* 0.5 to 1 ml P.O. b.i.d. to t.i.d.

## ADVERSE REACTIONS
**GI:** vomiting after ingestion of the dried plant.
**Respiratory:** allergic reaction, asthma, hayfever.

**Other:** rapid breathing after ingestion of the dried plant. Poisoning resulting from parasites, fungus, and rust in the dried plant may lead to weight loss, leg and abdominal edema, enlarged spleen, and GI hemorrhage.

## INTERACTIONS
**Herb-drug.** *Cephalosporins, disulfiram, metronidazole:* Disulfiram-like reaction caused by large amounts of alcohol in liquid preparations. Advise patient to avoid using together.
*Other CNS depressants including barbiturates, benzodiazepines:* Increased CNS depression. Advise patient to use together cautiously, if at all.

## CAUTIONS
Pregnant women should avoid use because of risk of miscarriage. Patients with edema from impaired cardiac or renal function shouldn't use irrigation therapy.

## NURSING CONSIDERATIONS
• Find out why patient is using the herb.
• If patient is using goldenrod to treat hypertension or kidney stones, he should consult his health care provider for proper evaluation and treatment.
• Liquid extracts and tinctures may contain up to 45% alcohol and may be unsuitable for children, alcoholics, and patients with liver disease.

## Patient teaching
• Advise patient to consult with his health care provider before using

an herbal preparation because a treatment with proven efficacy may be available.

• Tell patient to remind pharmacist of any herbal or dietary supplement that he's taking, when filling a new prescription.

• Recommend that patient seeks medical supervision if he's using goldenrod as a diuretic or as treatment for hypertension or kidney stones.

• If patient is pregnant or is planning pregnancy, advise her not to use goldenrod.

• If patient has allergies, advise him not to use this herb.

• If patient is taking other drugs that interact with alcohol, tell him to avoid use of the extract and tincture.

• Encourage patient to drink at least 2 qt of fluids per day.

• Tell patient to store the herb away from light and moisture.

## goldenseal

*Hydrastis canadensis,* eye balm, eye root, ground raspberry, Indian dye, Indian plant, Indian turmeric, jaundice root, orange root, turmeric root, yellow Indian paint, yellow puccoon, yellow root

### Common trade names
*Golden Seal Extract, Golden Seal Extract 4:1, Golden Seal Power, Golden Seal Root, Nu Veg Golden Seal Herb, Nu Veg Golden Seal Root*

## HOW SUPPLIED
Available as capsules, dried ground root powder, tablets, tea, tincture*, and water ethanol extracts*.
*Capsules, tablets:* 250 mg, 350 mg, 400 mg, 404 mg, 470 mg, 500 mg, 535 mg, 540 mg

## ACTIONS & COMPONENTS
Consists of the rhizome and roots of *H. canadensis*. Principal chemical constituents are the alkaloids hydrastine and berberine. Also contains other alkaloids, volatile oils, chlorogenic acid, phytosterols, and resins.

May have anti-inflammatory, antihemorrhagic, immunomodulatory, and muscle relaxant properties. Decreases hyperphagia and polydipsia associated with streptozocin diabetes in mice. Exhibits inconsistent uterine hemostatic properties. Hydrastine causes peripheral vasoconstriction. Berberine can decrease the anticoagulant effect of heparin. It stimulates bile secretion and exhibits some antineoplastic and antibacterial activity. Berberine can stimulate cardiac function in lower doses or inhibit it at higher doses.

## USES
Used to treat postpartum hemorrhage and to improve bile secretion. Also used as a digestive aid and expectorant. Used topically on wounds and herpes labialis lesions.

## DOSAGE & ADMINISTRATION
*Alcohol and water extract:* 250 mg P.O. t.i.d.

---

*Bold italic type* indicates that reaction may be life-threatening.

*Dried rhizome*: 0.5 to 1 g in 1 cup of water t.i.d.
*Expectorant:* 250 to 500 mg P.O. t.i.d.
*For symptomatic relief of mouth sores and sore throat:* 2 to 4 ml of tincture (1:10 in 60% ethanol), swished or gargled t.i.d.
*Topical use:* Small amount of cream, ointment, or powder applied to wound once daily. Wound should be cleaned at least once per day.

**ADVERSE REACTIONS**
**CNS:** sedation, reduced mental alertness, hallucinations, delirium, paresthesia, paralysis.
**CV:** hypotension, hypertension, *asystole, heart block.*
**EENT:** mouth ulceration.
**GI:** nausea, vomiting, diarrhea, GI cramping.
**Hematologic:** megaloblastic anemia from decreased vitamin B absorption, *leukopenia.*
**Respiratory:** *respiratory depression.*
**Skin:** contact dermatitis.

**INTERACTIONS**
**Herb-drug.** *Anticoagulants:* May reduce anticoagulant effect. Advise patient to avoid using together.
*Antidiabetics, insulin:* Increased hypoglycemic effects. Advise patient to use together cautiously.
*Antihypertensives:* May reduce or enhance hypotensive effect. Advise patient to avoid using together.
*Beta blockers, calcium channel blockers, digoxin:* May interfere or enhance cardiac effects. Advise patient to avoid using together.
*CNS depressants such as benzodiazepines:* May enhance sedative

effects. Advise patient to avoid using together.
*Disulfiram, metronidazole, cephalosporins:* Disulfiram-like reaction when taken with herbal liquid preparations. Advise patient to avoid using together.
**Herb-lifestyle.** *Alcohol:* May enhance sedative effects. Advise patient to avoid using together.

**CAUTIONS**
Patients with hypertension, heart failure, or arrhythmias should avoid use. Pregnant and breastfeeding patients and those with severe renal or hepatic disease should also avoid use. Goldenseal shouldn't be given to infants.

**NURSING CONSIDERATIONS**
• Find out why patient is using the herb.
• German Commission E hasn't endorsed the use of goldenseal for any condition because of the potential toxicity and lack of well-documented efficacy.
• Berberine increases bilirubin levels in infants and thus shouldn't be given to them.
• Goldenseal is less effective than ergot alkaloids in treating postpartum hemorrhage. Berberine can decrease the duration of diarrhea caused by various pathogens (*Vibrio cholerae, Shigella, Salmonella, Giardia,* some *Enterobacteriaceae*).
• Monitor patient for signs and symptoms of vitamin B deficiency such as megaloblastic anemia, paresthesia, seizures, cheilosis, glossitis, and seborrheic dermatitis.

*Liquid may contain alcohol.

• Monitor patient for adverse CV, respiratory, and neurologic effects. If patient has a toxic reaction, induce vomiting and perform gastric lavage. After lavage, instill activated charcoal and treat symptomatically.

**Patient teaching**

• Advise patient to consult with his health care provider before using an herbal preparation because a treatment with proven efficacy may be available.

• Tell patient to remind pharmacist of any herbal or dietary supplement that he's taking, when filling a new prescription.

• Advise patient not to use goldenseal because of its toxicity and lack of documented efficacy, especially if the patient has CV disease. ⚡ALERT: High doses may lead to vomiting, bradycardia, hypertension, respiratory depression, exaggerated reflexes, seizures, and death.

• Warn patient to avoid driving until he knows how goldenseal will affect his CNS.

## gossypol

American upland cotton, common cotton, cotton root, upland cotton, wild cotton

**Common trade names**
*None known*

**HOW SUPPLIED**
Available as liquid extracts* and tinctures*.

**ACTIONS & COMPONENTS**
Derived from the stems, roots, and seeds of plants from the Malvaceae family. The cotton plant (*Gossypium* species) is the most common source. Gossypol is the active ingredient found in seeds and other parts of the plant; however, content varies significantly from species to species.

Exerts antifertility action by inhibiting sperm production and motility. Possesses antitumorigenic activity and may also have anti-HIV properties.

**USES**
Used in China as a male contraceptive. Also used topically as a spermicide.

**DOSAGE & ADMINISTRATION**
*Contraceptive use:* 20 mg P.O. q.d. for 2 to 3 months until the sperm count is decreased to less than 4 million/ml. The dosage is reduced to a maintenance ranging from 50 mg weekly to 75 to 100 mg twice a month.

**ADVERSE REACTIONS**
**CNS:** paralysis.
**CV:** circulatory problems, *heart failure.*
**GI:** diarrhea, malnutrition.
**GU:** *nephrotoxicity.*
**Metabolic:** hypokalemia.
**Musculoskeletal:** muscle fatigue, muscle weakness.
**Other:** hair discoloration.

**INTERACTIONS**
**Herb-drug.** *Nephrotoxic drugs:* May increase risk of nephrotoxici-

---

*Bold italic type* indicates that reaction may be life-threatening.

ty. Advise patient to avoid using together.
*Potassium wasting diuretics:* Hypokalemia. Advise patient to avoid using together.

## CAUTIONS
Pregnant and breast-feeding patients should avoid use.

Patients with renal insufficiency should use cautiously.

## NURSING CONSIDERATIONS
- Find out why patient is using the herb.
- The contraceptive effect of gossypol in men is higher than 99%. Fertility usually returns to normal within 3 months of discontinuation; however, inhibition of spermatogenesis may persist in up to 20% of men 2 years after discontinuation.
- Monitor serum electrolyte levels, especially potassium, creatinine, and BUN levels.
- Monitor patients for muscle weakness and fatigue.
- If using formulation containing alcohol, avoid using in patients taking disulfiram, metronidazole, cephalosporins, or any CNS depressants.

### Patient teaching
- Advise patient to consult with his health care provider before using an herbal preparation because a treatment with proven efficacy may be available.
- Tell patient to remind pharmacist of any herbal or dietary supplement that he's taking, when filling a new prescription.

- If patient is pregnant or breast-feeding, advise her not to use gossypol.
- Inform men of the potential for permanent sterility after using oral gossypol.
- Advise women who are considering the use of gossypol as a topical spermicide about the lack of adequate information on safety and efficacy. Inform them of alternative, safe, and effective contraceptive methods.
- Warn patient to keep all herbal products away from children and pets.

## gotu kola

*Centella asiatica*, hydrocotyle, Indian pennywort, Indian water navelwort, marsh penny, talepetrako, TECA, thick-leaved pennywort, white rot

**Common trade names**
*Centalase, Centasium, Emdecassol, Gotu Kola Gold Extract, Gotu Kola Herb, Madecassol*

## HOW SUPPLIED
Available as ampules, capsules, ointment, powder, tablets, tinctures*, and extract.
*Ampule:* 10 mg/ml
*Capsules:* 221 mg, 250 mg, 435 mg, 439 mg, 441 mg
*Ointment:* 1%
*Powder:* 2%

## ACTIONS & COMPONENTS
Derived from the leaves, stem, and aerial parts of *C. asiatica*. Contains madecassol, madecassic acid, asiatic acid, asiaticentoic acid, cen-

tellic acid, centoic acid, isothanku-niside, flavonoids including quercetin and kaempferol, and various glycosides such as asiaticoside, brahminoside, brahmoside, centelloside, and madecassoid. Also contains fatty acids, amino acids, phytosterols, and tannin.

Asiaticoside promotes wound healing, brahminoside and brahmoside possess sedative properties, and madecassoid exerts anti-inflammatory action.

## USES
Used for its anticarcinogenic, anti-fertility, and antihypertensive effects. Also used to treat chronic venous insufficiency, chronic hypertension, and chronic hepatic disorders. Used topically to treat psoriasis and burns and to promote wound healing in patients with chronic lesions such as cutaneous ulcers, leprosy sores, fistulas, and surgical and gynecologic wounds.

## DOSAGE & ADMINISTRATION
*Capsules:* 450 mg once q.d.
*Creams, ointments:* Applied to affected area q.d. to b.i.d.
*Dried leaves:* 0.6 g of dried leaves or infusion P.O. t.i.d.
*Standardized extract (40% asiaticoside, 29% to 30% asiatic acid and madecassic acid, respectively, and 1% to 2% madecassoside):* 20 to 40 mg P.O. t.i.d.

## ADVERSE REACTIONS
**CNS:** sedation with higher doses.
**Metabolic:** hypercholesterolemia, hyperglycemia.
**Skin:** contact dermatitis, burning, pruritus.

## INTERACTIONS
**Herb-drug.** *Antidiabetics:* Large doses of gotu kola may interfere with the effect of these drugs. Advise patient to avoid using together. *Cholesterol-lowering drugs:* Large doses of gotu kola may interfere with the effect of these drugs. Advise patient to avoid using together.

## CAUTIONS
Pregnant patients, breast-feeding patients, young children, and patients with severe renal or hepatic disease should avoid use.

Patients with a history of contact dermatitis should use cautiously.

## NURSING CONSIDERATIONS
• Find out why patient is using the herb.
• Topical asiaticoside may cause cancer.
• Monitor patient for CNS depression including drowsiness and increased sleep time.
• Monitor blood glucose and serum cholesterol levels.

### Patient teaching
• Advise patient to consult with his health care provider before using an herbal preparation because a treatment with proven efficacy may be available.
• Tell patient to remind pharmacist of any herbal or dietary supplement that he's taking, when filling a new prescription.
• Warn patient of potential for sedation. Advise him to avoid driving until he knows how the herb affects him.

---

*Bold italic type* indicates that reaction may be life-threatening.

- If patient is using the herb for contraception, recommend another method.
- Recommend that patient not use the herb for longer than 6 weeks at a time.
- Tell patient to take capsules with meals.
- Advise patient to report planned or suspected pregnancy.

## grape seed

grape seed, grape seed extract, grape seed oil, muskat

**Common trade names**
*Grape Seed Extract (various manufacturers), Mega Juice, NutraPack*

### HOW SUPPLIED
Available as tablets, capsules, grape concentrate liquid, and antistax (capsules, drops, cream).

### ACTIONS & COMPONENTS
Obtained by grinding the seeds of red grapes. Grape seed extract contains procyanidins, also called proanthocyanidins, or flavonoids, which are free radical scavengers. The procyanidins inhibit proteolytic enzymes, including collagenase, elastase, beta-glucuronidase and hyaluronidase. By this mechanism, they help stabilize collagen.

Grape seed oil contains essential fatty acids and vitamin E. It has antioxidant properties that are said to be greater than those of vitamin C or vitamin E.

Grape seed extract also has anticarcinogenic effects. It prevents oxidative damage to cholesterol and may lower the serum cholesterol level. It protects collagen lining the walls of the arteries and stabilizes the vasculature. It also protects the eyes against oxidative damage and prevents diabetic retinopathy and macular degeneration.

Grape seed may also prevent dental caries by inhibition of *Streptococcus mutans* and glucan formation from sucrose.

### USES
Used for its antioxidant properties to prevent CV disease and cancer. Used to treat venous insufficiency, bruising, edema, and allergic rhinitis.

### DOSAGE & ADMINISTRATION
*Capsules or tablets:* Initially, 75 to 300 mg P.O. q.d. for 3 weeks, then 40 to 80 mg q.d.
*Liquid concentrate:* 1 tbs mixed in 1 cup of water P.O.

### ADVERSE REACTIONS
**Hepatic:** *hepatotoxicity.*

### INTERACTIONS
None reported.

### CAUTIONS
Patients with liver dysfunction should use cautiously.

### NURSING CONSIDERATIONS
- Find out why patient is using the herb.
- If patient has liver dysfunction, monitor liver enzyme tests.
- Grape seed may interfere with the intended therapeutic effect of conventional drugs.

---

*Liquid may contain alcohol.

- Grape seed extract may have antiplatelet effects. If a patient is having elective surgery, it may be prudent to stop the supplement 2 to 3 days before surgery. Monitor PT and INR.

**Patient teaching**
- Advise patient to consult with his health care provider before using an herbal preparation because a treatment with proven efficacy may be available.
- Tell patient to remind pharmacist of any herbal or dietary supplement that he's taking, when filling a new prescription.
- Warn patient not to treat symptoms of venous insufficiency or circulatory disorders before seeking appropriate medical evaluation because doing so may delay diagnosis of a potentially serious medical condition.
- Warn patient to keep all herbal products away from children and pets.

## green tea

*Camellia sinensis,* black tea, Chinese tea, Matsu-cha, tea

**Common trade names**
*Chinese Green Tea Bags, Green Tea (various manufacturers), Green Tea Extract, Green Tea Power, Green Tea Power Caffeine Free, Standardized Green Tea Extract*

**HOW SUPPLIED**
Available as capsules, dried extract, liquid, tablets, and teas.

*Capsules:* 100 mg, 150 mg, 175 mg, 333 mg, 383 mg, 500 mg
*Tablets:* 100 mg

**ACTIONS & COMPONENTS**
Prepared from the steamed and dried leaves of *C. sinensis.* Contains the polyphenols, epigallocatechin and epigallocatechin-3-gallate, some of the most potent anticarcinogenic substances found in nature.

Green tea's antioxidant activity and its ability to inhibit cell proliferation and induce apoptosis are what give it its anticarcinogenic effects. The caffeine can have stimulatory effects on the CNS. The tannins have astringent properties, which provide an antidiarrheal effect.

Green tea may also decrease serum cholesterol levels and have antibacterial properties.

**USES**
Used to prevent cancer, hyperlipidemia, atherosclerosis, dental caries, and headaches, and to treat wounds, skin disorders, stomach disorders, and infectious diarrhea. Also used as a CNS stimulant, a mild diuretic, an antibacterial and, topically, as an astringent.

**DOSAGE & ADMINISTRATION**
*Oral use:* A typical daily dose is 300 to 400 mg of polyphenols. (3 cups of green tea contain 240 to 320 mg of polyphenols.)

**ADVERSE REACTIONS**
**CNS:** nervousness, insomnia.
**CV:** tachycardia.

---

*Bold italic type* indicates that reaction may be life-threatening.

**GI:** hyperacidity, GI irritation, decreased appetite, constipation, diarrhea.
**Metabolic:** increased blood glucose and cholesterol levels.
**Respiratory:** asthma.
**Other:** allergic reactions.

## INTERACTIONS
**Herb-drug.** *Ephedrine, any drug that acts as a stimulant:* Increased stimulatory effects because of the caffeine component. Advise patient to avoid using together.

## CAUTIONS
Patients allergic to green tea and breast-feeding patients should avoid use. Green tea shouldn't be used in infants or small children. Pregnant women should avoid or minimize use because of the caffeine.

Patients with CV or renal disease, hyperthyroidism, spasms, and psychic disorders should use cautiously.

## NURSING CONSIDERATIONS
● Find out why patient is using the herb.
● Dosage varies with the form of the herb.
● Look for products standardized to 80% polyphenol and 55% epigallocatechin gallate.
● Daily consumption should be limited to fewer than 5 cups, or the equivalent of 300 mg of caffeine, per day to avoid the adverse effects of caffeine.
● Prolonged high caffeine intake may cause restlessness, irritability, insomnia, palpitations, vertigo,

headache, and adverse GI effects. Monitor patient's intake.
● The adverse GI effects of chlorogenic acid and tannin can be avoided if milk is added to the tea mixture.
● The tannin content in tea increases the longer it's left to brew; this increases the antidiarrheal properties of the tea.
● In children, administering green tea with iron supplements or multivitamins with iron prevents the absorption of iron.
● The first signs of a toxic reaction are vomiting and abdominal spasm.

**Patient teaching**
● Advise patient to consult with his health care provider before using an herbal preparation because a treatment with proven efficacy may be available.
● Tell patient to remind pharmacist of any herbal or dietary supplement that he's taking, when filling a new prescription.
● Instruct patient not to consume more than 5 cups a day, or 300 mg of caffeine, to avoid or minimize adverse effects.
● Advise patient that heavy consumption may be associated with esophageal cancer secondary to the tannin content in the mixture.
● Tell patient that the first signs of toxic reaction are vomiting and abdominal spasm.

## ground ivy

*Glechoma hederacea*, alehoof, catsfoot, creeping Charlie's cat's paw, gill-go-by-the-hedge, gill-go-over-the-ground, haymaids, hedgemaids, lizzy-run-up-the-hedge, robin-run-in-the-hedge, tun-hoof, turnhoof

**Common trade names**
*None known*

### HOW SUPPLIED
Available as a tea of leaves and flowers, liquid extract*, and tincture*.

### ACTIONS & COMPONENTS
Contains the volatile oil, pulegone, which has abortifacient, hepatotoxic, and irritant properties.

### USES
Used to dry secretions, to treat poorly healing wounds, and to treat upper respiratory tract complaints, including problems with the ears, nose, and throat. Used as a decongestant, an anti-inflammatory, and an astringent. May also help with problems in the GI tract, including diarrhea, gastritis, and hemorrhoids.

In Chinese medicine, it's used to treat irregular periods, lower abdominal pain, scabies, carbuncles, dysentery, and jaundice.

### DOSAGE & ADMINISTRATION
*Dried drug:* 2 to 4 g P.O. q.d.
*Fluidextract (1:1, 25% ethanol):* 14 to 28 grains P.O. t.i.d.
*Topical:* Crushed leaves are applied to affected area.

### ADVERSE REACTIONS
None reported.

### INTERACTIONS
None known.

### CAUTIONS
Pregnant and breast-feeding patients, children, and those with renal or hepatic impairment should avoid use.

### NURSING CONSIDERATIONS
• Find out why patient is using the herb.
• Ground ivy may interfere with the intended therapeutic effect of conventional drugs.
• Patients taking disulfiram, metronidazole, a cephalosporin, or a CNS depressant should avoid formulations containing alcohol.
• Horses grazing on this plant have experienced cyanosis, lung congestion, sweating, salivation, pupil dilation, and death.

### Patient teaching
• Advise patient to consult with his health care provider before using an herbal preparation because a treatment with proven efficacy may be available.
• Tell patient to remind pharmacist of any herbal or dietary supplement that he's taking, when filling a new prescription.
• Warn patient to keep all herbal products away from children and pets.

---

*Bold italic type* indicates that reaction may be life-threatening.

## guarana

*Paullinia cupana,* Brazilian cocoa, guarana bread, guarana gum, guarana paste, guarana seed paste, paullinia, zoom

**Common trade names**
*Guarana Plus, Guarana Rush, Guarana Seed, Superguarana*

### HOW SUPPLIED
Available as alcoholic extracts*, capsules, elixirs, syrups, tablets, and teas. Also available in various soft drinks, weight-loss products, energy drinks, and vitamin supplements.

### ACTIONS & COMPONENTS
Guarana is the dried paste made from the peeled, dried, roasted, and crushed seeds of *P. cupana.* Contains 3% to 7% caffeine, whereas coffee contains 1% to 2% caffeine; tannins, which provide an astringent taste; and theophylline and theobromine, which are alkaloids that are similar to caffeine.

Primarily used for its caffeine content. Stimulates the CNS, suppresses the appetite, and inhibits platelet aggregation. Also induces diuresis and relaxes bronchial smooth muscle.

### USES
Used to promote weight loss, to enhance athletic performance, to protect against malaria and dysentery, and to treat headaches, painful menstruation, and digestion problems. Used as a stimulant similar to coffee or tea, an aphrodisiac, and a tonic to quiet hunger or thirst. Also used as a flavoring agent and a source of caffeine in soft drinks.

### DOSAGE & ADMINISTRATION
*Capsules:* 1 to 2 capsules contain 200 to 800 mg of guarana extract. Dosage shouldn't exceed 3 g q.d.

### ADVERSE REACTIONS
**CNS:** insomnia, irritation, nervousness, anxiety, headache, *seizures.*
**CV:** rapid heart rate, *arrhythmias,* inhibited platelet aggregation.
**EENT:** tinnitus.
**GI:** abdominal spasms, vomiting.
**GU:** diuresis, painful urination, fibrocystic breast disease.

### INTERACTIONS
**Herb-drug.** *Adenosine:* Decreased antiarrhythmic effect. Patient may require additional doses or another drug.
*Anticoagulants, antiplatelet drugs:* May increase bleeding tendency. Monitor PT and INR.
*Caffeine-containing analgesics or nonprescription drugs such as NoDoz and Vivarin:* Potentiates the effects of caffeine. Advise patient to avoid using together.
*Cimetidine:* May decrease the clearance of caffeine from the body, increasing its effects. Monitor patient for toxic reaction.
*Ciprofloxacin:* May decrease the elimination of caffeine from the body, increasing its effects. Advise patient to use together cautiously.
*Ephedrine and phenylpropanolamine:* Increases stimulant effects; may increase blood pressure. Advise patient to avoid using together.

---

*Liquid may contain alcohol.

*Theophylline:* Large amounts of guarana and caffeine can increase the effects of theophylline. Monitor patient for toxic reaction.

**Herb-food.** *Other products containing caffeine, including coffee and cola beverages:* Additive effects. Advise patient to avoid using together.

**Herb-herb.** *Green and black tea, maté:* Additive effects. Advise patient to avoid using together.

## CAUTIONS

Pregnant and breast-feeding patients and those with cardiac arrhythmias should avoid use.

Patients sensitive to caffeine and patients with CV or renal disease, hyperthyroidism, spasms, and psychic disorders such as panic attacks or anxiety should use cautiously.

## NURSING CONSIDERATIONS

- Find out why patient is using the herb.
- High doses may cause caffeine-like adverse effects.
- If patient is sensitive to caffeine, monitor blood pressure and heart rate.
- If patient is taking an anticoagulant or an antiplatelet, monitor PT and INR.
- The first signs of a toxic reaction are dysuria, vomiting, and abdominal spasms.

## Patient teaching

- Advise patient to consult with his health care provider before using an herbal preparation because a treatment with proven efficacy may be available.

- Tell patient to remind pharmacist of any herbal or dietary supplement that he's taking, when filling a new prescription.
- Advise patient who is or wants to become pregnant not to use guarana.
- Tell patient that herb may increase blood pressure, cause arrhythmia, and aggravate hiatal hernia, peptic ulcer disease, gastroesophageal reflux disease, and anxiety or depressive disorders.
- Advise patient that the caffeine content in guarana is higher than in coffee.
- Warn patient to keep all herbal products away from children and pets.

## guggul

*Commiphora molmol,* guggal, guggal gum, gugulipid, gum guggulu

**Common trade names**
*Guggulow, Guggul Raj, Gugulmax, Gugulplus, Ultra Guggulow*

## HOW SUPPLIED

Available as capsules and tablets.

## ACTIONS & COMPONENTS

An extract of the plant, containing gugulipid and guggulsterone is used medicinally. May lower serum cholesterol levels by 24% and triglyceride levels by 23% by increasing the hepatic binding of LDL cholesterol. The herb has variable effects on HDL cholesterol levels, either increasing or decreasing it. Guggulsterone stimulates the thyroid gland, has anti-inflammatory properties, may help in weight reduction, and protects against myocardial necrosis resulting from drug toxicity.

## USES
Used primarily for its ability to decrease serum cholesterol levels. Used to treat atherosclerosis and high cholesterol and high triglyceride levels.

In Ayurvedic medicine, it's used to treat arthritis and to aid in weight loss.

## DOSAGE & ADMINISTRATION
*Oral use:* Daily dose of guggulsterone is 25 mg t.i.d. This is provided in a 500-mg tablet standardized to contain 5% guggulsterone.

## ADVERSE REACTIONS
**GI:** diarrhea, anorexia, abdominal pain.
**Skin:** rash.

## INTERACTIONS
**Herb-drug.** *Diltiazem, propranolol:* Potential reduction in the bioavailability of single doses. Monitor cardiac rhythm and vital signs if patient uses these together. *Thyroid drugs:* Altered effects because guggul stimulates the thyroid gland. Advise patient to avoid using together.
**Herb-herb.** *Garlic:* Increased lipid-lowering effect. This is a therapeutic effect.

## CAUTIONS
Package inserts of products sold in India recommend against using guggul in patients with liver or kidney disease. Pregnant and breast-feeding patients should also avoid use.

## NURSING CONSIDERATIONS
• Find out why patient is using the herb.
• Monitor patients with thyroid disease and those taking a thyroid supplement because guggul stimulates the thyroid gland.
• Guggul may interfere with the intended therapeutic effect of conventional drugs.
• Only preparations with standardized amounts of guggulsterone should be used.
• Use should be limited to 12 to 24 weeks.
• Monitor serum cholesterol level.

### Patient teaching

• Tell patient to remind pharmacist of any herbal or dietary supplement that he's taking, when filling a new prescription.
• If patient is pregnant or breast-feeding, or is planning to become pregnant, instruct her not to use guggul.
• Tell patient that herb isn't a substitute for healthy eating and exercise.
• Advise patient to keep guggul out of reach of children and pets.

---

*Liquid may contain alcohol.

# H

## hawthorn

*Crataegus laevigata, C. monogyna,* English hawthorn, haw, may, maybush, mayflower

**Common trade names**
*Hawthorne Berry, Hawthorne Extract, Hawthorne Formula, Hawthorne Power*

### HOW SUPPLIED
Available as dried leaves, liquid extract*, and tincture*.

### ACTIONS & COMPONENTS
The active compounds of hawthorn are obtained from the berries, flowers, and leaves of the *Crataegus* species, most commonly from *C. laevigata* or *C. monogyna.* The primary ingredients responsible for the pharmacologic effects of hawthorn include flavonoids and procyanidins.

The hawthorn flavonoids increase myocardial contraction by dilating coronary blood vessels, reducing peripheral resistance, and reducing oxygen consumption. They also lower blood pressure by inhibiting ACE. The procyanidins slow the heart rate, lengthening the refractory period, and also have mild CNS depressant effects. Hawthorn's pharmacologic effects usually develop slowly.

### USES
Used to regulate blood pressure and heart rate and to treat atherosclerosis. Used as a cardiotonic and as a sedative for sleep. Used in mild cardiac insufficiency, heart conditions not requiring digoxin, mild stable forms of angina pectoris, and mild forms of bradycardia and palpitations.

### DOSAGE & ADMINISTRATION
*Dried fruit:* 300 mg to 1,000 mg t.i.d. P.O.
*Liquid extract (1:1 in 25% alcohol):* 0.5 to 1 ml t.i.d. P.O.
*Oral use:* The average daily dose is 5 g or 160 to 900 mg of extract.
*Tincture (1:5 in 45% alcohol):* 1 to 2 ml t.i.d. P.O.

### ADVERSE REACTIONS
**CNS:** agitation, dizziness, fatigue, headache.
**CV:** circulatory disturbances, palpitations.
**GI:** GI complaints, nausea.
**Skin:** rash on hands.
**Other:** sweating.

### INTERACTIONS
**Herb-drug.** *Antiarrhythmics:* Herb's action is similar to that of a class III antiarrhythmic. Use of both could enhance this action. Advise patient to avoid using together.
*Antihypertensives, nitrates:* Increased risk of hypotension. Advise patient to avoid using together.
*Cardiac glycosides:* Increased risk of cardiac toxicity. Advise patient to avoid using together. If used together, monitor serum digoxin level.

*Liquid may contain alcohol.

*CNS depressants:* Additive depressant effects. Monitor patient closely.

**CAUTIONS**
Patients with hypersensitivity to hawthorn, severe renal or hepatic impairment, children, pregnant patients, and breast-feeding patients should all avoid hawthorn use.

**NURSING CONSIDERATIONS**
• Find out why patient is using the herb.
• High doses may cause hypotension and sedation. Monitor patient for CNS adverse effects, and monitor blood pressure.
• Hawthorn may interfere with digoxin's effects or serum monitoring.
• If patient has heart failure, he should only use hawthorn under close medical supervision and in combination with other standard treatments, only as directed.
• Observe patient closely for adverse reactions, especially adverse CNS reactions.

**Patient teaching**
• Advise patient to consult with his health care provider before using an herbal preparation because a treatment with proven efficacy may be available.
• Tell patient to remind pharmacist of any herbal or dietary supplement that he's taking, when filling a new prescription.
• Warn patient not to treat cardiac symptoms such as edema or angina before seeking appropriate medical evaluation because doing

so may delay diagnosis of a potentially serious medical condition.
• Advise patient to use hawthorn only under medical supervision.
• Advise patient to use caution when performing activities that require mental alertness because of potential CNS adverse effects.
• Warn patient that hawthorn won't stop an angina attack.
• Instruct patient to notify his health care provider if he experiences dizziness, excessive sedation, irregular heartbeats, or any other adverse reactions.
• Instruct patient to seek emergency medical help if he experiences shortness of breath or chest pain.

## hellebore, American

*Helleborus virdis,* bear's foot, bugbane, devil's bite, Earth gall, false hellebore, green hellebore, Indian poke, itchweed, swamp hellebore, tickleweed, white hellebore

**Common trade names**
*Cryptenamine*

**HOW SUPPLIED**
Available as liquid extract*, powder, and tincture*.

**ACTIONS & COMPONENTS**
The active ingredients of American hellebore are obtained from the dried rhizome and roots of *Veratrum viride*. The active components of American hellebore are steroid ester alkaloids that exert their physiologic effects by lowering arterial blood pressure and

---

*Bold italic type* indicates that reaction may be life-threatening.

heart and respiratory rates. They also inhibit inactivation of sodium-ion channels in excitable cells, therefore increasing nerve and muscle excitability, especially in the cardiac muscles.

## USES
Used to depress the action of the heart and reduce blood pressure. Also used as a diuretic, antispasmodic, antipyretic, and sedative.

## DOSAGE & ADMINISTRATION
*Tincture (1:10):* 0.3 to 2 ml P.O. q.d.

## ADVERSE REACTIONS
**CNS:** *seizure,* syncope, sedation, paralysis.
**CV:** *arrhythmias, bradycardia,* ECG changes, hypertension, hypotension.
**EENT:** blindness, burning sensations in the mouth and pharynx, lacrimation, salivation, sneezing.
**GI:** abdominal pain and distention, diarrhea, nausea, vomiting.
**Musculoskeletal:** muscular weakness.
**Respiratory:** *respiratory depression.*

## INTERACTIONS
**Herb-drug.** *Cardiac drugs (antiarrhythmics, antihypertensives, cardiac glycosides, and nitrates):* Potential for increased or decreased effects of these groups of drugs. Monitor patient closely if used together.
*CNS depressants:* Increased sedation, respiratory depression. Advise patient to use together cautiously.

## CAUTIONS
⚡**ALERT:** Medicinal use isn't recommended because of the herb's narrow therapeutic index and highly toxic adverse effects.

## NURSING CONSIDERATIONS
• Find out why patient is using the herb.
• Not for use in allopathic medicine because of high risk for toxic reaction.
• Signs and symptoms of toxic reaction include burning of mouth and throat, inability to swallow, abdominal pain, cardiac abnormalities, seizures, impaired vision, nausea, shortness of breath, loss of consciousness, and paralysis. Monitor patient closely for adverse reactions.
• If overdose occurs, perform gastric lavage and administer activated charcoal, I.V. diazepam to treat spasms, and sodium bicarbonate to counteract acidosis. Patient may need respiratory support with mechanical ventilation.

### Patient teaching
• Advise patient not to delay seeking appropriate medical evaluation because doing so may delay diagnosis of a potentially serious medical condition.
• Advise patient to consult with his health care provider before using an herbal preparation because a treatment with proven efficacy may be available.
• Tell patient to remind pharmacist of any herbal or dietary supplement that he's taking, when filling a new prescription.

---

*Liquid may contain alcohol.

• Advise patient to avoid use because of toxic adverse effects and narrow therapeutic index.
• Warn patient to keep all herbal products away from children and pets.

## hellebore, black

*Helleborus niger,* black hellebore, Christe herbe, Christmas rose, melampode

**Common trade names**
*None known*

### HOW SUPPLIED
Available as liquid extract, powder, and solid extract.

### ACTIONS & COMPONENTS
The active ingredients are obtained from the rhizome and root of the plant, *Helleborus niger.* The whole black hellebore plant is considered poisonous. Black hellebore root contains glycosides with cardio-active properties similar to digitalis. It also contains saponins that can cause irritation to the mucous membranes. Topical application of the plant may cause serious skin irritation.

### USES
Used to treat nausea, worm infestations, amenorrhea, and anxiety. Also used as a laxative and as an abortifacient. Because of its possible immunostimulatory effects, black hellebore is used as adjuvant therapy in cancer patients.

Used in homeopathy to treat eclampsia, epilepsy, meningitis, encephalitis, and mental disorders.

### DOSAGE & ADMINISTRATION
*Powder (medicine content 10%):*
The average daily dose in one source is 0.05 g, with a maximum single dose of 0.2 g.

### ADVERSE REACTIONS
**CNS:** dizziness.
**CV:** *arrhythmias, bradycardia,* irregular pulse.
**EENT:** burning sensations in the mouth and pharynx, increased salivation, sneezing.
**GI:** abdominal pain, diarrhea, nausea, vomiting.
**Respiratory:** shortness of breath, *respiratory failure.*

### INTERACTIONS
**Herb-drug.** *Cardiac drugs including antiarrhythmics, beta blockers, cardiac glycosides:* Potential for increased or decreased effects of these groups of drugs. Monitor patient closely if used together.
*CNS depressants:* Increased sedation, respiratory depression. Advise patient to use together cautiously.

### CAUTIONS
⚠ALERT: Medicinal use isn't recommended because of the poisonous nature of the plant and its highly toxic adverse effects.

### NURSING CONSIDERATIONS
• Find out why patient is using the herb.
• Herb is considered dangerous in allopathic doses.
• Patient should be monitored closely for toxic reaction.

---

*Bold italic type* indicates that reaction may be life-threatening.

## Patient teaching

- Advise patient to consult with his health care provider before using an herbal preparation because a treatment with proven efficacy may be available.
- Tell patient to remind pharmacist of any herbal or dietary supplement that he's taking, when filling a new prescription.
- Advise patient that black hellebore is unsafe for use because it's toxic.
- Advise patient not to delay seeking appropriate medical evaluation because doing so may delay diagnosis of a potentially serious medical condition.
- Warn patient to keep all herbal products away from children and pets.

## hops

*Humulus lupulus,* common hops, European hops, lupulin

**Common trade names**
*Ez, Re-X, Stress Free*

## HOW SUPPLIED

Available as liquid extract*, tea preparation, and tincture*.

## ACTIONS & COMPONENTS

The medicinal parts include the glandular hairs separated from the flowers, the fresh cones, and the fresh or dried female flowers.

The active ingredient 2-methy-3-butene-2-ol has sedative-hypnotic properties. The bitter acid constituents lupulone and humulone inhibit the growth of gram-positive organisms by disrupting the primary membrane of the bacteria. The flavonoglucosides have diuretic and antispasmodic activities. Estrogenic or hormone activities in hops haven't been proven in more recent studies.

## USES

Used to treat neuralgia, insomnia, nervous tension, restlessness, sleep disturbances, intestinal spasms, anxiety, mood disturbances, sleep disturbances such as insomnia, and digestive tract disorders involving spasms of the smooth muscle. Used as a mild diuretic, appetite stimulant, digestive aid, and an aphrodisiac. Topically, used as a mild antibacterial. Also used to preserve beer.

## DOSAGE & ADMINISTRATION

*As a sedative:* 500 to 1,000 mg of dried herb P.O. as a single dose. Or as tea, prepared by brewing dried herb in 5 oz of boiling water for 5 to 10 minutes, and then straining.
*Liquid extract (1:1 preparation in 45% alcohol):* 0.5 to 2 ml as a single dose P.O.
*Tincture (1:5 preparation in 60% alcohol):* 1 to 2 ml as a single dose P.O.

## ADVERSE REACTIONS

**CNS:** sedation.
**Respiratory:** bronchial irritation and bronchitis after inhalation.
**Skin:** contact dermatitis.
**Other:** *anaphylaxis,* allergic reaction.

---

*Liquid may contain alcohol.

## INTERACTIONS
**Herb-drug.** *CNS depressants:*
Possible additive effects when
used together. Advise patient to
avoid using together.
*Phenothiazine-type antipsychotics:*
Possible additive effects on hyperthermia. Advise patient to avoid
using together.

## CAUTIONS
Patients with hypersensitivity to
hops and patients with estrogenic-
dependent tumors such as breast,
uterine, or cervical cancer should
avoid use because of possible estrogenic effects.

Patients taking a CNS depressant or an antipsychotic should use
extremely cautiously.

## NURSING CONSIDERATIONS
• Find out why patient is using the
herb.
• Liquid extract and tincture contain alcohol. It may be inappropriate for patients with liver disease
or those taking metronidazole or
disulfiram.
• Monitor for adverse effects such
as increased sedation and respiratory difficulties.
• Patient shouldn't inhale smoke
from the plant.

## Patient teaching
• Advise patient to consult with his
health care provider before using
an herbal preparation because a
treatment with proven efficacy may
be available.
• Tell patient to remind pharmacist
of any herbal or dietary supplement that he's taking, when filling
a new prescription.

• Warn patient not to treat digestive problems or mood disturbances with hops before seeking
appropriate medical evaluation
because doing so may delay diagnosis of a potentially serious medical condition.
• Although hops is botanically related to marijuana, smoking the
plant as a substitute may be dangerous because of adverse effects.
• Warn patient to avoid hazardous
activities because of potential CNS
adverse effects.
• Advise patient to notify health
care provider immediately if he
develops a rash or if he experiences shortness of breath, wheezing, or itching.
• Warn patient to keep all herbal
products away from children and
pets.

## horehound

*Marrubium vulgare,* common
horehound, hoarhound,
houndsbane marrubium,
marvel, white horehound

**Common trade names**
*Horehound Herbs, Hore Hound
Tea*

## HOW SUPPLIED
The active ingredients are obtained
from the leaves and flowers of *M.
vulgare.* Available as dried herb,
liquid extract*, lozenges, powder,
syrup, and tea.

## ACTIONS & COMPONENTS
Horehound's active compound,
marrubiin, stimulates secretions in
the bronchioles and works as an

---

expectorant. It also contains anti-arrhythmic properties but is of limited use because large doses can also cause arrhythmias. Marrubin acid, derived from marrubin, stimulates bile secretion. An aqueous extract from horehound may have antagonistic activities toward serotonin. The horehound extract has hypoglycemic effects.

## USES
Used to treat acute or chronic bronchitis, whooping cough, and sore throat. Used as an expectorant for treating nonproductive coughs and as a digestive aid. Horehound also may be used for its transient bile secretion-stimulant properties.

## DOSAGE & ADMINISTRATION
*Dried herbs:* 1 to 2 g P.O. t.i.d. as an infusion. Prepared by pouring boiling water over 1 to 2 g of the herb and straining after 10 minutes.
*Liquid extract (1:1 preparation in 20% alcohol):* 2 to 4 ml P.O. t.i.d.
*Oral use:* Average daily dose is 4.5 g of the herb; 30 to 60 ml of the pressed juice.

## ADVERSE REACTIONS
**CV:** *arrhythmias.*
**GI:** diarrhea.
**Metabolic:** hypoglycemia.
**Skin:** contact dermatitis.

## INTERACTIONS
**Herb-drug.** *Antiarrhythmics, some antidepressants, antiemetics, and antimigraine drugs*: May potentiate the serotonergic effects when used with horehound. Advise patient to use cautiously.

*Antidiabetics and insulin:* Enhanced hypoglycemic effects. Monitor serum glucose level.

## CAUTIONS
Patients with arrhythmias or diabetes mellitus and patients who are pregnant or breast-feeding should avoid use.
   Patients with CV disease should use cautiously.

## NURSING CONSIDERATIONS
• Find out why patient is using the herb.
• Medicinal use isn't recommended. The FDA banned the use of horehound in the preparation of OTC cough remedies because of unconvincing evidence to support its effectiveness; however, horehound preparation is still available in sore throat products.
• Herb may interfere with the intended therapeutic effect of conventional drugs.
• Monitor serum glucose level.
• Monitor heart rate and rhythm.
• Monitor for changes in bowel habits.

### Patient teaching
• Advise patient to consult with his health care provider before using an herbal preparation because a treatment with proven efficacy may be available.
• Tell patient to remind pharmacist of any herbal or dietary supplement that he's taking, when filling a new prescription.
• Warn patient not to treat chronic cough and dyspepsia before seeking appropriate medical evaluation because doing so may delay diag-

nosis of a potentially serious medical condition.

• If patient has diabetes or cardiac problems, advise him not to use this herb.

• Advise patient to use less or to stop using horehound if he experiences upset stomach or diarrhea.

• Advise patient to seek medical help if cough doesn't improve significantly in 2 weeks, or if a cough brings up brown, black, or bloody phlegm.

• Warn patient to keep all herbal products away from children and pets.

## horse chestnut

*Aesculus hippocastanum,* buckeye, California buckeye, chestnut, Ohio buckeye, Spanish-chestnut

**Common trade names**
*Horse Chestnut (some products that contain varying amounts of horse chestnut include: Arthro-Therapy, Cell-U-Var Cream, Varicare, Varicosin, and VenoCare Ultra-Joint Response), Venastat*

**HOW SUPPLIED**
Available as capsules and as creams made from an aescin/cholesterol complex.
*Capsules (extract standardized for an aescin content of 16% to 21%):* 250 mg/300 mg

**ACTIONS & COMPONENTS**
Derived from the seeds and bark of the Aesculus tree. Aescin seems to provide some weak diuretic activity and may decrease the perme-

ability of venous capillaries. Also, it has a tonic effect on the veins and prevents collagen breakdown by inhibiting glycosaminoglycan hydrolases. Sterol content may have some anti-inflammatory activity. The toxic glycoside, aesculin, is a hydroxycoumarin with potential antithrombotic activity. However, the toxin is removed during preparation.

**USES**
Used to treat chronic venous insufficiency, varicose veins, leg pain, tiredness, tension, and leg swelling and edema. Extract is used as a conjunctive treatment for lymphedema, hemorrhoids, and enlarged prostate.

Horse chestnut has been used as an analgesic, anticoagulant, antipyretic, astringent, expectorant, and tonic. It has also been used to treat skin ulcers, phlebitis, leg cramps, cough, and diarrhea.

**DOSAGE & ADMINISTRATION**
*For symptomatic treatment of chronic venous insufficiency:* 250 mg P.O. q.d. to t.i.d. Some sources recommend taking 450 to 750 mg q.d. to decrease symptoms, and then decreasing dose to 175 to 350 mg q.d.
*Tincture formulation:* 1 to 4 ml P.O. t.i.d.

**ADVERSE REACTIONS**
**GI:** GI irritation, especially with immediate-release product.
**GU:** toxic nephropathy.
**Hepatic:** *hepatotoxicity.*
**Musculoskeletal:** calf cramps.

---

**Skin:** itching, skin cancer (topical skin cleansers).
**Other:** *anaphylaxis.*

## INTERACTIONS
**Herb-drug.** *Anticoagulants:* May increase anticoagulant effects with increased bleeding and bruising. Monitor PT and INR.
*Antidiabetic, insulin:* Increased hypoglycemic effects. Monitor serum glucose level.
*Drugs that are highly protein-bound:* Aescin binds to plasma proteins and may displace these drugs. Monitor for decreased clinical effect or toxicity.
**Herb-herb.** *Other herbs with anticoagulant or antiplatelet potential such as feverfew, garlic, ginkgo, and ginseng:* May increase anticoagulant effects with increased bleeding and bruising. Use together cautiously.
*Other herbs with hypoglycemic potential such as aconite, dong quai, and gotu kola:* Increased hypoglycemic effects. Monitor serum glucose level.

## CAUTIONS
The FDA considers whole horse chestnut to be an unsafe herb. Those with infectious or inflammatory GI conditions shouldn't use the herb because of the potential for GI tract irritation. Patients with severe renal or hepatic impairment, diabetic patients, and patients taking anticoagulants should also avoid the herb. Pregnant and breast-feeding women shouldn't use this herb either.

## NURSING CONSIDERATIONS
● Find out why patient is using the herb.
● The nuts, seeds, twigs, sprouts, and leaves of horse chestnut are poisonous. Standardized formulations remove most of the toxins and standardize the amount of aescin.
⚡ALERT: High doses and non-standardized forms can be lethal.
● Signs and symptoms of toxicity include loss of coordination, salivation, hemolysis, headache, dilated pupils, muscle twitching, seizures, vomiting, diarrhea, depression, paralysis, respiratory and cardiac failure, and death.
● Monitor patient for signs of toxicity and discontinue horse chestnut immediately if any occur.
● Monitor blood glucose level in patients taking antidiabetics for hypoglycemia.

**Patient teaching**
● Advise patient to consult with his health care provider before using an herbal preparation because a treatment with proven efficacy may be available.
● Tell patient to remind pharmacist of any herbal or dietary supplement that he's taking, when filling a new prescription.
● Inform patient that the FDA classifies horse chestnut as an unsafe herb and that deaths have occurred.
● Advise patient to use only a standardized extract containing 16% to 21% aescin, at recommended doses, and to discontinue use if he experiences signs of toxic reaction.

• Tell patient that this is only symptomatic treatment of chronic venous insufficiency and not a cure.

• Advise patient not to confuse horse chestnut with sweet chestnut, used as a food.

• Advise patient to keep the herb away from children. Consumption of amounts of leaves, twigs, and seeds equaling 1% of a child's weight may be lethal.

## horseradish

*Armoracia rusticana,* great raifort, mountain radish, pepperrot, red cole

**Common trade names**
*Horseradish*

## HOW SUPPLIED
Available as fresh or dried root, ointment with 2% mustard oil from pressed root, and tincture.

## ACTIONS & COMPONENTS
Topically, the mustard content irritates the skin and stimulates local blood flow, giving relief to minor muscle aches and inflamed joints or tissues. Both the mustard oil and the glucosinolate composition give the root its characteristic pungency, helping to decrease congestion and inflammation of the respiratory tract. Horseradish may also have some antimicrobial activity against both gram-negative and gram-positive bacteria.

## USES
Used orally to decrease sinus congestion, to relieve cough from congestion, and to treat edematous conditions; used as an adjunct for UTI and kidney stones. Used topically for respiratory congestion and minor muscle aches. Also used in foods as a flavoring agent.

## DOSAGE & ADMINISTRATION
*Oral use:* Typical doses range from 6 to 20 g q.d. of the root or equivalent preparations.
*Topical use:* Ointments contain a maximum of 2% mustard oil and are applied, as needed.

## ADVERSE REACTIONS
**EENT:** mucous membrane inflammation.
**GI:** GI irritation, abdominal pain, diarrhea, *bloody vomiting and diarrhea* with large doses.
**Metabolic:** decreased thyroid function.
**Skin:** skin irritation and blistering, topical allergic reaction.

## INTERACTIONS
**Herb-drug.** *Anticoagulants, antiplatelet drugs:* Increased bleeding tendencies. Monitor PT and INR.
*Levothyroxine or hypothyroid therapy:* Further decreased thyroid function. Monitor $T_4$ and thyroid-stimulating hormone and adjust drug dosages, as needed.
*NSAIDs:* May increase frequency of GI irritation in patients taking an NSAID. Advise patient to use together cautiously.

## CAUTIONS
Those with kidney inflammation should avoid use because of the herb's diuretic effect. Patients with infectious or inflammatory GI con-

ditions or stomach or intestinal ulcers and children younger than age 4 should avoid use. Pregnant patients should avoid taking large oral doses because of the toxic and irritating mustard oil components.

Patients with thyroid conditions and those taking an anticoagulant or an NSAID should use the herb cautiously.

**NURSING CONSIDERATIONS**
• Find out why patient is using the herb.
• Tincture doses taken regularly and in large amounts may have abortifacient effects.
• Before applying horseradish topically to a large area, the patient should test it on a small area first to see how he responds.

**Patient teaching**
• Advise patient to consult with his health care provider before using an herbal preparation because a treatment with proven efficacy may be available.
• Tell patient to remind pharmacist of any herbal or dietary supplement that he's taking, when filling a new prescription.
• If patient has hypothyroid disease, warn him about possible interaction with horseradish and any other plants from the cabbage family.
• Advise patient to stay within the recommended dose of 20 g per day and to take the herb with meals, to minimize GI irritation and upset.
• Tell patient to discontinue herb if he experiences adverse reactions such as GI irritation and pain.

• Warn patient to keep all herbal products away from children and pets.

## horsetail

*Equisetum arvense,* bottle-brush, corn horsetail, Dutch rushes, field horsetail, horsetail grass, horse willow, paddock-pipes, pewterwort, shave grass, toadpipe

**Common trade names**
*Alcohol Free Horsetail, Horsetail, Horsetail Grass, Springtime Horsetail, Wild Countryside*

**HOW SUPPLIED**
Available as dried extract in powdered form, dried or fresh stem of horsetail plant, infusion, liquid extract (1:1 in 25% alcohol),* and tea.

**ACTIONS & COMPONENTS**
Horsetail's mild diuretic action is probably the result of the equisetonin and flavonoid glycoside constituents. Horsetail also contains small amounts of pharmacologically active nicotine and inorganic silica components.

**USES**
Used orally to treat diuresis, edema, and general disturbances of the kidney and bladder. Used topically as supportive treatment for burns and wounds.

Horsetail has also been used to treat brittle fingernails, rheumatic diseases, gout, frostbite, and profuse menstruation.

## DOSAGE & ADMINISTRATION
*Diuresis:* 6 g of the dried stem P.O. q.d. with plenty of fluids; or 1 cup of tea made from the dried stem taken several times between meals; or 1 to 4 ml of liquid extract P.O. t.i.d.

*Infusion:* Prepared by placing 1.5 g of dried stem in 1 cup of water. May take 2 to 4 g P.O. q.d.

*Tea:* Prepared by pouring boiling water over 2 to 3 g of the herb, boiling for 5 minutes, and then straining after 10 to 15 minutes. To be consumed several times a day between meals.

*Topical support for burns or wounds:* Compress containing 10 g of stem/L of water.

## ADVERSE REACTIONS
**Metabolic:** electrolyte imbalance.
**Skin:** skin irritation from topical use.
**Other:** thiamine deficiency from long-term use; symptoms of nicotine poisoning and toxicity including nausea and vomiting, muscle weakness, abnormal pulse rate, fever, and ataxia.

## INTERACTIONS
**Herb-drug.** *Benzodiazepines, disulfiram, metronidazole:* May cause a disulfiram-like reaction. Advise patient to avoid using together.

*Digoxin:* May increase digitalis toxicity as a result of potassium loss with diuretic effect. Advise patient to avoid using together, if possible.

*Potassium-wasting drugs (including corticosteroids, diuretics, laxative stimulants):* May increase risk of hypokalemia. Advise patient to use together cautiously.

**Herb-herb.** *Licorice:* Overuse with horsetail may increase potassium depletion and risk of cardiac toxicity. Advise patient to avoid excessive use together.

**Herb-lifestyle.** *Alcohol:* Excessive alcohol use may lead to thiamine deficiency. Advise patient to avoid using horsetail.

## CAUTIONS
Pregnant patients, breast-feeding patients, those with impaired heart or kidney function, those with liver problems, those who are taking a cardiac glycoside, and those who have a history or potential of thiamine deficiency (for example, alcoholic patients) should avoid use.

## NURSING CONSIDERATIONS
• Find out why patient is using the herb.

⚡**ALERT:** The liquid extract contains 25% alcohol and so shouldn't be used with disulfiram, metronidazole, and benzodiazepines.

• Dosage varies with the formulation. The FDA lists horsetail on its "undetermined safety" list. Large amounts may cause a toxic reaction.

• The dried extract in powdered form is more concentrated than stem alone.

• Monitor serum potassium level.

• Assess patient for signs and symptoms of hypokalemia, including weakness, muscle flaccidity, and abnormal ECG results.

---

*Bold italic type* indicates that reaction may be life-threatening.

- Horsetail should be kept away from children because poisonings have occurred in those who have used the stems as blow guns or whistles.
- Herb should be used only for short-term effects because of potential for toxic reaction and thiamine depletion.

**Patient teaching**
- Advise patient to consult with his health care provider before using an herbal preparation because a treatment with proven efficacy may be available.
- Tell patient to remind pharmacist of any herbal or dietary supplement that he's taking, when filling a new prescription.
- Tell patient to limit his use of the herb to short-term use.
- Instruct patient to immediately stop taking the herb if he experiences signs or symptoms of nicotine toxicity—including muscle weakness, abnormal pulse rate, fever, ataxia, and cold extremities—or symptoms of potassium depletion—including muscle cramping, irritability, or weakness.
- If patient is pregnant or breastfeeding or if she's taking a potassium-wasting diuretic, a cardiac glycoside (Lanoxin), a corticosteroid, or licorice, advise her not to use the herb.

## hyssop

*Hyssopus officinalis*

**Common trade names**
*Hyssop, Hyssop Herb*

**HOW SUPPLIED**
Available as capsules and extracts.
*Capsules:* 445 mg
*Extract:* 0.03% dried plant

**ACTIONS & COMPONENTS**
Obtained from the dried aboveground parts including leaves and flowering tops of *H. officinalis.* The oil used in flavorings and extracts is also made from the aboveground parts of the plant.

The plant contains numerous components that make up the essential oil. One of the glycoside components, marrubiin, stimulates bronchiole secretions. Hyssop has strong antiviral effects, probably because of the caffeic acid, tannin, and high-molecular-weight components present. It may have some activity against HIV-1 replication and the herpes simplex virus.

**USES**
Used orally to treat upset stomach, liver and gallbladder complaints, indigestion, colds, fevers, respiratory and chest ailments, sore throat, asthma, urinary tract inflammation, gas, and colic. Also used as an expectorant and as an appetite and circulation stimulant.

Used topically in a salve or compress to treat skin irritations, burns, bruises, and frostbite. The oil is used as fragrance in soaps and perfumes.

Used in other foods and extracts and as a flavoring in alcoholic beverages, at a maximum level of 0.06% dried herb and 0.004% volatile oil. Also used in soaps and cosmetics.

*Liquid may contain alcohol.

## DOSAGE & ADMINISTRATION
*Capsules:* Two 445-mg capsules P.O. t.i.d.
*Extract:* 10 to 15 gtt in water P.O. b.i.d. to t.i.d.
*Tea:* To be gargled or consumed t.i.d., 1 to 2 tsp dried hyssop tops in 5 oz boiling water.

## ADVERSE REACTIONS
**CNS:** *tonic-clonic seizures, neurotoxicity.*
**GU:** uterine stimulation.

## INTERACTIONS
**Herb-drug.** *Anticonvulsants:* May counteract antiseizure effects. Advise patient to avoid using together.

## CAUTIONS
Pregnant patients should avoid use because of possible uterine stimulation leading to miscarriage and hemorrhaging. Children should avoid use because of reports that 2 to 3 gtt of volatile oil over several days may cause tonic-clonic seizures. Also, patients with seizure disorders shouldn't use hyssop.

## NURSING CONSIDERATIONS
- Find out why patient is using the herb.
- Only standardized dose forms should be used.
- Internal use of oil is associated with seizures and possible neurotoxicity.
- Herb may alter the intended therapeutic effect of conventional drugs.

## Patient teaching
- Advise patient to consult with his health care provider before using an herbal preparation because a treatment with proven efficacy may be available.
- Tell patient to remind pharmacist of any herbal or dietary supplement that he's taking, when filling a new prescription.
- If patient is pregnant or breast-feeding or is planning to become pregnant, advise her not to use this herb.
- Advise patient to use this herb only at the recommended dosages and to avoid long-term use.
- Inform patient that several other plants have variations of the name "hyssop"; however, these plants are not related to the genus *Hyssopus*.

---

*Bold italic type* indicates that reaction may be life-threatening.

# I

## Iceland moss

*Cetraria islandica,* eryngo-leaved liverwort, Iceland lichen, lichen

**Common trade names**
*Iceland Moss*

### HOW SUPPLIED
Available as dried whole plant of *C. islandica* and as powdered herb extracts*.

### ACTIONS & COMPONENTS
The mucilage components lichenin and isolichenin may have soothing effects on the oral and pharyngeal membranes. The bitter organic components may stimulate the appetite and promote gastric secretion.

### USES
Used to soothe oral and pharyngeal membranes, to relieve dry cough, to stimulate appetite, and to prevent infection, the common cold, dyspeptic complaints, and fevers.

The alcoholic extract is used as a flavoring agent in alcoholic beverages.

### DOSAGE & ADMINISTRATION
*For cough and sore throat:* Tea is prepared by simmering 1.5 to 3 g dried plant in 5 oz of boiling water, and then straining. Maximum dose of the extract is 4 to 6 g q.d. because of potential lead contamination.

### ADVERSE REACTIONS
**GI:** GI irritation.

### INTERACTIONS
**Herb-drug.** *Aspirin, NSAIDs:* May exacerbate irritation of the gastric mucosa by these medicines. Advise patient to use together cautiously.
*Oral drugs:* The fiber in Iceland moss can impair the absorption of oral drugs. Instruct patient to separate administration times by at least 2 hours.

### CAUTIONS
Patients with gastroduodenal ulcers or GI distress or disease should avoid use because of potential for mucosal irritation. Pregnant and breast-feeding patients should also avoid use because of potential lead contamination. Herb shouldn't be used in children.

### NURSING CONSIDERATIONS
• Find out why patient is using the herb.
• Warn patient not to treat symptoms of respiratory infection before seeking appropriate medical evaluation because doing so may delay diagnosis of a potentially serious medical condition.

### Patient teaching
• Advise patient to consult with his health care provider before using an herbal preparation because a treatment with proven efficacy may be available.

---

*Liquid may contain alcohol.

- Tell patient to remind pharmacist of any herbal or dietary supplement that he's taking, when filling a new prescription.
- Tell patient to only take recommended doses and to discontinue if he experiences any GI distress.
- Advise patient to take this herb at least 1 hour before or 2 hours after any other drugs.
- Inform patient that taking herb with food may help prevent GI upset.
- Advise patient not to delay treatment of an illness that doesn't respond after taking this herb.
- Warn patient to keep all herbal products away from children and pets.

## indigo

common indigo, Indian indigo, pigmentum indicum

**Common trade names**
*None known*

### HOW SUPPLIED
Available as the blue dye that's extracted from the leaves and branches of numerous species of *Indigofera* (for example, *I. tinctoria, I. suffruticosa, I. aspalathoides, I. spicata, I. enneaphylla*).

### ACTIONS & COMPONENTS
During fermentation of the leaves, indigo is derived from indican, a glucoside constituent of several *Indigofera* species. Little is known about the pharmacologic effects of the herb. Indigo has emetic, anti-inflammatory, and antipyretic properties.

### USES
Used as an emetic. *I. tinctoria*, in particular, is used to treat nematodal infections and malignancies of the ovaries or stomach.

In traditionalChinese medicine, herb was used to detoxify the liver and the blood, reduce inflammation and fever, and relieve pain. Throughout the world, indigo is still used commercially for dyeing wool and cotton.

### DOSAGE & ADMINISTRATION
Not well documented.

### ADVERSE REACTIONS
**EENT:** mild ocular irritation.
**Hepatic:** *hepatotoxicity.*

### INTERACTIONS
None reported.

### CAUTIONS
Pregnant patients should avoid use because some species of *Indigofera* have teratogenic effects; breast-feeding patients should also avoid use.

Any patient using indigo should use it cautiously because data regarding its effects are lacking.

### NURSING CONSIDERATIONS
- Find out why patient is using the herb.
- With the exception of *I. tinctoria*, many of the other *Indigofera* species are hepatotoxic. *I. spicata* has caused cleft palate and embryonic death.
- **ALERT:** Don't confuse this herb with false, wild, or bastard indigo (*Baptisia tinctoria*).

---

*Bold italic type* indicates that reaction may be life-threatening.

## Patient teaching
• Advise patient to consult with his health care provider before using an herbal preparation because a treatment with proven efficacy may be available.
• Tell patient to remind pharmacist of any herbal or dietary supplement that he's taking, when filling a new prescription.
• If patient is pregnant or breast-feeding, advise her not to use this herb.
• Advise patient to use this herbal product with caution because of the risk of liver toxicity.
• Warn patient to keep all herbal products away from children and pets.

## Irish moss

*Chondrus crispus,* carragennan, carragheen, carrahan, chondrus extract

**Common trade names**
*None known*

### HOW SUPPLIED
Available as dried jellied fruit, jellies, puddings, raw leaves, and teas.

### ACTIONS & COMPONENTS
Irish moss is obtained from the dried thallus of *C. crispus.* Considered to be a seaweed and consists of polysaccharides, vitamins, minerals, and iodine. The extract is known as carrageenin, a starchlike substance. This extract can be further differentiated into two types, k-carrageenin and l-carrageenin. The former type is the gelling fraction; the latter form is the non-gelling component.

The herb has expectorant, demulcent, anti-inflammatory, anticoagulant, antihypertensive, immunosuppressive, and antidiarrheal properties. Irish moss also interferes with the absorption of food. Irish moss may reduce serum cholesterol and possess antiviral activity.

### USES
Used to soothe irritating coughs that result from various respiratory infections and to produce bulky stools in patients with chronic diarrhea. Because of its demulcent properties, this herb is also used to treat gastritis and peptic ulcer disease. Used as a nutritional supplement to facilitate recuperation in those with debilitating diseases. Irish moss can also be found as an ingredient in weight-loss products.

Used as a skin softener in commercial cosmetic products and lotions. Used topically to treat anorectal symptoms.

In manufacturing, Irish moss can be used as a binder, emulsifier, thickener, and as a stabilizer in drugs, foods, and toothpaste.

### DOSAGE & ADMINISTRATION
*Decoction:* Prepared by boiling 1 oz of dried plant in 1 to 1½ pints of water for 10 to 15 minutes, and then straining. Dosage is 1 cup b.i.d. to t.i.d. Lemon, honey, ginger, or cinnamon may be added to enhance the flavor.

*Liquid may contain alcohol.

## ADVERSE REACTIONS
**CV:** bleeding, hypotension.
**GI:** cramping, diarrhea.
**Other:** infection.

## INTERACTIONS
**Herb-drug.** *Anticoagulants:* Increased risk of bleeding. Advise patient to avoid administering together.
*Antihypertensives:* Potentiated hypotensive effects of these drugs. Advise patient to use together cautiously.
*Drugs:* Irish moss may decrease the absorption of drugs. Advise patient to separate administration times by at least 2 hours.

## CAUTIONS
Pregnant or breast-feeding patients should avoid use. Infants shouldn't be given this herb because it may suppress the immune system.

Patients with underlying bleeding disorders or hypotension should use this herb cautiously.

## NURSING CONSIDERATIONS
• Find out why patient is using the herb.
• Monitor blood pressure regularly during the course of therapy. Patients should also be monitored for signs and symptoms of bleeding.
• In patients receiving warfarin, closely monitor PT and INR.

## Patient teaching
• Advise patient to consult with his health care provider before using an herbal preparation because a treatment with proven efficacy may be available.

• Tell patient to remind pharmacist of any herbal or dietary supplement that he's taking, when filling a new prescription.
• If patient is pregnant or breast-feeding, advise her not to use this herb.
• Tell patient to avoid taking Irish moss within 2 hours of other drugs.
• If patient is taking this herb with an antihypertensive, instruct him to notify his health care provider if he experiences dizziness, light-headedness, or syncope.
• If patient is using this herb to treat diarrhea, advise him to consult with his health care provider if the diarrhea persists for longer than 3 to 4 days.
• Warn patient to keep all herbal products out of the reach of children and pets.

---

# J

## jaborandi

*Pilocarpus microphyllus*, arruda brava, arruda do mato, jamguarandi, juarandi, maranhao jaborandi

**Common trade names**
*None known*

## HOW SUPPLIED
Obtained from dried leaves of *P. microphyllus.*

## ACTIONS & COMPONENTS
Contains volatile oils and three alkaloids: pilocarpine, isopilocarpine, and pilocarpidine. Pilocarpine, a parasympathomimetic, is the primary constituent and contributes to the herb's cholinergic properties, including salivation, perspiration, miosis, and increased GI tract motility.

## USES
Previously used to induce sweating and diarrhea. Currently used to produce pilocarpine, and approved by the FDA for treating glaucoma.

## DOSAGE & ADMINISTRATION
Oral use of jaborandi is unsafe. Pilocarpine, a jaborandi constituent, is commercially available by prescription as an ophthalmic solution in various strengths.

## ADVERSE REACTIONS
**CNS:** *seizures*.
**CV:** *bradycardia, cardiac arrest,* hypotension.
**GI:** nausea, vomiting, diarrhea.

**Respiratory:** *bronchospasm,* dyspnea.
**Other:** increased sweating, hypersalivation.

## INTERACTIONS
None reported.

## CAUTIONS
Because jaborandi has teratogenic effects and promotes uterine stimulation, pregnant women shouldn't use it. Breast-feeding women should avoid it, as well.

## NURSING CONSIDERATIONS
● Find out why patient is using the herb.
● Patients with cardiac and circulatory diseases are particularly sensitive to adverse CV reactions.
● Because of potential toxicity, jaborandi isn't recommended for oral or topical use.
● Symptoms of toxicity can develop after ingestion of 60 mg or more of jaborandi, which is equivalent to 5 to 10 mg of pilocarpine.
⚡ALERT: Contact the health care provider if patient shows signs and symptoms of toxicity: bradycardia, bronchospasm, cardiac arrest, seizures, hypotension, dyspnea, nausea, vomiting, diarrhea, increased sweating, and hypersalivation. If toxicity develops, prepare for gastric lavage followed by administration of activated charcoal and atropine. Expect to give diazepam if seizures develop. Give I.V. fluids as directed if hypotension occurs.

Patient also may undergo hemodialysis.

• Don't confuse this herbal product with *P. jaborandi* (Pernambuco jaborandi) or *P. pennatifolius* (Paraguay jaborandi).

**Patient teaching**

• Advise patient to consult with his health care provider before using an herbal preparation because a treatment with proven efficacy may be available.

• Tell patient to remind pharmacist of any herbal and dietary supplements that he's taking, when filling a new prescription.

• Because of the risk of toxicity, warn patient to avoid using jaborandi.

• Advise pregnant and breast-feeding patients to avoid using this herb.

• Warn patient not to take herb before seeking medical attention because doing so may delay diagnosis of a potentially serious medical condition.

## Jamaican dogwood

*Piscidia piscipula*, dogwood, fishfuddle, fish poison bark, fish poison tree, Jamaica dogwood, West Indian dogwood

**Common trade names**
*None known*

**HOW SUPPLIED**
Obtained from the root bark of *P. piscipula* or *P. communis*. Available as dried bark and liquid extract.

**ACTIONS & COMPONENTS**
Jamaican dogwood contains isoflavones, organic acids, ichthynone, rotenones, and tannins. Both rotenone and ichthynone have produced toxic effects; rotenone may be carcinogenic. The liquid extract possesses sedative, hypnotic, antitussive, antipyretic, anti-inflammatory, and antispasmodic properties.

**USES**
Used for anxiety, neuralgia, migraines, insomnia, and dysmenorrhea.

**DOSAGE & ADMINISTRATION**
Because of its rotenone and ichthynone components, this herb is toxic and should be avoided. Root bark and liquid extract are no longer used.

**ADVERSE REACTIONS**
**CNS:** numbness, tremors.
**GI:** salivation.
**Skin:** sweating.

**INTERACTIONS**
**Herb-drug.** *CNS depressants:* May enhance sedative effects. Advise patient to avoid using together.
**Herb-herb.** *Herbs with sedative properties such as calamus, calendula, California poppy, capsicum, catnip, celery, couch grass, elecampane, goldenseal, gotu kola, hops, kava-kava, lemon balm, sage, sassafras, shepherd's purse, Siberian ginseng, skullcap, St. John's wort, valerian, wild lettuce, and yerba maté:* Possible enhanced sedation. Advise patient to avoid using together.

---

***Bold italic type*** indicates that reaction may be life-threatening.

## CAUTIONS
Children shouldn't use Jamaican dogwood because neuromuscular depressant effects are potentiated in this age group. Pregnant and breast-feeding patients should avoid use, as well.

## NURSING CONSIDERATIONS
• Find out why patient is using the herb.

⚠**ALERT:** Patients should avoid Jamaican dogwood because of its potential toxicity and the lack of data regarding its efficacy. Suspect toxicity and contact the health care provider if patient complains of numbness, tremors, salivation, and sweating.

• Geriatric patients are more sensitive to this herb's toxic effects.
• Don't confuse this herbal product with American dogwood *(Cornus florida)*.

### Patient teaching
• Advise patient to consult with his health care provider before using an herbal preparation because a treatment with proven efficacy may be available.
• Tell patient to remind pharmacist of any herbal and dietary supplements that he's taking, when filling a new prescription.
• Advise patients to avoid this herbal product because of the risk of toxicity.
• Warn patient not to take herb for anxiety, migraine, or insomnia before seeking medical attention because doing so may delay diagnosis of a potentially serious medical condition.

• Warn patient to keep all herbal products away from children and pets.

## jambolan

*Syzygium cumini, Syzygium cumini* semen (seed), jambul, jamum, java plum, rose apple

**Common trade names**
*None known*

## HOW SUPPLIED
Derived from dried bark and seeds of *S. cumini* or *S. jambolana.* Available as dried bark, powdered seeds, and liquid extract.

## ACTIONS & COMPONENTS
Bark contains gallic and ellagic acid derivatives, flavonoids, and tannins. Tannins in the bark cause astringent effects. Bark also has antibacterial, hypoglycemic, and sedative activity. Seeds contain fatty oils and tannins and possess hypoglycemic, anti-inflammatory, antipyretic, antispasmodic, sedative, tonic, antidepressant, and aphrodisiac properties.

## USES
Jambolan bark is taken orally for nonspecific acute diarrhea. It's also applied to the skin, mouth, or pharynx to decrease mild inflammation. The bark has been used to treat bronchitis, asthma, and dysentery through oral administration, and for ulcers through topical application.

Jambolan seed is used for diabetes, flatulence, constipation, pancreatic and gastric disorders, muscle spasms, fatigue, depression, and anxiety. The seed is also used as an aphrodisiac or diuretic. In India, jambolan seed is used to manage diabetes-induced polydipsia.

## DOSAGE & ADMINISTRATION
*Dried bark:* 3 to 6 g P.O. q.d.
*Liquid extract containing jambolan seed:* 4 to 8 ml P.O. q.d.
*Powdered seeds:* 0.3 to 2 g P.O. q.d.
*Tea:* Prepared by simmering 1 to 2 tsp of dried bark in 5 oz of boiling water for 5 to 10 minutes, and then straining before use.
*Topical:* A warm compress is made from jambolan bark tea.

## ADVERSE REACTIONS
**Metabolic:** hypoglycemia.

## INTERACTIONS
**Herb-drug.** *Insulin, oral hypoglycemics:* Jambolan seed may enhance hypoglycemic effects. Monitor blood glucose level closely.

## CAUTIONS
Pregnant and breast-feeding patients should avoid use because herb's effects are unknown.

Diabetic patients should use jambolan seed cautiously because no data exist to support its use.

## NURSING CONSIDERATIONS
• Find out why patient is using the herb.
• Although no known chemical interactions have been reported in clinical studies, advise patient that the herb may interfere with the therapeutic effect of conventional drugs.
• Monitor blood glucose level closely in diabetic patients who use

jambolan seed because it may cause hypoglycemia.

## Patient teaching
• Advise patient to consult with his health care provider before using an herbal preparation because a treatment with proven efficacy may be available.
• Tell patient to remind pharmacist of any herbal and dietary supplements that he's taking, when filling a new prescription.
• Advise patient taking jambolan seed for diabetes that other drugs of known efficacy and safety are available.
• Instruct diabetic patients to routinely monitor their blood glucose level if they take jambolan seed.
• Advise patient to consult with his health care provider if diarrhea persists for longer than 3 or 4 days.
• Inform pregnant and breast-feeding patients to avoid using this herb.
• Warn patient not to take herb for a GI disorder before seeking medical attention because doing so may delay diagnosis of a potentially serious medical condition.

## jimson weed

*Datura stramonium*, datura, devil's apple, devil's trumpet, Jamestown weed, mad-apple, nightshade, Peru-apple, stinkweed, stinkwort, Stramonium, thorn-apple

**Common trade names**
*None known*

---

*Bold italic type* indicates that reaction may be life-threatening.

## HOW SUPPLIED
Most commonly used as dried leaves, with or without tips of flowering branches. Also used as ripe seeds and flowers without leaves. Seeds are small, long, flat, and dark yellow to brown.

## ACTIONS & COMPONENTS
Primary action is anticholinergic caused by 0.1% to 0.6% atropine, hyoscyamine, and scopolamine. All parts of the plant contain these compounds, but highest concentration is in the seeds. Anticholinergic levels in other plant parts vary from year to year and from plant to plant. The alkaloids are readily absorbed across GI mucous membranes and across the respiratory tract. Anticholinergic effects usually occur within 60 minutes and may last 24 to 48 hours because of impaired GI motility.

## USES
Used to treat asthma and cough from bronchitis or influenza, usually by smoking cigarettes made from the leaves. Also used to treat disorders of the autonomic nervous system. Little data exist to support routine therapeutic use of jimson weed.

Illicitly, the seeds have been chewed, the leaves smoked as cigarettes, and a tea brewed and ingested to cause hallucinations and euphoria.

## DOSAGE & ADMINISTRATION
Not well documented.

## ADVERSE REACTIONS
**CNS:** headache, confusion, hallucinations, agitation, emotional lability, motor incoordination, restlessness, *seizures,* loss of consciousness, hyperthermia.
**CV:** tachycardia, hypertension leading to hypotension, *arrhythmias.*
**EENT:** dilated pupils, blurred vision, photophobia, dry mucous membranes.
**GI:** nausea, vomiting, decreased GI tract motility, excessive thirst.
**GU:** urine retention.
**Respiratory:** tachypnea, *respiratory depression, respiratory arrest.*
**Skin:** dry, flushed skin.

## INTERACTIONS
**Herb-drug.** *Anticholinergics, such as amantadine; antihistamines, such as diphenhydramine; atropine; phenothiazines, such as prochlorperazine and promethazine; tricyclic antidepressants, such as amitriptyline and imipramine; scopolamine:* Additive effects. Advise patient to avoid using together.
**Herb-herb.** *Deadly nightshade:* Additive anticholinergic toxicity. Advise patient to avoid using together.

## CAUTIONS
Women who are pregnant or breastfeeding should avoid use. Those with glaucoma, BPH, urine retention, tachycardia, or hypersensitivity to herb should also avoid use.

## NURSING CONSIDERATIONS
• Find out why patient is using the herb.
• Listed as an unsafe herb by the FDA. Not recommended for routine therapeutic use.
▨ ALERT: Fatal poisonings resulting from respiratory depression

---

and circulatory collapse have been reported from adult doses equal to 10 mg of atropine (15 to 100 g of dried leaves or about 100 [15 to 25 g] seeds). Fatal doses in children may be much smaller.

• Don't confuse this herb with deadly nightshade *(Atropa belladonna),* which has similar effects.

• Although no known chemical interactions have been reported in clinical studies, advise patient that herb may interfere with therapeutic effects of conventional drugs.

• Monitor patient for signs and symptoms of anticholinergic toxicity: mydriasis, blurred vision, photophobia, tachycardia, hypertension or hypotension, confusion, agitation, hallucinations, and motor incoordination.

• Avoid using sedatives or phenothiazines to treat toxicity because they may have additive anticholinergic effects.

• The antidote for anticholinergic toxicity is physostigmine. To avoid profound cholinergic effects, use it only for severe toxicity, including seizures, severe hypertension, severe hallucinations, arrhythmias, or life-threatening respiratory depression.

**Patient teaching**
• Advise patient to consult with his health care provider before using an herbal preparation because a treatment with proven efficacy may be available.

• Tell patient to remind pharmacist of any herbal and dietary supplements that he's taking, when filling a new prescription.

• Warn patient that herb isn't recommended for routine therapeutic use.

• Tell patient to report signs and symptoms of anticholinergic toxicity: dilated pupils, impaired vision, dry mouth, heart palpitations, dizziness, confusion, hallucinations, and incoordination.

• Warn patient to keep all herbal products away from children and pets.

## jojoba

*Simmondsia californica, S. chinesis,* deernut, goatnut, pignut

**Common trade names**
*None known*

**HOW SUPPLIED**
Available as soap, shampoo, conditioner, and other skin care products.
*Shampoos and conditioners:* 1% to 2%
*Skin care products:* 5% to 10%
*Soaps:* 0.5% to 3%

**ACTIONS & COMPONENTS**
Wax (commonly called oil) from the seeds is odorless and colorless to light yellow. It readily penetrates the skin. Taken orally, it's absorbed, not digested, and stored in intestinal and liver cells. The oil contains 14% erucic acid, which in higher doses has been reported to cause myocardial fibrosis. Seeds are dark brown, about the size of coffee beans or peanuts.

---

*Bold italic type* indicates that reaction may be life-threatening.

## USES
Used topically to treat acne, psoriasis, and sunburn. Also used to unclog hair follicles in the scalp, preventing buildup of sebum, which is believed to contribute to hair loss.

Commonly used in shampoos, conditioners, cosmetics, lotions, sunscreens, and cleaning products. Used as an industrial lubricant because it doesn't break down at high temperatures.

## DOSAGE & ADMINISTRATION
No information available.

## ADVERSE REACTIONS
**Skin:** contact dermatitis (with shampoos, hair conditioners, and pure oil application).

## INTERACTIONS
None reported.

## CAUTIONS
Contraindicated in patients hypersensitive to herb.

## NURSING CONSIDERATIONS
• Find out why patient is using the herb.
• Minimal toxicity reported, particularly after topical application.
• Symptoms of contact dermatitis include itching, erythema, and occasional vesicle formation.
• Herb shouldn't be taken orally because of inadequate information.
• No routine monitoring after topical application is needed.

### Patient teaching
• Advise patient to consult with his health care provider before using an herbal preparation because a treatment with proven efficacy may be available.
• Tell patient to remind pharmacist of any herbal and dietary supplements that he's taking, when filling a new prescription.
• Warn patient to avoid taking the herb orally.
• Tell patient to report any skin irritation from jojoba-containing products.
• Teach proper skin care for the prevention of acne.
• Teach patient to avoid excessive sun exposure.

## juniper

*Baccae juniperi, Juniperi fructus, Juniperus communis,* enebro, Genievre, ginepro, juniper berry, Wacholderbeeren, zimbro

**Common trade names**
*Euro Quality Juniper Berries, Juniper, Juniper Berry. Also numerous combination products.*

## HOW SUPPLIED
Available as ripe berry, also called *berry-like cones* or *mature female cones,* fresh or dried. Also available as powder, tea, tincture*, oil*, or liquid extract*. Immature berries are green, taking 2 to 3 years to ripen to a purplish blue-black.

## ACTIONS & COMPONENTS
Active component is a volatile oil, which is 0.2% to 3.4% of the berry. The best described effect is diuresis caused by terpinene-4-ol, which results from a direct irrita-

*Liquid may contain alcohol.

tion to the kidney, leading to increased GFR.

Other reported effects of juniper are hypoglycemia, hypotension or hypertension, anti-inflammatory and antiseptic effects, and stimulation of uterine activity leading to decreased implantation and increased abortifacient effects.

## USES
Used to treat UTI and kidney stones. Also used as a carminative and for multiple nonspecific GI tract disorders, including dyspepsia, flatulence, colic, heartburn, anorexia, and inflammatory GI disorders.

The herb is applied topically to treat small wounds and relieve muscle and joint pain caused by rheumatism. It's inhaled as steam to treat bronchitis. The oil is used as a fragrance in many soaps and cosmetics. It's the principal flavoring agent in gin, as well as some bitters and liqueurs.

As a food, maximum flavoring concentrations are 0.01% of the extract or 0.006% of the volatile oil. At these concentrations, neither therapeutic nor adverse effects should be experienced.

## DOSAGE & ADMINISTRATION
The patient shouldn't take juniper preparations for longer than 4 weeks.
*Dried ripe berries:* 1 to 2 g P.O. t.i.d. Maximum, 10 g dried berry q.d., equaling 20 to 100 mg essential oil.
*Liquid extract (1:1 in 25% alcohol):* 2 to 4 ml P.O. t.i.d.
*Oil (1:5 in 45% alcohol):* 0.03 to 0.2 ml P.O. t.i.d.

*Tea:* Prepared by placing 1 tbs crushed berries in 5 oz boiling water, steeping 10 minutes, then straining. Taken t.i.d.
*Tincture (1:5 in 45% alcohol):* 1 to 2 ml P.O. t.i.d.

## ADVERSE REACTIONS
**CNS:** *seizures.*
**GI:** local irritation.
**GU:** *kidney failure.*
**Skin:** local irritation.

## INTERACTIONS
**Herb-drug.** *Antidiabetics, such as chlorpropamide, glipizide, and glyburide:* May potentiate hypoglycemic effects. Monitor patient closely.
*Antihypertensives:* May interfere with blood pressure. Monitor patient closely.
*Diuretics:* May potentiate the effects of diuretics such as furosemide, leading to additive hypokalemia. Monitor potassium levels frequently.
*Disulfiram:* Disulfiram-like reaction could occur because of alcohol content of the herb. Advise patient to avoid using together.
**Herb-herb.** *Asian ginseng, dandelion, fenugreek, Siberian ginseng:* Possible additive hypoglycemic effects with other herbs that lower blood glucose level. Monitor blood glucose level closely.
*Cowslip, cucumber, dandelion, horsetail:* May have additive effects with other herbs causing diuresis. Monitor patient closely.
**Herb-lifestyle.** *Alcohol:* Various preparations are made with alcohol; additive effects may occur.

---

*Bold italic type* indicates that reaction may be life-threatening.

Advise patient to avoid using together.

**CAUTIONS**

Women who are pregnant or breast-feeding should avoid this herb because of its uterine stimulant and abortifacient properties. Juniper shouldn't be used by those with renal insufficiency, inflammatory disorders of the GI tract (such as Crohn's disease), seizure disorders, or known hypersensitivity. It shouldn't be used topically on large ulcers or wounds because it may cause local irritation.

**NURSING CONSIDERATIONS**

- Find out why patient is using the herb.
- Juniper should be used cautiously by patients with urinary problems, bronchitis, and GI disorders.

⚡**ALERT:** Kidney damage may occur in patients taking juniper for extended periods. This effect may stem from prolonged kidney irritation caused by terpinene-4-ol or by turpentine oil contamination of juniper products.

- Overdose may cause seizures, tachycardia, hypertension, and renal failure with albuminuria, hematuria, and purplish urine. Monitor blood pressure and potassium, BUN, creatinine, and blood glucose level.
- Don't confuse with *cade oil*, derived from juniper wood.

**Patient teaching**

- Advise patient to consult with his health care provider before using an herbal preparation because a treatment with proven efficacy may be available.

- Tell patient to remind pharmacist of any herbal and dietary supplements that he's taking, when filling a new prescription.
- Advise women to report planned or suspected pregnancy before using this herb.
- Warn patient not to use herb for longer than 4 weeks.
- Inform patient that urine may turn purplish with higher doses.
- Tell patient to avoid applying to large ulcers or wounds because local irritation (burning, blistering, redness, and edema) may occur.
- Caution patient against using alcohol while taking this herb.
- Recommend that patient seek medical diagnosis before taking juniper. Unadvised use of juniper could worsen urinary problems, bronchitis, GI disorders, and other conditions if medical diagnosis and proper treatment are delayed.

---

*Liquid may contain alcohol.

# K

## karaya gum

*Sterculia tragacanth, S. urens,
S. villosa,* Bassora tragacanth,
Indian tragacanth, kadaya,
karaya, kullo, mucara, Sterculia
gum

**Common trade names**
*None known*

### HOW SUPPLIED
Soft gum obtained from *Sterculia,*
a softwood tree cultivated in India
and Pakistan. Available as a dry
powder or paste.

### ACTIONS & COMPONENTS
Absorbs more than 100 times its
weight in water. Forms a viscous
solution in low concentrations in
water and a gel or paste in higher
concentrations. When taken orally,
it isn't digested or systemically absorbed. In the GI tract, it acts as a
bulk-forming laxative to stimulate
peristalsis.

Dried bark may have astringent
properties. Paste is reputedly antibacterial when applied topically
to wounds.

### USES
Used industrially as a thickener in
pharmaceuticals, cosmetics, hair-
sprays, lotions, and denture adhesives. Herb is also used as a binder
or stabilizer in foods and beverages. Used orally as bulk-forming
laxative akin to psyllium. Applied
topically as powder or paste to
treat pressure sores or care for
ileostomies or colostomies.

### DOSAGE & ADMINISTRATION
No information available for use as
a bulk laxative. Herb is generally
recognized as safe for ingestion as
a food additive.

### ADVERSE REACTIONS
**GI:** constipation, abdominal distention, bloating.
**Respiratory:** dyspnea, cough,
wheezing.

### INTERACTIONS
**Herb-drug.** *Oral drugs:* May decrease absorption. Advise patient
to separate administration times.

### CAUTIONS
Patients with bowel obstruction
should avoid using karaya or any
other bulk-forming laxative.

### NURSING CONSIDERATIONS
• Find out why patient is using the
herb.
• No information is available on
use by pregnant or breast-feeding
women.
• As with other bulk-forming laxatives, karaya gum may decrease absorption of drugs taken together.
This effect should be clinically in-
significant with amounts found in
food and pharmaceuticals.
• To maximize laxative effect, patient needs adequate fluid intake.
• May cause pain when applied
topically to wounds.

## Patient teaching

- Advise patient to consult with his health care provider before using an herbal preparation because a treatment with proven efficacy may be available.
- Tell patient to remind pharmacist of any herbal and dietary supplements that he's taking, when filling a new prescription.
- Encourage adequate fluid intake, and teach patient about increasing fiber in his diet.
- Instruct patient to separate intake of oral drugs by 2 hours.

## kava-kava

*Piper methysticum,* ava, awa, kava, kew, sakau, tonga, yagona

### Common trade names
*Contained in a variety of products including, but not limited to, the following: Alcohol-Free Kava-Kava, Kavacin, Kava Kava Plus, Kava Kava Root, Kava Tone, St. John's Plus Kava Kava, and Standardized Kava Extract*

### HOW SUPPLIED
Obtained from dried rhizome and root of *Piper methysticum,* a member of the black pepper family (Piperaceae). Available as capsules, soft gel caps, liquid spray, Veggie-Capsules, and tea bags.

### ACTIONS & COMPONENTS
The herb contains seven major and several minor kava lactones, both aqueous and lipid soluble. Pharmacologic effects result from lipid-soluble lactones. Their mechanism of action differs from that of benzodiazepines and opiate-agonists. Kava-kava affects the limbic system, modulating emotional processes to produce anxiolytic effects. Kava lactones inhibit MAO type B, producing psychotropic effects. They also inhibit voltage-gated calcium and sodium channels, producing anticonvulsant and skeletal muscle relaxant effects. The kava lactone kawain inhibits cyclooxygenase and thromboxane synthase, producing antithrombotic effects on human platelets.

### USES
Used to treat nervous anxiety, stress, and restlessness. It's used orally to produce sedation, to promote wound healing, and to treat headaches, seizure disorders, the common cold, respiratory tract infection, tuberculosis, and rheumatism. It's also used to treat urogenital infections, including chronic cystitis, venereal disease, uterine inflammation, menstrual problems, and vaginal prolapse. Some herbal practitioners consider kava-kava an aphrodisiac. Kava juice is used to treat skin diseases, including leprosy. It's also used as a poultice for intestinal problems, otitis, and abscesses.

### DOSAGE & ADMINISTRATION
*Anxiety:* 50 to 70 mg purified kava lactones t.i.d., equivalent to 100 to 250 mg of dried kava root extract per dose. (By comparison, the traditional bowl of raw kava beverage contains about 250 mg of kava lactones.)

---

*Bold italic type* indicates that reaction may be life-threatening.

*Restlessness:* 180 to 210 mg of kava lactones taken as a tea 1 hour before h.s. The typical dose in this form is 1 cup t.i.d. Prepared by simmering 2 to 4 g of the root in 5 oz boiling water for 5 to 10 minutes and then straining.

## ADVERSE REACTIONS

**CNS:** mild euphoric changes characterized by feelings of happiness, fluent and lively speech, and increased sensitivity to sounds; morning fatigue.
**EENT:** visual accommodation disorders, pupil dilation, and disorders of oculomotor equilibrium.
**GI:** mild GI disturbances, mouth numbness.
**GU:** hematuria.
**Hematologic:** increased RBC count, decreased platelets and lymphocytes.
**Respiratory:** pulmonary hypertension.
**Skin:** scaly rash.
**Other:** reduced levels of albumin, total protein, bilirubin and urea; increased HDL cholesterol level.

## INTERACTIONS

**Herb-drug.** *Antiplatelet drugs, MAO type B inhibitors:* Possible additive effects. Monitor patient closely.
*Barbiturates, benzodiazepines:* Kava lactones potentiate the effects of CNS depressants, leading to toxicity. Advise patient to avoid using together.
*Levodopa:* Possible reduced effectiveness of levodopa therapy in patients with Parkinson's disease, apparently because of dopamine antagonism. Advise patient to use cautiously.
**Herb-herb.** *Calamus, calendula, California poppy, capsicum, catnip, celery, couch grass, elecampane, German chamomile, goldenseal, gotu kola, hops, Jamaican dogwood, lemon balm, sage, sassafras, shepherd's purse, Siberian ginseng, skullcap, stinging nettle, St. John's wort, valerian, wild lettuce, yerba maté:* Additive sedative effects may occur. Monitor patient closely.
**Herb-lifestyle.** *Alcohol:* Increased risk of CNS depression and liver damage. Warn patient to avoid using together.

## CAUTIONS

Patients hypersensitive to kava-kava or any of its components should avoid this herb. Depressed patients should avoid the herb because of possible sedative activity; those with endogenous depression should avoid it because of possible increased risk of suicide. Pregnant women should avoid the herb because of possible loss of uterine tone; those who are breast-feeding should also avoid it. Children younger than age 12 shouldn't use this herb.

## NURSING CONSIDERATIONS

• Find out why patient is using the herb.
• Patient shouldn't use kava with conventional sedative-hypnotics, anxiolytics, MAO inhibitors, other psychopharmacologic drugs, levodopa, or antiplatelet drugs without first consulting a health care provider.

---

*Liquid may contain alcohol.

• Adverse effects of kava-kava are mild at suggested dosages. They may occur at start of therapy but are transient.
• Oral use is probably safe for 3 months or less; use for longer than 3 months may be habit forming.
• Kava-kava can cause drowsiness and may impair motor reflexes.
• Patients should avoid taking herb with alcohol because of increased risk of CNS depression and liver damage.
• Periodic monitoring of liver function tests and CBC may be needed.
• Heavy kava-kava users are more likely to complain of poor health: 20% are underweight with reduced levels of albumin, total protein, bilirubin, urea, platelets, and lymphocytes; increased HDL cholesterol and RBCs; hematuria; puffy faces; scaly rashes; and some evidence of pulmonary hypertension. These symptoms resolve several weeks after the herb is stopped. Toxic doses can cause progressive ataxia, muscle weakness, and ascending paralysis, all of which resolve when herb is stopped. Extreme use (more than 300 g per week) may increase gamma-glutamyl transferase levels.

**Patient teaching**
• Advise patient to consult with his health care provider before using an herbal preparation because a treatment with proven efficacy may be available.
• Tell patient to remind pharmacist of any herbal and dietary supplements that he's taking, when filling a new prescription.

• Encourage patients to seek medical diagnosis before taking kava-kava.
• Advise patient that usual doses can affect motor function; caution him against performing hazardous activities.
• Tell patient oral use is probably safe for 3 months or less, but use for longer than 3 months may be habit forming.
• Warn patient to avoid taking herb with alcohol because of increased risk of CNS depression and liver damage.

## kelp

*Laminariae stipites,* seaweed, tangleweed

**Common trade names**
*Kelp, Kelp Liquid, Kelp Norwegian. Contained in a variety of products including, but not limited to, the following: Activex 40 Plus, Cellbloc, Fat-Solv, Herbal Diuretic Complex, Kelp Plus 3, Plantiodine Plus, PMT Complex, Vitaforce 21-Plus, and Vitaforce Forti-Plus*

**HOW SUPPLIED**
Kelp is a dried preparation of various species of seaweed. It's also an ingredient of several dietary supplements and herbal preparations.

**ACTIONS & COMPONENTS**
Not well defined.

**USES**
Used for regulating thyroid function, for goiter, as a bulk laxative, and for obesity. Also used as an iodine source.

---

*Bold italic type* indicates that reaction may be life-threatening.

**DOSAGE & ADMINISTRATION**
Not well documented.

**ADVERSE REACTIONS**
**CNS:** restlessness, insomnia.
**CV:** palpitations.
**Metabolic:** hyperthyroidism.
**Other:** allergic reaction.

**INTERACTIONS**
**Herb-drug.** *Diuretics:* Possible decreased effectiveness of diuretics caused by high sodium content. Monitor diuretic response closely.
*Iron:* Prolonged ingestion can reduce iron absorption. Monitor patient closely.
*Lithium:* Possible enhanced hypothyroid activity caused by high iodine content. Monitor patient for evidence of hypothyroidism.
*Thyroid hormone:* May interfere with thyroid hormone replacement therapy. Monitor patient for evidence of hypothyroidism.
**Herb-food.** *Foods high in iron:* Prolonged kelp ingestion can reduce iron absorption. Advise patient that iron replacement may be needed.

**CAUTIONS**
Patients hypersensitive to kelp or any of its components, including iodine, shouldn't use it. Children and women who are pregnant or breast-feeding should avoid kelp as well.

**NURSING CONSIDERATIONS**
• Find out why patient is using the herb.
• Kelp can worsen hyperthyroidism and acne. The high sodium content can worsen conditions that need sodium restriction. Because it in-

hibits iron absorption, kelp can worsen iron deficiency anemia. Kelp should be used cautiously by patients with hyperthyroidism, those who need sodium restriction, and those with iron deficiency anemia.
• Use of kelp has been linked to heavy metal poisoning.
• Kelp may increase serum thyroid-stimulating hormone level, $T_4$ level, and results of thyroid function tests using radioactive iodine uptake.
• Patients sensitive to iodine should avoid kelp.
• Toxicity may cause palpitations, restlessness, insomnia, and other changes.

**Patient teaching**
• Advise patient to consult with his health care provider before using an herbal preparation because a treatment with proven efficacy may be available.
• Tell patient to remind pharmacist of any herbal and dietary supplements that he's taking, when filling a new prescription.
• Encourage patient to seek medical diagnosis before taking kelp.
• Tell women to notify health care provider about suspected, planned, or known pregnancy if they take kelp.
• Caution patient to avoid kelp if he takes a diuretic, lithium, thyroid replacement hormones, anticoagulants, or an iron supplement.
• Warn patient to keep all herbal products away from children and pets.

## kelpware

*Fucus vesiculosus, Quercus marina,* black-tang, bladder focus, bladderwrack, blasentang, cutweed, fucus, knotted wrack, rockweed, rockwrack, seawrack, tang

**Common trade names**
*Contained in a variety of products including, but not limited to, the following: Advantage, Aqua Greens, Atkins Dieters Better Living Multi Vitamins, Daily Essentials, Doctor's Choice, Osteosupport*

### HOW SUPPLIED
Available as dried brown algae plant, liquid extract*, tablets, capsules, and soft gel caps.

### ACTIONS & COMPONENTS
Limited information is available for kelpware, but pharmacologic activities are recognized for the individual constituents and other brown seaweed species. Kelpware contains more than 600 mcg of iodine per gram of seaweed. A constituent, algin, has bulk laxative and soothing effects. An isolated fraction, fucoidin, has 40% to 50% of the anticoagulation activity of heparin. Live *Fucus* can concentrate heavy metals from sea water.

### USES
Used to treat thyroid disorders, iodine deficiency, lymphadenoid goiter, myxedema, obesity, arthritis, and rheumatism. Used for arteriosclerosis, digestive disorders, blood cleansing, constipation, bronchitis, emphysema, GU disorders, anxiety, skin diseases, burns, and insect bites.

### DOSAGE & ADMINISTRATION
*Dried plant:* Usual dose is 5 to 10 g P.O. t.i.d.
*Liquid extract:* Typical dose of liquid extract (1:1) is 4 to 8 ml P.O. t.i.d.
*Tea:* Prepared by soaking 5 to 10 g in 5 oz of boiling water for 5 to 10 minutes and then straining. Tea is taken t.i.d.

### ADVERSE REACTIONS
**CNS:** restlessness, insomnia.
**CV:** palpitations.
**Hematologic:** anemia.
**Metabolic:** hyperthyroidism or thyrotoxicosis.
**Skin:** acne.
**Other:** allergic reactions.

### INTERACTIONS
**Herb-drug.** *Diuretics:* Possible decrease in diuretic effectiveness because of high sodium content. Monitor diuretic response closely.
*Heparin, low-molecular-weight heparin, warfarin:* Increased risk of bleeding. Monitor INR, PT, and PTT closely.
*Iron preparations:* Prolonged kelpware ingestion can reduce iron absorption. Monitor patient closely.
*Lithium:* May enhance hypothyroid activity because of high iodine content. Monitor patient for signs of hypothyroidism.
*Thyroid hormone:* High iodine content may interfere with thyroid hormone replacement therapy. Monitor patient for signs of hypothyroidism.
**Herb-food.** *Foods high in iron:* Prolonged kelpware ingestion can

---

*Bold italic type* indicates that reaction may be life-threatening.

reduce iron absorption. Advise patient that iron replacement may be needed.

## CAUTIONS
Patients hypersensitive to kelpware or any of its components, including iodine, shouldn't use kelp. Kelpware should be used cautiously by patients with hyperthyroidism, those who need sodium restriction, and those with iron deficiency anemia. Children and women who are pregnant or breast-feeding should avoid using kelpware.

## NURSING CONSIDERATIONS
• Find out why patient is using the herb.
• Kelpware may increase PTT test results, serum thyroid-stimulating hormone level, $T_4$ level, and results of thyroid function tests that use radioactive iodine uptake.
• A case of heavy metal (arsenic) poisoning has been reported from ingestion of contaminated kelpware.
⚡ALERT: Signs and symptoms of toxicity include palpitations, restlessness, and insomnia.
• Don't confuse bladderwrack (kelpware) with bladderwort *(Utricularia)*, a freshwater pond plant.

### Patient teaching
• Advise patient to consult with his health care provider before using an herbal preparation because a treatment with proven efficacy may be available.
• Tell patient to remind pharmacist of any herbal and dietary supplements that he's taking, when filling a new prescription.
• Encourage patient to seek medical diagnosis before taking kelpware.
• Tell women to notify health care provider about planned, suspected, or known pregnancy.
• Caution patient to avoid using kelpware if he takes a diuretic, lithium, thyroid replacement hormones, an anticoagulant, or an iron supplement.

## khat

*Catha edulis,* Abyssinian tea, Arabian tea, chaat, gat, kat, Kus es Salahin, qut, Somali tea, tchaad, tohai, tohat, tschut

**Common trade names**
*None known*

## HOW SUPPLIED
Available as leaves wrapped in plastic, damp paper, or false banana leaves to avoid wilting and drying. Khat is a tree *(Catha edulis)* cultivated in southwestern Arabia and eastern Africa.

## ACTIONS & COMPONENTS
Contains mainly sympathomimetic alkaloids cathinone and cathine (norpseudoephedrine). Cathinone and cathine antagonize the actions of physostigmine, but not those of tubocurarine. Chewing khat causes psychotropic effects from amphetamine-like compounds, which interact with the dopaminergic pathway. Both cathinone and cathine decrease appetite and increase locomotor activity.

## USES
Leaf is used for treating depression, fatigue, obesity, and gastric ulcers. The leaf and stem are chewed by some people in East Africa and the Arabian countries as a euphoriant or appetite suppressant.

## DOSAGE & ADMINISTRATION
Usually, khat leaves are chewed and the juice is swallowed; the residues are kept in the cheek for up to 2 hours and then expectorated. Sometimes the chewed leaves are also swallowed. Occasionally, khat is brewed as a tea or crushed and mixed with honey to make a paste.

## ADVERSE REACTIONS
**CNS:** euphoria, increased alertness, garrulousness, hyperactivity, excitement, aggressiveness, anxiety, manic behavior, insomnia, malaise, lack of concentration, psychotic reactions, migraine, *cerebral hemorrhage.*
**CV:** tachycardia, palpitations, increased blood pressure, *MI,* pulmonary edema.
**EENT:** pupil dilation and decreased intraocular pressure.
**GI:** stomatitis, esophagitis, gastritis, constipation, periodontal disease, keratosis of the buccal mucosa.
**GU:** increased libido in men, followed by loss of sexual drive, spermatorrhea, and impotence; increased sexual desire and improved performance in women.
**Hepatic:** *cirrhosis.*
**Musculoskeletal:** temporomandibular joint dysfunction.
**Respiratory:** increased respiratory rate.

**Other:** hyperthermia, sweating.

## INTERACTIONS
None known.

## CAUTIONS
Patients hypersensitive to khat or any of its components should avoid use. Pregnant women should avoid it because it may reduce birth weight. Breast-feeding mothers should avoid khat because it contains norpseudoephedrine, which passes into breast milk.

## NURSING CONSIDERATIONS
- Find out why patient is using the herb.
- Advise cautious use in patients with diabetes, hypertension, tachyarrhythmias, glaucoma, migraines, GI disorders, or underlying psychotic disorders.
- Although khat doesn't cause physical dependence, it does cause psychological dependence and can cause serious physical and psychological adverse effects.
- Long-term use may lead to hypertension in young adults, increased susceptibility to infection, insomnia, and disturbed circadian rhythms.
- Khat suppresses the appetite, causing users to skip meals, decrease adherence to dietary advice, and increase consumption of sweetened beverages, potentially leading to hyperglycemia.

## Patient teaching
- Advise patient to consult with his health care provider before using an herbal preparation because a

---

*Bold italic type* indicates that reaction may be life-threatening.

treatment with proven efficacy may be available.

• Tell patient to remind pharmacist of any herbal and dietary supplements that he's taking, when filling a new prescription.

• Tell patient that the leaf isn't physically addicting but may cause psychological dependence.

• Warn patient to keep all herbal products away from children and pets.

• Inform patient that long-term use may cause hypertension in young adults.

• Caution women to notify health care provider about planned, suspected, or known pregnancy.

## khella

*Ammi daucoides, A. visnaga,* bishop's weed, greater Ammi, khella fruits, visnaga, visnaga fruit

**Common trade names**
*Doctor's Choice for Heart Health*

### HOW SUPPLIED
Derived from fruits and seeds of *Ammi visnaga,* a member of the carrot family. Available as capsules, tablets, and tea. One standardized form contains a minimum of 10% gamma-pyrones, calculated as 100 mg khellin.

### ACTIONS & COMPONENTS
One constituent, visnadin, acts as a mild positive inotrope by dilating coronary vessels and increasing coronary and myocardial circulation. Another component, khellin, is commercially available and used as a vasodilator in treating bronchial asthma and angina pectoris.

### USES
Used orally for angina pectoris, cardiac insufficiency, paroxysmal tachycardia, extrasystoles, hypertonia, asthma, whooping cough, and cramp-like complaints of the abdomen. Extracts are used topically for psoriasis.

### DOSAGE & ADMINISTRATION
*Capsules or tablets:* Average daily dose is 20 mg gamma-pyrones P.O.
*Tea:* Rarely used as a tea, but prepared by pouring boiling water over the powdered fruits, soaking for 10 to 15 minutes, then straining.

### ADVERSE REACTIONS
**CNS:** dizziness, headache, insomnia.
**GI:** nausea, constipation, lack of appetite.
**Hepatic:** elevated liver transaminases and gamma-glutamyl transferase, cholestatic jaundice.
**Skin:** phototoxicity, skin cancer.
**Other:** itching.

### INTERACTIONS
**Herb-drug.** *Hepatotoxic drugs:* Additive effects. Advise patient to avoid using together.
**Herb-herb.** *St. John's wort:* Increased photosensitivity risk. Patient should avoid unprotected sunlight exposure.
**Herb-lifestyle.** Alcohol: May lead to hepatotoxicity. Discourage use.
*Sunlight:* Photosensitivity may occur. Advise patient to take precautions.

*Liquid may contain alcohol.

## CAUTIONS

Patients hypersensitive to khella or any of its components should avoid the herb. It shouldn't be used by women who are pregnant or breast-feeding, by patients with liver disease, or by people who are prone to skin cancer.

## NURSING CONSIDERATIONS

• Find out why patient is using the herb.
• Oral use may raise liver enzyme levels.

### Patient teaching

• Advise patient to consult with his health care provider before using an herbal preparation because a treatment with proven efficacy may be available.
• Tell patient to remind pharmacist of any herbal and dietary supplements that he's taking, when filling a new prescription.
• Although chemical interactions haven't been reported in clinical studies, tell patient that herb may interfere with therapeutic effect of conventional drugs.
• Warn patient not to take herb for cardiac failure before seeking appropriate medical evaluation because doing so may delay diagnosis of a potentially serious medical condition.
• Warn patient to keep all herbal products away from children and pets.
• Warn patient against taking herb with alcohol or with hepatotoxic drugs.
• Tell patient taking this herb to protect himself against sun exposure.

• Advise women to notify health care provider about planned, suspected, or known pregnancy before taking this herb.

---

*Bold italic type* indicates that reaction may be life-threatening.

# L

## lady's mantle

*Alchemilla vulgaris*, bear's foot, dew cup, leontopodium, lion's foot, nine hooks, stellaria

**Common trade names**
*None known*

### HOW SUPPLIED
Obtained from stem, seeds, leaves, and flowers of *Alchemilla vulgaris.* Available as tea, tablets, tincture, and ointment.

### ACTIONS & COMPONENTS
Above-ground parts of *Alchemilla* contain tannins, mainly ellagic acid glycosides (6% to 8%), various flavonoids, such as quercitrin, and salicylic acid in trace amounts. Tannins impart a mild topical astringent action for use as a styptic and in treating mild diarrhea. Salicylic acid amount isn't enough to provide any therapeutic effect. Lady's mantle is an aquaretic herb causing loss of water rather than electrolytes.

### USES
Used as a topical astringent or as a styptic for wounds. Also used as a tea to control mild diarrhea and in women to reduce uterine bleeding, ease menstrual cramps, and regulate the menstrual cycle.

### DOSAGE & ADMINISTRATION
*Ointment:* Applied to wounds q.d. or b.i.d.

*Tablets:* 1 tablet P.O. every 30 to 60 minutes for acute diarrhea or 1 to 3 times P.O. q.d. for chronic diarrhea.
*Tea:* 2 to 4 g of dried herb added to 5 oz of boiling water and steeped for 10 minutes; prepared q.d. Tea is divided and taken t.i.d.
*Tincture:* 5 gtt of tincture P.O. every 30 to 60 minutes for acute diarrhea or 1 to 3 times P.O. q.d. for chronic diarrhea.

### ADVERSE REACTIONS
**Hepatic:** liver damage.

### INTERACTIONS
None reported.

### CAUTIONS
Because safety hasn't been determined, pregnant and breast-feeding patients shouldn't consume herb. Patients with liver dysfunction should also avoid use.

### NURSING CONSIDERATIONS
- Find out why patient is using the herb.
- Long-term use may lead to liver dysfunction. Monitor patient's liver function tests.
- No data exist to support any claims for this herb.
- Don't confuse herb with Alpine lady's mantle *(A. alpina),* which is unapproved by the German Commission E because of lack of documented effectiveness and safety.

### Patient teaching
- Advise patient to consult with his health care provider before using

an herbal preparation because a treatment with proven efficacy may be available.

● Tell patient to remind pharmacist of any herbal and dietary supplements that he's taking, when filling a new prescription.

● Warn patient not to take herb for a GI disturbance before seeking medical attention because doing so may delay diagnosis of a potentially serious medical condition.

● Tell patient not to take herb for longer than 4 days if he's taking it to control mild diarrhea. Tell patient to consult with his health care provider if diarrhea persists or worsens.

## lady's slipper

*Cypripedium calceolus,* American valerian, bleeding heart, golden slipper, moccasin flower, monkey flower, nerve root, Noah's ark, slipper root, venus shoe, whippoorwill's shoe, yellow Indian shoe, yellows

**Common trade names**
*None known*

### HOW SUPPLIED
Obtained from *C. calceolus,* a member of the Orchid family. Because this species may be protected, collecting native specimens may be forbidden. It's usually available in combination with other herbs, especially valerian, as liquid extract*, powdered root, dried root, tea, and tincture.

### ACTIONS & COMPONENTS
Not reported. Some *Cypripedium* species contain allergens and phenanthrene quinones, which are skin irritants.

### USES
Used as a tea for nervousness, headaches (especially stress-related headaches), and emotional tension. It's a mild sedative, a mild hypnotic, and a GI antispasmodic.

### DOSAGE & ADMINISTRATION
*Dried root:* 2 to 4 g P.O. t.i.d.
*Extract (1:1 water or 1:45% ethanol):* 2 to 4 ml P.O. t.i.d.

### ADVERSE REACTIONS
**CNS:** sedation, giddiness, headache, hallucinations, restlessness.
**Skin:** contact dermatitis.

### INTERACTIONS
**Herb-drug.** *Disulfiram:* May react to alcohol content of extract. Advise patient to avoid using together. *Dopamine agonists:* Increased risk of hallucinations. Advise patient to avoid using together.

### CAUTIONS
Herb shouldn't be used by patients allergic to members of the Orchid family or by patients prone to headaches or mental illness unless under medical supervision. Not recommended for use while pregnant or breast-feeding.

### NURSING CONSIDERATIONS
● Find out why patient is using the herb.
● Monitor patient for psychotic behavior or headaches.

---

***Bold italic type*** indicates that reaction may be life-threatening.

• Because clinical and safety data are lacking, use of this herb can't be recommended.

**Patient teaching**
• Advise patient to consult with his health care provider before using an herbal preparation because a treatment with proven efficacy may be available.
• Tell patient to remind pharmacist of any herbal and dietary supplements that he's taking, when filling a new prescription.
• Warn patient that little data exist to support this herb's use or establish its safety.
• Although no chemical interactions have been reported in clinical studies, caution patient that herb may interfere with therapeutic effects of conventional drugs.
• Because sedation is possible, advise patient not to drive or perform hazardous tasks while taking herb.
• Discourage alcohol use.
• Have patient report signs of contact dermatitis to a health care provider.
• Warn patient not to take herb for headaches or anxiety before seeking appropriate medical evaluation because doing so may delay diagnosis of a potentially serious medical condition.

## lavender

*Lavandula angustifolia,* aspic, English lavender, French lavender, garden lavender, lavandin, spike lavender, true lavender

**Common trade names**
*Lavender Liquid Extract, Lavender Flowers*

### HOW SUPPLIED
Available as a volatile oil distilled from flowers of *Lavandula officinalis* and other species, collected just before they open. Also available as dried, unopened flowers, tincture, and lavender spirits.

### ACTIONS & COMPONENTS
Volatile oil of lavender (0.5 to 1.0%) contains more than 100 monoterpene components, up to 40% linalyl acetate and linalool and less than 1% camphor. Several coumarins, ursolic acid, flavonoids, and tannins are also found in the plant. Monoterpenes account for reported antiseptic actions of the oil—cineole and linalool for the hypotensive action, and linalool and linalyl acetate for CNS depression. Lavender oil's sedative effects have been recorded from oral, topical, and inhaled doses.

True lavender oil *(L. officinalis)* isn't toxic at oral doses of up to 5 g/kg; it's rarely toxic dermally and seldom causes sensitization. Spike lavender oil *(L. stoechas)* is neurotoxic because of its high camphor content (15% to 30%). Lavendin is an oil from the hybrid. *Lavandula*

*Liquid may contain alcohol.

*X intermedia* may be toxic because of its 5% to 15% camphor content.

## USES
By direct topical application, the oil is used as an antiseptic to treat psoriasis, minor scrapes, cuts, and burns. Orally, topically, or by inhalation, the oil is used for a calming, mild sedative effect. As an aid to relaxation, oil is added to warm baths. Orally, the flowers have been used as a tea to calm a "nervous stomach."

## DOSAGE & ADMINISTRATION
*Dried flowers:* 20 to 100 g dried flowers added to a bath.
*Oil:* 1 to 4 gtt P.O. on a sugar cube, or diluted in a carrier oil (2% to 5%) as a topical massage, or a few drops added to a bath for psoriasis, wounds, or burns.
*Tea:* Prepared by adding 1 to 2 tsp dried flowers in 5 oz hot water.

## ADVERSE REACTIONS
**CNS:** CNS depression, confusion, dizziness, syncope, drowsiness, headache, neurotoxicity.
**CV:** hypotension.
**GI:** nausea, vomiting, constipation.
**Respiratory:** *respiratory depression.*

## INTERACTIONS
**Herb-drug.** *CNS depressants:* Oil may potentiate the effects of other sedative drugs. Monitor patient closely for oversedation.
*Disulfiram:* Forms that contain alcohol may cause a disulfiram-like reaction. Advise patient to avoid using together.

**Herb-lifestyle.** *Alcohol:* Oral, topical, or inhalation use of oil may potentiate CNS depressant effects of alcohol. Advise patient to avoid using together.

## CAUTIONS
Pregnant patients, breast-feeding patients, and patients hypersensitive to lavender should avoid using this herb.

## NURSING CONSIDERATIONS
● Find out why patient is using the herb.
● Massaging with diluted oil is unlikely to be toxic.
● Some people may be allergic to lavender-containing perfumes, although its allergenic potential is low.
● Don't confuse true lavender oil with lavandin or spike lavender oil; the latter two contain high enough levels of camphor to elicit neurotoxicity.

## Patient teaching
● Advise patient to consult with his health care provider before using an herbal preparation because a treatment with proven efficacy may be available.
● Tell patient to remind pharmacist of any herbal and dietary supplements that he's taking, when filling a new prescription.
● Although no chemical interactions have been reported in clinical studies, advise patient that lavender may interfere with therapeutic effects of conventional drugs.
● Advise patient that excessive inhalation of the oil may lead to dizziness, nausea, and syncope.

---

*Bold italic type* indicates that reaction may be life-threatening.

• Teach patient that oil should be purchased in dropper-tipped amber glass bottles and stored away from light, heat, and small children.
• Warn patient about the possibility of CNS depression, and tell him to avoid hazardous activities until full effects of herb are known.

## lemon

*Citrus limon,* limon

**Common trade names**
*None known*

### HOW SUPPLIED
Available as fruit, fruit juice, expressed peel oil, dried peel, and lemon peel tincture.

### ACTIONS & COMPONENTS
Expressed oil comprises 2.5% of the peel, and consists mainly of monoterpenes (up to 70% limonene); some sesquiterpenes, such as bisabolol; several coumarins and furanocoumarins; citrus bioflavonoids, such as hesperidan, rutin, naringoside; and others. The juice contains bioflavonoids plus vitamin C. Pectin is mainly found in the white endocarp of the peel. The bioflavonoids are used to treat vascular insufficiency and problems with capillary fragility by decreasing porosity. Bisabolol possesses some anti-inflammatory activity. The coumarins and furanocoumarins are photodermatotoxic. Various monoterpenes produce antispasmodic (1, 8 cineole) antimutagenic (limonene), antitumor or chemopreventive (limonene), antioxidant (myrcene), irritant (terpinene-4-ol), and antiviral (α-pinene) actions.

### USES
Lemon is used as a food and a flavor. The oil is used as a carminative. It's also used as a mild anti-inflammatory and diuretic. It's found as a scenting agent in many soaps, cleaners, and cosmetics. Nutritionally, the juice and pulp are a good source of vitamin C, potassium, and bioflavonoids.

### DOSAGE & ADMINISTRATION
Lemon is taken internally as an oil, as a tincture, or as fresh fruit.

### ADVERSE REACTIONS
**Skin:** phototoxicity from expressed oil.

### INTERACTIONS
None reported.

### CAUTIONS
Oral ingestion of expressed oil by pregnant or breast-feeding patients isn't recommended because of the toxicity of its furanocoumarin constituents. Patients hypersensitive to members of the citrus family should avoid lemon preparations as well.

### NURSING CONSIDERATIONS
• Find out why patient is using the herb.
• Patient should avoid topical application of expressed oil and application to mucous membranes because of its irritant qualities.
• Direct application of the oil to skin exposed to sunlight can cause photodermatotoxicity.

*Liquid may contain alcohol.

• Topical products for application to the skin should contain no more than 2% expressed oil because it contains photodermatotoxic furanocoumarins. Distilled lemon oils are inferior smelling and aren't phototoxic.

• Lemon petitgrain oil is the distilled oil from lemon leaf. Advise patient not to confuse with or substitute for lemon peel oil.

**Patient teaching**

• Advise patient to consult with his health care provider before using an herbal preparation because a treatment with proven efficacy may be available.

• Tell patient to remind pharmacist of any herbal and dietary supplements that he's taking, when filling a new prescription.

• Caution women not to consume expressed oil when pregnant or breast-feeding.

• Warn patient not to apply expressed oil to the skin or mucous membranes.

• If patient uses oil, recommend appropriate precautions against prolonged or unprotected sun exposure.

• Advise patient to discontinue use if skin reactions occur.

## lemon balm

*Melissa officinalis,* balm, common balm, cure-all, dropsy plant, honey plant, Melissa, sweet balm, sweet Mary

**Common trade names**
*Melissa Lemon Balm Herb, Quanterra Sleep*

**HOW SUPPLIED**
Available as leaf or powder, volatile oil, liquid extract, or "Spirits of Melissa" (75% alcohol). Often combined with other sedative herbs.

**ACTIONS & COMPONENTS**
Action results from volatile oil consisting of 0.1% to 0.2% citral a (geranial) and b (neral), limonene, small amounts of flavonoids, tannins, protocatechuic and caffeic acids, and ursolic and pomolic acids. The latter, along with the distinctly lemon-scented volatile oil, may account for its use as a carminative to settle the stomach. The volatile oil components also account for the herb's diaphoretic actions. Limonene, oleanolic acid, and geranial have demonstrated sedative actions. Citral has an estrogenic effect. Rosmarinic acid has antiviral actions.

Lemon balm has shown *Herpes simplex* antiviral activity when applied topically. Minor beneficial effects in treating some psychiatric disorders have been reported. Lemon balm also exerts antithyroid effects by inhibiting thyroid-stimulating hormone and the enzyme iodothyronine deiodinase in vitro. Several components of the volatile oil cause skin sensitization, and some are teratogenic.

**USES**
Used as a sedative, usually in combination with other herbal sedatives for nervous sleeping disorders or as a carminative to settle the stomach. Also used for nervous gastric complaints, chronic bronchial catarrh, palpitations related to anxiety or

nervousness, vomiting, migraine, headache, and high blood pressure. Externally, herbal compresses are used to relieve stiff neck, nerve pain, and rheumatism.

## DOSAGE & ADMINISTRATION
*Tea:* 1.5 to 4.5 g of the herb per cup of tea p.r.n., or the equivalent in other preparations.

## ADVERSE REACTIONS
None reported.

## INTERACTIONS
**Herb-drug.** *Disulfiram:* Forms that contain alcohol may cause a disulfiram-like reaction. Advise patient to avoid using together.

## CAUTIONS
Patients with glaucoma and patients hypersensitive to lemon balm shouldn't use this herb. Activity of volatile oil components warrants cautious use by pregnant and breast-feeding women, and by patients with BPH, thyroid disorders, and allergies to lemon- or citrus-scented perfumes.

## NURSING CONSIDERATIONS
• Find out why patient is using the herb.
• Patients with thyroid disorders should use herb cautiously. Monitor thyroid-stimulating hormone levels, as needed.
• Oral use of the volatile oil isn't recommended.

**Patient teaching**
• Advise patient to consult with his health care provider before using an herbal preparation because a treatment with proven efficacy may be available.
• Tell patient to remind pharmacist of any herbal and dietary supplements that he's taking, when filling a new prescription.
• Although no chemical interactions have been reported in clinical studies, advise patient that herb may interfere with therapeutic effects of conventional drugs.
• Urge patient to discontinue use of herb or its oil if ocular pain or rash develops.
• Tell patient not to use herb if he's allergic to lemon-scented perfumes or products.
• Caution patient against oral use of oil. If needed, mention that brewed tea is usually well tolerated.
• Warn patient to take precautions until sedative effects of the herb are known.
• Advise patient not to take herb for anxiety or a sleep disorder before seeking medical attention because doing so may delay diagnosis of a potentially serious medical condition.

## lemongrass

*Cymbopogon citratus*, capim-cidrao, citronella, fevergrass, Indian melissa, Indian verbena

**Common trade names**
*Carmol (lemongrass oil)*

## HOW SUPPLIED
Available as leaves and oil.

## ACTIONS & COMPONENTS
Lemongrass contains alkaloids, a saponin fraction, and cymbopogo-

nol. Fresh leaves contain 0.4% to 0.5% volatile oil that contains citral, myrcene, and geranial, and several other fragrant compounds. Myrcene may have some peripheral analgesic activity similar to peripherally acting opiates that directly downregulate sensitized receptors.

## USES
Leaves are used as an antispasmodic, an analgesic, and a treatment for nervous and GI disorders. Crushed leaves are used topically as a mosquito repellant. Essential oil is used as a food additive and in perfumes.

## DOSAGE & ADMINISTRATION
*Oil:* Applied topically for pain, arthritis, ringworm.
*Tea:* 2 to 4 g of fresh or dried leaves boiled in 5 oz water.

## ADVERSE REACTIONS
**GI:** dry mouth.
**GU:** polyuria.

## INTERACTIONS
None known.

## CAUTIONS
Patients who are pregnant or hypersensitive to herb shouldn't use this herb.

## NURSING CONSIDERATIONS
● Find out why patient is using the herb.
● Herb may cause increased frequency of urination.

## Patient teaching
● Advise patient to consult with his health care provider before using an herbal preparation because a treatment with proven efficacy may be available.
● Tell patient to remind pharmacist of any herbal and dietary supplements that he's taking, when filling a new prescription.
● Inform patient that animal and human studies haven't supported claimed uses for herb.
● Caution patient not to take herb at bedtime because it may increase frequency of urination.

## licorice

*Glycyrrhiza glabra,* Chinese licorice, licorice root, Persian licorice, Russian licorice, Spanish licorice, sweet root, sweet wood, sweet wort

### Common trade names
*Herbal Booster, Herbal Laxative, Herbal Nerve (Canada), Honey and Molasses (UK), Licorice Power, Lightning Cough Remedy, Phyto Power, Standardized Licorice, Wild Countryside Licorice Root*

## HOW SUPPLIED
Obtained from dried, unpeeled roots of *Glycyrrhiza glabra.* Available as liquid and capsules.
*Capsules:* 100 mg, 200 mg, 400 mg, 444 mg, 445 mg, 450 mg, 500 mg, 520 mg

## ACTIONS & COMPONENTS
Licorice contains 7% to 10% glycyrrhizin (glycyrrhizic acid), as well as natural sugars, glucose, mannose, sucrose, flavonoids, isoflavonoids, and sterols (beta-

---

*Bold italic type* indicates that reaction may be life-threatening.

sitosterol and stigmasterol). Glycyrrhizin is a glycoside 50 times sweeter than sugar, which helps to mask the bitter taste of quinine and similar drugs. The active ingredient for treating stomach ulcers is carbenoxolone, a semisynthetic ester of glycyrrhetic acid.

Licorice has shown antiinflammatory and antarthritic effects by inhibiting prostaglandin activity. This activity may make it useful in treating pain and inflammation from arthritis.

The active ingredient, glycyrrhetinic acid, inhibits 11-beta-hydroxydehydrogenase, an enzyme that prevents cortisol from acting as a mineralocorticoid. Inhibiting this enzyme allows increased mineralocorticoid activity, or aldosterone-like activity, leading to sodium and water retention and potassium excretion. Many reports have been made about severe toxicity caused by these effects.

### USES
Licorice is used to treat stomach ulcers and as an expectorant. It's also used in sweets, soft drinks, medicines, and chewing tobacco.

### DOSAGE & ADMINISTRATION
*Capsules:* Doses vary from 5 to 15 g/day of licorice root (200 to 600 mg glycyrrhizin) q.d. Daily intake of more than 50 g of the herb is considered toxic.

### ADVERSE REACTIONS
**CNS:** numbness or tingling, paralysis.
**CV:** hypertension, *heart failure, arrhythmias.*

**Metabolic:** hypernatremia, hypokalemia.
**Musculoskeletal:** myopathy, muscle cramps.

### INTERACTIONS
**Herb-drug.** *Antiarrhythmics, such as procainamide, quinidine:* Hypokalemia and torsades de pointes. Advise patient to avoid using together.
*Antihypertensives:* May be rendered less effective. Monitor blood pressure closely.
*Corticosteroids:* May have additive effects. Advise patient to use cautiously.
*Digoxin:* Hypokalemia increases the risk of digoxin toxicity. Advise patient to avoid using together.
*Diuretics:* May worsen hypokalemia. Advise patient to avoid using together.
**Herb-lifestyle.** *Smoking:* Possible reduced metabolism of herb because of reported licorice toxicity. Monitor patient closely.

### CAUTIONS
Patients who are pregnant, who are hypersensitive to herb, or who have arrhythmias, diabetes, glaucoma, cerebrovascular accident, or renal, hepatic, or cardiac disease should avoid using this herb.

### NURSING CONSIDERATIONS
• Find out why patient is using the herb.
• Toxicity can occur with long-term use or with single large doses of licorice. Licorice shouldn't be used for longer than 4 weeks at a time.
• Monitor patient for symptoms of hypokalemia or hypernatremia.

*Liquid may contain alcohol.

- Assess patient's drug profile for use of diuretics, antihypertensives, corticosteroids, or digoxin.
- Monitor patient's blood pressure closely.

**Patient teaching**
- Advise patient to consult with his health care provider before using an herbal preparation because a treatment with proven efficacy may be available.
- Tell patient to remind pharmacist of any herbal and dietary supplements that he's taking, when filling a new prescription.
- Warn patient not to take herb for worrisome symptoms before seeking medical attention because doing so may delay diagnosis of a potentially serious medical condition.
- Caution patient not to take large doses of licorice or use it for longer than 4 weeks at a time because of the risk of toxicity.
- Tell patient to notify his health care provider if he develops swelling, muscle cramps, tiredness, or weakness.

## lily-of-the-valley

*Convallaria majalis,* convall-lily, Jacob's ladder, ladder to heaven, lily constancy, maiblume, maiglöckchenkraut, may bells, mayflower, may lily, muguet, Our Lady's tears

**Common trade names**
*None known*

**HOW SUPPLIED**
Obtained from all parts of the plant of *Convallaria majalis.*

**ACTIONS & COMPONENTS**
Lily-of-the-valley has a positive inotropic effect on the heart through natural cardioactive glycosides, including convallatoxin, convalloside, and convallatoxol.

**USES**
Used for mild exertional failure, age-related cardiac complaints, chronic cor pulmonale.

**DOSAGE & ADMINISTRATION**
No dosage is recommended because of plant's toxic potential. Dose of 0.6 g standardized lily-of-the-valley powder contains 0.2% to 0.3% content of cardioactive glycosides.

**ADVERSE REACTIONS**
**CV:** *cardiac arrythmias.*
**GI:** nausea, vomiting, abdominal pain, cramping, diarrhea.
**Metabolic:** hyperkalemia.

**INTERACTIONS**
**Herb-drug.** *Beta blockers, calcium channel blockers:* Increased risk of bradycardia or heart block. Advise patient to avoid using together.
*Calcium salts, digoxin, glucocorticoids, laxatives, quinidine:* Possible additive effects and increased risk of adverse reactions. Advise patient to avoid using together.

**CAUTIONS**
This herb is not recommended for use.

**NURSING CONSIDERATIONS**
✍ALERT: The FDA considers lily-of-the-valley an unsafe and

---

*Bold italic type* indicates that reaction may be life-threatening.

poisonous plant because of the level of toxins present.
- Find out why patient is using the herb.
- Monitor patient for serious adverse effects, such as increased potassium levels or heart arrhythmias.

**Patient teaching**
- Advise patient to consult with his health care provider before using an herbal preparation because a treatment with proven efficacy may be available.
- Tell patient to remind pharmacist of any herbal and dietary supplements that he's taking, when filling a new prescription.
- ⚠ALERT: Discourage use of this herb. Warn patient that it's considered poisonous and unsafe by the FDA.
- Inform patient about the serious adverse effects, especially when used with digoxin, beta blockers, or calcium channel blockers.
- Tell patient to notify his health care provider if he develops nausea, vomiting, muscle cramps, or a change in heartbeat. They may warn of serious adverse effects.

## linden

*Tilia cordata, T. platyphyllos,* and *T. tomentosa,* basswood, European linden, lime flower, lime tree

**Common trade names**
*Linden Capsules*

## HOW SUPPLIED
Obtained from fresh and dried flowers and leaves of *Tilia* trees.

## ACTIONS & COMPONENTS
Linden extract contains flavonoid compounds, including kaempferol and quercitin; *p*-coumaric, caffeic, and chlorogenic acids; and amino acids. The plant contains 0.02% to 0.1% volatile oils, including citral, eugenol, and limonene. The ratio of tannins to mucilage polysaccharides contained in various *Tilia* species accounts for differences in the flavor of teas made from this herb. Quercitin, *p*-coumaric acid, and kaempferol may cause diaphoretic action.

## USES
Used to induce sweating and to treat various nervous disorders, feverish colds, throat irritation, nasal congestion, infections, and cold-related cough.

## DOSAGE & ADMINISTRATION
*Liquid extract:* 2 to 4 ml of 1:1 preparation with 25% alcohol.
*Tea:* 2 to 4 g/day.

## ADVERSE REACTIONS
**CNS:** drowsiness.
**Skin:** contact allergies.

## INTERACTIONS
**Herb-drug.** *Disulfiram:* Alcohol in extract may cause disulfiram-like reaction. Advise patient to avoid using together.
**Herb-lifestyle.** *Alcohol:* Possible additive effects. Discourage use.

## CAUTIONS
Patients hypersensitive to herb and those with a history of heart disease shouldn't use herb.

## NURSING CONSIDERATIONS
• Review patient's drug history and herb usage. Find out why patient is using the herb.
• Although no chemical interactions have been reported in clinical studies, consider the herb's pharmacologic properties and the risk that it will interfere with the intended therapeutic effects of conventional drugs.
• Some patients may be allergic to linden. If signs or symptoms develop, patient should discontinue herb and consult a health care provider.

### Patient teaching
• Advise patient to consult with his health care provider before using an herbal preparation because a treatment with proven efficacy may be available.
• Tell patient to remind pharmacist of any herbal and dietary supplements that he's taking, when filling a new prescription.
• Caution patients with a history of heart disease not to use linden. Frequent use may damage cardiac tissue.
• Warn patient to contact a health care provider if he develops a rash, swelling, or trouble breathing.
• Warn patient to avoid hazardous activities until full effects of herb are known. It may cause drowsiness.
• Warn patient not to take herb for worrisome symptoms before seeking appropriate medical evaluation because doing so may delay diagnosis of a potentially serious medical condition.

## lobelia

*Lobelia inflata,* asthma weed, bladderpod, cardinal flower, emetic herb, emetic weed, eyebright, gagroot, Indian pink, Indian tobacco, pukeweed, vomitroot, vomitwort, wild tobacco

**Common trade names**
*Lobelia Compound, Lobelia Extract*

### HOW SUPPLIED
Obtained from the dried leaves of *Lobelia inflata.* Available as tablets and tincture.

### ACTIONS & COMPONENTS
Contains 6% alkaloids. Lobeline accounts for most of the herb's effects. Lobelanine, lobelanidine, norlobelanine, and isolobinine are also present. Lobelia acts like nicotine and interacts at the nicotine receptor, stimulating respiratory and emetic centers of the brain.

### USES
Used as an antasthmatic, an emetic, and a smoking cessation aid.

### DOSAGE & ADMINISTRATION
Lobelia is used as a constituent of some homeopathic preparations. Doses of 600 to 1,000 mg of the leaves are considered toxic. Some sources consider a dose of lobeline sulfate above 20 mg daily to be toxic. Others warn that a 4-g dose may be fatal.

---

*Bold italic type* indicates that reaction may be life-threatening.

## ADVERSE REACTIONS
**CNS:** anxiety, dizziness, headache, paresthesias, shivering, sweating, *seizures.*
**CV:** increased heart rate or *bradycardia,* increased or decreased blood pressure.
**GI:** dry mouth, mouth irritation, abdominal pain, diarrhea, nausea, vomiting.
**GU:** burning of the urinary tract.
**Respiratory:** cough, tickling or choking sensation, pain or burning, decreased respiration, *paralysis of the respiratory center* with overdose.
**Skin:** contact allergies.

## INTERACTIONS
**Herb-drug.** *GI or respiratory irritants, nicotine-containing cessation products:* Possible additive toxicity. Advise patient to avoid using together.

## CAUTIONS
Patients with heart disease or hypersensitivity to tobacco or lobelia should avoid using this herb. Women who are pregnant or breastfeeding should also avoid it.

## NURSING CONSIDERATIONS
• Find out why patient is using the herb.
• Several studies of lobeline, the active ingredient in lobelia, for smoking cessation have found little evidence to support its efficacy.
• Lobelia shouldn't be used for longer than 6 weeks.
• Antacids may decrease the adverse GI effects of lobeline.
• Monitor patient's blood pressure, heart rate, and respirations.

## Patient teaching
• Advise patient to consult with his health care provider before using an herbal preparation because a treatment with proven efficacy may be available.
• Tell patient to remind pharmacist of any herbal and dietary supplements that he's taking, when filling a new prescription.
• Warn patient not to use lobelia for longer than 6 weeks.
• Tell patient not to take lobelia while smoking or chewing tobacco. Offer other tobacco-cessation options.
• Advise patient that antacids may decrease adverse GI effects.

## lovage

*Aetheroleum levistici, Angelica levisticum, Hipposelinum levisticum, Levisticum officinale, L. radix,* lavose, maggi plant, sea parsley, smellage

**Common trade names**
*None known*

## HOW SUPPLIED
Obtained from roots and seeds of *Levisticum officinale* and *L. radix.* Available as a tea.

## ACTIONS & COMPONENTS
The root contains several compounds that contribute to its aromatic odor and flavor, including butylidenephthelide, butylthalide, and ligustilide; coumarins; terpenoids; and volatile acids, such as caffeic and benzoic acids. Other compounds include camphene, bergapten, and psoralen. Lovage

exerts weak diuretic, spasmolytic, and sedative effects; it also stimulates salivation and gastric secretion.

## USES
Used for its diuretic properties in treating pedal edema. In Germany, it's approved for irrigation in urinary tract inflammation and for renal calculus prophylaxis. Also used as a spasmolytic, a sedative, a mucolytic, a carminative (to relieve gastric discomfort and flatulence), and a remedy for menstrual complaints.

## DOSAGE & ADMINISTRATION
*Tea:* Prepared by pouring 1 cup boiling water over 1.5 to 3 g of finely cut root and draining after 15 minutes. Dosage is 4 to 8 g P.O. q.d., taken between meals.

## ADVERSE REACTIONS
**Skin:** photosensitivity, dermatitis.

## INTERACTIONS
**Herb-drug.** *Warfarin, other anticoagulants:* May potentiate effects. Advise patient to avoid using together.
**Herb-lifestyle.** *Sunlight:* Photosensitivity may occur. Advise patient to take precautions.

## CAUTIONS
Patients with acute renal inflammation or dysfunction should avoid using this herb, as should women who are pregnant or breast-feeding.

## NURSING CONSIDERATIONS
- Find out why patient is using the herb.
- Patients with a history of photosensitivity reactions and those with plant allergies should use lovage cautiously.
- Monitor serum electrolyte, BUN, and serum creatinine values periodically while patient is taking herb.
- Make sure the patient maintains adequate fluid intake.
- Herb may prolong INR and PT if patient also receives an anticoagulant.

### Patient teaching
- Advise patient to consult with his health care provider before using an herbal preparation because a treatment with proven efficacy may be available.
- Tell patient to remind pharmacist of any herbal and dietary supplements that he's taking, when filling a new prescription.
- If patient takes lovage for pedal edema, recommend a complete medical evaluation by a health care provider. Explain that pedal edema may indicate a serious underlying CV or renal disorder that needs medical treatment.
- Discuss other proven diuretics currently available.
- Tell patient to notify health care provider about any skin changes or photosensitivity reactions. Emphasize need to avoid prolonged exposure to sunlight while using lovage.
- Caution patient to avoid using herb with anticoagulants.

---

*Bold italic type* indicates that reaction may be life-threatening.

# lungwort

*Pulmonaria officinalis,* dage of Jerusalem, Jerusalem cowslip, lungmoss, spotted comfrey

**Common trade names**
*Lungwort Compound*

## HOW SUPPLIED
Available as tablets, syrup, juice, drops, and extracts.

## ACTIONS & COMPONENTS
Lungwort leaves contain allantoin, which may contribute to its emollient action. Tannins and flavonoids contained in the plant may exert astringent and anti-inflammatory action, and mucilage may act as an antitussive. Other components include ascorbic acid, saponins, potassium and iron salts, and salicylic acid.

## USES
Used as an antitussive, expectorant, and anti-irritant in bronchitis, cough, influenza, and tuberculosis. Also used for its astringent properties in treating diarrhea, hemorrhoids, GI ulceration, kidney and urinary tract conditions, and excessive menstrual flow. Used topically to encourage wound healing.

## DOSAGE & ADMINISTRATION
*Infusion:* 1.5 g of dried herb, finely cut. Placed in cold water and brought to a rapid boil. Or, herb is steeped in boiling water for 5 to 10 minutes, then taken t.i.d.
*Tincture:* 1 to 4 ml P.O. t.i.d.

## ADVERSE REACTIONS
**GI:** nausea.
**Skin:** contact dermatitis.
**Other:** bleeding time may be prolonged.

## INTERACTIONS
**Herb-drug.** *Warfarin, other anticoagulants:* Possible potentiation of effect. Advise patient to avoid using together.

## CAUTIONS
Patients with a history of contact allergies, patients who receive an anticoagulant, and patients who are pregnant or breast-feeding should avoid using this herb.

## NURSING CONSIDERATIONS
● Find out why patient is using the herb.
● Monitor patient's INR and PT, as needed, because herb may prolong bleeding indexes. Monitor patient for occult blood.

### Patient teaching
● Advise patient to consult with his health care provider before using an herbal preparation because a treatment with proven efficacy may be available.
● Tell patient to remind pharmacist of any herbal and dietary supplements that he's taking, when filling a new prescription.
● If patient has a respiratory disorder, tell him to discuss conventional medical treatments with a health care provider before using the herb.
● Inform patient that insufficient data exist to support therapeutic use of this herb.

• Warn patient to avoid using herb with an anticoagulant, such as warfarin.

• Tell patient to notify a health care provider about signs and symptoms of increased bleeding time, such as bruising, bleeding gums, or dark stools.

## madder

*Rubia tinctorum*, dyer's madder,
madder root, robbia

**Common trade names**
*Madder Whole Root*

### HOW SUPPLIED
Available as dried root, extract, and
capsules.

### ACTIONS & COMPONENTS
Contains 2% to 4% anthraquinone
derivatives and glycosides. Principal components are ruberythric
acid, alizarin, pseudopurpurin, ru-
biadin, lucidin, and lucidin 3-O-
primeveroside. Mechanism of action stems from the $Ca^{2+}$ chelating
properties of anthraquinones. Herb
may also be mutagenic and carcinogenic because of the lucidin component.

### USES
Used as an antispasmodic, a diuretic, and a prophylactic and
treatment for kidney stones. Also
added to foods as a colorant.

### DOSAGE & ADMINISTRATION
*Capsules:* 1 capsule P.O. t.i.d. for
up to 2 months.
*Extract:* 20 gtt P.O. t.i.d. for up to 2
months.
*Infusion:* 1 to 2 g P.O. q.i.d. for up
to 2 months.

### ADVERSE REACTIONS
**Skin:** contact dermatitis.

**Other:** *cancer,* red discoloration
of perspiration, saliva, tears, urine
and bone.

### INTERACTIONS
None known.

### CAUTIONS
Because of the risk of toxicity, no
one should take madder. Patients
who do take it should be supervised by a knowledgeable health
care provider. Pregnant or breast-
feeding women should avoid this
herb because of possible mutagen-
icity and carcinogenicity. Patients
hypersensitive to madder should
also avoid it.

### NURSING CONSIDERATIONS
● Find out why patient is using
herb.

### Patient teaching
● Advise patient to consult with his
health care provider before using
an herbal preparation because a
treatment with proven efficacy may
be available.
● Tell patient to remind pharmacist
of any herbal and dietary supplements that he's taking, when filling
a new prescription.
● Warn patients about possible mutagenic and carcinogenic effects of
madder.
● If patient has suspected kidney
stones, tell him to discuss conventional treatments with health care
provider before using this herb.
● Advise women to avoid madder
while pregnant or breast-feeding.

- Instruct women who take madder to notify health care provider about planned, suspected, or known pregnancy.
- Inform patient that madder may discolor body fluids and items he touches, such as contact lenses.

## male fern

*Dryopteris filix-mas,* bear's paw root, knotty brake, male shield fern, marginal fern, sweet brake, wurmfarn

**Common trade names**
*Aspidium Oleoresin, Bontanifuge, Extractum Filicis, Extractum Filicis Aethereum, Extractum Filicis Maris Tenue, Male Fern Oleoresin, Paraway Plus*

### HOW SUPPLIED
Available as extract (1.5% to 22% filicin), draught (4 g of male fern extract), and capsules.

### ACTIONS & COMPONENTS
Filicic and flavaspidic acids are the main active components responsible for herb's anthelmintic properties. Other components include volatile oils, tannin, paraspidin, and desaspidin. Desaspidin and aspidin may have antitumor activity.

### USES
Long used as an anthelmintic against pork tapeworm *(Taenia solium),* beef tapeworm *(T. saginata),* and fish tapeworm *(Diphyllobothrium latum).* Also applied topically for muscle pain, arthritis, sciatica, neuralgia, earache, and toothache.

### DOSAGE & ADMINISTRATION
*Draught:* 50 ml given by duodenal tube. Treatment may be repeated in 7 to 10 days, p.r.n.
*Extract:* For adults, 3 to 6 ml P.O. after fasting. For children older than age 4, 0.25 to 0.5 ml P.O. per year of age. Maximum, 4 ml P.O. in divided doses.

### ADVERSE REACTIONS
**CNS:** headache, *seizures,* queasiness, psychosis, paralysis, *coma.*
**CV:** *heart failure.*
**EENT:** optic neuritis, permanent visual disorders.
**GI:** severe abdominal cramps, diarrhea, nausea, vomiting.
**Hepatic:** *hepatotoxicity,* jaundice.
**Respiratory:** dyspnea, *respiratory failure.*
**Other:** hyperbilirubinemia, albuminuria.

### INTERACTIONS
**Herb-drug.** *Antacids, H₂-blockers (such as famotidine and ranitidine), proton pump inhibitors (including lansoprazole and omeprazole), other alkalinizing drugs:* The acid components of male fern are inactivated in an alkaline pH. Advise patient to separate administration times by several hours.
*Drugs that increase liver enzyme levels, such as HMG-CoA (atorvastatin, simvastatin):* Increased risk of hepatocellular damage. Advise patient to avoid using together.
**Herb-food.** *Fats and oils, including castor oil:* Increased absorption and risk of toxicity. Advise patient to avoid using together.

---

***Bold italic type*** indicates that reaction may be life-threatening.

## CAUTIONS

Pregnant women should avoid using this herb because it may stimulate uterine muscle. Patients who are breast-feeding, infants and children younger than age 4, geriatric patients, and debilitated patients should avoid use as well, along with patients who are hypersensitive to male fern or its components and those with anemia, GI ulceration, CV disease, diabetes, and hepatic or renal failure.

## NURSING CONSIDERATIONS

⚠ALERT: Male fern is toxic. Ingestion isn't recommended. In poisoning or overdose, optic neuritis, blindness, seizures, psychosis, paralysis, respiratory and cardiac failure, coma, and death may ensue. The patient should seek emergency medical care. Poisoning should be treated with activated charcoal; fatty and oily cathartics should be avoided. Patients may need benzodiazepines for seizure control along with respiratory and cardiac support. Vision should be tested during and after exposure.

• Find out why patient is using herb

• Male fern has a narrow window of intended activity; toxic effects can occur in that window.

• Draught is considered a more effective anthelmintic than capsule form.

• Patients being treated with drugs that affect bilirubin conjugation or alter liver enzyme levels should use herb cautiously or avoid it.

• Patient may take a laxative the evening before herb treatment and a second laxative dose with the herb the next morning before eating.

• Monitor patient's liver function tests and renal function.

• Monitor fluid intake and electrolyte loss in patients who develop vomiting and diarrhea.

**Patient teaching**

• Advise patient to consult with his health care provider before using an herbal preparation because a treatment with proven efficacy may be available.

• Tell patient to remind pharmacist of any herbal and dietary supplements that he's taking, when filling a new prescription.

• Inform patient that toxic effects can occur with normal doses.

• If patient takes an antacid, $H_2$-blocker, or proton pump inhibitor, tell him to avoid using this herb.

• Tell patient to avoid fats and oils while taking herb.

• Advise patient that conventional anthelmintics for tapeworms are safer than male fern.

• Urge patient to seek medical care for suspected tapeworm before using this herb.

• If patient has persistent abdominal pain or yellowing of the skin and eyes, stress that he should obtain medical care.

• If patient is pregnant or breast-feeding or has anemia, a GI condition, or cardiac, hepatic, or renal impairment, caution against using herb.

## mallow

*Malva sylvestris*, blue mallow, cheeseflower, high mallow, mallow flower (*Malvae flos*), mallow leaf (*Malvae folium*), mauls

**Common trade names**
*Malvedrin, Malveol*

### HOW SUPPLIED
Available as an extract and as dried herb.

### ACTIONS & COMPONENTS
Mallow contains glycosides, flavonoids, mucilage, anthocyanin, and tannins. The mucilage component, made up largely of glucuronic acid, galacturonic acid, rhamnose, and galactose, is responsible for emollient and demulcent action. Mallow may also act as an astringent and expectorant.

### USES
Used as demulcent to treat oral and pharyngeal mucosal irritation, cough, hoarseness, bronchitis, laryngitis, and tonsillitis. Used topically as an emollient for skin irritation and swelling. Also used as a laxative, for the pain of teething in children and, when combined with yarrow, as a vaginal douche.

### DOSAGE & ADMINISTRATION
*Dried herb:* 5 g q.d.
*Infusion:* For mallow flower (*Malvae flos*), 1.5 to 2 g of dried flower added to cold water, boiled, then strained after 10 minutes. For mallow leaf (*Malvae folium*), 5 oz of boiling water poured over 3 to 5 g and steeped for 2 to 3 hours; stirred occasionally.

### ADVERSE REACTIONS
**Musculoskeletal:** muscle tremors.

### INTERACTIONS
None reported.

### CAUTIONS
Mallow should be avoided by pregnant or breast-feeding patients and by those hypersensitive to it.

### NURSING CONSIDERATIONS
• Find out why patient is using herb.
• Don't confuse mallow with the sound-alike herb, marshmallow.
• No clinical data support the use of this herb.

### Patient teaching
• Advise patient to consult with his health care provider before using an herbal preparation because a treatment with proven efficacy may be available.
• Tell patient to remind pharmacist of any herbal and dietary supplements that he's taking, when filling a new prescription.
• Advise patient to consult a health care provider about a persistent cough and throat or mouth pain or irritation.
• Inform patient that little medicinal data support the use of this herb.
• Advise patient to report suspected pregnancy, if using this herb.

---

*Bold italic type* indicates that reaction may be life-threatening.

## marigold

*Calendula officinalis,* garden marigold, goldbloom, golds, holligold, marigold, marybud, marygold, mary gowles, pot marigold, ruddes

**Common trade names**
*Calendula Gel, Calendula Ointment, California Candula Gel, Kneipp's Calendula Ointment*

### HOW SUPPLIED
Available as ointment, cream, gel, shampoo, tincture*, tea, and mouth-wash; obtained from powdered flowers, shoots, and leaves of the marigold plant *(Calendula officinalis).*

### ACTIONS & COMPONENTS
Contains lutein, volatile oils, flavo-noids, carotenoid pigments, and sterols. Topical use of extracts pro-motes wound healing. The herb has antibacterial, antifungal, antiviral, antimitotic, antimutagenic, antioxi-dant, cancerostatic, and immuno-stimulating properties. The ex-tracts also have a systemic anti-inflammatory effect.

### USES
Ointments are used for wounds, burns, chapped lips, nipples cracked by breast-feeding, skin in-flammation, furunculosis, eczema, acne, and varicose veins; tinctures or teas, for peptic ulcers, dysmen-orrhea, and sore throat; and ex-tracts, as cancer therapy and as im-munostimulants in viral and bacte-rial infections. Other reported uses include diuresis and treatment of fever, toothache, and eye inflam-mation. Volatile oil is used in per-fumes, and plant pigments are used in cosmetics.

### DOSAGE & ADMINISTRATION
*Ointment:* 2 to 5 g powdered herb in 100 g ointment for external use.
*Tea:* 1 to 2 g per cup of water q.d., ingested or used as a gargle.
*Tincture:* 1:9 with 20% alcohol/wa-ter mixture for external use.

### ADVERSE REACTIONS
None known.

### INTERACTIONS
None known.

### CAUTIONS
Women who are pregnant or breast-feeding should avoid using the herb, along with patients who have a history of environmental al-lergies or hypersensitivity to herb.

### NURSING CONSIDERATIONS
• Find out why patient is using herb.
• Don't confuse marigold *(C. offici-nalis)* with African, Inca, or French marigolds *(Tagetes),* often used in gardens to repel insects.

### Patient teaching
• Advise patient to consult with his health care provider before using an herbal preparation because a treatment with proven efficacy may be available.
• Tell patient to remind pharmacist of any herbal and dietary supple-ments that he's taking, when filling a new prescription.
• Warn patient about the risk of al-lergic reaction.

---

*Liquid may contain alcohol.

• Advise women to avoid use while pregnant or breast-feeding. Tell women to notify health care provider about planned, suspected, or known pregnancy.
• Warn patient not to take herb for worrisome symptoms before seeking appropriate medical evaluation because doing so may delay diagnosis of a potentially serious medical condition.

## marjoram

*Origanum majorana,* common marjoram, knotted marjoram, sweet marjoram, wild marjoram

**Common trade names**
*Marjoram, Marjoram Essential Oil, Sweet Marjoram*

**HOW SUPPLIED**
Available as tea from dried leaves and flowers of *Origanum marjorana,* and as essential oil of marjoram (extracted by distillation).

**ACTIONS & COMPONENTS**
Marjoram contains thymol, carvacrol, tannins, flavonoids, hydroquinone, and phenolic glycosides. Extracts decrease response to acetylcholine, histamine, serotonin, and nicotine. Antiviral, bactericidal, antiseptic, and antifungal effects are attributed to thymol, carvacrol, and the essential oil.

**USES**
Used to treat headaches, depression, dizziness, insomnia, motion sickness, conjunctivitis, and GI complaints, such as gastritis, flatulence, and colic. Also used for symptomatic treatment of rhinitis and colds. Essential oil is used externally for musculoskeletal pain and aromatherapy.

**DOSAGE & ADMINISTRATION**
*Essential oil:* Apply externally, p.r.n.
*Tea:* 1 to 2 tsp dried leaves in 1 cup water, q.d. to t.i.d.

**ADVERSE REACTIONS**
**GI:** nausea, vomiting, or diarrhea.

**INTERACTIONS**
None reported.

**CAUTIONS**
Pregnant or breast-feeding women shouldn't use herb in amounts larger than those used in cooking. Children shouldn't use the essential oil. Patients with a history of allergic reaction to oregano or thyme shouldn't use this herb.

**NURSING CONSIDERATIONS**
• Find out why patient is using herb.
• There are no reported cases of toxicity. However, marjoram essential oils contain thymol, arbutin, and hydroquinone in low concentrations, which may be toxic during extended use.
• Patients should avoid using essential oil internally.

**Patient teaching**
• Advise patient to consult with his health care provider before using an herbal preparation because a treatment with proven efficacy may be available.

- Tell patient to remind pharmacist of any herbal and dietary supplements that he's taking, when filling a new prescription.
- Warn patient not to take herb for headaches, insomnia, or depression before seeking medical attention because doing so may delay diagnosis of a potentially serious medical condition.
- Advise patient to stop taking herb if he develops nausea, vomiting, or diarrhea. Tell him to notify his health care provider if symptoms last longer than 2 or 3 days. This may be a sign of toxicity.
- Advise patient to avoid use of volatile oils. If he uses them anyway, tell him to keep them away from eyes.
- Counsel patients not to use more of the herb than is normally used for cooking.
- Safety in children hasn't been established for amounts greater than those used for cooking.
- Discourage prolonged use.

## marshmallow

*Althaea officinalis,* althea, cheeses, mallards, Moorish mallow, mortification root, Schloss tea, sweet weed, white maoow, wymote

**Common trade names**
*Marshmallow Root*

### HOW SUPPLIED
Available as whole dried root, dried leaves or flowers, capsules, extracts, syrup, and tea.

### ACTIONS & COMPONENTS
Contains mucilage, pectin, and starch. Herb has emollient, demulcent, urinary analgesic, anti-inflammatory, and anticomplement activity. Inhibits mucociliary activity and stimulates phagocytosis and immune activity.

### USES
Used as a cough suppressant to alleviate irritation of oral and pharyngeal tissue. Also used to treat inflammation and burns and to relieve mild gastric inflammation, irritable bowel syndrome, diarrhea, and constipation.

### DOSAGE & ADMINISTRATION
*Leaf:* 5 g P.O. q.d.
*Root:* 6 g P.O. q.d.
*Syrup:* 10 g single dose.
*Tea:* 10 to 15 g in 5 oz cold water, freshly prepared several times q.d.

### ADVERSE REACTIONS
None reported.

### INTERACTIONS
**Herb-drug.** *Insulin, sulfonylureas:* May enhance hypoglycemic activity. Advise patient to avoid using together; monitor blood glucose level closely.
*Other drugs:* May delay absorption of other drugs. Advise patient to separate administration times.

### CAUTIONS
Patients who are pregnant or breast-feeding should avoid use of herb, along with patients hypersensitive to herb.

*Liquid may contain alcohol.

## NURSING CONSIDERATIONS
• Find out why patient is using herb.
• Diabetic patients should use herb cautiously and monitor closely for hypoglycemia.

**Patient teaching**
• Advise patient to consult with his health care provider before using an herbal preparation because a treatment with proven efficacy may be available.
• Tell patient to remind pharmacist of any herbal and dietary supplements that he's taking, when filling a new prescription.
• Although no chemical interactions have been reported in clinical studies, advise patient that herb may interfere with therapeutic effect of conventional drugs.
• Caution women to avoid using herb during pregnancy and while breast-feeding because effects aren't known.
• Inform patient that no data exist to support the use of marshmallow.
• Counsel diabetic patient to avoid use of marshmallow. If he uses it anyway, tell him to frequently monitor blood glucose level.
• Tell patient to separate administration times of marshmallow and drugs.
• Advise patient to store herb away from light.

## mayapple

*Podophyllum peltatum,* devil's apple, duck's foot, ground lemon, hog apple, Indian apple, mandrake, raccoon berry, umbrella plant, vegetable mercury, wild lemon

**Common trade names**
*Condylox, Podocon-25, Podofilm, Podofin, Warix, Wartex*

### HOW SUPPLIED
Available as dried roots and rhizomes, powder, and extracted resin.
*Concentrated tincture:* 5% to 25% in alcohol or benzoin available by prescription for topical use
*Resinous extract:* 0.5% in alcohol available by prescription for topical use

### ACTIONS & COMPONENTS
Contains podophyllic acid, picropodophyllin, alpha- and beta-peltatin, and podophyllotoxin. These components demonstrate antimitotic effects, thereby inhibiting tumor growth. Some components decrease mitochondrial cytochrome activity as well. Various anticancer drugs contain a synthetic component of the plant (podophyllin). Dried root irritates colonic mucosa, acting as purgative cathartic.

### USES
Mayapple extracts are included in prescription keratolytics used to treat condylomata acuminata, external and perianal warts, keratoses, laryngeal papilloma, and plan-

---

tar warts. Some plant components are included in anticancer drugs used to treat testicular, ovarian, and small-cell lung cancer. Mayapple is used as a stimulant laxative, cathartic, purgative, counterirritant, and vermifuge. It's also used to treat tinea capitis, rheumatoid arthritis, and amenorrhea. Topical tincture and extract are FDA approved for treating warts. Podophyllum is recommended by the Centers for Disease Control and Prevention as an alternative to cryotherapy for external warts.

### DOSAGE & ADMINISTRATION

*Dried root:* 1.5 to 3 g P.O. q.d.
*Tincture (25% in benzoin):* Applied to dry skin with dropper or applicator. A health care provider should apply the solution. To avoid toxicity, the treated area shouldn't exceed 25 cm². Dried resin is removed with soap and water after 1 to 4 hours.
*Topical solution (0.5%):* Applied b.i.d. with cotton-tipped applicator to wart surface for 3 days and then discontinued for 4 days. Repeat cycle up to four times.

### ADVERSE REACTIONS

**CNS:** mental status changes, *seizures,* stupor, dizziness, hallucinations, decreased reflexes, peripheral neuropathy, *coma.*
**CV:** hypotension, tachycardia.
**EENT:** conjunctivitis, keratitis.
**GI:** nausea, vomiting, diarrhea, abdominal pain, paralytic ileus.
**GU:** *nephrotoxicity,* urine retention.
**Hematologic:** anemia, *leukopenia, thrombocytopenia, myelosuppression.*

**Hepatic:** *hepatotoxicity.*
**Metabolic:** hypokalemia.
**Respiratory:** shortness of breath, tachypnea.
**Skin:** hair loss, ulcerative skin lesion.
**Other:** pyrexia.

### INTERACTIONS

None reported.

### CAUTIONS

Women who are pregnant or breastfeeding shouldn't take this herb. Patients with diabetes mellitus, circulatory problems, inflamed surrounding tissue, or open warts should avoid using the herb as well, along with patients hypersensitive to mayapple.

### NURSING CONSIDERATIONS

🖉 **ALERT:** This entire herb is considered toxic and should be used only under the supervision of a qualified health care provider. Only the ripe fruits are edible.
• Find out why patient is using herb.
• Patients shouldn't use topically for areas larger than 25 cm² because of the risk of resorptive poisoning.
• Resin extracts are for external use only.
• Topical solutions should be washed off genital and perianal warts in 1 to 4 hours.
• Solution should be washed off meatal warts in 1 to 2 hours.
• Patients should apply occlusive dressing or urea around treated area to avoid contact with healthy skin.

---

*Liquid may contain alcohol.

**Patient teaching**
- Advise patient to consult with his health care provider before using an herbal preparation because a treatment with proven efficacy may be available.
- Tell patient to remind pharmacist of any herbal and dietary supplements that he's taking, when filling a new prescription.
- Advise patient to report any irritation or increase in bleeding or bruising to his health care provider.
- Warn patient not to use mayapple near the eyes.
- Caution patient about ingesting large amounts of the dried root to avoid excess cathartic effects and poisoning.
- Warn patient to keep all herbal products away from children and pets.

## meadowsweet

*Filipendula ulmaria, Spireaea ulmaria,* bridewort, dolloff, dropwort, lady of the meadow, meadow queen, meadow-wort, meadsweet, meadwort, queen of the meadow

**Common trade names**
*Arkocaps, Artival, Neutracalm, Rheuma-Tee, Rheumex, Santane, Spireadosa*

### HOW SUPPLIED
Available as dried flowers, stems, leaves, and roots; tablets, infusion, powder, liquid extract, and tincture.
*Tablets:* 300 mg

### ACTIONS & COMPONENTS
Meadowsweet contains flavonoids, salicylates, coumarins, tannins, methyl salicylate, mucilage, ascorbic acid, and carbohydrates. It displays analgesic, antipyretic, antiemetic, antiulcer, antirheumatic, antiflatulent, laxative, sedative, diuretic, and anti-inflammatory actions. A heparin complex found in the plant demonstrates in vitro fibrinolytic and anticoagulant properties. Extracts from the flower exhibit in vitro bacteriocidal activity against *Staphylococcus aureus, S. epidermidis, Escherichia coli, Pseudomonas aeruginosa,* and *Proteus vulgaris.* Astringent properties have been attributed to the tannins in the plant. Extracts demonstrate antitumor, sedative, and urinary antiseptic properties as well.

### USES
Used as an analgesic and anti-inflammatory for conditions such as toothache, rheumatoid arthritis, headache, tendinitis, and sprains. Also used for GI complaints such as gastritis, diarrhea, peptic ulcer, heartburn, and irritable bowel syndrome. Also used as a diuretic or astringent and to relieve cough, colds, and bronchitis.

### DOSAGE & ADMINISTRATION
*Dried flowers:* 2.5 to 3.5 g P.O. q.d.
*Dried herb:* 4 to 5 g P.O. q.d.
*Infusion:* 3 to 6 g prepared with 100 ml boiling water, strained after 10 minutes, taken P.O. t.i.d., p.r.n.
*Liquid extract (1:1 in 25% alcohol):* 1.5 to 6 ml P.O. t.i.d.
*Powder:* ½ tsp in a small amount of water P.O. t.i.d.

*Tincture (1:5 in 25% alcohol):* 2 to 4 ml P.O. t.i.d.

**ADVERSE REACTIONS**
**GI:** nausea.
**Respiratory:** *bronchospasm.*

**INTERACTIONS**
**Herb-drug.** *Disulfiram:* Herbal products prepared with alcohol may cause a disulfiram-like reaction. Advise patient to avoid using together.
*Salicylate and salicylate derivatives:* May result in additive salicylates. Advise patient to avoid using together.
*Warfarin:* May have additive effect. Advise patient to avoid using together.

**CAUTIONS**
Meadowsweet shouldn't be used by patients with a history of salicylate or sulfite sensitivity, patients taking warfarin, or patients with cardiac conditions who take aspirin. It also shouldn't be used by children or by pregnant or breast-feeding patients.

**NURSING CONSIDERATIONS**
• Find out why patient is using herb.
• Asthmatic patients should use herb cautiously.
⚡**ALERT:** This product contains methyl salicylate, which is fatal in high doses.

**Patient teaching**
• Advise patient to consult with his health care provider before using an herbal preparation because a

treatment with proven efficacy may be available.
• Tell patient to remind pharmacist of any herbal and dietary supplements that he's taking, when filling a new prescription.
• Although no chemical interactions have been reported in clinical studies, advise patient that herb may interfere with therapeutic effect of conventional drugs.
• Caution patient to avoid use if he has a history of asthma or sensitivity to aspirin.
• Tell patient to stop using salicylates if using meadowsweet.
• Warn patient not to take herb for chronic or unexplained pain before seeking appropriate medical evaluation because doing so may delay diagnosis of a potentially serious medical condition.
• Advise women to avoid use during pregnancy and while breast-feeding.
• Tell patient to keep herb out of reach of children because of risk of salicylate poisoning.

## melatonin

MEL

**Common trade names**
*Circadian (controlled-release, not available in U.S.), Mela-T, Melatonex*

**HOW SUPPLIED**
Available as synthetic or animal-derived (pineal tissue) products.
*Tablets:* 300 mcg, 1.5 mg, 3 mg. Also available as lozenges.

## ACTIONS & COMPONENTS
Melatonin is a hormone produced by the pineal gland. Secretion is stimulated by darkness and inhibited by light. Secretion peaks between 2:00 a.m. and 4:00 a.m., and the extent of excretion diminishes with advancing age. Melatonin administration may regulate circadian rhythms and may also help regulate body temperature, CV function, and reproduction. It may also protect cells against oxidation caused by free-radical formation.

## USES
Used for treating insomnia, jet lag, shift-work disorder, blind entrainment, immune system enhancement, tinnitus, depression, and benzodiazepine withdrawal in geriatric patients with insomnia. Also used as a cancer therapy adjuvant, antiaging product, contraceptive, and as prophylactic therapy for cluster headaches. Topically, it's used for skin protection against ultraviolet light.

## DOSAGE & ADMINISTRATION
*Adjunctive therapy for metastatic lung cancer:* 10 mg P.O. h.s.
*Benzodiazepine withdrawal in geriatric patients with insomnia:* 2 mg of controlled-release P.O. h.s. for 6 weeks while benzodiazepine dosage is reduced by 50% during week 2, 75% during weeks 3 and 4, and discontinued during weeks 5 and 6; may continue for up to 6 months for insomnia.
*Jet lag:* 5 mg P.O. h.s. for 1 week, beginning 3 days before the flight.
*Sleep disturbance:* 0.3 to 5 mg P.O. h.s.

*Topical use:* Dosage not well documented.

## ADVERSE REACTIONS
**CNS:** headache, depression, daytime fatigue and drowsiness, dizziness, irritability, reduced alertness.
**GI:** abdominal cramps.
**Other:** increased hormone levels.

## INTERACTIONS
**Herb-drug.** *Atenolol:* May reverse negative sleep effects caused by atenolol. Monitor patient.
*CNS depressants:* Possible additive sedation. Warn patient of potential hazards.
*Fluoxetine:* May reduce sleep disturbance in patients with major depressive disorder who take fluoxetine. Monitor patient for effect.
*Immunosuppressants:* Melatonin may interfere with immunosuppressant therapy by improving immune function. Advise patient to avoid using together.
*Verapamil:* May increase melatonin secretion. Monitor for increased adverse melatonin effects.
**Herb-herb.** *Sedating herbs or supplements, such as 5-HTP, kava-kava, valerian:* May contribute to additive sedation. Advise patient to avoid using together.
**Herb-lifestyle.** *Alcohol:* Additive sedative effects may occur. Advise patient to avoid using together.

## CAUTIONS
Because melatonin may worsen depression, it shouldn't be used by depressed patients taking CNS depressants. It shouldn't be taken by patients using immunosuppressants or by women who are preg-

---

*Bold italic type* indicates that reaction may be life-threatening.

nant or breast-feeding. It also shouldn't be used by children because melatonin may inhibit gonadal development.

## NURSING CONSIDERATIONS
• Find out why patient is using herb.
• Monitor patient for excessive daytime drowsiness.
• May increase human growth hormone levels.

### Patient teaching
• Advise patient to consult with his health care provider before using an herbal preparation or supplement because a treatment with proven efficacy may be available.
• Tell patient to remind pharmacist of any herbal and dietary supplements that he's taking, when filling a new prescription.
• Warn patient to avoid hazardous activities until full extent of CNS depressant effects are known.
• If patient wishes to conceive, tell her that melatonin may have a contraceptive effect. However, herb shouldn't be used as a form of birth control.
• Although no chemical interactions have been reported in clinical studies, tell patient that melatonin may interfere with therapeutic effects of conventional drugs.
• Warn patient about possible additive effects if taken with alcohol.
• Advise patient to use only the synthetic form (not the animal-derived product) because of concerns about contamination and viral transmission.

• Advise patient not to use melatonin for prolonged periods because safety data aren't available.

## methylsulfonylmethane

MSM, dimethyl sulfone, crystalline DMSO, $DMSO_2$, methyl sulfonyl methane, sulfonyl sulfur

**Common trade names**
*None known*

### HOW SUPPLIED
Available as capsules, tablets, powder, and liquid. Cream, lotion, nasal spray, EENT drops, shampoo, and conditioner formulations are also available.
*Capsules:* 500 mg, 750 mg, 1,000 mg
*Liquid:* 390 mg/5 ml
*Powder:* 2,600 mg/0.5 tsp
*Tablets:* 500 mg, 750 mg, 1,000 mg

### ACTIONS & COMPONENTS
Methylsulfonylmethane is found naturally in foods, but heat or dehydration destroys it. It's found in green plants such as field horsetail *(Equisetum arvense),* some algae species, fruits, vegetables, grains, and some animal products such as adrenal cortex of cattle, milk, and urine. It's a possible source of sulfur for formation of amino acids cysteine and methionine.

### USES
Used to treat GI upset, inflammatory disorders, musculoskeletal pain, arthritis, allergies, autoimmune diseases, cancer, and intersti-

---

*Liquid may contain alcohol.

tial cystitis. Also used as an anti-microbial and an immune system stimulant.

**DOSAGE & ADMINISTRATION**
Dosages vary from 250 to 3,000 mg P.O. daily with meals. Dosages for topical use aren't well documented.

**ADVERSE REACTIONS**
**CNS:** headache, fatigue.
**GI:** nausea, diarrhea.

**INTERACTIONS**
None reported.

**CAUTIONS**
Women who are pregnant or breast-feeding should avoid this supplement, as should patients who are hypersensitive to it.

**NURSING CONSIDERATIONS**
● No important toxicities or contraindications have been reported.

**Patient teaching**
● Advise patient to consult with his health care provider before using an herbal preparation or supplement because a treatment with proven efficacy may be available.
● Tell patient to remind pharmacist of any herbal and dietary supplements that he's taking, when filling a new prescription.
● Tell patient to avoid use during pregnancy and lactation.
● Urge patient to report adverse effects to a health care provider.
● Because heat destroys methylsulfonylmethane, advise patient to store it in a cool, dry place.

## milk thistle

*Silybum marianum,* cardui mariae fructus, holy thistle, lady's thistle, Marian thistle, Mary thistle, silymarin, St. Mary thistle

**Common trade names**
*Liver Formula with Milk Thistle, Milk Thistle Extract, Milk Thistle Phytosome, Milk Thistle Plus, Milk Thistle Power, Milk Thistle Super Complex, Silybin Phytosome, Silymarin Milk Thistle, Simply Milk Thistle, Thisilyn*

**HOW SUPPLIED**
Obtained from seeds of *Silybum marianum.* Available as capsules, soft gels, liquid, extract*, and I.V. silbinin (I.V. form unavailable in the United States).
*Capsules:* 120 mg, 175 mg, 280 mg, 350 mg, 525 mg
*Liquid caps:* 75 mg, 150 mg
*Softgels:* 100 mg, 150 mg

**ACTIONS & COMPONENTS**
Contains silymarin, which consists of hepatoprotective flavonolignans, including silibinin (silybin), silidyanin, and silychristin. Silymarin alters liver cell walls to prevent toxin entry and acts as an antioxidant by scavenging free radicals. It also stimulates protein synthesis in the liver, promoting liver cell generation. Silymarin's anti-inflammatory and immunomodulatory activity may add to its protective actions on the liver. Milk thistle components reduce histamine release from basophils through membrane stabilization, inhibit T-lymphocyte acti-

vation, increase neutrophil motility, and alter polymorphonuclear leukocyte function. Silibinin administration decreases biliary cholesterol levels. Milk thistle reduces insulin resistance in alcoholic cirrhosis patients.

**USES**
Used for dyspepsia, liver damage from chemicals, *Amanita* mushroom poisoning, supportive therapy for inflammatory liver disease and cirrhosis, loss of appetite, and gallbladder and spleen disorders. It's also used as a liver protectant.

**DOSAGE & ADMINISTRATION**
*Dried fruit or seed:* 12 to 15 g P.O. q.d.
*Injection (not available in the United States), for Amanita phalloides mushroom poisoning:* 20 to 50 mg/kg I.V. over 24 hours, divided into four doses infused over 2 hours each.
*Oral:* Doses of milk thistle extract vary from 200 to 400 mg of silibinin (70% silymarin extract) P.O. q.d.
*Tea:* 3 to 5 g freshly crushed fruit or seed steeped in 5 oz of boiling water for 10 to 15 minutes. 1 cup of tea P.O. t.i.d. to q.i.d., 30 minutes before meals.

**ADVERSE REACTIONS**
**GI:** nausea, vomiting, diarrhea.

**INTERACTIONS**
**Herb-drug.** *Aspirin:* May improve aspirin metabolism in patients with liver cirrhosis. Advise patient to discuss use with health care provider.

*Cisplatin:* May prevent kidney damage by cisplatin. Advise patient to discuss use with health care provider.
*Disulfiram:* Products that contain alcohol may cause a disulfiram-like reaction. Advise patient to avoid using together.
*Hepatotoxic drugs:* May prevent liver damage from butyrophenones, phenothiazines, phenytoin, acetaminophen, and halothane. Advise patient to discuss use with health care provider.
*Tacrine:* Silymarin reduces adverse cholinergic effects when given together. Advise patient to discuss use with health care provider.

**CAUTIONS**
Milk thistle shouldn't be used by patients who are pregnant or breast-feeding or by patients hypersensitive to it. Use in decompensated cirrhosis isn't recommended.

**NURSING CONSIDERATIONS**
● Find out why patient is using herb.
● Mild allergic reactions may occur, especially in people allergic to members of the Asteraceae family, including ragweed, chrysanthemums, marigolds, and daisies.
● Don't confuse milk thistle seeds or fruit with other parts of the plant or with blessed thistle *(Cnictus benedictus)*.
● Silymarin has poor water solubility; therefore, efficacy when prepared as a tea is questionable.

---

*Liquid may contain alcohol.

**Patient teaching**

• Advise patient to consult with his health care provider before using an herbal preparation because a treatment with proven efficacy may be available.

• Tell patient to remind pharmacist of any herbal and dietary supplements that he's taking, when filling a new prescription.

• Although no chemical interactions have been reported in clinical studies, advise patient that herb may interfere with therapeutic effect of conventional drugs.

• Warn patient not to take this herb while pregnant or breast-feeding.

• Tell patient to stay alert for possible allergic reactions, especially if allergic to ragweed, chrysanthemums, marigolds, or daisies.

• Warn patient not to take herb for liver inflammation or cirrhosis before seeking appropriate medical evaluation because doing so may delay diagnosis of a potentially serious medical condition.

• Warn patient to keep all herbal products away from children and pets.

## mistletoe

*Phoradendron serotinum, Viscum album,* all-heal, American mistletoe, birdlime, devil's fuge, European mistletoe, mistelkraut, mystyldene, visci

**Common trade names**
*Helixor, Iscador, Plenosol*

**HOW SUPPLIED**
Available as dried leaves, stems, flowers, and fruit; extract*, and injectable (I.V. form unavailable in the United States) are obtained from American mistletoe *(Phoradendron* species*)* and European mistletoe *(Viscum* species*)*.

**ACTIONS & COMPONENTS**
Phoratoxins and viscotoxins are toxic proteins isolated from American and European mistletoe, respectively. Phoratoxins from American mistletoe can cause hypertension, hypotension, bradycardia, and increased uterine and intestinal motility. Phoratoxins may also cause depolarization of skeletal muscle, smooth muscle contraction, vasoconstriction, and cardiac arrest. Lectins and viscotoxins from European mistletoe may possess anticancer and immunostimulation activity. Other effects include hypotension, bradycardia, and sedation. As an immunomodulator, *V. album* may stimulate DNA repair through lymphokines and cytokines in cancer patients. A lectin from mistletoe extract increases secretion of tumor necrosis factor, interleukin-1, and interleukin-6.

**USES**
American mistletoe is used as a smooth muscle stimulant for increasing blood pressure and uterine and intestinal contractions. European mistletoe is used to treat hypertension, cancer, as well as internal bleeding, major blood loss, blood purification, arteriosclerosis, epilepsy, gout, and hysteria.

## DOSAGE & ADMINISTRATION
Not well documented.

## ADVERSE REACTIONS
**CNS:** delirium, hallucinations.
**CV:** *bradycardia,* hypertension, vasoconstriction, *cardiac arrest.*
**EENT:** double vision.
**GI:** nausea, vomiting, diarrhea, acute gastroenteritis.
**Hepatic:** *hepatitis.*
**Skin:** infiltration after S.C. injection.

## INTERACTIONS
**Herb-drug.** *Anticoagulants, coagulants:* European mistletoe may alter efficacy of either drug type. Advise patient to avoid using together.
*Antidepressants:* European mistletoe may interfere with therapy. Advise patient to avoid using together.
*Blood pressure-modifying drugs:* Blood pressure may be lowered by European mistletoe. Monitor blood pressure frequently.
*Immunosuppressants:* European mistletoe may interfere with therapy. Advise patient to avoid using together.

## CAUTIONS
All components of mistletoe, including berries, are considered toxic and shouldn't be taken by anyone.

## NURSING CONSIDERATIONS
• Find out why patient is using herb.
🗲ALERT: Signs and symptoms of toxicity include nausea, bradycardia, gastroenteritis, hypertension, delirium, and hallucinations. Diarrhea and vomiting can lead to serious dehydration, hypovolemic shock, and CV collapse. Monitor blood pressure and heart rate closely. If any berries are ingested, rapid gastric emptying should be used. Adverse effects seem to be dose related.
• American mistletoe (*Phoradendron* species) and European mistletoe (*Viscum* species) may have varying pharmacologic effects. Ask patient which one he's taking.

## Patient teaching
• Advise patient to consult with his health care provider before using an herbal preparation because a treatment with proven efficacy may be available.
• Tell patient to remind pharmacist of any herbal and dietary supplements that he's taking, when filling a new prescription.
🗲ALERT: Inform patient that the FDA has forbidden marketing of this herb as a food additive until proven safe and has seized or barred the sale of commercial products known to contain mistletoe.
• Tell patient to notify health care provider about adverse effects, especially chest pain or tightness, nausea, vomiting, diarrhea, hallucinations, double vision, or slowed heart rate.

## monascus

red rice yeast, red yeast, xuezhikang, zhitai

**Common trade names**
*Cholester-Reg, CholesteSure, Cholestin, Ruby Monascus*

---

*Liquid may contain alcohol.

## HOW SUPPLIED
Obtained from a yeast, *Monascus purpureus,* grown on cooked, non-glutinous rice. Available as capsules and extract.
*Capsules:* 500 mg, 600 mg (0.4% or 2.4 mg of HMG-CoA reductase inhibitors)
*Ethanol extract:* 1.1% HMG-CoA reductase inhibitors

## ACTIONS & COMPONENTS
Yeast contains 3-hydroxy-3-methyl-glutaryl-coenzyme A (HMG-CoA) reductase inhibitors, primarily lovastatin (or monacolin K). Lovastatin is available as a prescription cholesterol-lowering drug. Monacolin K is converted in the body to mevinolinic acid, which competitively binds to HMG-CoA reductase in place of the endogenous substance, HMG-CoA, inhibiting cholesterol formation.

## USES
Used to reduce total cholesterol, low-density lipoprotein cholesterol, and triglyceride levels; to increase high-density lipoprotein levels in patients with hypercholesterolemia; and to sustain desirable cholesterol levels in healthy people. Also used for indigestion and diarrhea, and for improving blood circulation and promoting stomach and spleen health.

## DOSAGE & ADMINISTRATION
*Hypercholesterolemia:* 1,200 mg (7.2 mg Lovastatin, 9.6 mg total HMG Co-A reductase inhibitors) P.O. b.i.d. with food. One manufacturer recommends 600 mg q.d. and another recommends 1,000 mg q.d.

## ADVERSE REACTIONS
**GI:** gastritis, abdominal discomfort.
**GU:** *nephrotoxicity.*
**Hepatic:** elevated liver enzyme levels.
**Musculoskeletal:** *rhabdomyolysis,* muscle pain, tenderness, weakness.

## INTERACTIONS
**Herb-drug.** *Cholesterol-lowering drugs, including gemfibrozil, niacin:* To limit adverse effects and determine whether combination therapy is more effective, monitor patient closely if patient is taking drug and monascus concurrently.
*Cytochrome P450-3A-inhibiting drugs, such as fluconazole, itraconazole, ketoconazole, theophylline:* May increase serum levels and adverse effects from monascus. Monitor patient for adverse effects and efficacy.
*HMG-CoA reductase inhibitors:* May increase risk of adverse effects without added benefit. Advise patient to avoid using together.
*Levothyroxine:* Rarely, may alter thyroid function. Monitor thyroid function tests if patient is taking drug and monascus together.
**Herb-food.** *Grapefruit juice:* Increased bioavailability of lovastatin, increasing the risk of adverse effects. Monitor patient closely for adverse effects.
**Herb-lifestyle.** *Alcohol:* May increase risk of liver toxicity. Advise patient to avoid using together.

---

*Bold italic type* indicates that reaction may be life-threatening.

## CAUTIONS

Patients at risk for liver disease, with active liver disease, or with a history of liver disease shouldn't take monascus. Pregnant women should avoid monascus because cholesterol is important for fetal development. Women should also avoid use while breast-feeding. Maker of Cholestin brand of monascus warns patients not to take product if they consume more than two alcoholic drinks per day, have a serious infection, have undergone an organ transplant, have had recent major surgery, or have a serious disease or physical disorder.

Patients younger than age 18 should use cautiously because safety hasn't been established.

## NURSING CONSIDERATIONS

- Find out why patient is using herb.
- Monitor lipid panel for efficacy and liver function tests for liver toxicity at regular intervals.
- If patient develops muscle pain or weakness, check creatine kinase to test for rhabdomyolysis.
- Review patient's current drug list. Many drugs, especially cytochrome P450-3A inhibitors, may cause drug interactions.

### Patient teaching

- Advise patient to consult with his health care provider before using an herbal preparation because a treatment with proven efficacy may be available.
- Tell patient to remind pharmacist of any herbal and dietary supplements that he's taking, when filling a new prescription.

- Tell patient to take herb with food.
- Warn patient with liver disease not to take this drug.
- Recommend that patient abstain from alcohol or limit its use.
- Caution patient against using herb while pregnant or breast-feeding.
- Urge patient to seek medical attention if he experiences brown urine, muscle pain, or weakness.
- Teach patient the importance of laboratory monitoring for efficacy and toxicity.

## morinda

*Morinda citrifolia,* ba ji tian, hog apple, Indian mulberry, mengkudu, mora de la India, noni, pain killer, ruibardo caribe, wild pine

**Common trade names**
*Morinda, Morinda Citrifolia Capsules, Noni, Noni Nectar, Noni Juice, Tahitian Noni Juice*

## HOW SUPPLIED

Obtained from root of *Morinda citrifolia*; leaves, fruit, and juice also are used. Available in many forms, including fruit leather, capsules, oil, fiber, and combination foods, such as protein wafers, juices, and nutritional supplements.

## ACTIONS & COMPONENTS

Above-ground portions contain essential oils with hexoic and octoic acids, paraffin and esters of methyl, and ethyl alcohols. Root contains anthraquinones, alizarin, morindone, xeronine, and damnacanthal.

Xeronine, a digestive enzyme, may be responsible for herb's action in repairing damaged cells in digestive, respiratory, and skeletal systems, possibly by affecting shape of protein molecules and by enhancing immune function.

Damnacanthal exerts antitumor activity by inhibiting the reticular activating system oncogene, a protein partially responsible for cell proliferation. Alcoholic extracts have anthelmintic and central analgesic activity. Tannins contained in morinda may have hypoglycemic properties.

## USES
Used to treat diabetes, high blood pressure, and GI and liver conditions. Also used as a sedative and for chronic fatigue syndrome, premenstrual syndrome, and ankylosing spondylitis. Also used topically for soothing headaches and arthritic joints by wrapping leaves around affected areas. Other uses include immunostimulant, anticancer, and anthelmintic effects.

## DOSAGE & ADMINISTRATION
Dosage can range from 3 to 6 g daily in two divided doses P.O. on an empty stomach.
*Tea:* Prepared by adding 5 to 9 g herb to 3 to 4 cups of water, boiling until volume is reduced by half, and cooling. Taken in two divided doses on empty stomach.
*Tincture:* 30 to 60 g steeped in 1 L of ethanol for 2 to 3 months. 30 ml taken P.O. b.i.d. on empty stomach in afternoon and h.s.

## ADVERSE REACTIONS
**Metabolic:** *hyperkalemia* in patients with chronic renal failure.

## INTERACTIONS
**Herb-drug.** *ACE inhibitors, angiotensin II receptor antagonists, beta blockers, potassium-sparing diuretics, trimethoprim-sulfamethoxazole:* Additive effects of hyperkalemia. Monitor patient closely for potassium accumulation when herb and drug are used together.
*Immunosuppressants:* May counteract the effects of immunosuppressants. Advise patient to avoid using together.

## CAUTIONS
Pregnant women and those who are breast-feeding shouldn't use morinda. It also shouldn't be used by patients with end-stage renal disease (noni juice form contains potassium) or those hypersensitive to it. It shouldn't be used in organ transplant recipients because of the increased risk of rejection raised by herb's immune system-enhancing properties.

## NURSING CONSIDERATIONS
- Find out why patient is using herb.
- Morinda shouldn't replace conventional therapies that are known to be effective in the treatment of different cancers and CV and endocrine disorders.
- Carefully monitor patient for adverse effects.

---

*Bold italic type* indicates that reaction may be life-threatening.

**Patient teaching**

• Advise patient to consult with his health care provider before using an herbal preparation because a treatment with proven efficacy may be available.

• Tell patient to remind pharmacist of any herbal and dietary supplements that he's taking, when filling a new prescription.

• Although no chemical interactions have been reported in clinical studies, advise patient that herb may interfere with therapeutic effect of conventional drugs.

• Teach patient that anthraquinone content in the product may turn urine a pink or rust color.

• Instruct patient to take herb on an empty stomach so intestines may activate the enzyme.

• Because sedation is possible, advise patient not to perform hazardous tasks while taking herb.

• Advise patient with kidney failure that noni juice is a source of potassium and that he shouldn't use it.

• Warn pregnant or breast-feeding patients to avoid using this herb.

• Warn patient not to take herb for worrisome symptoms before seeking appropriate medical evaluation because doing so may delay diagnosis of a potentially serious medical condition.

## motherwort

*Leonurus cardiaca,* lion's ear, lion's tail, Roman motherwort, throw-wort

**Common trade names**
*Motherwort Flowering Tops, Motherwort Flowers, Motherwort Herb—Organic Alcohol*

### HOW SUPPLIED
Obtained from above-ground parts of *Leonurus cardiaca.* Available as powdered herb, leaf and flowering tops\*, flowering tops\*, fluidextract\*, solid extract, and alcohol extracts.

### ACTIONS & COMPONENTS
Contains leocardin, ajugoside (leonuride), ajugol, galiridoside, reptoside and other constituents including flavonoids, leonurin, betaine, caffeic acid derivative, tannins, and traces of volatile oil. Alkaloids responsible for major herb activity include stachydrine, betonicine, turicin, leonurine, leonuridin, and leonurinine. Herb has mild negative chronotropic properties, and hypotonic, cardiac-inhibitory, antispasmodic, and sedative actions. Leonurine may stimulate uterine tone and blood flow, and stachydrine may stimulate oxytocin release. Ursolic acid may have antiviral, tumor-inhibiting, and cytotoxic activity. "K substance," an extract of motherwort, may decrease blood viscosity through platelet aggregation inhibition and inhibitory effects on cardiac function.

---

\*Liquid may contain alcohol.

## USES

Used for hyperthyroidism, management of mild to moderate cardiac insufficiency (New York Heart Association classes I and II), arrhythmias such as tachycardia, and other nervous cardiac conditions. Also used for flatulence, amenorrhea, itching, and shingles; used topically to improve eyesight and as a generalized tonic and antiplatelet agent. Used in combination with other herbs to treat symptoms of BPH.

## DOSAGE & ADMINISTRATION

*Acute conditions:* 5 gtt, 1 tablet, 10 pellets P.O. every 30 to 60 minutes.
*Dietary supplement:* Fluidextract 1:1 (g/ml) 1 to 2 ml P.O. t.i.d. (extract contains 12% to 15% organic alcohol).
*Dried above-ground parts:* 2 g P.O. t.i.d.
*Infusion for internal use:* Average total daily dose, 4.5 g herb.
*Long-term use:* 5 gtt, 1 tablet, 10 pellets, P.O. q.d. to t.i.d.
*Tea:* Prepared by steeping 2 g dried above-ground part in 5 oz boiling water for 5 to 10 minutes, then straining. 1 cup taken t.i.d.
*Tincture:* 1:5 (g/ml) 22.5 ml (tincture contains 56% to 62 % grain alcohol).

## ADVERSE REACTIONS

**GI:** diarrhea, stomach irritation.
**GU:** uterine bleeding.
**Skin:** contact dermatitis, photosensitivity reaction.
**Other:** allergic reactions.

## INTERACTIONS

**Herb-drug.** *Antihistamines, CNS depressants:* Possible increased sedation. Monitor patient.
*Cardiac glycosides:* Additive effects and possible cardiac glycoside toxicity. Advise patient to avoid using together.
*Disulfiram or metronidazole:* Disulfiram-like reaction may result from alcohol content of herb preparations. Advise patient to avoid using together.
**Herb-herb.** *Herbs containing cardiac glycosides, such as black hellebore, Canadian hemp roots, digitalis leaf, figwort, hedge mustard, lily-of-the-valley roots, oleander leaf, pheasant's-eye plant, pleurisy root, squill bulb leaf scales, strophanthus seeds, and uzara:* Additive effects and possible cardiac glycoside toxicity. Advise patient to avoid using together.
**Herb-lifestyle.** *Alcohol:* May potentiate sedative effects. Discourage using together.
*Sunlight:* Photosensitivity reaction may occur. Advise patient to take precautions.

## CAUTIONS

Herb shouldn't be used by pregnant women because of possible uterine-stimulating properties. Effects in breast-feeding patients are unknown; use should be avoided. Patients currently receiving treatment for cardiac dysfunction or arrhythmias shouldn't use motherwort because of the risk of increased toxicity.

---

*Bold italic type* indicates that reaction may be life-threatening.

## NURSING CONSIDERATIONS
• Find out why patient is using herb.
• Because of effects of sedatives, geriatric patients should be monitored closely and full precautions taken.
• Tinctures, fluidextracts, and flowering tops contain a large amount of alcohol and shouldn't be used by children, alcoholic patients, or patients taking disulfiram or metronidazole.

### Patient teaching
• Advise patient to consult with his health care provider before using an herbal preparation because a treatment with proven efficacy may be available.
• Tell patient to remind pharmacist of any herbal and dietary supplements that he's taking, when filling a new prescription.
• Advise patient that motherwort has an unpleasant odor.
• Tell patient to notify health care provider about planned, suspected, or known pregnancy. Discourage breast-feeding while taking herb.
• Tell patient that doses higher than recommended may cause diarrhea, stomach irritation, or uterine bleeding.
• Warn patient that herb may cause sedation and that he should avoid hazardous activities.
• Tell patient to keep fluidextract, tincture, and flowering tops out of the reach of children.
• Teach patient that motherwort may make him sensitive to the effects of sunlight; explain the need for adequate sunscreen when going outdoors.

# mugwort

*Artemisiae vulgaris radix, Artemisia vulgaris,* artemisia, carline thistle, felon herb, hierba de San Juan, sailor's tobacco, St. John's plant, wormwood

**Common trade names**
*Mugwort, Wormwood*

## HOW SUPPLIED
Obtained from leaves and roots of *Artemisia vulgaris.* Available as leaves, tablets, fluidextract, and powder. Also used in food products, such as pasta.
*Mugwort tincture:** (1:5, 50% alcohol)

## ACTIONS & COMPONENTS
Contains volatile oils (including 1,8-cineol, camphor, linalool, or thujone), sesquiterpene lactones, lipophilic flavonoids, polyenes, umbelliferone, aesculetin, and hydroxycoumarins. Aqueous extract and essential oil have antimicrobial activity. Thujone may be responsible for uterine stimulant activity.

## USES
Used for many GI complaints, such as colic, diarrhea, constipation, cramps, weak digestion, and persistent vomiting. Also used as a laxative for obesity, to stimulate gastric juice and bile secretion, as a therapeutic hand soak, and as a tonic for asthenia. Also used for worm infestations, epilepsy, poor circulation, sedation, and menstrual problems. Used in combination with other herbs for psychoneuroses, neurasthenia, depression,

hypochondria, autonomic neuroses, general irritability, restlessness, insomnia, and anxiety states.

## DOSAGE & ADMINISTRATION

*Hand soak:* 2 handfuls of dried mugwort steeped in 10 oz raw apple cider vinegar. Then, 1 to 2 tbs of this infusion added to warm water; hands are soaked for 10 minutes.
*Tea:* 15 g of the dried herb steeped in 16 oz of boiling water and strained. 2 to 3 cups of tea taken q.d. before meals.
*Tincture:* Dosages vary depending on formulation and reason for treatment.

## ADVERSE REACTIONS

**Skin:** rarely, sensitization through skin contact.

## INTERACTIONS

**Herb-drug.** *CNS depressants:* Increased sedative effects. Monitor patient.
*Disulfiram or metronidazole:* Disulfiram-like reaction may occur because of alcohol content. Advise patient to avoid using together.
**Herb-lifestyle.** *Alcohol:* May potentiate sedative effects. Advise patient to avoid using together.

## CAUTIONS

Women who are pregnant or breast-feeding should avoid using this herb; mugwort has abortifacient properties via uterine stimulation. Patients hypersensitive to members of the Asteraceae family (such as ragweed, chrysanthemums, marigolds, daisies, sage, wormwood) may have an allergic reaction to mugwort and should use the herb with caution. Allergic reactions may also occur in people allergic to tobacco, honey, or royal jelly.

## NURSING CONSIDERATIONS

- Find out why patient is using herb.
- Allergic IgE-mediated reactions via histamine release may occur in patients with allergies to plants of the same family.
- Tincture contains significant amounts of alcohol and shouldn't be used by children, alcoholic patients, or those taking disulfiram or metronidazole.

## Patient teaching

- Advise patient to consult with his health care provider before using an herbal preparation because a treatment with proven efficacy may be available.
- Tell patient to remind pharmacist of any herbal and dietary supplements that he's taking, when filling a new prescription.
- Advise patient that mugwort root has a pleasant, tangy taste; aboveground parts are aromatic and bitter.
- Caution patient that he may become sensitized to the herb with skin contact.
- If patient is allergic to herbs of the Asteraceae family (ragweed, chrysanthemums, marigolds, daisies, sage, wormwood), tobacco, honey, or royal jelly, warn of a possible hypersensitivity reaction to mugwort.
- Warn patient to keep all herbal products away from children and pets.

---

*Bold italic type* indicates that reaction may be life-threatening.

• Instruct women taking this herb to notify a health care provider about planned, suspected, or known pregnancy. Advise against taking herb while breast-feeding.

## mullein

*Verbascum densiflorum,* Aaron's rod, Adam's flannel, ag-leaf, ag-paper, American mullein, beggar's blanket, blanket herb, blanket-leaf, bouillon blanc, candleflower, candlewick plant, clot-bur, clown's lungwort, cuddy's lungs, duffle, European mullein, feltwort, flannelflower, fluffweed, golden rod, hag's taper, hare's beard, hedge-taper, Jacob's staff, Jupiter's staff, longwort, orange mullein, Our Lady's flannel, rag paper, shepherd's club, shepherd's staff, torches, torch weed, velvet plant, verbasci flos, wild ice leaf, woollen

**Common trade names**
*Alcohol-Free Mullein Leaves, Mullein Extract, Mullein Leaf, Mullein Tea*

### HOW SUPPLIED
Obtained from dried flowers and leaves. Available as extracts, dried herb, capsules, teas, and oil. Available in many tea preparations and in combination with other herbs.
*Capsules:* 330 mg dried leaf
*Extracts in grain alcohol (45% to 55%):* 250 mg dry leaves = 1 ml liquid extract
*Leaves in vegetable glycerin (alcohol-free)*
*Oil:* Fresh flowers in pure virgin oil

### ACTIONS & COMPONENTS
Contains mucilage, triterpene saponins (including songarosaponin D, E, and F) iridoide monoterpenes, tannins, caffeic acid derivatives, flavonoids, and invert sugar. Tannins, saponins, and mucilage are responsible for herb's effects. Saponins have expectorant actions, mucin has antibiotic actions, and the combination alleviates irritation from colds. Demulcent properties may be useful for the treatment of sore throats. Mullein extract may have activity against influenza types A and B and against herpes simplex virus type I.

### USES
Used for respiratory tract inflammation, cough, sore throat, bronchitis, and respiratory tract inflammation. Also used internally as a diuretic, sedative, and narcotic; as an antirheumatic; and for croup, asthma, and tuberculosis. Used topically for hemorrhoids, burns, bruises, frostbite, and erysipelas. Oil is used to soothe earaches, and leaves are used to soften and protect the skin. Mullein is also used as a flavoring agent in alcoholic beverages.

### DOSAGE & ADMINISTRATION
*Capsules (330 mg):* 2 to 3 capsules P.O. b.i.d. with meals.
*Decoction:* 1.5 to 2 g of herb placed in 5 to 8 oz cold water and boiled for 10 minutes. Taken b.i.d.
*Fluidextract:* 1:1 (g/ml) 1.5 to 2 ml P.O. b.i.d. (contains 45% to 55% grain alcohol).
*Mullein extract:* 3 to 4 ml P.O. t.i.d. Use half this dose in children.

*Liquid may contain alcohol.

*Mullein flower oil:* 5 to 10 gtt extract in a little water P.O. b.i.d. to t.i.d.

*Mullein leaves liquid:* 4 to 8 gtt in a little water P.O. b.i.d.; liquid is alcohol-free.

*Tea:* Prepared by pouring boiling water over 1.5 to 2 g (1 tsp = 0.5 g drug) finely cut petals, steeping for 10 to 15 minutes, then straining. 1 cup taken q.d.

*Tincture:* 1:5 (g/ml) 7.5 to 10 ml P.O. b.i.d. May dilute in warm water.

## ADVERSE REACTIONS
None reported.

## INTERACTIONS
**Herb-drug.** *CNS depressants:* May potentiate sedative effects. Monitor patient.
*Disulfiram or metronidazole:* Disulfiram-like reaction may occur because of alcohol content. Advise patient to avoid using together.
**Herb-lifestyle.** *Alcohol:* May potentiate sedative effects. Advise patient to avoid using together.

## CAUTIONS
Herb shouldn't be used by patients who are pregnant or breast-feeding and by those who are hypersensitive to it.

## NURSING CONSIDERATIONS
• Find out why patient is using herb.
• Extracts may contain large amounts of alcohol and shouldn't be used by children, alcoholic patients, or those taking disulfiram or metronidazole.

• Don't confuse mullein with golden rod (*Solidago* species), which is also known as Aaron's rod.

## Patient teaching
• Advise patient to consult with his health care provider before using an herbal preparation because a treatment with proven efficacy may be available.
• Tell patient to remind pharmacist of any herbal and dietary supplements that he's taking, when filling a new prescription.
• Although no chemical interactions have been reported in clinical studies, advise patient that herb may interfere with therapeutic effect of conventional drugs.
• Tell patient to store herb in cool, dry place protected from light. If herb comes into contact with light or moisture, it discolors to brown or dark brown.
• Warn patient that mullein extracts contain alcohol and should be kept away from children.
• Advise patient to refrigerate mullein extract after opening it.
• Instruct women taking herb to notify a health care provider about planned, suspected, or known pregnancy. Caution against breast-feeding while taking this herb.

---

*Bold italic type* indicates that reaction may be life-threatening.

## mustard

Black mustard, brown mustard, Chinese mustard, Indian mustard, mustard oil, synapis alba, white mustard, yellow mustard

**Common trade names**
*Dr. Singha's Mustard Bath, Dr. Singha's Mustard Rub, Mustard, Essence of Mustard*

### HOW SUPPLIED

Mustard preparations extracted from the dried ripe seeds of *Sinapis alba* or *Brassica alba* (white mustard) or *Brassica nigra* (black mustard), powder. Also available as essential oil of mustard and essence of mustard* (27% alcohol).

### ACTIONS & COMPONENTS

The therapeutic action of mustard is achieved when the glucosinolates are hydrolyzed by the enzyme myrosin, and the active components are released, which occurs upon chewing or grinding the seeds and mixing them with warm water. Sinalbin is the glucosinolate found in white mustard and sinigrin in black or brown mustard. Sinalbin is hydrolyzed to p-hydroxybenzyl isothiocyanate or p-hydroxybenzylamine while sinigrin is hydrolyzed to allyl isothiocyanate. These substances, which are the active constituents responsible for the characteristic pungent odor, are potent skin irritants and bacteriostatic agents, and may possess anticarcinogenic properties. Mustard also contains fatty oil,

proteins, and phenylpropane derivatives. Mustard acts as a counterirritant when diluted to a 1:50 ratio. Mustard oil is absorbed through the skin and eliminated through the lungs.

### USES

Mustard has been used for upper respiratory tract conditions including the common cold, cough, bronchitis, fevers and colds, and inflammation of the mouth and pharynx. It's also used in a poultice for catarrhs of the respiratory tract, hyperemization of the skin, and chronic degenerative disorders. Black mustard oil or mustard seed is used topically for pulmonary congestion, rheumatism, and arthritis; as a counterirritant; in footbaths for aching feet; and as a bath for soothing paralytic conditions. Black mustard oil is used as a flavoring agent in foods and drinks, a lubricant and illuminant in soaps, and in cat and dog repellents. Mustard seed, a culinary spice, is also a flavoring agent in many foods including condiments and beverages. White mustard is used to clear the voice and for those with tendency for infection.

### DOSAGE & ADMINISTRATION

Average daily doses of mustard range from 60 to 240 g.
*For external use:* Mix 50 to 70 g (4 tbs) of powdered seeds with warm water, wrap in gauze and apply to affected area for 10 to 15 minutes for adults and 5 to 10 minutes for children older than age 6.

---

*Liquid may contain alcohol.

*For tired, aching feet:* Place 20 to 30 g of mustard flour in 1 L of water for footbath.

*Mustard plaster:* For adults, 100 g of black mustard flour (ground mustard) is mixed with warm water to form a paste. The paste is packed in linen and applied to the affected area for 10 to 15 minutes.

*To clear the voice:* Mix mustard flour with honey, form into balls and take 1 to 2 balls P.O. on an empty stomach q.d.

*To soothe paralytic symptoms:* Place 150 g of mustard flour in a pouch and drop into bathwater.

## ADVERSE REACTIONS

**CNS:** nerve damage, *coma,* somnolence.
**CV:** *heart failure.*
**GI:** vomiting, diarrhea, stomach pain.
**Respiratory:** breathing difficulties.
**Skin:** blistering, urticaria, ulceration, necrosis.
**Other:** goiter, *anaphylactic reactions, angioedema.*

## INTERACTIONS

**Herb-drug.** *Antacids, $H_2$ antagonists, sucralfate, and proton pump inhibitors:* Effects of these drugs may be diminished because of increased stomach acid production. Monitor patient for increased abdominal symptoms if used together.

## CAUTIONS

Patients with gastric or duodenal ulcers and reflux conditions shouldn't use mustard because of the irritant GI effects. Patients with inflammatory kidney diseases should avoid use because of the potential for irritant poisoning. Mustard shouldn't be used in children younger than age 6. Pregnant women shouldn't use mustard because of possible abortifacient actions. Breast-feeding patients should avoid use because of lack of information. Patients with allergies to coriander and curry should use with caution. Patients allergic to mustard shouldn't use herbal mustard preparations.

## NURSING CONSIDERATIONS

• Find out why patient is using herb.
• Small amounts of mustard can cause allergic reactions ranging from contact dermatitis to anaphylaxis.
• Patients with eczema may experience an exacerbation with external use.
• Don't confuse with Hedge mustard.
🗲 **ALERT:** Irritant poisoning may occur if mustard oil is used in its undiluted form.

### Patient teaching

• Explain that to release the active component, the patient must rub the powder on with warm water. Hot water will destroy the active enzymes.
• Advise patient to store the herb in a cool, dry place and protect it from light.
• Warn patient to wash hands after preparing herb and not to touch eyes, mouth, or nose until hands are washed.
• Tell patient not to use externally on open wounds or cuts.

---

*Bold italic type* indicates that reaction may be life-threatening.

- Inform patient that mustard oil is highly irritating and shouldn't be tasted or inhaled undiluted.
- Tell patient that herb may cause pain and increased inflammation of the skin when applied topically.
- Tell patient not to use herb topically for longer than 2 weeks and not to apply it for longer than 15 to 30 minutes.
- Caution patients with sensitive skin to shorten application time.
- Warn patient that he may experience coughing or sneezing when handling mustard flour.
- Tell patient results of a soak or bath may be improved if followed by a brief, cold shower.
- Warn patient to keep all herbal products away from children and pets.

## myrrh

*Commiphora molmol,* Balsamodendron myrrha, comniphora, commiphora myrrha(nees), African myrrh, Somali myrrh, arabian myrrh, Yemen myrrh, Guggal gum, guggal resin, didin, didthin, bola, heerabol

**Common trade names**
*Myrrh Gum Commiphora, Myrrh Extract Liquid, Myrrh Gum Capsules, Myrrh Gum Extract, Myrrh Gum Resin, Myrrh Tincture, Medicinol*

### HOW SUPPLIED
The active constituent of myrrh is obtained from the oleo-gum resin, which is exuded from the stems of *Commiphora molmol.* This resin is air dried and then crushed into a powder or dissolved in liquid. Myrrh can also originate from other Commiphora species if the chemical composition is comparable to the official drug. Forms include oil, tincture, mouth rinse, liquid extract, gum capsules (1 g), dental powder (10%), and home antifungal lotion.

### ACTIONS & COMPONENTS
The active constituents of myrrh are obtained from the resin, gum, and volatile oils. Myrrh is reported to have mild astringent properties on mucous membranes. The phenol component of the volatile oils may account for the antimicrobial activity in vitro. In animal studies, anti-inflammatory and antipyretic actions are well documented for *Commiphora molmol.* A hypoglycemic effect was reported in both normal and diabetic rats. Myrrh was found to be an active component in a multi-plant extract that exhibited antidiabetic activity. The mode of action is thought to involve a decrease in gluconeogenesis and an increase in peripheral glucose use.

### USES
Myrrh is used for mouth and throat ulcers, pharyngitis, laryngitis, respiratory and sinus congestion, the common cold, sore throats, and as an anti-flatulent. Myrrh is also used topically in the treatment of decubitus ulcers, muscle pain, wounds, and abrasions. Other uses include canker sores, herpes, athlete's foot, and gingivitis.

## DOSAGE & ADMINISTRATION
*Athlete's foot:* Applied topically to affected area b.i.d. to q.i.d.
*Capsules:* 1 g P.O. t.i.d.
*Dental powder (10%):* Applied topically to affected area b.i.d. to q.i.d.
*Undiluted tincture as a rinse or gargle:* 5 to 10 gtt in a glass of water.

## ADVERSE REACTIONS
**CNS:** apprehension, restlessness.
**GI:** diarrhea, hiccups.
**Skin:** dermatitis.

## INTERACTIONS
**Herb-drug.** *Hypoglycemics:* Action of hypoglycemic drugs may be enhanced. Discourage patient from using together.

## CAUTIONS
Contraindicated in patients with diabetes. Pregnant and breast-feeding patients should avoid use. Large doses may stimulate the uterus.

## NURSING CONSIDERATIONS
● Find out why patient is using herb.
● Myrrh is an active ingredient in many multi-herbal combination products. Patients may not realize that they are using a product that contains myrrh.
● Myrrh at excessive doses may produce hiccups, diarrhea, restlessness, and apprehension.

## Patient teaching
● Advise patient to consult his health care provider before using an herbal preparation because a treatment with proven efficacy may be available.
● Advise patient to report prolonged diarrhea immediately to a health care provider.
● Tell patient to protect herb from light and moisture and to store it in a sealed container away from exposure to water.

## myrtle

*Myrtus communis, Myrti folium, Myrti aetheroleum,* myrtle oil

**Common trade names**
*Myrtle Essential Oil*

## HOW SUPPLIED
The medicinal parts of myrtle are obtained from the leaves and the branches. *Myrti folium* are the dried leaves of *Myrtus coomunis; Myrti aetheroleum* is the essential oil of *Myrtus communis.* The essential oil is extracted from the leaves and branches by steam distillation; the percentage extracted ranges from 0.1% to 0.5%. Other preparations are available; however, information is limited.

## ACTIONS & COMPONENTS
The chief components of myrtle are volatile oils, tannins, and acetylphloroglucinols. Myrtol is the active constituent. It's absorbed in the intestine, stimulates the mucous membranes of the stomach, and deodorizes the breath. This component also possesses fungicidal, disinfectant, and antibacterial effects.

---

*Bold italic type* indicates that reaction may be life-threatening.

## USES
Internally, myrtle is used in the treatment of acute and chronic infections of the respiratory tract such as bronchitis, whooping cough, and tuberculosis. Other uses include bladder conditions, diarrhea, worm infestation, muscle spasms, and hemorrhoids. Externally, myrtle is used to treat acne and varicose veins.

## DOSAGE & ADMINISTRATION
Dosage varies according to manufacturer and indication. Dosage may be as high as 200 mg P.O. q.i.d.

## ADVERSE REACTIONS
**GI:** nausea, vomiting, diarrhea. **Respiratory:** *glottal and bronchial spasm.*

## INTERACTIONS
None reported.

## CAUTIONS
Patients with GI, biliary, or liver disease shouldn't use myrtle. Pregnant and breast-feeding women should avoid use. Topical use in children may stimulate an asthmalike response.

## NURSING CONSIDERATIONS
● Find out why patient is using herb.
**⚡ALERT:** Overdose of myrtle oil (more than 10 g) can lead to a rapid fall in blood pressure, and circulatory and respiratory collapse. Vomiting shouldn't be induced because of the danger of aspiration. Following administration of activated charcoal, give diazepam and atropine to treat symptoms. Intubation and oxygen may be needed.

## Patient teaching
● Advise patient to consult his health care provider before using an herbal preparation because a treatment with proven efficacy may be available.
● Tell patient to remind pharmacist of any herbal and dietary supplements that he's taking, when filling a new prescription.
● Tell patient to report worrisome symptoms to health care provider before using treatments that haven't been adequately studied.
● Warn patient not to use the herb topically on the face of children because this may cause glottal and bronchial spasm.
● Advise patient that this product should be stored away from light and children.

---

*Liquid may contain alcohol.

# N

## nettle

*Urtica dioica, Urticae herba, Urticae radix,* annual nettle, brennesselkraut, nettle herb, nettle root, nettle weed, small nettle, stinging nettle

**Common trade names**
*Freeze-Dried Nettle Capsules, Fresh Nettle Leaf, Nettle Blend, Nettle Leaf, Nettle Leaf Tea, Nettle Organic Tea, Nettle Root, Nettle Seed*

### HOW SUPPLIED
Available as tea, tablets, capsules, tincture*, and liquid extract.
*Capsules:* 50 mg, 100 mg

### ACTIONS & COMPONENTS
Obtained from fresh or dried roots and above-ground parts of *Urtica dioica, U. urens,* and hybrids of these species. Contains acids, amines, flavonoids, choline acetyltransferase, and lectins. Aqueous extract yields five immunologically active polysaccharides and some lectins, which may also have antiinflammatory and immunostimulant properties. The lectin agglutinin has antifungal activity. Two of the five polysaccharides have antihemolytic effects. Nettle leaves have diuretic, analgesic, and immunomodulating pharmacologic actions in vivo.

### USES
Used to treat allergic rhinitis, osteoarthritis, rheumatoid arthritis, kidney stones, asthma, and BPH.

Also used as a diuretic, an expectorant, a general health tonic, a blood builder and purifier, a pain reliever and anti-inflammatory, and a lung tonic for ex-smokers. Also used for eczema, hives, bursitis, tendinitis, laryngitis, sciatica, and premenstrual syndrome. Nettle is being investigated for treatment of hay fever and irrigation of the urinary tract.

### DOSAGE & ADMINISTRATION
*Allergic rhinitis:* 600 mg freeze-dried leaf P.O. at onset of symptoms.
*BPH:* 4 g root extract P.O. q.d., or 600 to 1,200 mg P.O. encapsulated extract q.d.
*Fresh juice:* 5 to 10 ml P.O. t.i.d.
*Infusion:* 1.5 g powdered nettle in cold water; heated to boiling for 1 minute, then steeped covered for 10 minutes and strained (1 tsp = 1.3 g herb).
*Liquid extract (1:1 in 25% alcohol):* 2 to 6 ml P.O. t.i.d.
*Osteoarthritis:* 1 leaf applied to affected area q.d.
*Rheumatoid arthritis:* 8 to 12 g leaf extract P.O. q.d.
*Tea:* 1 tbs fresh young plant steeped in 1 cup boiled water for 15 minutes. 3 or more cups taken q.d.
*Tincture (1:5 in 45% alcohol):* 2 to 6 ml P.O. t.i.d.

### ADVERSE REACTIONS
**CV:** edema.
**GI:** gastric irritation, gingivostomatitis.
**GU:** decreased urine formation; oliguria; increased diuresis in pa-

---

*Liquid may contain alcohol.

tients with arthritic conditions and those with myocardial or chronic venous insufficiency.
**Skin:** topical irritation, burning sensation, urticaria.

**INTERACTIONS**
**Herb-drug.** *Disulfiram:* Possible disulfiram-like reaction if taken with liquid extract or tincture. Advise patient to avoid using together.
**Herb-lifestyle.** *Alcohol:* Possible additive effect from liquid extract and tincture. Discourage alcohol use.

**CAUTIONS**
Patients with fluid retention caused by reduced cardiac or renal activity, patients hypersensitive to herb, and patients who are pregnant or breast-feeding shouldn't use this herb.

**NURSING CONSIDERATIONS**
• Find out why patient is using the herb.
• Nettle is reported to be an abortifacient and may affect the menstrual cycle.
• Allergic adverse effects from internal use are rare.

**Patient teaching**
• Advise patient to consult with his health care provider before using an herbal preparation because a treatment with proven efficacy may be available.
• Tell patient to remind pharmacist of any herbal and dietary supplements that he's taking, when filling a new prescription.
• Recommend caution if patient takes an antihypertensive or antidiabetic.

• Warn patient that external adverse effects result from skin contact and include burning and stinging that may persist for 12 hours or longer.
• Inform patient that capsules and extracts should be stored at room temperature, away from heat and direct light.
• Instruct women taking herb to notify health care provider about planned, suspected, or known pregnancy.
• Advise patient not to breast-feed while taking this herb.

## night-blooming cereus

*Cactus grandiflorus, Selenicereus grandiflorus,* large-flowered cactus, sweet-scented cactus, vanilla cactus

**Common trade names**
*Liquid Extract of Cereus, Tincture of Cereus*

**HOW SUPPLIED**
Available as liquid extract* and tincture*.

**ACTIONS & COMPONENTS**
Obtained from fresh or dried flowers and fresh young stems or shoots of *Selenicereus grandiflorus,* a cactus cultivated in greenhouses. Contains flavonoids, amines (mainly tyramine, which produces a digitalis effect), and betacyans. May induce a positive inotropic effect, causing cardiac stimulation and coronary and peripheral vessel dilation. May also stimulate motor neurons of the spinal cord.

## USES
Used for nervous cardiac disorders, angina pectoris, stenocardia, urinary ailments, hemoptysis, menorrhagia, dysmenorrhea, and hemorrhage. Juice of whole plant is used for cystitis, shortness of breath, and edema. Used externally as astringent for rheumatism.

## DOSAGE & ADMINISTRATION
*Liquid extract:* 0.06 ml to 6 ml P.O. 1 to 10 times q.d.
*Tincture of cereus:* 0.12 ml to 2 ml P.O. b.i.d. to t.i.d.
*Tincture in sweetened water (1:10):* 10 gtt P.O. 3 to 5 times q.d.

## ADVERSE REACTIONS
**CV:** decreased heart rate.
**GI:** nausea, vomiting, diarrhea.
**Skin:** burning sensation, irritation.

## INTERACTIONS
**Herb-drug.** *Digoxin:* Possible increased effect. Monitor digoxin levels.
*MAO inhibitors, OTC cold and flu drugs:* Possible additive effect. Advise patient to use cautiously.

## CAUTIONS
Patients who take MAO inhibitors and those with cardiac disorders shouldn't take this herb.

Women who are pregnant or breast-feeding should avoid using this herb, as should patients who are hypersensitive to it.

## NURSING CONSIDERATIONS
• Find out why patient is using the herb.
• Overdose with cereus may cause severe nausea, vomiting, and diarrhea.
• Herb may decrease heart rate. Monitor patient.

## Patient teaching
• Advise patient to consult with his health care provider before using an herbal preparation because a treatment with proven efficacy may be available.
• Tell patient to remind pharmacist of any herbal and dietary supplements that he's taking, when filling a new prescription.
• Although no chemical interactions have been reported in clinical studies, advise patient that herb may interfere with therapeutic effect of conventional drugs.
• Caution patient to immediately notify health care provider about prolonged nausea, vomiting, or diarrhea.
• Instruct women taking herb to notify health care provider about planned, suspected, or known pregnancy.

## nutmeg
*Myristica fragrans,* mace, moschata, Myristicea nux

**Common trade names**
*Nutmeg Essential Oil, Nutmeg Tincture, Oil of Nutmeg, Powdered Nutmeg, Spirits of Nutmeg*

## HOW SUPPLIED
Available as essential oil, spirit, dried seeds, powder, pressed seed cake, and fluidextract.

## ACTIONS & COMPONENTS
Obtained from nuts and seeds of an evergreen tree *(Myristica fragrans)*. Nutmeg oil, also known as myristica oil, is distilled from the nuts. The dried aril of the nutmeg seed produces another herbal product, known as mace. Nuts contain 20% to 40% of a fixed oil called nutmeg butter. Oil contains myristic acid and glycerides of laureic, tridecanoic, stearic, and palmitic acids. Also present are starch, protein, saponin, and catechins. The nut also contains 8% to 15% of an aromatic oil believed to be partially responsible for nutmeg intoxication. This aromatic oil contains d-camphene (60% to 80%), dipentene (8%), and myristicin (4% to 8%). Nutmeg is known for its psychoactive and hallucinogenic properties resulting from CNS effects. Nutmeg may play a role in inhibiting prostaglandin synthesis and platelet aggregation.

## USES
Used internally for diarrhea, indigestion, loss of appetite, colic, flatulence, and insomnia. It's also used as a larvicidal and as an hallucinogen. Used externally for rheumatoid arthritis. Nutmeg butter also is used in soaps and perfumes.

## DOSAGE & ADMINISTRATION
*Dried seed powder:* 300 mg to 1,000 mg P.O. q.d.
*Fluidextract:* 10 to 30 gtt P.O. up to q.i.d.
*Powder:* 5 to 20 grains applied topically to affected area up to t.i.d.
*Spirits:* 5 to 20 gtt P.O. up to q.i.d.

## ADVERSE REACTIONS
**CNS:** hallucinations, giddiness, fear of impending death, disorientation, loss of feeling in limbs, depolarization.
**CV:** tachycardia, decreased pulse, feeling of pressure in chest.
**EENT:** dry mouth.
**Skin:** flushing, allergic contact dermatitis.
**Other:** hypothermia.

## INTERACTIONS
**Herb-drug.** *MAO inhibitors, psychoactive drugs:* May potentiate effects of these drugs via the herb's mild MAO-inhibiting action. Advise patient to avoid using together.

## CAUTIONS
Pregnant patients, breast-feeding patients, and patients with cardiac disorders should avoid using this herb, as should patients who are hypersensitive to it.

## NURSING CONSIDERATIONS
• Find out why patient is using the herb.
• Misuse and abuse of nutmeg is a growing problem.
🖉ALERT: Ingestion of several tablespoons of nutmeg can lead to a stuporous intoxication that may be severe. Symptoms of overdose (nausea and violent vomiting) occur 3 to 8 hours after ingestion of the herb. Episodes are characterized by weak pulse, hypothermia, disorientation, giddiness, and a feeling of pressure in the chest or lower abdomen. For up to 24 hours, an extended period of alternating delirium and stupor persists, ending in heavy sleep. The patient

---

*Bold italic type* indicates that reaction may be life-threatening.

may have a sensation of loss of limbs and a terrifying fear of death. Gastric lavage and supportive therapy, such as haloperidol, may be warranted. Recovery usually occurs within 24 hours but may take several days.

**Patient teaching**
• Advise patient to consult with his health care provider before using an herbal preparation because a treatment with proven efficacy may be available.
• Tell patient to remind pharmacist of any herbal and dietary supplements that he's taking, when filling a new prescription.
⚠ALERT: Caution patient to use nutmeg in moderation because intoxication and death can occur after ingestion of large doses.
• Warn patient not to use this spice if he has cardiac problems; women shouldn't use it if pregnant or breast-feeding.
• Warn patient not to take herb for diarrhea, indigestion, or chronic GI distress before seeking appropriate medical evaluation because doing so may delay diagnosis of a potentially serious medical condition.

# O

## oak bark

*Quercus alba,* oak, stave oak, stone oak, tanner's oak, white oak

**Common trade names**
*Products containing oak are commercially available under names such as: Alvita White Bark Tea, Conchae Compound, Eichen-rinden-Ekstrakt, Entero-Sanol, Hamon N0. 14, Kernosan Elixir, Menodoron, Nature's Way White Oak Bark Capsules and Powders, Peerless Composition Essence, Pektan N, Silvapin, Tisanes de l'Abbe, Tonsilgon-N and Traxton*

### HOW SUPPLIED
Available as chopped or powdered bark, capsules, liquid extracts, teas, compress, decoction, extract, gargles, lotions, mouthwash, and poultices.

### ACTIONS & COMPONENTS
White oak bark contains the tannin, quercitannic acid, which is thought to have astringent, antiseptic, and anti-inflammatory properties.

### USES
Used to treat inflammatory skin diseases, mild oropharyngeal inflammation, inflammation of genital and anal areas, and acute diarrhea.

### DOSAGE & ADMINISTRATION
*Baths:* 5 g of herb or 1 to 3 tsp of bark extract to every 1 L of water.

*For diarrhea:* 3 g P.O. q.d. of powdered oak bark, or 1 cup of tea t.i.d. Tea is prepared by adding 1 g of powdered bark or 1 to 2 tsp of chopped bark to 500 ml of water, boiling for 15 minutes, straining, then cooling. Taken undiluted. Herb shouldn't be used for longer than 3 days.
*Rinses, compresses, and gargles:* 20 g of bark boiled in 1 L of water for 10 to 15 minutes; the liquid is taken strained, and undiluted.

### ADVERSE REACTIONS
**GI:** constipation, nausea or vomiting, stomach upset, abdominal pain.
**GU:** renal damage.
**Hepatic:** liver damage.
**Respiratory:** *respiratory failure.*

### INTERACTIONS
**Herb-drug.** *Atropine, digoxin, heavy metal salts (such as iron or gold), morphine, nicotine, quinine:* May reduce absorption of these drugs. Advise patient to avoid using together.

### CAUTIONS
Patients allergic to oak bark pollen shouldn't use any products containing oak. Those with skin damage over large areas shouldn't use topical oak products. Those with weeping eczema, febrile or infectious disease, asthma, COPD, renal or hepatic insufficiency, or New York Heart Association class III or IV heart failure shouldn't take full baths containing oak.

*Liquid may contain alcohol.

## NURSING CONSIDERATIONS
● Find out why patient is using the herb.
● Oak and other tannin-containing herbs shouldn't be used for prolonged periods because of poorly understood cancer risks.
● Short-term external use of oak preparations may be effective for skin conditions; however, safety and efficacy of internal use hasn't been studied.
● Geriatric patients may be more sensitive to adverse effects.

### Patient teaching
● Advise patient to consult with his health care provider before using an herbal preparation because a treatment with proven efficacy may be available.
● Tell patient to remind pharmacist of any herbal and dietary supplements that he's taking, when filling a new prescription.
● Warn patient not to apply topical oak bark preparations on large areas of damaged skin.
● Advise patient to stop taking herb and contact a health care provider if diarrhea lasts longer than 3 days.
● Tell patient to keep oak preparation out of eyes. If contact occurs, advise flushing eyes with water for at least 15 minutes.

## oats

*Avena sativa, Avenae fructus,* oat herb, wild oat herb

**Common trade names**
*Aveeno Cleansing Bar, Aveeno Colloidal, Aveeno Dry, Aveeno Lotion, Aveeno Oilated Bath, Aveeno Regular Bath, Oat Bran, Oats and Honey, Oatstraw, Oat Straw Tea, Quaker Oat Bran, Wild Oats*

### HOW SUPPLIED
Available as tablets, whole grains, cereals, wafers, teas, soaps, gels, powders, lotions, creams, colloidal oatmeal, and bath preparations.
*Tablets:* 850 mg, 1,000 mg

### ACTIONS & COMPONENTS
Contains fresh or dried aboveground parts or flowers of *Avena sativa.* Foods are made from the grains (seeds) of the plant, and oat bran is made from the inner husks of the seeds. Oats contain gluten, which forms a sticky mass that holds moisture in skin when mixed with liquid. Oat bran also contains beta-glucan, which may have serum lipid-reducing properties.

### USES
Used to treat dry, itchy skin. Dietary oat bran may lower serum cholesterol levels. Also used to treat opium and cigarette addiction, but mechanism is unknown.

### DOSAGE & ADMINISTRATION
*Baths:* Follow package labeling.
*Cholesterol reduction:* 3 to 5 g soluble oat fiber P.O. q.d.

---

*Bold italic type* indicates that reaction may be life-threatening.

## ADVERSE REACTIONS
**GI:** increased stool bulk, increased defecation, flatulence, abdominal bloating.

## INTERACTIONS
None reported.

## CAUTIONS
Patients allergic to the *Avena sativa* plant should avoid using oat products. Because gluten damages digestive and absorptive cells in the intestines in those with celiac disease, oats should be avoided by these patients. Patients with dermatitis herpetiformis should avoid diets high in gluten because they may cause intestinal abnormalities.

## NURSING CONSIDERATIONS
• Find out why patient is using the herb.
• Patients with intestinal problems should use oat products cautiously.
• As with all fiber products, oats should be taken with plenty of fluids to ensure adequate hydration and dispersion of fiber in the GI tract.
• Patients may experience frequent bowel movements, resulting in anogenital irritation.

## Patient teaching
• Advise patient to consult with his health care provider before using an herbal preparation because a treatment with proven efficacy may be available.
• Tell patient to remind pharmacist of any herbal and dietary supplements that he's taking, when filling a new prescription.

• Tell patient to drink plenty of water to help regulate bowel movements.
• Caution patient that skin care products shouldn't be used near eyes or on inflamed skin.

## octacosanol

octacosanol, 1-octacosanol, 14c-octacosanol, n-octacosanol, octacosyl alcohol, and policosanol

**Common trade names**
*Enduraplex, Octacosanol Capsules, Octacosanol Concentrate, Octa Power, Super Octacosanol; in combination with other dietary supplements such as Boost, Prometol, and Stamiplex*

## HOW SUPPLIED
Available as capsules, soft gels, and tablets.
*Capsules:* 60 mcg, 2,000 mcg, 3,000 mcg, 8,000 mcg
*Softgel capsules:* 3,000 mcg
*Tablets:* 1,000 mcg, 6,000 mcg

## ACTIONS & COMPONENTS
Octacosanol is a type of long-chain alcohol that can be extracted from wheat germ oil, sugar cane wax, and other vegetable oils. Octacosanol may have ergogenic effects and is thought to increase oxygen use by tissues during workouts; it also may improve glycogen storage in muscles.

## USES
Used by athletes to improve cardiac function, stamina, strength, and reaction time. Also used to

treat Parkinson's disease and amy-otrophic lateral sclerosis (Lou Gehrig's disease), although little evidence exists to support its use for these disorders. Octacosanol is also being studied as an antiviral for herpes and as a treatment for inflammatory skin disorders.

## DOSAGE & ADMINISTRATION
*For Parkinson's disease:* 5 mg P.O. t.i.d. with meals.
*To enhance athletic performance:* 40 to 80 mg P.O. q.d.

## ADVERSE REACTIONS
**CNS:** dizziness; jerky, involuntary movements; nervousness.
**CV:** orthostasis.

## INTERACTIONS
**Herb-drug.** *Levodopa-carbidopa:* Potential additive effects. Advise patient to avoid using together.

## CAUTIONS
Patients allergic to wheat germ oil or sugar cane shouldn't take octa-cosanol.

## NURSING CONSIDERATIONS
• Find out why patient is using the supplement.
• Patients with Parkinson's disease should use it cautiously.
▧ALERT: The combination of octacosanol and levodopa-carbidopa may worsen dyskinesias.
• Patients allergic to wheat germ oil or sugar cane shouldn't take oc-tacosanol.
• Although no chemical interac-tions have been reported in clinical studies, consideration must be giv-en to the pharmacologic properties of the supplement and their poten-tial to interfere with the intended effect of conventional drugs.

## Patient teaching
• Advise patient to consult with his health care provider before using an herbal preparation because a treatment with proven efficacy may be available.
• Tell patient to remind pharmacist of any herbal and dietary supple-ments that he's taking, when filling a new prescription.
• If patient is considering taking oc-tacosanol as part of a new exercise routine, recommend that he consult his health care provider first.
• Advise patient with Parkinson's disease or any undiagnosed tremor to consult a health care provider be-fore taking octacosanol.

## oleander

*Nerium oleander,* adelfa, laurier rose, rosa fancesca, rose laurel, rosebay

**Common trade names**
*None known*

## HOW SUPPLIED
Available as leaf extract and tinc-ture.

## ACTIONS & COMPONENTS
Obtained from a flowering orna-mental shrub *(Nerium oleander)* grown widely throughout the southern and southwestern United States and Hawaii. Oleander is a natural cardiac glycoside that has positive inotropic and negative

---

*Bold italic type* indicates that reaction may be life-threatening.

chronotropic effects on cardiac muscle. Its actions mimic digoxin.

## USES
Reported uses include treating heart and skin diseases, but oleander's effectiveness hasn't been proven.

## DOSAGE & ADMINISTRATION
Oleander isn't recommended for use. Dosages aren't well documented.

## ADVERSE REACTIONS
**CNS:** enlarged pupils, *seizures.*
**CV:** irregular pulse, *heart failure.*
**GI:** abdominal pain, appetite loss, nausea, vomiting, bloody diarrhea.
**Respiratory:** *respiratory paralysis.*

## INTERACTIONS
**Herb-drug.** *Beta blockers, calcium channel blockers, digoxin:* Potential for additive effects. Oleander shouldn't be used while taking these drugs.

## CAUTIONS
The use of oleander in any form should be avoided.

## NURSING CONSIDERATIONS
• Find out why patient is using the herb.
⚡**ALERT:** All plant parts are toxic and shouldn't be used. Adults and children have died after ingesting flowers, nectar, and leaves—even from using oleander branches to roast foods. Ingesting water that the plant has soaked in and inhaling smoke from burning oleander wood also can be toxic.

• Patients who ingest oleander may need immediate medical attention. Accidental poisonings may require gastric lavage, activated charcoal, and ipecac syrup. Digoxin-specific Fab fragments (Digibind) used in digoxin overdoses have been used with some success in oleander poisonings. Patients should have continuous ECG monitoring, and respiratory resuscitation equipment should be close at hand.
• Don't confuse oleander *(Nerium oleander)* with yellow oleander *(Thevetia peruviana)*, which may also be toxic.

### Patient teaching
• Advise patient to consult with his health care provider before using an herbal preparation because a treatment with proven efficacy may be available.
• Tell patient to remind pharmacist of any herbal and dietary supplements that he's taking, when filling a new prescription.
• Patients who ingest any part of the oleander plant should be advised to contact a poison control center or seek immediate medical attention.
• Warn patient to keep all herbal products away from children, pets, and livestock. Plants should be clearly labeled.
• Advise patients not to burn oleander branches and leaves in poorly ventilated areas because smoke is toxic.

## olive (oil and leaf)

*Oleae folium, Olivae oleum*

### Common trade names
*Bertolli Olive Oil, Colavita Olive Oil, East Park D-Lenolate Olive Leaf Extract Capsules, Italica Olive Oil, Natrol Olive Leaf Extract, Nature's Herb Olive Leaf Powder, Olive Leaf PE 10%, Pompeian Olive Oil, Solar Ray Olive Leaf Extract Capsules, Solgar Olive Leaf Extract Capsules, Villa Blanca Olive Oil, Virtane, Wellness Olive Leaf*

### HOW SUPPLIED
Available as oil, capsules, and powder.
*Olive leaf extract capsules:* 60 mg to 500 mg

### ACTIONS & COMPONENTS
Obtained from leaves and fruits of *Olea europaea.* Contains phenolic compound oleuropein, which has anti-inflammatory and antioxidant properties. Oleuropein may exert its anti-inflammatory activity by damping the expression of intercellular adhesion molecule-1, involved in adhesion of leukocytes to endothelial cells. The antioxidant properties of oleuropein may prevent the oxidative modification of low-density lipoprotein cholesterol. Olive oil also inhibits platelet aggregation. All of these mechanisms indicate that olive-derived products may help prevent atherosclerosis.

Oleuropein may also have vasodilatory, hypoglycemic, and antimicrobial properties. Although the exact mechanism of vasodilation is unknown, the hypoglycemic activity may result from either a potentiation of insulin release or increased peripheral uptake of glucose. Olive polyphenols have antimicrobial activity against certain gram-positive and gram-negative bacteria.

### USES
Used as an emollient and topical lubricant, to treat skin irritations (such as burns and psoriasis), to soften ear wax, and to relieve constipation. Also used for dry hair and itchy scalp and to prevent stretch marks caused by pregnancy. Recent evidence suggests that olive oil, when part of a diet high in monounsaturated fats, may lower serum cholesterol levels.

Olive leaf preparations have been used to lower blood pressure, reduce blood glucose level in diabetic patients, and treat various bacterial, viral, and fungal infections.

### DOSAGE & ADMINISTRATION
*Cholesterol reduction:* Used in moderation as part of a diet low in saturated fats.
*Hair and skin problems:* Rub undiluted oil into affected area, p.r.n.
*Infections:* 60 to 500 mg olive leaf preparation P.O. every 6 hours.
*Laxative:* 1 to 2 oz oil P.O. p.r.n.

### ADVERSE REACTIONS
**CV:** hypotension.
**GI:** stomach irritation.
**Metabolic:** hypoglycemia.

---

*Bold italic type* indicates that reaction may be life-threatening.

## INTERACTIONS
**Herb-drug.** *Antihypertensives:* Potential additive effects. Monitor blood pressure closely.
*Hypoglycemic drugs:* Potential additive effects. Monitor blood glucose level closely.

## CAUTIONS
Patients allergic to any part of the olive plant shouldn't use these products.

## NURSING CONSIDERATIONS
• Find out why patient is using the herb.
• Patients who are immunocompromised shouldn't use olive leaf products because safety and efficacy data are lacking.
• Diabetic patients who choose to use olive leaf preparations should check blood glucose level more frequently because of the risk of hypoglycemia.
• Olive oil should be part of a diet that's low in saturated fat and cholesterol.
• Monitor blood pressure closely for hypotension.

**Patient teaching**
• Advise patient to consult with his health care provider before using an herbal preparation because a treatment with proven efficacy may be available.
• Tell patient to remind pharmacist of any herbal and dietary supplements that he's taking, when filling a new prescription.
• Tell patient that olive leaf preparations should be taken with food to avoid stomach upset.

⚡ **ALERT:** Caution patient to consult a health care provider if he has HIV or another condition that weakens the immune system, diabetes, or blood pressure abnormalities.
• Remind patient to consult a health care provider if he thinks he has diabetes because it's a serious condition and its management should be overseen by a professional.
• Review the signs of hypoglycemia, including a fast heart rate, sweating, nausea, and hunger.

## onion

Allii cepae bulbus, allium cepa

**Common trade names**
*None known*

## HOW SUPPLIED
Available as leaves and bulbs.

## ACTIONS & COMPONENTS
Contains essential oils, organosulfur compounds, cysteine sulfoxide, quercetin glycosides, thiosulfinates, and diphenylamine. The organosulfur compound may have antimicrobial and anticancer effects. Cysteine sulfoxide is responsible for flavor and lacrimation effects. Quercetin glycosides impart antioxidant properties. Thiosulfinates inhibit mediators of bronchoconstriction such as leukotriene and thromboxane; extracts containing the compound have reduced bronchial constriction in patients with asthma. The herb inhibits platelet aggregation, lowers serum cholesterol levels, decreases blood pressure, enhances fibrinolysis, and has hypoglycemic and antifungal effects.

*Liquid may contain alcohol.

## USES
Used as raw herb for anemia, exhaustion, appetite loss, stomach gas, furuncles, warts, bruises, bronchitis, asthma, atherosclerosis, diabetes, dyspepsia, fever, colds, hypertension, hypercholesterolemia, infection, inflammation, angina, dehydration, and menstruation. Also used as a mucolytic agent, an anthelmintic, a diuretic, and a gallbladder stimulant. Onion water is used as tea to relieve sore throat and cough.

Used topically as a poultice for sores, bites, and burns. Fishermen have used onion to treat stingray and fish-spine wounds. Onion is also used as a food flavoring.

## DOSAGE & ADMINISTRATION
*Externally:* Onion slices or poultices containing onion juice are placed on the skin and covered with a cloth.
*Internally:* Typically, 50 g fresh onion or juice from 50 g of fresh onion P.O. q.d.; 20 g of dried onion q.d. can also be used. Maximum recommended dose of diphenylamine is 35 mg q.d. if use is intended over several months.

## ADVERSE REACTIONS
**EENT:** excessive tearing.
**GI:** nausea.
**Skin:** eczema.

## INTERACTIONS
**Herb-drug.** *Antilipemics:* May alter serum cholesterol levels. Monitor cholesterol panel.
*Antiplatelet drugs:* May increase bleeding risk. Monitor hematologic panel; advise patient at risk of bleeding to use herb cautiously. Observe and monitor patient for evidence of bleeding.
*Hyperglycemics:* May affect blood glucose control. Monitor blood glucose level.
**Herb-herb.** *Other herbs with antiplatelet and anticoagulant properties:* Increased risk of bleeding. Advise caution.
*Other herbs with hypoglycemic effects:* Increased risk of hypoglycemia. Advise caution, and monitor blood glucose level in diabetic patients.

## CAUTIONS
Patients hypersensitive to onions should avoid these products.

## NURSING CONSIDERATIONS
• Find out why patient is using the herb.
• Should be used cautiously by patients with diabetes, bleeding disorders, and eczema.
• Monitor blood glucose control carefully in diabetic patients.
• Observe patient for evidence of bleeding.

### Patient teaching
• Advise patient to consult with his health care provider before using an herbal preparation because a treatment with proven efficacy may be available.
• Tell patient to remind pharmacist of any herbal and dietary supplements that he's taking, when filling a new prescription.
• Tell patient that information on the use of onion during pregnancy and lactation is lacking, and that

---

*Bold italic type* indicates that reaction may be life-threatening.

amounts greater than those used in foods should be avoided.

• Urge diabetic patient to monitor blood glucose level carefully and to stay alert for signs of hypoglycemia, such as sweating, a racing heart, hunger, and nausea.

• Warn patient of potential for flare of eczema.

• Instruct patient to wash hands after handling onion.

• If patient takes an antiplatelet drug or an anticoagulant, warn him about the increased risk of bleeding caused by onion.

## oregano

*Origani vulgaris herba,* dostenkraut, mountain mint, orgianum, origano, wild marjoram, winter marjoram, wintersweet

**Common trade names**
*Oil of Oregano, Oregamax, Oregano, Oregano Powder*

### HOW SUPPLIED
Available as oil and dried herb.
*Oil:* 0.15% to 1.0%

### ACTIONS & COMPONENTS
Obtained from leaves of *Origanum vulgare.* Chief components of oil are carvacrol 40% to 70%, gamma-terpinene 8% to 10%, p-cymene 5% to 10%, alpha-pinene, myrcene, and thymol. Other species may contain linalool, caryophyllene, or germacren D. Carvacrol has antifungal and antibacterial action against gram-positive and gram-negative bacteria and against yeast. Oregano also has anthelmintic, antispasmod-

ic, irritant, diuretic, bile stimulant, and expectorant properties. It also has antioxidant effects and may act at progesterone receptors in intact human breast cancer cells.

### USES
Used for urinary tract disorders, respiratory tract ailments, cough, painful menstruation, arthritis, diuresis, scrofulosis, GI disorders, dyspepsia, and bloating. Also used as an expectorant, a sedative, a diaphoretic, and a stimulant of appetite, digestion, and bile excretion.

### DOSAGE & ADMINISTRATION
*Bath:* 1 L of water poured over 100 g of oregano; strained after 10 minutes and added to a full bath.
*Tea:* 8 oz of boiling water poured over 1 heaping tsp and strained after 10 minutes; tea may be sweetened with honey. Unsweetened tea may be used as a gargle and a mouthwash.

### ADVERSE REACTIONS
**Other:** systemic allergic reactions.

### INTERACTIONS
**Herb-drug.** *Iron:* May decrease iron absorption. Advise patient to separate administration of oregano and iron supplements by at least 2 hours.

### CAUTIONS
Patients hypersensitive to oregano or other members of the Mint family should avoid using this herb. Pregnant women should also avoid use because of its possible abortifacient and menstruation-stimulant effects.

---

*Liquid may contain alcohol.

## NURSING CONSIDERATIONS
• Find out why patient is using the herb.
• Stay alert for evidence of an allergic reaction.
• Patients should take oregano and iron supplements at least 2 hours apart.
• Oregano may cause systemic allergic reactions, and patients allergic to other plants in the same plant family may show cross-sensitivity. Other herbs that belong to the Mint family include thyme, hyssop, basil, marjoram, mint, sage, and lavender.

### Patient teaching
• Advise patient to consult with his health care provider before using an herbal preparation because a treatment with proven efficacy may be available.
• Tell patient to remind pharmacist of any herbal and dietary supplements that he's taking, when filling a new prescription.
⚠ALERT: Tell patient to notify a health care provider if he experiences a serious allergic reaction to oregano because he may need immediate medical care. Symptoms include difficulty breathing, speaking, or swallowing. Other symptoms may include facial swelling and itching.
• Tell patient to notify his health care provider if he takes an iron supplement.
• Counsel pregnant women to avoid excessive use of tea and not to use herb in the bath.

## Oregon grape

barberry, blue barberry, creeping barberry, holly barberry, holly-leaved berberis, holly mahonia, mahonia aquifolium, mountain grape, Oregon barberry, Oregon grapeholly, trailing mahonia, water-holly

**Common trade names**
*Oregon Grape Root, Prime Relief*

### HOW SUPPLIED
Available as capsules, powder, tincture, ointment, and creams.
*Capsules:* 400 mg

### ACTIONS & COMPONENTS
Obtained from rhizome and root of Oregon grape *(Mahonia aquifolium).* Physiologic activity stems from alkaloids berberine, berbamine, and oxyacanthine. Berberine and oxyacanthine have antibacterial properties. Berberine also has activity against amoebas and trypanosomes, as well as anticonvulsant, sedative, and uterine-stimulant properties. Berbamine and berberine may have anticancer activity. Berbamine has a hypotensive effect. Berbamine and oxyacanthine are potent lipoxygenase inhibitors. Herb may also have anti-inflammatory and antifungal activity.

### USES
Used topically for psoriasis. Also used in small doses for ulcers, heartburn, and stomach problems. Larger doses have a cathartic effect. Used for dry skin rashes, for

---

*Bold italic type* indicates that reaction may be life-threatening.

general debility, and to improve appetite.

**DOSAGE & ADMINISTRATION**
*Powder:* 0.5 to 1 g P.O. t.i.d.
*Tincture:* 2 to 4 ml P.O. t.i.d.
*Topical:* Apply bark extract (10%) ointment to affected areas b.i.d. or t.i.d. for psoriasis. Massage root extract (10%) cream into affected areas t.i.d. or as directed by a health care provider.

**ADVERSE REACTIONS**
**CNS:** lethargy.
**CV:** hypotension, *cardiac damage.*
**EENT:** epistaxis, skin and eye irritation.
**GI:** stomach upset.
**GU:** kidney irritation, *hemorrhagic nephritis.*
**Respiratory:** dyspnea, *respiratory spasm and arrest.*
**Skin:** itching, burning, skin irritation.
**Other:** allergic reactions.

**INTERACTIONS**
**Herb-drug.** *Antihypertensives:* Potential additive effect. Advise patient to avoid using together.
**Herb-herb.** *Other herbs containing berberine, including amur cork tree, bloodroot, celandine, Chinese corktree, Chinese goldthread, European barberry, goldenseal, and goldthread:* Possible increased risk of toxicity. Advise patient to avoid using together.

**CAUTIONS**
Pregnant and breast-feeding women shouldn't use Oregon grape. Berberine may cause or worsen kidney irritation. It also can induce nephri-

tis. Patients hypersensitive to Oregon grape or to related plants shouldn't use it.

**NURSING CONSIDERATIONS**
• Find out why patient is using the herb.
• This herb should be used cautiously by patients with kidney problems.
• Don't confuse Oregon grape with "European barberry" *(Berberis vulgaris).*

**Patient teaching**
• Advise patient to consult with his health care provider before using an herbal preparation because a treatment with proven efficacy may be available.
• Tell patient to remind pharmacist of any herbal and dietary supplements that he's taking, when filling a new prescription.
• Tell patient not to use Oregon grape if she's pregnant or breast-feeding.
• Advise patient that poisoning and death have resulted from excessive doses of berberine.

---

*Liquid may contain alcohol.

# P

## pansy

*Viola tricolor, Violae tricoloris herba,* European wild pansy, heartsease, heart's ease herb, Johnny-jump-up, stiefmütterchenkraut, wild pansy

**Common trade names**
*None known*

### HOW SUPPLIED
Available as extract, tea, and poultice.

### ACTIONS & COMPONENTS
Obtained from dried and fresh leaves, stems, and flowers of *Viola tricolor.* Contains flavonoids (0.2%), mucilage (10%), tannins (2% to 5%), and hydroxycoumarins. Pansy has antioxidant and anti-inflammatory properties.

### USES
Used orally to promote metabolism, treat respiratory disorders, and provide mild laxative effect. Used topically for mild seborrheic skin and scalp disorders, warts, skin inflammation, acne, exanthema, eczema, impetigo, and pruritus vulvae.

### DOSAGE & ADMINISTRATION
*Poultice:* Applied t.i.d.
*Tea:* 1 cup t.i.d. Prepared by steeping 1.5 g of herb in 5 oz of boiling water for 5 to 10 minutes and then straining.

### ADVERSE REACTIONS
None reported.

### INTERACTIONS
None reported.

### CAUTIONS
Pregnant and breast-feeding women shouldn't use this herb.

### NURSING CONSIDERATIONS
• Find out why patient is using the herb.
• Pansy may be effective for mild seborrheic disorders, but information on its use for other conditions is lacking.
• Although no chemical interactions have been reported in clinical studies, herb may interfere with therapeutic effect of conventional drugs.

**Patient teaching**
• Advise patient to consult with his health care provider before using an herbal preparation because a treatment with proven efficacy may be available.
• Tell patient to remind pharmacist of any herbal and dietary supplements that he's taking, when filling a new prescription.
• Tell patient to avoid use while pregnant or breast-feeding.
• Advise patient to store herb in well-sealed container to limit exposure to moisture and light.

---

*Liquid may contain alcohol.

## papaya

*Carica papaya, Caricae papayae folium,* baummelonenblätter, mamaerie, melon tree, papaw, pawpaw

**Common trade names**
*Papaya Digestive Enzyme, Papaya Digestive Enzyme–Double Strength, Papaya Enzyme, Papaya Enzyme with Chlorophyll, Papaya Leaf, Papaya with Papain, Super Papaya Enzyme, Super Papaya–Plex*

**HOW SUPPLIED**
Available as tablets, tea, and as combination products.
*Chewable tablets:* 25 mg
*Tablets:* 5 mg

**ACTIONS & COMPONENTS**
Obtained from leaves and fruits of *Carica papaya.* Leaf contains 2% papain and carpain. Papain is a mixture of proteolytic enzymes found in the fruit latex and the leaf; it has a fairly broad spectrum of activity. It hydrolyzes proteins, peptides, amides, and some esters. Carpain may have amebicidal properties. Other components of the enzyme blend hydrolyze fats and carbohydrates. Papaya has bacteriostatic and antioxidant activity and may also have antisickling properties.

**USES**
Used to promote digestion, to expel intestinal parasites, and to treat inflammation, gastroduodenal ulcers, pancreatic excretion insufficiency, chronic infected ulcers, and keloid scars. Also used as a sedative and a diuretic. Used in preparations to control edema and inflammation from surgical, accidental, or sports trauma. Chymo-papain, obtained from papain, is used to treat intervertebral disc hernia in a procedure called chemonucleolysis. Papain is also used as a meat tenderizer.

**DOSAGE & ADMINISTRATION**
*For enhancing digestion:* 10 to 50 mg papain tablets P.O. Or, chewable tablets containing 250 mg papaya powder, 150 mg pineapple juice powder, 10 mg of papain P.O. t.i.d. after meals.

**ADVERSE REACTIONS**
**GI:** gastritis, esophageal perforation (with ingestion of large amounts of papain).
**Respiratory:** asthma attacks.
**Other:** allergic reactions.

**INTERACTIONS**
**Herb-drug.** *Anisindione, dicumarol, warfarin:* Possible increased INR. Advise patient to avoid using together.
**Herb-herb.** *Papain:* Potentiates effects. Advise patient to avoid using together.

**CAUTIONS**
Pregnant and breast-feeding women shouldn't use this herb because papain may be teratogenic and embryotoxic, and it may cause menstruation. Patients allergic to papaya and those with a history of Crohn's disease or chronic gastritis should avoid this herb as well.

**NURSING CONSIDERATIONS**
● Find out why patient is using the herb.

---

*Bold italic type* indicates that reaction may be life-threatening.

- Monitor patient for allergic reactions to papaya.
- Although no chemical interactions have been reported in clinical studies, herb may interfere with therapeutic effect of conventional drugs.

**Patient teaching**
- Advise patient to consult with his health care provider before using an herbal preparation because a treatment with proven efficacy may be available.
- Tell patient to remind pharmacist of any herbal and dietary supplements that he's taking, when filling a new prescription.
- Instruct pregnant women to avoid papaya because it can cause menstruation. Urge breast-feeding women to avoid it as well.
- If patient takes warfarin, tell him to consult with his health care provider before taking papaya.

## pareira

*Chondrodendron tomentosum,* ice vine, pareira brava, velvet leaf

**Common trade names**
*None known*

## HOW SUPPLIED
Available as powder, granules, and in various combination products. Not commercially available in the United States.

## ACTIONS & COMPONENTS
Obtained from fresh or dried bark, roots, and stems of *Chondrodendron tomentosum.* Effects of pareira depend on the toxic derivatives that enter the bloodstream and cause systemic effects. Pareira contains dibenzoyl isoquinoline alkaloids, such as D-tubocurarine, chondrocurarine, curine, chondrofoline, chondrocurine, and isochondrodendrine. These alkaloids have emmenagogic, diuretic, and muscle-relaxing effects. Tubocurarine chloride is used medicinally as a muscle relaxant during anesthesia. It works as a nondepolarizing (competitive) neuromuscular blocker by competing with acetylcholine for cholinergic receptors, thus decreasing the response to acetylcholine and inhibiting skeletal muscle contraction. This effect doesn't occur with oral administration unless the amount absorbed is increased because of cuts or ulcers in the mouth or GI tract.

## USES
Used as a laxative, tonic, and diuretic. Also used to relieve kidney inflammation and induce menstruation. Brazilians use pareira for snakebites; they drink an infusion of the plant and apply bruised leaves to the bite. The herb is also used to make a curare, a paralyzing arrow poison used during hunting.

## DOSAGE & ADMINISTRATION
Not commercially available in the United States. Dosages not well documented.

## ADVERSE REACTIONS
**CNS:** sedation.
**CV:** flushing, hypotension, tachycardia.
**EENT:** blurred vision.

**GI:** decreased GI motility, nausea.
**Musculoskeletal:** skeletal muscle relaxation, jaw weakness.
**Respiratory:** *bronchospasm, apnea.*

### INTERACTIONS
**Herb-drug.** *Calcium channel blockers, such as diltiazem and verapamil; skeletal muscle relaxants, including vecuronium; anticonvulsants, such as phenytoin; ketamine; quinidine; procainamide; other drugs containing tubocurarine:*
May potentiate neuromuscular blocking action of pareira. Advise patient to avoid using together.

### CAUTIONS
The plant is considered poisonous and shouldn't be consumed.

### NURSING CONSIDERATIONS
● Find out why patient is using the herb.
● The FDA doesn't recommend this product for use.
● Nausea and heavy urine flow have been observed in patients poisoned with tubocurare.

### Patient teaching
⚡ALERT: Advise patients not to use this poisonous herb.
● Tell patient to consult with his health care provider before using an herbal preparation because a treatment with proven efficacy may be available.
● Tell patient to remind pharmacist of any herbal and dietary supplements that he's taking, when filling a new prescription.

## parsley

*Petroselinum crispum,* garden parsley, Hamburg parsley, persely, petersylinge, rock parsley

**Common trade names**
*Parsley Herb, Parsley Leaf*

### HOW SUPPLIED
Available as dried herb, seeds, liquid extract, capsules, tincture, and tea. Also available in combination with other herbs, such as garlic.
*Leaf and root:* 430-mg capsules
*Leaf extract:* In vegetable glycerin and grain neutral spirit (12% to 14%)
*Leaves:* 450-mg, 455-mg capsules

### ACTIONS & COMPONENTS
Obtained from leaves, roots, and seeds of *Petroselinum crispum.*
Contains carotene and vitamins B, C, E, and K; iron and calcium; flavonoids with anti-inflammatory and antioxidant activity; coumarins with anticoagulant properties; psoralens; and two volatile oils, apiole and myristicin. The volatile oils are the most active components. Leaves contain 0.3% to 0.5% and seeds contain 2% to 7% oils.
    Myristicin and apiole act as diuretics and strong uterine stimulants. They may act as MAO inhibitors, causing decreased intracellular metabolism of norepinephrine, serotonin, and other biogenic amines. Sympathetic activity of myristicin and renal irritation of apiole contribute to diuretic effects. Myristicin may be metabolized to compounds with stimulat-

---

ing effects in the body, explaining the CNS effects seen with higher doses.

## USES
Used for indigestion, flatulence, dyspepsia, colic, kidney ailments, diuresis, cystitis, liver and spleen disorders, functional amenorrhea, uterine contraction, and dysmenorrhea. Used to increase milk production, freshen breath, promote hair growth, and provide antiseptic effects. Also used as an antirheumatic, analgesic, antispasmodic, expectorant, and decongestant.

## DOSAGE & ADMINISTRATION
*Breath freshener:* Sprigs are dipped into vinegar and chewed slowly before swallowing.
*Decoction:* 1 to 2 tsp of dried leaves or root or 1 tsp of bruised seeds dissolved in a cup of water.
*Diuresis:* 6 g q.d. of root or leaves P.O.; 1 tsp, chopped, equals 2 g.
*Dried root:* 2 to 4 g P.O. or by oral infusion t.i.d.
*Hair growth promoter:* Crushed parsley leaves are rubbed over scalp.
*Leaf:* 2 to 4 g P.O. t.i.d.
*Leaf capsules:* 2 capsules (450 mg each) P.O., b.i.d. or t.i.d.; 3 capsules (455 mg each) P.O. t.i.d.
*Leaf extract in vegetable glycerin and grain neutral spirit (12% to 14%):* 10 to 15 gtt with water P.O. b.i.d. or t.i.d.
*Liquid extract (1:1 in 25% alcohol):* 2 to 4 ml P.O. t.i.d.
*Seeds:* 1 to 2 g P.O. t.i.d.
*Uterine contractions:* Parsley juice (85%).

## ADVERSE REACTIONS
**CNS:** sedation, headache, loss of balance, *seizures,* giddiness, hallucinations.
**CV:** hypotension, *bradycardia,* flushing, tachycardia, hypotension, *ventricular arrhythmias, shock.*
**EENT:** deafness.
**GI:** nausea, vomiting, irritation of stomach and intestines.
**GU:** menstruation, miscarriages, irritation of the kidneys, nephrosis.
**Hematologic:** hemolytic anemia, *thrombocytopenic purpura.*
**Hepatic:** fatty degeneration of the liver, hepatic dysfunction.
**Musculoskeletal:** paralysis, neuropathy.
**Skin:** pruritus, pigmentation, photosensitivity.

## INTERACTIONS
**Herb-drug.** *Antidepressants, hormonal drugs:* May cause phytotoxicity. Advise patient to avoid using together.
*Disulfiram, metronidazole:* Herbal products that contain alcohol may cause a disulfiram-like reaction. Advise patient to avoid using together.
*MAO inhibitors, such as isocarboxazid, moclobemide, phenelzine, selegiline, tranylcypromine:* May potentiate these drugs. Advise patient to avoid using together.
*Warfarin:* Decreased anticoagulant effects. Advise patient to avoid using together.

## CAUTIONS
Pregnant and breast-feeding women shouldn't use this herb. Patients should avoid consuming high doses of seed products because of the

---

* Liquid may contain alcohol.

high volatile oil content. High doses may also potentiate MAO inhibitor therapy. Patients with kidney and liver disease shouldn't use this herb because some forms may contain alcohol.

## NURSING CONSIDERATIONS
• Find out why patient is using the herb.
• Some products may contain alcohol and may not be suitable for use by children, alcoholic patients, patients with liver failure, or patients who take disulfiram or metronidazole.
• Consumption of high amounts can cause serious adverse effects.
• If patient takes warfarin, monitor him closely for decreased warfarin effects.
• Psoralens raises the risk of photosensitivity.
• Parsley seeds may cause a higher risk of adverse reactions because they contain higher amounts of volatile oils.

### Patient teaching
• Advise patient to consult with his health care provider before using an herbal preparation because a treatment with proven efficacy may be available.
• Tell patient to remind pharmacist of any herbal and dietary supplements that he's taking, when filling a new prescription.
• Advise patient not to delay treatment for an illness that doesn't resolve after taking this herb.
• Instruct patient that parsley seeds contain the highest amount of volatile oils and should be used cautiously. Tell patient to avoid high

doses or prolonged use of parsley because of the risk of adverse reactions.
• Advise patient that parsley components may cause uterine stimulation and may complicate pregnancy or cause miscarriage.
• Warn patient not to use alcohol-containing forms if he takes disulfiram, metronidazole, or any other drug that interacts with alcohol.

## parsley piert

*Aphanes arvensis,* field lady's mantle, parsley breakstone, parsley piercestone

**Common trade names**
*None known*

### HOW SUPPLIED
Available as dried herb, liquid extract, tincture, and infusion.
*Liquid extract:* 1:1 in 25% alcohol
*Tincture:* 1:5 in 45% alcohol

### ACTIONS & COMPONENTS
Obtained from *Aphanes arvensis.* Contains tannin—a styptic and astringent—similar to a related species, *Alchemilla vulgaris* (lady's mantle). May have diuretic and demulcent properties.

### USES
Used as a diuretic and demulcent, and for dissolving kidney or bladder calculi. Also used for dysuria, edema of renal or hepatic origin, bladder inflammation, and recurrent UTI.

## DOSAGE & ADMINISTRATION
*Dried herb:* 2 to 4 g P.O. t.i.d.
*Infusion:* 1 cup t.i.d. or q.i.d. Prepared by boiling 1 oz dried herb in 1 pint of water, simmering for 1 minute, cooling, and straining.
*Liquid extract (1:1 in 25% alcohol):* 2 to 4 ml P.O. t.i.d.
*Tincture (1:5 in 45% alcohol):* 2 to 10 ml P.O. t.i.d.

Parsley piert is also combined with other products, such as mullein flowers, sweet flag root, marshmallow root, comfrey root, slippery elm, gravel root, and pellitory.

## ADVERSE REACTIONS
**CNS:** headache.
**CV:** flushing, tachycardia, hypotension, *ventricular arrhythmias.*
**GI:** nausea, vomiting.
**Other:** *shock.*

## INTERACTIONS
**Herb-drug.** *Disulfiram:* Herbal products that contain alcohol may cause a disulfiram-like reaction. Advise patient to avoid using together.

## CAUTIONS
Pregnant and breast-feeding women shouldn't use this herb because published information is lacking. Liquid extract and tincture contain alcohol and shouldn't be used by patients with liver disease or alcoholism.

## NURSING CONSIDERATIONS
• Find out why patient is using the herb.
• Some products may contain alcohol and may not be suitable for use by children, alcoholic patients, those with liver failure, or those taking disulfiram or metronidazole.
• Taking disulfiram with an herbal product that contains alcohol can inhibit the aldehyde dehydrogenase enzyme, which inhibits conversion of acetaldehyde to acetate. The accumulation of acetaldehyde can produce a disulfiram-like reaction, such as flushing, headache, nausea, vomiting, tachycardia, hypotension, ventricular arrhythmias, and shock leading to death.
• Don't confuse parsley piert with the true parsley used in cooking.

### Patient teaching
• Advise patient to consult with his health care provider before using an herbal preparation because a treatment with proven efficacy may be available.
• Tell patient to remind pharmacist of any herbal and dietary supplements that he's taking, when filling a new prescription.
• Warn patient not to use parsley piert tincture or liquid extracts with disulfiram, metronidazole, or any other drugs that interact with alcohol.
• Advise patient not to exceed recommended doses.

*Liquid may contain alcohol.

## passion flower

*Passiflora incarnata,* grenadille, maypop, passiflora, passion vine, purple passion flower, wild passionflower

**Common trade names**
*Passion Flower, Alcohol Free Passion Flower Liquid*

### HOW SUPPLIED
Available as fruits, flowers, extracts, capsules, tincture, and tea.
*Capsules:* 400 mg
*Liquid:* 1:1 alcohol free

### ACTIONS & COMPONENTS
Obtained from leaves, fruits, and flowers of *Passiflora incarnata.* Contains indole alkaloids, including harman and harmine, flavonoids, and maltol. Indole alkaloids are the basis of many biologically active substances, such as serotonin and tryptophan. Exact effect of these alkaloids is unknown; however, they can cause CNS stimulation via MAO inhibition, thereby decreasing intracellular metabolism of norepinephrine, serotonin, and other biogenic amines. Flavonoids can reduce capillary permeability and fragility. Maltol can cause sedative effects and potentiate hexobarbital and anticonvulsive activity.

### USES
Used as a sedative, a hypnotic, an analgesic, and an antispasmodic for treating muscle spasms caused by indigestion, menstrual cramping, pain, or migraines. Also used for neuralgia, generalized seizures, hysteria, nervous agitation, and insomnia. Crushed leaves and flowers are used topically for cuts and bruises.

### DOSAGE & ADMINISTRATION
*Dried herb:* 250 mg to 1 g P.O., two to three 100-mg capsules P.O. b.i.d., or one 400-mg capsule P.O. q.d.
*Extract in vegetable glycerin base (alcohol free):* 10 to 15 gtt P.O., b.i.d. or t.i.d.
*For cuts and bruises:* Crushed leaves and flowers are applied topically, p.r.n.
*For hemorrhoids:* Prepared by soaking 20 g dried herb in 200 ml of simmering water, straining, then cooling before use. Applied topically, as indicated.
*Infusion:* 150 ml of hot water poured over 1 tsp of herb. Strained after standing for 10 minutes. Taken b.i.d. or t.i.d., with a final dose about 30 minutes before h.s.
*Liquid extract (1:1 in 25% alcohol):* 0.5 to 1 ml P.O. t.i.d.
*Solid extract:* Taken in doses of 150 to 300 mg/day P.O.
*Tincture (1:8 in 45% alcohol):* 0.5 to 2 ml P.O. t.i.d. or ½ to 1 tsp P.O. t.i.d.

### ADVERSE REACTIONS
**CNS:** drowsiness, headache, flushing, agitation, confusion, psychosis.
**CV:** tachycardia, hypotension, *ventricular arrhythmias.*
**GI:** nausea, vomiting.
**Respiratory:** asthma.
**Other:** allergic reactions, *shock.*

### INTERACTIONS
**Herb-drug.** *Disulfiram, metronidazole:* Herbal products that

---

*Bold italic type* indicates that reaction may be life-threatening.

contain alcohol may cause a disulfiram-like reaction. Advise patient to avoid using together.
*Hexobarbital:* Increased sleeping time and other barbiturate effects may be potentiated. Monitor patient's level of consciousness carefully.
*Isocarboxazid, moclobemide, phenelzine, selegiline, and tranylcypromine:* Actions can be potentiated by passion flower. Advise patient to avoid using together.

## CAUTIONS
Excessive doses may cause sedation and may potentiate MAO inhibitor therapy. Pregnant patients shouldn't take this herb. Those with liver disease or a history of alcoholism should avoid products that contain alcohol.

### NURSING CONSIDERATIONS
- Find out why patient is using the herb.
- Monitor patient for possible adverse CNS effects.
- No adverse effects have been observed with recommended doses.
- A disulfiram-like reaction may produce nausea, vomiting, flushing, headache, hypotension, tachycardia, ventricular arrhythmias, and shock leading to death.
- Patients with liver disease or alcoholism shouldn't use herbal products that contain alcohol.

### Patient teaching
- Advise patient to consult with his health care provider before using an herbal preparation because a treatment with proven efficacy may be available.

- Tell patient to remind pharmacist of any herbal and dietary supplements that he's taking, when filling a new prescription.
- Because sedation is possible, caution patient to avoid hazardous activities.
- Warn patient not to take herb for chronic pain or insomnia before seeking medical attention because doing so may delay diagnosis of a potentially serious medical condition.
- Caution pregnant patients to avoid this herb.

## pau d'arco

*Tabebuia avellanedae, Tabebuia impetiginosa,* ipe roxo, lapacho, tabebuia ipe, taheebo, tahuari, tajy, queshua

**Common trade names**
*Amazon Support, Antifungal Formula, BP-X, Caprylimune, Pau d'Arco Power Pack, Red Clover Blend Defense Maintenance*

### HOW SUPPLIED
Available as capsules, extracts*, and tea.
*Capsules:* 300 mg

### ACTIONS & COMPONENTS
Obtained from bark and heartwood of *Tabebuia avellanedae.* Contains anthraquinones, naphthoquinones (such as lapachol), flavonoids, alkaloids, and traces of saponins. Lapachol compounds may be effective against psoriasis. Compounds of the lapachol fraction block electron transport in the mitochondria and have shown activity against

*Liquid may contain alcohol.

colon, breast, and lung cancer cells. Lapachol may also interact directly with nucleic acids, thereby blocking DNA replication. A constituent of the extract, beta-lapachone, stimulates lipid peroxidation, producing toxic derivatives that further weaken cell proliferation.

Herb is active against *Bacillus subtilis, Mycobacterium pyogenes aureus, Trypanosoma cruzi*, and certain viruses, such as herpesvirus, avian myeloblastosis, Rous sarcoma, and murine leukemia virus. Lapachol acts as a mild sedative; it has hypotensive action and may be blended with other decongestants.

## USES
Used to treat ulcers, diarrhea, rheumatism, cancers, vaginal infections with *Candida albicans* or *Trichomonas vaginalis*, inflammation, and other infections, such as colds, flu, and bladder infections. Also used to kill vaginal parasites and to reduce fever and arthritis pain.

## DOSAGE & ADMINISTRATION
Duration of treatment may exceed 3 weeks but is usually shorter than 6 months.
*Alcoholic tincture:* 1.2 to 1.5 ml diluted in ½ cup of warm water P.O. t.i.d.
*Bark decoction:* ½ to 1 cup taken once daily to t.i.d. Prepared by adding bark to 1 cup of water, bringing to a boil, and simmering for 5 minutes.
*Capsules:* Average daily dose is 250 mg to 1 g P.O. Five capsules usually equal 2 cups of tea.

*Colds and flu:* 1 or 2 cups of tea q.d. as a preventive measure.
*Tea:* Should be freshly prepared and taken at least b.i.d.
*Vaginal infections:* Gauze tampons soaked in the extract inserted vaginally and changed every 12 hours to heal swollen mucous membranes and kill parasites.

## ADVERSE REACTIONS
**GI:** nausea, diarrhea.
**Hematologic:** anemia, anticoagulation.

## INTERACTIONS
**Herb-drug.** *Warfarin, other anticoagulants:* Possible additive effect. Advise patient to avoid using together.
**Herb-herb.** *Yerba maté:* May potentiate pau d'arco products. Advise patient to avoid using together.
**Herb-food.** *Iodine:* Inhibits absorption. Monitor patient's thyroid function.

## CAUTIONS
Pregnant patients and those with thyroid disorders shouldn't use this herb.

## NURSING CONSIDERATIONS
• Find out why patient is using the herb.
• Overdose may cause changes in blood values. Advise anemic patients and those whose WBC count changes during lapachol treatment to stop taking the drug.
• Monitor patient's thyroid function because lapachol can interfere with iodine utilization.
• Adverse reactions occur mainly at higher-than-recommended doses.

---

*Bold italic type* indicates that reaction may be life-threatening.

- Herb may act against vitamin K, causing symptoms of anemia.

**Patient teaching**
- Advise patient to consult with his health care provider before using an herbal preparation because a treatment with proven efficacy may be available.
- Tell patient to remind pharmacist of any herbal and dietary supplements that he's taking, when filling a new prescription.
- If patient has thyroid problems, tell him to consult his health care provider before taking pau d'arco because lapachol may inhibit iodine utilization. If he takes the herb, tell him to have his thyroid function checked regularly.
- Advise women who are pregnant or breast-feeding to avoid this herb.

## peach

*Prunus persica,* amygdalin, laetrile, vitamin $B_{17}$

**Common trade names**
*Laetrile, Vitamin $B_{17}$*

**HOW SUPPLIED**
Available as persic oil, peach kernel oil, seeds, dried bark, leaves, and flowers.

**ACTIONS & COMPONENTS**
Obtained from *Prunus persica.* Mechanism of action is unknown. Contains cyanogenic glycosides (amygdalin), volatile oils that are carminatives and GI irritants, and phloretin. A 1-g peach seed also contains about 2.6 mg of hydro-cyanic acid. Phloretin may have antibacterial activity against gram-positive and gram-negative organisms.

**USES**
Used for constipation, cough, bad breath, blisters, boils, bronchitis, bruises, burns, dysentery, earache, eczema, edema, headache, hemorrhage, hypertension, locked jaw, menstrual pain, minor wounds, nervousness, pain, pinworm, tapeworm, pneumonia, scurvy, shingles, skin irritation and inflammation, sore throat, stomach upset, warts, and kidney or liver problems. Peach seed was thought to be a cancer remedy; however, studies performed by the National Cancer Institute failed to show clinical effectiveness.
⚡ALERT: Laetrile, also known as amygdalin or vitamin $B_{17}$, touted as an anticancer agent, has been banned by the FDA because of its high cyanide content and potential for overdosing or poisoning.

**DOSAGE & ADMINISTRATION**
*Indigestion and bladder inflammation:* Tea is prepared from 0.5 oz dried bark or 1 oz dried leaves in 16 oz boiling water, steeped for 15 minutes, then taken t.i.d.
*Sores and wounds:* Peach leaves applied as a poultice, p.r.n.

**ADVERSE REACTIONS**
**CNS:** peripheral neuropathy.
**EENT:** deafness.
**Musculoskeletal:** muscle spasms.
**Other:** *cyanide poisoning.*

*Liquid may contain alcohol.

## INTERACTIONS
None reported.

## CAUTIONS
Pregnant patients and those hypersensitive to herb shouldn't use it. Herb should be used cautiously because seeds contain cyanogenic glycosides.

## NURSING CONSIDERATIONS
● Find out why patient is using the herb.

⚡ALERT: Monitor patient for signs and symptoms of cyanide poisoning, such as vomiting, severe stomach pain, fainting, drowsiness, seizures, or coma.

● If cyanide toxicity is suspected, expect to give sodium thiosulfate immediately and to obtain laboratory confirmation of cyanide levels.

### Patient teaching
● Advise patient to consult with his health care provider before using an herbal preparation because a treatment with proven efficacy may be available.

● Tell patient to remind pharmacist of any herbal and dietary supplements that he's taking, when filling a new prescription.

● Warn patient that laetrile is banned by the FDA. Warn patient against high doses or long-term use of seeds because of risk of cyanide poisoning.

● Review signs and symptoms of cyanide poisoning, such as vomiting, severe stomach pain, fainting, drowsiness, seizures, and coma.

## pennyroyal

*Mentha pulegium,* American pennyroyal, European pennyroyal, lurk-in-the-ditch, mosquito plant, piliolerial, pudding grass, pulegium, run-by-the-ground, squaw balm, squawmint tickweed

### Common trade names
*Pennyroyal, Pennyroyal Extract, Pennyroyal Tea*

## HOW SUPPLIED
Available as tea, tincture*, loose dried herb, and capsules.

## ACTIONS & COMPONENTS
Leaves and flowering tops contain pennyroyal oil. The oil contains D-pulegione (60% to 90%), methone, isomethone, tannins, and flavonoids. Pulegione depletes glutathione in the liver. In high doses, it has abortifacient properties.

## USES
Used for digestive disorders, liver and gallbladder disorders, bowel disorders, pneumonia, gout, and colds. Used topically for skin diseases. Also used as an abortifacient, insect repellent, antiseptic, flavoring agent, and fragrance in detergents, soaps, and perfumes.

## DOSAGE & ADMINISTRATION
*Dried herb:* 1 to 4 g P.O. t.i.d.
*Insect repellant:* Oil is applied sparingly to skin, p.r.n.
*Tea:* 1 cup P.O. q.d.

---

*Bold italic type* indicates that reaction may be life-threatening.

## ADVERSE REACTIONS
**CNS:** lethargy, delirium, unconsciousness, *seizures,* hallucinations.
**CV:** hypertension, tachycardia, shock.
**GI:** abdominal pain, nausea, vomiting.
**GU:** irreversible renal damage.
**Hepatic:** *hepatotoxicity, severe liver damage.*
**Skin:** dermatitis.

## INTERACTIONS
**Herb-drug.** *Disulfiram, metronidazole:* Herbal products that contain alcohol may cause a disulfiram-like reaction. Advise patient to avoid using together.

## CAUTIONS
Pregnant patients and those with liver or kidney disease shouldn't use this herb.

## NURSING CONSIDERATIONS
● Find out why patient is using the herb.
🖉**ALERT:** Severe acute poisonings have been reported after consumption of 5 g of oil as an abortifacient. Overdose may cause vomiting, hypertension, anesthetic-like paralysis, and respiratory failure.
● Tincture contains alcohol and should be avoided by patients who take metronidazole or disulfiram.

### Patient teaching
● Advise patient to consult with his health care provider before using an herbal preparation because a treatment with proven efficacy may be available.
● Tell patient to remind pharmacist of any herbal and dietary supplements that he's taking, when filling a new prescription.
● Caution patient against internal use of herb because of its toxic effects on the liver. If he takes herb internally, tell him to do so only with close supervision by a health care provider.
● If patient is using the oil as a flavoring, warn him to use only small amounts.
● Advise pregnant women not to use this herb because it has abortifacient properties.
● Although no chemical interactions have been reported in clinical studies, tell patient that herb may interfere with therapeutic effects of conventional drugs.
● Warn patient to keep all herbal products away from children and pets.

## pepper, black

*Piper nigrum,* pepper bark, pimenta, piper

**Common trade names**
*None known*

## HOW SUPPLIED
Available as dried berries, powder, and ointment for external use.

## ACTIONS & COMPONENTS
Obtained from berries of *Piper nigrum.* The shell is removed, and the green fruit is sun-dried or roasted. This yields volatile oils (1.2% to 2.6%), limonene (15% to 20%), sabinene (15% to 25%), caryophyllene (10% to 15%), betaphinene (10% to 12%), alpha-pinene (8% to 12%), acid amides

(pungent substances), and fatty oils. Pepper stimulates thermal receptors and increases secretion of saliva and gastric mucus. May have abortifacient, analgesic, diaphoretic, diuretic, sedative, emetic, hypnotic, mydriatic, narcotic, sudorific, insecticidal, and antimicrobial effects.

## USES
Used for constipation, gonorrhea, dyspepsia, colic, headache, cholera, diarrhea, scarlatina, paralytic disorders, asthma, bronchitis, delirium, dysmenorrhea, insomnia, pertussis, tuberculosis, flatulence, nausea, vertigo and arthritic conditions. Also used to ease nicotine withdrawal symptoms during smoking cessation. Used externally for neuralgia and scabies. Used extensively as a domestic spice and flavoring ingredient.

## DOSAGE & ADMINISTRATION
*Scabies:* Ointment applied externally, p.r.n.
*To improve digestive function:* 1.5 g P.O. q.d.; divided doses 0.3 to 0.6 g P.O. per dose.

## ADVERSE REACTIONS
**CNS:** tremors, numbness.
**EENT:** eye irritation, mucous membrane irritation, salivation.
**GI:** nausea, gastric pain.
**Skin:** skin irritation.
**Other:** sweating.

## INTERACTIONS
**Herb-drug.** *Drugs metabolized by cytochrome P-450 system, such as acetaminophen, erythromycin, ibuprofen, ketoconazole, naproxen:* Possible reduced drug effects. Mon-

itor patient, and advise him to avoid using together.
*Phenobarbital, phenytoin, propranolol, rifampin, theophylline:* Possible increased absorption. Monitor patient closely for adverse reactions and toxic effects of these drugs. Advise patient to avoid using together.
*Warfarin:* Warfarin metabolism may be altered by pepper. Monitor INR closely to maintain therapeutic value. Advise patient to avoid using together.

## CAUTIONS
Pregnant patients and those hypersensitive to black pepper shouldn't use it.

## NURSING CONSIDERATIONS
● Find out why patient is using the herb.
● Black pepper is an irritant when inhaled or allowed into the eyes. Flush eyes with water to lessen the irritation.
● Exceeding recommended internal dose may cause GI irritation.
● No health hazards or adverse effects have been reported with proper use of standard amounts.

### Patient teaching
● Advise patient to consult with his health care provider before using an herbal preparation because a treatment with proven efficacy may be available.
● Tell patient to remind pharmacist of any herbal and dietary supplements that he's taking, when filling a new prescription.
● Advise patient to be careful of nasal or eye irritation if using powder.

---

*Bold italic type* indicates that reaction may be life-threatening.

• Tell patient not to exceed recommended amounts without consulting health care provider. Explain that higher-than-recommended amounts can cause GI irritation.

## peppermint

*Mentha x piperita*, brandy mint, lamb mint, Menthae piperitae folium (leaves), Menthae piperitae aetheroleum (oil)

**Common trade names**
*Peppermint Capsules, Peppermint Plus Menthoril, Peppermint Tea*

### HOW SUPPLIED
Available as essential oil, ointment, liniment, extract, tincture*, leaves, dried herb, and capsules.
*Aqueous alcohol preparation:* 5% to 10% essential oil
*Enteric-coated capsules:* 0.2/0.02 ml
*Ointment:* 1% to 5% essential oil
*Semisolid and oily preparations:* 5% to 20% essential oil
*Tincture:* 1:10

### ACTIONS & COMPONENTS
Obtained from dried leaves and flowering branch tips of *Mentha x piperita*. The oil contains more than 100 components, including menthol (29% to 48%), methyl acetate (3% to 10%), menthone (20% to 31%), caffeic acid, azulene, and flavonoids. Actions include antibacterial, antiviral, and spasmolytic effects on smooth muscles. When taken as enteric-coated capsules, peppermint oil may have antispasmodic effects on smooth muscle of the intestines; antispasmodic activity results from calcium antagonist effect of menthol. Flavonoids may cause bile-stimulating effect. Azulene may have anti-inflammatory and antiulcer action.

### USES
Used for irritable bowel syndrome, colitis, ileitis, Crohn's disease, and other spasmodic conditions of the bowel. Also used for liver and gallbladder complaints, cramps of the upper GI tract and bile ducts, menstrual cramps, colds and flu, inflammation of the oral and pharyngeal mucosa, loss of appetite, dyspepsia, flatulence, and gastritis. Used externally for myalgia, neuralgia, itching, and skin irritation. Oil is applied to forehead to relieve tension and migraine headaches.

### DOSAGE & ADMINISTRATION
*Dry normalized extract:* 0.44 to 0.57 g P.O. b.i.d. or t.i.d.
*Enteric-coated capsules:* 0.6 ml essential oil in enteric-coated capsules P.O. q.d. for irritable bowel syndrome.
*Essential oil:* 0.2 ml P.O. q.d.
*Fluidextract:* 2 ml P.O. b.i.d. or t.i.d.
*Infusion:* 2 g dried leaf in 150 ml water P.O. b.i.d. or t.i.d.; 3 to 6 g q.d. of cut leaf for infusions and extracts.
*Liniment:* 5% to 20% essential oil in vegetable oil, applied with friction to area of joint or bone pain.
*Nasal ointment:* 1% to 5% essential oil, applied topically, p.r.n.
*Ointment:* 5% to 20% essential oil in petroleum or lanolin used topically, p.r.n.
*Tincture:* 10 ml P.O. b.i.d. or t.i.d. For topical use, aqueous-alcoholic preparation of 5% to 10% essential oil.

*Liquid may contain alcohol.

## ADVERSE REACTIONS
**CNS:** headache.
**CV:** flushing.
**EENT:** spasm of tongue, eye irritation, *glottal spasm*.
**GI:** gastroesophageal reflux.
**Respiratory:** *bronchospasm, respiratory arrest.*
**Skin:** contact dermatitis, irritation.
**Other:** allergic reactions.

## INTERACTIONS
**Herb-drug.** *Calcium channel blockers, such as amlodipine, bepridil, diltiazem, felodipine, isradipine, nicardipine, nifedipine, nimodipine, nitrendipine, verapamil:* Decreased drug effects. Monitor patient closely.

## CAUTIONS
Patients with gallstones, obstructed bile ducts, gallbladder inflammation, and severe liver damage shouldn't take this herb. Peppermint oil shouldn't be applied to the face or nasal passages of infants or children because of the risk of tongue spasms or respiratory arrest.

## NURSING CONSIDERATIONS
● Find out why patient is using the herb.
● If patient has a hiatal hernia, monitor him closely because peppermint weakens the esophageal sphincters.
● When used for irritable bowel syndrome or other intestinal disorders, the enteric-coated capsule must be used; otherwise the peppermint oil will not reach the intestines in its active form.
● Contact dermatitis may result from use of oil.

### Patient teaching
● Advise patient to consult with his health care provider before using an herbal preparation because a treatment with proven efficacy may be available.
● Tell patient to remind pharmacist of any herbal and dietary supplements that he's taking, when filling a new prescription.
● Advise parents not to use peppermint products containing oil on the face, especially around nares, of infants and children. It may cause glottal or bronchial spasm.
● If patient may have a hiatal hernia, tell him to contact a health care provider before using peppermint internally.
● If patient takes peppermint for irritable bowel syndrome or other bowel disorders, make sure he uses enteric-coated capsules.
● Stress that patient should consult his health care provider if symptoms don't improve in a reasonable length of time.
● Warn patient that contact dermatitis can occur with topical administration of peppermint oil.

## peyote

*Lophophora williamsii,* devil's root, dumpling cactus, mescal buttons, mescaline, pellote, sacred mushroom

**Common trade names**
*None known*

## HOW SUPPLIED
Available as buttons, extracts, and tinctures.

---

*Bold italic type* indicates that reaction may be life-threatening.

## ACTIONS & COMPONENTS
Root and hair tufts of the cactus *Lophophora williamsii* are removed and the mescaline-rich center is sliced and dried, making mescaline buttons. A button contains up to 7% mescaline (trimethoxyphenethylamine), the main active ingredient. It has an emetic and hallucinogenic effect. Mescaline may cause visual, auditory, gustatory, kinesthetic, and synesthetic hallucinations.

## USES
Peyote isn't currently used as a medicinal herb. It's illegally used for psychogenic and hallucinogenic effects.

## DOSAGE & ADMINISTRATION
No dosages are available for internal ingestion because herb has no medicinal use.

## ADVERSE REACTIONS
**CNS:** visual, aural, kinesthetic, and synesthetic hallucinations.
**CV:** hypotension, *bradycardia,* vasodilation.
**Respiratory:** *bronchospasm.*

## INTERACTIONS
**Herb-drug.** *Drugs with sedative properties:* Increased sedation. Warn patient not to take peyote.

## CAUTIONS
Peyote is categorized as controlled substance schedule I and has no proven medicinal use.

## NURSING CONSIDERATIONS
✍ALERT: Mescaline doses above 20 mg may cause hypotension, bradycardia, vasodilation, and respiratory depression. Nausea and vomiting may occur 30 to 60 minutes after ingestion.
● Find out why patient is using the herb.
● Peyote isn't taken for any legitimate reason. It's mainly ingested illegally for its hallucinogenic action.

### Patient teaching
● Advise patient to consult with his health care provider before using an herbal preparation because a treatment with proven efficacy may be available.
● Tell patient to remind pharmacist of any herbal and dietary supplements that he's taking, when filling a new prescription.
● Advise patient that peyote shouldn't be taken for any reason.

## pill-bearing spurge

*Euphorbia ceritera, Euphorbia pilulifera,* asthma weed, Euphorbia, garden spurge, milkweed, snakeweed

**Common trade names**
*Available as combination products*

## HOW SUPPLIED
Available as dried herb, extract*, and tincture*.
*Liquid extract:* 1:1 in 45% alcohol
*Tincture:* 1:5 in 50% alcohol

## ACTIONS & COMPONENTS
Contains 0.4% of a glycosidal substance, tannin, fatty acids, phorbic acid, sterols, euphosterol, jambulol, melissic acid, and sugars.

*Liquid may contain alcohol.

## USES
Used for upper respiratory catarrh, bronchial asthma, bronchitis, laryngeal spasm, and intestinal amoebiasis.

## DOSAGE & ADMINISTRATION
*Dried herb:* 120 to 300 mg infusion P.O.
*Liquid extract:* 0.12 to 0.3 ml P.O.
*Tincture:* 0.6 to 2 ml P.O.

## ADVERSE REACTIONS
**GI:** nausea, vomiting.
**Respiratory:** *respiratory failure.*
**Skin:** contact dermatitis.

## INTERACTIONS
**Herb-drug.** *ACE inhibitors, such as clonidine, enalapril, quinapril:* Potentiated hypotension. Monitor patient's blood pressure closely. Advise patient to avoid using together.
*Anticholinergics, such as atropine, ipratropium, scopolamine:* Decreased drug effects. Advise patient to avoid using together.
*Anticholinesterases, such as donepezil, edrophonium:* Additive effects. Monitor patient for adverse reactions. Advise patient to avoid using together.
*Arecoline, methacholine, muscarine, and muscarinic agonists:* Additive effects. Monitor patient for adverse reactions. Advise patient to avoid using together.
*Disulfiram, metronidazole:* Herbal products that contain alcohol may cause a disulfiram-like reaction. Advise patient to avoid using together.
*Drugs metabolized by the CYP3A enzyme system, such as cyclospor-*
*ine, erythromycin:* Decreased absorption. Advise patient to avoid using together.
*Barbiturates, such as phenobarbital:* Increased central hypnotic effects. Advise patient to avoid using together.
*Warfarin:* Potentiated effects. Monitor patient's INR. Advise patient to avoid using together.

## CAUTIONS
Pregnant and breast-feeding patients shouldn't use this herb. Pill-bearing spurge may decrease platelet aggregation and should be used cautiously by alcoholic patients, patients who take anticoagulants, and patients with bleeding disorders or liver disease.

## NURSING CONSIDERATIONS
● Find out why patient is using the herb.
● The FDA doesn't recognize this herb as a safe and effective treatment for asthma.
● The tincture and extract contain more than 40% alcohol.
● Use cautiously in patients with liver disease or alcoholism because of the alcohol content of the preparation.
● Alcohol-containing form of the herb shouldn't be used if patient takes metronidazole or disulfiram.

## Patient teaching
● Advise patient to consult with his health care provider before using an herbal preparation because a treatment with proven efficacy may be available.
● Tell patient to remind pharmacist of any herbal and dietary supple-

---

*Bold italic type* indicates that reaction may be life-threatening.

ments that he's taking, when filling a new prescription.

• Advise patient that tincture and extract contain alcohol. If he takes disulfiram or metronidazole, or if he's an alcoholic or has liver disease, warn him not to use these forms.

• If patient has a bleeding disorder and takes an anticoagulant, tell him not to take herb without consulting his health care provider.

• Tell pregnant and breast-feeding women to avoid this herb.

## pineapple

*Ananas comosus,* bromelainum, pineapple enzyme

**Common trade names**
*Ananas, Bromelain, Mega Bromelain*

### HOW SUPPLIED
Available as capsules, syrup, extracts, juices, candy, and whole fruit.

### ACTIONS & COMPONENTS
Contains bromelain, a proteolytic enzyme used commercially as a meat tenderizer and medically for its soft tissue anti-inflammatory effect. Bromelain prolongs PT and bleeding time because it enhances fibrinolytic activity. It also lowers serum bradykinin and kininogen levels. It may influence prostaglandin synthesis, thus explaining its effect in burn debridement and wound healing. It's also active against nematodes and may reduce the risk of cancer.

### USES
Used for acute postoperative and posttraumatic swelling, especially in nasal and paranasal sinuses. When combined with trypsin, amylase, and lipase enzymes, it's used for dyspepsia and exocrine hepatic insufficiency. Also used for constipation, jaundice, edema, inflammation, and wound debridement.

### DOSAGE & ADMINISTRATION
*Capsules:* For acute postoperative or posttraumatic swelling, 80 to 320 mg P.O. b.i.d. to t.i.d. for 8 to 10 days unless instructed otherwise.

### ADVERSE REACTIONS
**GI:** nausea, vomiting, diarrhea, stomatitis.
**GU:** menorrhagia, uterine contractions.
**Skin:** rash, loss of fingerprints after prolonged contact.
**Other:** *allergic reactions.*

### INTERACTIONS
**Herb-drug.** *ACE inhibitors, such as clonidine, enalapril, quinapril:* May alter bradykinin levels. Monitor patient. Advise patient to avoid using together.
*Tetracycline:* Increased plasma and urine drug levels. Advise patient to avoid using together.
*Warfarin:* Potentiated effect. Monitor INR levels closely. Advise patient to avoid using together.

### CAUTIONS
Pregnant patients, patients who intend to become pregnant, patients who take anticoagulants, and patients hypersensitive to pineapple shouldn't use this herb.

*Liquid may contain alcohol.

## NURSING CONSIDERATIONS
● Find out why patient is using the herb.
● Fruit packers who cut pineapple have reported a loss of their fingerprints because of bromelain's keratolytic effects.

### Patient teaching
● Advise patient to consult with his health care provider before using an herbal preparation because a treatment with proven efficacy may be available.
● Tell patient to remind pharmacist of any herbal and dietary supplements that he's taking, when filling a new prescription.
● If patient takes an anticoagulant, tell him not to take this herb because it's also an anticoagulant.
● Caution patient not to take pineapple when taking aspirin.
● If patient is taking tetracycline, advise him not to use pineapple unless advised by his health care provider.
● Warn patient not to take pineapple for constipation, inflammation, or edema before seeking medical attention because doing so may delay diagnosis of a potentially serious medical condition.

## pipsissewa

*Chimaphila umbellata,* bitter wintergreen, butter winter, ground holly, King's cure, love in winter, Prince's pine, rheumatism weed, wintergreen

**Common trade names**
*Pipsissewa*

## HOW SUPPLIED
Available as decoction, tincture, extract, and syrup.

## ACTIONS & COMPONENTS
Obtained from above-ground parts of *Chimaphila umbellata.* Active components include ericolin, chimaphilin, ursolic acid, tannin, gallic acid, and arbutin, a hydroquinone glycoside. Arbutin and chimaphilin are reported to function as urinary antiseptics. May also have hypoglycemic activity.

## USES
Used to treat tuberculosis of the lymph nodes, cardiac and kidney disease, and as a diuretic and astringent. Also used to treat chronic gonorrhea, catarrh of the bladder, gallstones, kidney stones, and ascites. Combined with other treatments, herb is used for dropsy. Used topically as a rubefacient. Also used as a flavoring agent in beverages.

## DOSAGE & ADMINISTRATION
*Syrup:* 1 or 2 tbs, as directed, P.O.
*Tincture:* 1 to 5 grains per dose, P.O.
*Tubercular sores:* Decoction applied topically to external sores, p.r.n.

## ADVERSE REACTIONS
**Hepatic:** *hepatotoxicity.*
**Skin:** redness, vesication, irritation.

## INTERACTIONS
None reported.

---

*Bold italic type* indicates that reaction may be life-threatening.

## CAUTIONS
Women who are pregnant or breast-feeding shouldn't take this herb. Because it contains the hydroquinone glycoside arbutin, this herb isn't recommended for long-term use because of risk of hepatotoxicity.

### NURSING CONSIDERATIONS
• Find out why patient is using the herb.
• Although no known chemical interactions have been reported in clinical studies, herb may potentially interfere with therapeutic effect of conventional drugs.
• Topical application may cause skin irritation, redness, and vesication.

### Patient teaching
• Advise patient to consult with his health care provider before using an herbal preparation because a treatment with proven efficacy may be available.
• Tell patient to remind pharmacist of any herbal or dietary supplements that he's taking, when filling a new prescription.
• Advise patient not to take this herb internally for prolonged periods because of potential liver damage.
• Tell patient that topical applications can cause skin irritation.
• Warn patient to keep all herbal products away from children and pets.

## plantain

*Plantago lanceolata, P. ovata, P. psyllium,* black psyllium, blond plantago, broad leaf plantain, common plantain, flea seed, French psyllium, greater plantain, Indian plantago, lance leaf plantain, narrow leaf plantain, psyllium seed, ribwort plantain, Spanish psyllium

### Common trade names
*Effer-Syllium, Ground Psyllium, Hydrocil, Konsyl, Metamucil, Perdiem, Psyllium, Psyllium Seed*

### HOW SUPPLIED
Available as powder, seeds, extract, infusion, pressed juice, and poultice.
*Extract:* 1 g:1 ml

### ACTIONS & COMPONENTS
Obtained from seed of *Plantago ovata, P. psyllium,* and other species. When seeds are mixed with water, a mucilaginous mass is formed. Seeds provide bulk to aid in treating constipation while the mucilage—2% to 6% of glucomannans, arabinogalactane, and rhamnogalacturontane—acts as a mild laxative. Taken in dry form, it decreases intestinal motility, and is useful in treating diarrhea and irritable bowel syndrome. Plantain also contains aglycone and aucubigenin, which give psyllium an antimicrobial action. Cholesterol-lowering action is caused by a polyphenolic compound contained in the herb.

## USES
Used as a bulk-forming laxative for constipation. For irritable bowel syndrome or diarrhea, plantain is taken without large amounts of water to decrease intestinal motility. Regular use may modestly reduce cholesterol levels. Also used to treat respiratory catarrh tract and oropharyngeal inflammation, and topically for skin inflammation.

## DOSAGE & ADMINISTRATION
*Compress:* Applied to affected area, p.r.n. Prepared by soaking 1.4 g cut herb in 5 oz cold water for 1 to 2 hours, stirring often.
*Infusion:* 1 cup P.O. t.i.d. to q.i.d. Prepared by steeping 1.4 g of herb in 5 oz boiled water for 10 to 15 minutes.
*Powder:* 3 to 6 g P.O. q.d.
*Rinse or gargle:* Swished t.i.d. to q.i.d.; not swallowed. Prepared by soaking 1.4 g cut herb in 5 oz cold water for 1 to 2 hours, stirring often.
*Tincture (1 g:5 ml):* 7 ml P.O. t.i.d. to q.i.d.

## ADVERSE REACTIONS
**EENT:** watery eyes.
**GI:** diarrhea, flatulence, GI obstruction.
**Respiratory:** sneezing, chest congestion.
**Other:** *anaphylaxis.*

## INTERACTIONS
**Herb-drug.** *Carbamazepine, lithium:* Decreased absorption. Advise patient to avoid using together.

*Feosol, iron supplements:* Decreased iron absorption. Advise patient to avoid using together.

## CAUTIONS
Patients hypersensitive to plantain products shouldn't use this herb.

## NURSING CONSIDERATIONS
• Find out why patient is using the herb.
• Lack of water when taking plantain can cause constipation because of the removal of liquid from the GI tract by the herb.
• Plantain may cause allergic reactions when first started.
• Don't confuse the herb plantain with the edible plantain or banana, *Musa paradisiacal.*

## Patient teaching
• Advise patient to consult with his health care provider before using an herbal preparation because a treatment with proven efficacy may be available.
• Tell patient to remind pharmacist of any herbal or dietary supplements that he's taking, when filling a new prescription.
• Advise patient to separate herb ingestion from other oral drugs by at least 2 hours to prevent decreased drug absorption caused by the increased gastric motility.
• Tell patient taking lithium and carbamazepine to speak to his health care provider before taking plantain.
• Warn patient to drink proper amount of water with each dose if using as a bulk laxative or increased constipation will occur.

---

**Bold italic type** indicates that reaction may be life-threatening.

• Inform patient that if allergic symptoms occur, including sneezing, itching, and swollen eyes, he should stop using product and consult his health care provider.

## pokeweed

*Phytolacca americana,* American nightshade, American spinach, Bear's grape, branching phytolacca, cancer-root, cankerroot, coakumchongras, crowberry, garget, inkberry, jalap, pigeon berry, poke, poke berry, red-ink plant, scoke, Virginian poke

**Common trade names**
*Pokeweed*

### HOW SUPPLIED
Available as powder, liquid, extract*, and tincture.

### ACTIONS & COMPONENTS
Contains triterpene, saponins, esculinic acid, and pokeweed mitogen. Mechanisms of action aren't known. Pokeweed mitogen has been linked to blood cell abnormalities. Extracts containing pokeweed mitogens may alter T and B lymphocytes. May also have antiinflammatory, antirheumatic, and digestive activity.

### USES
Used as an emetic because of its saponin content. Under investigation for its antiviral effects in flu, herpes simplex virus 1, and polio. Also used to treat rheumatism, cough, tonsillitis, itching, laryngitis, and swollen glands. Berries are used as a food coloring. Young spring plant shoots are used as an edible vegetable, but only after careful boiling.

### DOSAGE & ADMINISTRATION
*Emetic:* Dried root 60 to 300 mg P.O.
*Extract (1:1 in 45% alcohol):* 0.1 to 0.5 ml P.O.

### ADVERSE REACTIONS
**CNS:** dizziness, somnolence, *seizures.*
**CV:** hypotension, tachycardia.
**GI:** nausea, vomiting, severe stomach cramping, diarrhea.
**Respiratory:** *bronchospasm, apnea.*

### INTERACTIONS
None reported.

### CAUTIONS
Roots, berries, and purple bark of stems are poisonous. Because of its high toxicity, this herb shouldn't be used for any medical conditions. The FDA has classified pokeweed as an herb of undefined safety with demonstrated narcotic effects.

### NURSING CONSIDERATIONS
• Find out why patient is using the herb.
🗹 ALERT: Even properly prepared, pokeweed has caused toxicity. Symptoms of poisoning or overdose include nausea, vomiting, diarrhea, stomach cramps, and dizziness. Mild overdose usually subsides within 24 hours, but severe poisoning may last up to 48 hours. Gastric lavage, emesis, and symp-

*Liquid may contain alcohol.

tomatic and supportive treatment have been suggested.
• Because of blood cell alterations caused by pokeweed mitogens, gloves should be worn when handling this herb.

**Patient teaching**
• Advise patient to consult with his health care provider before using an herbal preparation because a treatment with proven efficacy may be available.
• Tell patient to remind pharmacist of any herbal and dietary supplements that he's taking, when filling a new prescription.
• Caution patient not to ingest any part of this herb because of its high toxicity.
• Advise patient to discuss alternative therapy with a knowledgeable health care provider.
• Warn patient to keep all herbal products away from children and pets.

## pomegranate

*Punica granatum,* grenadier

**Common trade names**
*Pomegranate*

**HOW SUPPLIED**
Available as juice, powder, and bark extract.

**ACTIONS & COMPONENTS**
Obtained from flowers, stems, bark, and rhizomes of *Punica granatum.* Contains tannins (20% to 25%) and piperidine alkaloids (0.4%). Piperidine alkaloids are the basis for use in treating tape-

worm. Tannins may be beneficial in treating hemorrhoids when applied externally.

**USES**
Used to treat tapeworm and other worm infestations. Also used as a gargle rinse for sore throat and topically for hemorrhoids. Herb may have abortifacient properties.

**DOSAGE & ADMINISTRATION**
*Hemorrhoids:* Juice or extract applied topically, p.r.n.
*Tapeworm:* 20 g bark juice extract P.O. as a single dose. Or, prepared by adding 60 parts herb and 400 parts water, then macerating for 12 hours to half initial volume. 65 ml extract instilled via duodenal probe every 30 minutes for three doses, followed by a laxative 1 hour after the third dose.

**ADVERSE REACTIONS**
**CNS:** dizziness, chills.
**CV:** *circulatory collapse.*
**EENT:** vision disorders.
**GI:** gastric irritation, vomiting.
**Respiratory:** *apnea.*

**INTERACTIONS**
None reported.

**CAUTIONS**
Women who are pregnant or breast-feeding shouldn't use this herb.

**NURSING CONSIDERATIONS**
• Find out why patient is using the herb.
• Although no chemical interactions have been reported in clinical studies, herb may interfere with

---

*Bold italic type* indicates that reaction may be life-threatening.

therapeutic effect of conventional drugs.

• Patients who use pomegranate to treat tapeworm need medical supervision and follow-up by a health care provider.

⌸ ALERT: Overdoses of rind, stem, or root may lead to vomiting (possibly bloody), dizziness, chills, visual disturbances (including blindness), circulatory collapse, and death. Treatment includes induced emesis (if patient is conscious) or gastric lavage and instillation of activated charcoal. Provide supportive treatment for shock. Patient may need intubation. Monitor renal function closely.

**Patient teaching**

• Advise patient to consult with his health care provider before using an herbal preparation because a treatment with proven efficacy may be available.

• Tell patient to remind pharmacist of any herbal and dietary supplements that he's taking, when filling a new prescription.

• Caution patient that respiratory, visual, and GI problems can occur with ingestion of higher doses of pomegranate. If they develop, advise patient to seek medical attention from a health care provider immediately.

• Warn patient to keep all herbal products away from children and pets.

## poplar

*Populus alba, P. gileadensis, P. nigra, P. tremuloides,* black poplar, Canadian poplar, European aspen, poplar bud (balm of Gilead buds), Populi cortex et folium, Populi gemma, quaking aspen, trembling poplar, white poplar

**Common trade names**
*None known*

### HOW SUPPLIED
Available as buds, ointment, extract*, powder, and dried bark (in combination products).

### ACTIONS & COMPONENTS
Obtained from bark and leaves of *Populus* species. Contains essential oil, flavonoids, phenol glycosides, and salicylate glycosides. Volatile oil has expectorant properties. Leaves of *P. alba* may contain up to 6% of glycosides and esters that yield salicylic acid. Populus bark contains about 2% salicylate compounds such as salicortin and salicin. Salicylate compounds contribute to herb's analgesic, anti-inflammatory, and antispasmodic properties. Caffeic acid, found in poplar buds, provides antibacterial properties. Zinc lignins contained in poplar may have a beneficial effect on micturition in prostatic hyperplasia.

### USES
Used for pain, rheumatism, and micturition complaints in prostatic hyperplasia. Used topically for superficial skin injuries, external he-

morrhoids, frostbite, and sunburn. Also used as an antiseptic and to stimulate wound healing. Used for respiratory tract infections and as a gargle for laryngitis.

## DOSAGE & ADMINISTRATION
*Dried bark:* 1 to 4 g, or as a tea P.O. t.i.d.
*Ground drug and galenic preparations of Populi cortex et folium:* As directed. Maximum, 10 g q.d.
*Liquid bark extract (1:1 in 25% alcohol):* 1 to 4 ml (20 to 80 gtt) P.O. t.i.d.
*Topical, semisolid, or ointment preparations containing 5 g of drug or 20% to 30% of drug:* Applied as directed.

## ADVERSE REACTIONS
**Hematologic:** depression of clotting factors.
**Skin:** rash.

## INTERACTIONS
**Herb-drug.** *Antarthritics:* Possible increased bleeding time. Monitor patient for signs of bleeding. Advise patient to avoid using together.
*Aspirin:* Possible increased bleeding time. Monitor patient for bruising and bleeding. Advise patient to avoid using together.
*Feosol and other iron supplements:* Possible reduced iron absorption. Advise patient to avoid using together.
*Warfarin and other anticoagulants:* Possible increased bleeding time. Monitor patient's laboratory values. Advise patient to avoid using together.

## CAUTIONS
Patients hypersensitive to poplar products, salicylates, or Peruvian balsam shouldn't take this herb. Herb should be used cautiously by patients with heart disease or a history of bleeding disorders.

## NURSING CONSIDERATIONS
• Find out why patient is using the herb.
• Closely monitor PT and INR if patient takes aspirin, an arthritis medicine, or an anticoagulant.

### Patient teaching
• Advise patient to consult with his health care provider before using an herbal preparation because a treatment with proven efficacy may be available.
• Tell patient to remind pharmacist of any herbal and dietary supplements that he's taking, when filling a new prescription.
• Tell patient to stop using topical preparation if it causes a rash or skin irritation.
• Inform patient that poplar contains aspirin-like compounds that can increase the risk of bleeding when taken orally with other drugs.
• Advise patient not to take iron supplements with poplar tea.

## prickly ash

*Zanthoxylum clava-herculis, Z. americanum, Z. facara,* northern prickly ash, suterberry, toothache tree, yellow wood

**Common trade names**
*Prickly Ash Autumn-Harvested*

---

*Bold italic type* indicates that reaction may be life-threatening.

## HOW SUPPLIED
Available as extract, tablets, dried bark, and in various combination products.
*Extract:* 65% to 70% grain alcohol

## ACTIONS & COMPONENTS
Obtained from bark and berries of the *Zanthoxylum clava-herculis* tree. Contains pyranocoumarins, such as xanthoxyletin; isoquinoline alkaloids, including berberine and N-methyl-isocorydin; volatile oil; and resins. Prickly ash has anti-inflammatory, antirheumatic, diaphoretic, and circulatory stimulant properties.

## USES
Used for cramps, hypotension, rheumatism, soreness, toothache, poor leg circulation, fever, and inflammation. Also used topically for treating indolent ulcers and wound healing.

## DOSAGE & ADMINISTRATION
*Dried bark:* 1 to 2 g as a tea, P.O. t.i.d.
*For toothache:* Dried bark or berries, chewed p.r.n.
*Liquid extract (1:1 in 45% alcohol):* 1 to 3 ml (20 to 60 gtt) of extract in a little water P.O. t.i.d.
*Tincture (1:5 in 45% alcohol):* 2 to 5 ml (40 to 100 gtt) P.O. t.i.d.

## ADVERSE REACTIONS
None reported.

## INTERACTIONS
**Herb-drug.** *Antihypertensives:* May potentiate effects. Monitor blood pressure, and advise patient to avoid using together.

*Iron supplements, such as ferrous sulfate:* Decreased iron absorption. Advise patient to avoid using together.
*Scopolamine and other muscle relaxants:* May potentiate effects. Advise patient to avoid using together.

## CAUTIONS
Pregnant and breast-feeding women shouldn't use this herb. Patients with cardiac disease should use it cautiously, especially those who take antihypertensives. Some prickly ash extracts contain 65% to 70% grain alcohol and should be avoided by alcoholic patients and those with liver disease.

## NURSING CONSIDERATIONS
• Find out why patient is using the herb.
• If patient has cardiac disease or takes an antihypertensive, monitor vital signs, particularly blood pressure, during and after use of prickly ash.
• Don't confuse true species of prickly ash trees *(Z. americanum, Z. clava-herculis, Z. fagara)* with Devil's walkingstick *(Aralia spinosa),* a shrub also commonly known as prickly ash.

## Patient teaching
• Advise patient to consult with his health care provider before using an herbal preparation because a treatment with proven efficacy may be available.
• Tell patient to remind pharmacist of any herbal and dietary supplements that he's taking, when filling a new prescription.

---

*Liquid may contain alcohol.

• If patient has cardiac disease or takes an antihypertensive, tell him to monitor his blood pressure during and after use of prickly ash.
• If patient has liver disease or alcoholism, warn him to avoid extracts because they may contain 65% to 70% grain alcohol.
• Tell patient to seek medical attention if his symptoms last longer than 7 days or if they worsen.

## pulsatilla

*Anemone pulsatilla, Pulsatilla pratensis, P. vulgaris,* Easter flower, meadow anemone, passe flower, pasque flower, pulsatillae herba, wild flower

**Common trade names**
*Boiron Pulsatilla 9c, Pulsatilla 200ck, Pulsatilla Nig. 30c; also available in combination products*

### HOW SUPPLIED
Available as dried herb, pellets, extracts*, tincture*, and tablets.

### ACTIONS & COMPONENTS
Obtained from dried above-ground parts of *Anemone pulsatilla (Pulsatilla vulgaris)* and *P. pratensis.* Contains protoanemonin, ranunculin, and degradation products of ranunculin, including anemonin, anemoninic acid, and anemonic acid. Protoanemonin may cause stimulation and paralysis of the CNS; its alkylating action may inhibit cell regeneration, leading to kidney irritation. Protoanemonin also has anti-infective activity. Abortion and birth defects have been reported among grazing animals who consumed large amounts of protoanemonin-containing plants.

### USES
Used for inflammatory and infectious diseases of the skin and mucosa, diseases and functional disorders of the GI tract, and functional urogenital disorders. Also used for neuralgia, migraine, and general restlessness.

### DOSAGE & ADMINISTRATION
*Dried herb:* 100 to 300 mg as a tea P.O. t.i.d.
*Liquid extract (1:1 in 25% alcohol):* 0.1 to 0.3 ml (2 to 6 gtt) P.O. t.i.d.
*Oral tablets and pellets:* P.O., as directed.
*Tincture (1:10 in 40% alcohol):* 0.5 to 3 ml (10 to 60 gtt) P.O. t.i.d.

### ADVERSE REACTIONS
**GI:** irritation of mucous membranes, nausea, vomiting, abdominal pain, colic, diarrhea.
**GU:** irritation of kidneys and urinary tract.
**Respiratory:** *asphyxiation.*
**Skin:** rash.

### INTERACTIONS
None reported.

### CAUTIONS
Pregnant and breast-feeding women shouldn't use this herb. Alcoholic patients and those with liver disease shouldn't use forms that contain alcohol.

## NURSING CONSIDERATIONS

- Find out why patient is using the herb.

⚡**ALERT:** Fresh pulsatilla plant parts can cause severe skin and mucosal irritation in susceptible patients. Irrigate affected area with dilute potassium permanganate solution, and then apply mucilage preparation. Overdose may cause renal and urinary tract irritation and severe stomach irritation with colic and diarrhea. Urge patient to go to the emergency room, where he may undergo gastric lavage with activated charcoal.

- Tincture contains alcohol and shouldn't be used in patients with liver disease or alcoholism.

## Patient teaching

- Advise patient to consult with his health care provider before using an herbal preparation because a treatment with proven efficacy may be available.
- Tell patient to remind pharmacist of any herbal and dietary supplements that he's taking, when filling a new prescription.
- Tell patient that fresh pulsatilla is considered poisonous and shouldn't be ingested or placed on the skin. If patient uses pulsatilla, it should be dried.
- Warn patient that kidney and urinary tract irritation can occur at higher-than-recommended doses.
- If patient is pregnant or planning pregnancy, caution her not to use this herb.
- If patient has liver disease or alcoholism, tell him to avoid forms that contain alcohol.

- Tell patient to consult a licensed health care provider if symptoms last longer than 7 days or if they worsen.

## pumpkin

*Cucurbita pepo,* field pumpkin, pompion, semina cucurbitae, yellow pumpkin

**Common trade names**
*None known; available in combination products*

## HOW SUPPLIED

Available as extract and seeds.
*Extract:* Water, coconut glycerin, 12% to 15% certified organic alcohol

## ACTIONS & COMPONENTS

Contains cucurbitacin, tocopherol, and selenium. Seeds contain fatty acids (50%). Curcubitacin may provide anthelmintic activity. Tocopherol and selenium may inhibit oxidative degradation of lipids, vitamins, hormones, and enzymes. Pumpkin also has anti-inflammatory, diuretic, antioxidative, and anti-androgenic actions. Delta-7 sterols in the fatty oils of the seeds may block dihydrotestosterone from androgen receptors and prevent hyperproliferation of prostate cells in an enlarged prostate.

## USES

Used for irritable bladder and micturition problems associated with BPH stages I and II. Also used as a diuretic and to treat childhood nocturnal enuresis and intestinal worms.

## DOSAGE & ADMINISTRATION

*As a dietary supplement:* 2 to 4 ml of liquid extract (about 56 to 112 gtt) P.O. t.i.d.

*As a diuretic:* 200 to 400 g of unpeeled seeds pounded or ground into a pulp. Mixed with milk and honey to form a porridge. Ingested orally on an empty stomach in 2 doses in the morning, followed by castor oil 2 to 3 hours later.

*Whole and coarse-ground seeds:* Average daily dose is 10 g of ground seeds P.O., half in the morning and half in the evening with 1 to 2 heaping tsp of fluid. Outer covering from hard seeds is removed before consumption.

## ADVERSE REACTIONS
None known.

## INTERACTIONS
None known.

## CAUTIONS
Patients hypersensitive to pumpkin or any of its components shouldn't take this herb.

## NURSING CONSIDERATIONS
• Find out why patient is using the herb.
• Although no adverse reactions are known, diuretics may cause fluid and electrolyte imbalances. Monitor patient appropriately.
• Monitor patient's renal status. Irritable bladder symptoms may signal a more serious problem.

## Patient teaching
• Advise patient to consult with his health care provider before using an herbal preparation because a treatment with proven efficacy may be available.
• Tell patient to remind pharmacist of any herbal and dietary supplements that he's taking, when filling a new prescription.
• Inform patient that although pumpkin may relieve irritable bladder and micturition problems caused by BPH stages I and II, it doesn't reduce prostate enlargement and its use requires medical supervision.
• Advise patient to store pumpkin preparations away from light and moisture.
• Tell patient to contact a licensed medical practitioner if symptoms last longer than 7 days or if they worsen.

---

**Q**

## Queen Anne's lace

*Daucus carota,* bees' nest, bird's nest, carrot, wild carrot

**Common trade names**
*None known*

### HOW SUPPLIED
Available as tea, seeds, dried herb, infusion, oil, and liquid extract*.

### ACTIONS & COMPONENTS
Obtained from all plant parts of *Daucus carota.* Contains a volatile oil that may have diuretic and hypotensive properties.

### USES
Used for kidney stones, bladder infections, gout, and swollen joints. Seeds are used for flatulence, windy colic, hiccups, dysentery, renal calculi, bowel obstruction, edema, and chronic coughs. Poultices of roots are used for pain of cancerous ulcers.

### DOSAGE & ADMINISTRATION
*Bruised seeds:* ⅓ tsp P.O. p.r.n. for flatulence, windy colic, hiccups, dysentery, and chronic cough.
*Dried herb:* 2 to 4 g as a tea P.O. t.i.d.
*Infusion:* 1 oz of herb in 1 pint of water. 1 wineglassful taken b.i.d. in morning and evening.
*Liquid extract (1:1 in 25% alcohol):* 2 to 4 ml (40 to 80 gtt) P.O. t.i.d.
*Seeds:* ⅓ to 1 tsp P.O. p.r.n.

*Tea:* Brewed from the whole root and taken P.O. b.i.d. morning and evening for gout.

### ADVERSE REACTIONS
**Skin:** rash.
**Other:** photosensitivity.

### INTERACTIONS
**Herb-drug.** *Antihypertensives, cardiac drugs:* Possible additive effects. Monitor patient's blood pressure closely. Advise patient to avoid using together.
**Herb-lifestyle.** *Sun exposure:* Possible additive photosensitivity risk. Advise patient to avoid prolonged or unprotected exposure to sunlight.

### CAUTIONS
Pregnant and breast-feeding women shouldn't use this herb.

### NURSING CONSIDERATIONS
• Find out why patient is using the herb.
• Essential oil may cause skin rash and photosensitivity.

**Patient teaching**
• Advise patient to consult with his health care provider before using an herbal preparation because a treatment with proven efficacy may be available.
• Tell patient to remind pharmacist of any herbal and dietary supplements that he's taking, when filling a new prescription.

• Inform patient that essential oil may cause a skin rash and increase the risk of sunburn. Advise precautions.

• Encourage patient to monitor his blood pressure during and after consuming Queen Anne's lace.

• Teach patient the symptoms of hypotension, including fatigue, light-headedness, and rapid heart rate.

• Advise pregnant patients or those planning pregnancy to avoid using excessive amounts of this herb.

## quince

*Cydonia oblongata*

**Common trade names**
*None known*

### HOW SUPPLIED
Available as powder, lotion, extract, fruit syrup, and Decoctum Cydoniae, B.P. (decoction from seeds).

### ACTIONS & COMPONENTS
Obtained from fruits and seeds of *Cydonia oblongata.* Fresh fruits and syrup have astringent properties. Seeds contain mucilage and a small amount of amygdalin, a cyanogenic glycoside. When soaked in water, the seeds swell to form a mucilaginous mass or gum that has demulcent properties.

### USES
Used as a demulcent in digestive disorders and diarrhea. Raw fruits are used for diarrhea. Decoction of seeds are used internally for dysentery, diarrhea, gonorrhea, thrush, and mucous membrane irritation. Decoction is also used as an adjunct to boric acid eye lotions and as a compress or poultice for skin wounds and injuries or inflammation of the joints and nipples.

### DOSAGE & ADMINISTRATION
*Decoctum Cydoniae:* Prepared by boiling 2 drams of seed in 1 pint of water in a tightly covered container for 10 minutes and then straining. Amount of liquid to be ingested varies and should be supervised by a health care provider.
*For external use:* Poultice is prepared from ground macerated seeds.

### ADVERSE REACTIONS
None reported.

### INTERACTIONS
None reported.

### CAUTIONS
Pregnant and breast-feeding women shouldn't use this herb. Geriatric patients and those with a history of immune disorders or peptic ulcers should use it cautiously.

### NURSING CONSIDERATIONS
• Find out why patient is using the herb.
⚠ALERT: Seeds may be toxic because they contain cyanogenic glycoside.

### Patient teaching
• Advise patient to consult with his health care provider before using an herbal preparation because a treatment with proven efficacy may be available.

---

*Bold italic type* indicates that reaction may be life-threatening.

- Tell patient to remind pharmacist of any herbal and dietary supplements that he's taking, when filling a new prescription.
- Warn patient not to eat the seeds because of the possible toxic effects.
- Warn patient not to take herb for digestive disorders before seeking medical attention because doing so may delay diagnosis of a potentially serious medical condition.
- Tell breast-feeding patients not to use this herb.
- Advise patient to store herb away from heat and direct sunlight, and to keep all herbal products away from children and pets.

# R

## ragwort

*Senecio jacoboea,* cankerwort, dog standard, ragweed, staggerwort, stammerwort, stinking nanny, St. James wort

**Common trade names**
*None known*

### HOW SUPPLIED
Available as fresh and dried herb, and lotion*.

### ACTIONS & COMPONENTS
Contains pyrrolizidine alkaloids (0.1% to 0.9%) and a volatile oil. The juice has cooling and astringent properties.

### USES
Used as a wash in burns, eye inflammation, sores, bee stings, and cancerous ulcers. Also used for rheumatism, painful menstruation, chronic cough, urinary tract inflammation, anemia, anemic headaches, sciatica, and gout. Leaves made into a poultice are applied to painful joints to reduce inflammation and swelling. Ragwort is gargled, but not swallowed, for ulcers of the throat and mouth. A decoction of the root has been used for inward bruises and wounds.

### DOSAGE & ADMINISTRATION
*Rheumatic arthritis:* Lotion is made from 1 part herb and 5 parts 10% alcohol. Applied topically, p.r.n.

### ADVERSE REACTIONS
**Hepatic:** *hepatotoxicity.*

### INTERACTIONS
None reported.

### CAUTIONS
Pregnant and breast-feeding women shouldn't use this herb.

### NURSING CONSIDERATIONS
• Find out why patient is using the herb.
**ALERT:** Ragwort may have hepatotoxic and carcinogenic properties from pyrrolizidine alkaloid content.
• Although no chemical interactions have been reported in clinical studies, herb may interfere with therapeutic effects of conventional drugs.
• For external use only; herb shouldn't be taken internally.

### Patient teaching
• Advise patient to consult with his health care provider before using an herbal preparation because a treatment with proven efficacy may be available.
• Tell patient to remind pharmacist of any herbal and dietary supplements that he's taking, when filling a new prescription.
• Tell patient the herb is for external use only. Caution patient about the risk of liver failure and cancer if herb is taken internally.
• Warn patient to keep all herbal products away from children and pets.

---

*Liquid may contain alcohol.

## raspberry

*Rubus idaeus,* bramble of
Mount Ida, hindberry, raspbis

**Common trade names**
*Alcohol-Free Red Raspberry Leaf,
Certified Organic Red Raspberry,
Red Raspberry, Red Raspberry
Leaves, Red Raspberry Leaves
Glycerine, Wild Countryside Red
Raspberry Leaves*

### HOW SUPPLIED
Available as tea, extract*, dried leaf,
and infusion.

### ACTIONS & COMPONENTS
Obtained from leaves and fruits of
*Rubus idaeus.* Contains tannins,
flavonoids, vitamin C, crystalliz-
able fruit sugar, fragrant volatile
oil, pectin, manganese, citric acid,
malic acid, and mineral salts. Tannins have astringent activity.

### USES
Leaves are used as a gargle for
sore mouths and canker sores and
as a wash for wounds and ulcers.
Infusion of leaves, taken cold, is
used to treat diarrhea. Herb is also
used to normalize blood glucose
level and to treat various disorders
of GI, CV, and respiratory systems.
Leaf tea is taken regularly during
pregnancy to prevent complications and tone the uterus in preparation for childbirth. Raspberry is
reputed to relieve heavy menstrual
bleeding and increase milk production in breast-feeding mothers.

### DOSAGE & ADMINISTRATION
*Dried leaf:* 4 to 8 g P.O. t.i.d.

*Liquid extract (1:1 in 25% alco-
hol):* 4 to 8 ml (80 to 160 gtt) P.O.
t.i.d.
*Tea:* Prepared by scalding 1.5 g
finely cut herb (1 tsp = 0.8 g herb),
steeping for 5 minutes, then straining. Taken t.i.d.

### ADVERSE REACTIONS
None reported.

### INTERACTIONS
**Herb-drug.** *Iron supplements,
such as ferrous sulfate:* Decreased
iron absorption. Advise patient to
avoid using together.

### CAUTIONS
Pregnant and breast-feeding women and patients hypersensitive to
raspberry products shouldn't use
this herb.

### NURSING CONSIDERATIONS
• Find out why patient is using the
herb.
• Safety in pregnant women,
breast-feeding women, young children, and patients with severe liver
or kidney disease hasn't been established.
• If patient has trouble breathing or
develops a rash, he may be allergic
to raspberry. He should immediately stop taking the herb and seek
medical attention.

### Patient teaching
• Advise patient to consult with his
health care provider before using
an herbal preparation because a
treatment with proven efficacy may
be available.
• Tell patient to remind pharmacist
of any herbal and dietary supple-

---

*Bold italic type* indicates that reaction may be life-threatening.

ments that he's taking, when filling a new prescription.
- Advise patient taking red raspberry for GI symptoms that other treatments with known safety and efficacy data are available.
- Inform patient that little evidence exists to support the use of herbal raspberry during pregnancy, childbirth, or menstruation.
- Warn patient to keep all herbal products away from children and pets, and to store them away from heat and direct sunlight.

## rauwolfia

*Rauwolfia serpentina,* Indian snakeroot, snakeroot

**Common trade names**
*None known*

### HOW SUPPLIED
Available as dried root, powder, and extracts.

### ACTIONS & COMPONENTS
Contains reserpine, ajmalicine, and numerous other alkaloids. The herb exerts hypotensive and antiarrhythmic effects. The whole extract is more easily tolerated with reserpine than the isolated substance, indicating the importance of the accompanying substances, or coeffectors.

### USES
Used internally to treat nervousness, insomnia, anxiety, tension states, and other psychometric disorders. Also used for flatulence, vomiting, liver disease, hypertension, and eclampsia. Also used to assist with contractions during childbirth. Used topically to treat wounds, snakebite, dysuria, and colic.

### DOSAGE & ADMINISTRATION
*Daily dose:* 600 mg (equivalent to 6 mg total alkaloids), P.O.

### ADVERSE REACTIONS
**CNS:** depression, fatigue, drowsiness, nightmares.
**EENT:** nasal congestion.
**GI:** nausea, vomiting.
**GU:** erectile dysfunction, decreased libido.

### INTERACTIONS
**Herb-drug.** *Antihypertensives:* Increased hypotension. Monitor patient's blood pressure. Advise patient to avoid using together.
*Barbiturates, neuroleptic drugs:* Synergistic effect. Monitor patient's laboratory values and advise against using together.
*Cardiac glycosides:* Severe bradycardia. Advise patient to avoid using together.
*Levodopa:* Decreased effect. Advise patient to avoid using together.
*OTC cold medicines, flu remedies, and appetite suppressants:* Increased blood pressure. Advise patient to avoid using together.
*Sympathomimetics:* Initial significant increase in blood pressure. Advise patient to avoid using together.
**Herb-lifestyle.** *Alcohol:* Increased impairment of motor reactions. Encourage patient taking rauwolfia not to consume foods or beverages that contain alcohol.

## CAUTIONS
Patients hypersensitive to rauwolfia products should avoid this herb, as should pregnant patients, breast-feeding patients, and patients with depression, ulceration, or pheochromocytoma.

## NURSING CONSIDERATIONS
• Find out why patient is using the herb.
• Monitor patient's blood pressure closely.

### Patient teaching
• Advise patient to consult with his health care provider before using an herbal preparation because a treatment with proven efficacy may be available.
• Tell patient to remind pharmacist of any herbal and dietary supplements that he's taking, when filling a new prescription.
• Warn patient to use caution when taking herb with OTC cough and flu drugs or appetite suppressants.
• Advise patient not to drink alcohol while taking this herb.
• Warn patient not to take herb for insomnia before seeking medical attention because doing so may delay diagnosis of a potentially serious medical condition.
• Warn patient to keep all herbal products away from children and pets.
• Tell patient to store herb away from heat and direct sunlight.

## red clover

*Trifolium pratense,* purple clover, trefoil, wild clover

### Common trade names
*EuroQuality Red Clover Blossoms, NuVeg Red Clover Concentrate, Promensil, Red Clover Blossom, Red Clover Herb, Red Clover Liquid*

### HOW SUPPLIED
Available as liquid extract*, tinctures*, and tea.

### ACTIONS & COMPONENTS
Obtained from dried and fresh flowerheads of *Trifolium pratense.* Contains volatile oil, isoflavones, coumarin derivatives, and cyanogenic glycosides. It has antispasmodic and expectorant effects and promotes skin healing. It also has hormonal effects similar to estrogen caused by isoflavones.

### USES
Used internally for some cancers and for coughs and respiratory problems in which mucus is lacking—as in whooping cough. It's also used to relieve menopausal symptoms. Used externally to treat chronic skin diseases such as eczema and psoriasis.

### DOSAGE & ADMINISTRATION
*Dried flowerheads:* 4 g P.O., or as a tea, up to t.i.d.
*Liquid extract (1:1 in 25% alcohol):* 1.5 to 3 ml (30 to 60 gtt) P.O. t.i.d.
*Tincture (1:10 in 45% alcohol):* 1 to 2 ml (20 to 40 gtt) P.O. t.i.d.

---

***Bold italic type*** indicates that reaction may be life-threatening.

## ADVERSE REACTIONS
**GU:** breast tenderness, breast enlargement.
**Metabolic:** weight gain.
**Respiratory:** dyspnea.
**Other:** allergic reaction including hives, swelling, itching.

## INTERACTIONS
**Herb-drug.** *Heparin, warfarin:* Possible increased INR. Monitor laboratory values and patient closely for bleeding. Advise patient to avoid using together.
*Hormone replacement therapy, oral contraceptives:* Possible enhanced estrogen effects. Advise patient to avoid using together.

## CAUTIONS
Pregnant and breast-feeding women should avoid this herb, as should patients hypersensitive to red clover products. Patients shouldn't use this herb for breast or uterine cancer because of possible hormonal effects, which may increase the metabolism of cancer cells. Safety in young children or patients with severe liver or kidney disease hasn't been established.

## NURSING CONSIDERATIONS
• Find out why patient is using the herb.
• Monitor patient for evidence of bleeding, especially if he takes warfarin or aspirin.

### Patient teaching
• Advise patient to consult with his health care provider before using an herbal preparation because a treatment with proven efficacy may be available.

• Tell patient to remind pharmacist of any herbal and dietary supplements that he's taking, when filling a new prescription.
• Caution patient to watch for signs and symptoms of bleeding, including easy bruising, bleeding gums, black tarry stools, and tea-colored urine, especially when taking large amounts of herb with warfarin.
• Advise women to watch for estrogen-like effects, such as breast tenderness, breast enlargement, and weight gain.
• Warn patient to keep all herbal products away from children and pets, and to store them away from heat and direct sunlight.

## red poppy

*Papaver rhoeas,* copperose, corn poppy, corn rose, cuppuppy, headache poppy, headwark, rheados flos

**Common trade names**
*None known*

## HOW SUPPLIED
Available as dried flower petals, powder, and teas.

## ACTIONS & COMPONENTS
Obtained from flowers of *Papaver rhoeas.* Contains small amounts of isoquinoline alkaloids (0.1%) and anthocyanin glycosides. Mechanism of action isn't well defined.

## USES
Used for respiratory tract diseases and discomforts, for disturbed sleep, for sedation, and for pain relief. Also used in children's cough

---

*Liquid may contain alcohol.

syrup, as a tea for insomnia, and as a colorant.

## DOSAGE & ADMINISTRATION

*Bronchial irritation:* Prepared by steeping 2 tsp dried petals in 1 cup boiling water for 5 to 10 minutes, then straining. 1 cup taken b.i.d. to t.i.d. May be sweetened with honey. 1 tsp = about 8 g of herb.

## ADVERSE REACTIONS

**GI:** vomiting, stomach pain.

## INTERACTIONS

None reported.

## CAUTIONS

Children and pregnant and breast-feeding women shouldn't use this herb.

## NURSING CONSIDERATIONS

• Find out why patient is using the herb.

⚡**ALERT:** Poisoning has occurred in children who consumed fresh leaves and blossoms, with symptoms including vomiting and stomach pain. The powdered herb has a low alkaloid content and is considered nontoxic.

### Patient teaching

• Advise patient to consult with his health care provider before using an herbal preparation because a treatment with proven efficacy may be available.

• Tell patient to remind pharmacist of any herbal and dietary supplements that he's taking, when filling a new prescription.

• Advise women to avoid use of red poppy while pregnant and breast-feeding.

• Warn patient to keep all herbal products away from children and pets.

## rhatany

*Krameria triandra,* krameria root, mapato, Peruvian rhatany, ratanhiae radix, ratanhiawurzel, red rhatany, rhatania

**Common trade names**
*None known*

## HOW SUPPLIED

Available as powder, tincture*, and tea.

## ACTIONS & COMPONENTS

Obtained from dried root of *Krameria triandra.* Contains high levels of proanthocyanidin tannins, which give the herb astringent properties.

## USES

Used internally as an antidiarrheal for enteritis. Used externally for mild inflammation of the oral and pharyngeal mucosa and gums, as well as fissures of the tongue, stomatitis, pharyngitis, noninfectious canker sores, chilblains, hemorrhoids, and leg ulcers.

## DOSAGE & ADMINISTRATION

*Decoction:* 1 g of powdered root in 1 cup of water.
*For external sores and ulcers:* Undiluted tincture painted on affected area, b.i.d. to t.i.d.
*Mouthwash and gargle:* Prepared by simmering 1 to 1.5 g powdered

root in 5 oz boiling water for 10 to 15 minutes, then straining. Swished, not swallowed, b.i.d. to t.i.d.
*Tea:* Prepared by scalding 1.5 to 2 g coarsely powdered rhatany in 1 cup boiling water for 10 to 15 minutes, then straining. 1 tsp = about 3 g of powdered rhatany.
*Tincture:* 5 to 10 gtt in 1 glass of water. Swished, not swallowed, b.i.d. to t.i.d.

## ADVERSE REACTIONS
**GI:** digestive complaints.
**Other:** allergic mucous membrane reactions.

## INTERACTIONS
**Herb-drug.** *Disulfiram:* Herbal products that contain alcohol may cause a disulfiram-like reaction. Advise patient to avoid using together.
*Iron supplements, such as ferrous sulfate:* Decreased absorption if taken with rhatany tea. Advise patient to avoid using together.
*Tretinoin:* Possible skin irritation if used with topical rhatany. Advise patient to avoid using together.
**Herb-herb.** *Echinacea:* May potentiate antibiotic activity of echinacea. Monitor patient closely. Advise patient to avoid using together.
**Herb-food.** *Milk or cream:* May inactivate tannins in rhatany tea. Advise patient to avoid using together.

## CAUTIONS
Rhatany shouldn't be used longer than 2 weeks if taken without medical advice. Pregnant and breast-feeding women shouldn't use this herb.

## NURSING CONSIDERATIONS
• Find out why patient is using the herb.
• Rhatany is difficult to find, and adulteration with other *Krameria* species is common.

**Patient teaching**
• Advise patient to consult with his health care provider before using an herbal preparation because a treatment with proven efficacy may be available.
• Tell patient to remind pharmacist of any herbal and dietary supplements that he's taking, when filling a new prescription.
• Advise women to avoid use of rhatany while pregnant and breast-feeding.
• Advise patient not to use rhatany for longer than 2 weeks without a health care provider's advice.

## rose hip

*Rosa canina, R. centifolia,* brier hip, brier rose, dog rose, heps, hip, hipberry, hip fruit, hip sweet, hopfruit, rose hip and seed, rosehips, sweet brier, wild boar fruit, witches' brier

**Common trade names**
*Ascorbate-C, Ester-C 1000, Hi-Potent-C, Honey C Chew Chewable C, Mega-Stress Complex, Vitamin C 500 mg (special)*

## HOW SUPPLIED
Available as capsules, tablets, powder, and tea, and in combination products.

---

*Liquid may contain alcohol.

## ACTIONS & COMPONENTS
Obtained from fruits (hips) and seeds of various species of *Rosa*. Contains pectins and fruit acids, such as malic and citric acids, which are responsible for diuretic and laxative effects, as well as tannins, vitamin C, carotenoids, and flavonoids. Fresh rose hip contains 0.5% to 1.7% vitamin C but, because it deteriorates in processing, many natural vitamin supplements have some vitamin C added to them. Rose hip also contains vitamins A, $B_1$, $B_2$, $B_3$, and K.

## USES
Used to treat diarrhea, respiratory disorders such as colds and flu, vitamin C deficiency (scurvy), gastric spasms and inflammation, intestinal diseases, edema, gout, arthritis, sciatica, diabetes, metabolic disorders of uric acid metabolism (including gout), lower urinary tract and gallbladder ailments, gallstones, kidney stones, and inadequate peripheral circulation. Also used as a diuretic, a laxative, an astringent, and a booster of immune function during exhaustion. Has recently been used to treat osteogenesis imperfecta in children.

## DOSAGE & ADMINISTRATION
*Osteogenesis imperfecta:* 250 to 600 mg/day, P.O.
*Tea:* Prepared by steeping 1 to 2.5 g of crushed rose hip in 5 oz boiling water for 10 to 15 minutes and then straining; 1 tsp = 3.5 g of herb. Taken as a diuretic, p.r.n.

## ADVERSE REACTIONS
**CNS:** insomnia, headache, fatigue.
**CV:** flushing.
**GI:** nausea, vomiting, abdominal cramps, esophagitis, gastroesophageal reflux, diarrhea.
**GU:** kidney stones.
**Respiratory:** severe respiratory allergies (after exposure to herb dust).
**Skin:** itching, prickly sensations.
**Other:** *anaphylaxis.*

## INTERACTIONS
**Herb-drug.** *Aluminum-containing antacids:* Possible increased aluminum absorption. Advise patient to avoid using together.
*Aspirin, salicylates:* Possible increased excretion of ascorbic acid and decreased excretion of salicylates. Monitor patient for salicylate toxicity. Advise patient to avoid using together.
*Barbiturates, estrogens, oral contraceptives, tetracyclines:* May increase vitamin C requirements. Advise patient to avoid using together.
*Iron:* May increase iron absorption. Advise patient to avoid using together.
*Tretinoin:* Possible additive effect. Advise patient to avoid using together.
*Warfarin:* Possible decreased effect. Monitor patient's INR. Advise patient to avoid using together.
**Herb-herb.** *Echinacea:* May potentiate antibiotic activity of echinacea. Monitor patient closely. Advise patient to avoid using together.
**Herb-food.** *Milk or cream:* May inactivate rose hip tea. Advise patient to avoid using together.

---

*Bold italic type* indicates that reaction may be life-threatening.

## CAUTIONS
Pregnant and breast-feeding women shouldn't use more of this herb than is found in foods. Patients with asthma should avoid this herb.

## NURSING CONSIDERATIONS
• Find out why patient is using the herb.
• Rose hip is nontoxic in recommended amounts; most people don't have adverse effects from ingesting small quantities.
• Rose hip interactions depend on the amount of vitamin C present.
• *The German Commission E Monographs* lists no known risks of using rose hip, but there have been reports of severe respiratory allergies with mild to moderate anaphylaxis in production workers exposed to rose hip dust during the manufacturing process. Plant fibers may also cause itching and a prickly sensation caused by mechanical irritation rather than allergic reaction.
• Herb may cause precipitation of urate, oxalate, or cysteine stones or drugs in the urinary tract causing kidney stones.
• Rose hip may cause false negative results for occult blood tests.
• The following tests may result in false increases: AST that uses color reactions (redox reactions) and Technicon SMA 12/60, bilirubin measured by colorimetric methods or Technicon SMA 12/60, carbamazepine (Tegretol) measured by Ames ARIS method, urine glucose level measured by Clinitest, serum or urine creatinine.
• The following tests may result in false decreases: lactic dehydrogenase measured by Technicon SMA 12/60 and Abbott 100 methods, theophylline measured by ARIS system or Ames Seralyzer photometer, and blood glucose level measured by Clinistix.

## Patient teaching
• Advise patient to consult with his health care provider before using an herbal preparation because a treatment with proven efficacy may be available.
• Tell patient to remind pharmacist of any herbal and dietary supplements that he's taking, when filling a new prescription.
• Warn patient with asthma to use rose hip with caution and to stop immediately and consult a health care provider if any wheezing or shortness of breath occurs.
• Inform patient that many rose hip-derived natural vitamin C supplements are fortified with synthetic vitamin C.
• Tell patient to take rose hip with vitamin C 2 hours before or 4 hours after taking antacids.

## rosemary

*Rosmarinus officinalis,* compass plant, compassweed, old man, polar plant, romero, rosmarinblätter

### Common trade names
*Barlean's Flax Oil, Breast Health Formula, Bright-Eyes, Complete Cleanse, Easy Now, Female Sage, Respi-Oil, RoseOx*

### HOW SUPPLIED
Available as dried leaves, essential oil, lotion, extracts*, and tea.

*Liquid may contain alcohol.

*Capsules:* 250 mg, 300 mg
*Extracts:* 1:1 in 45% alcohol

## ACTIONS & COMPONENTS

Obtained from leaves of *Rosmarinus officinalis*. Contains 1% to 2.5% of a volatile oil, composed of monoterpene hydrocarbons, camphor, borneol, and cineol. Leaves also contain rosmaricine; the flavonoid pigments diosmin, diosmentin, genkwanin, and related compounds; and various volatile and aromatic components. Diosmin decreases capillary permeability and fragility. Herb exerts some antibacterial activity, as well as spasmolytic effects on smooth muscle. It also may have a positive inotropic effect, increasing coronary blood flow. Rosemary may also have antifungal, antioxidant, anticancer, and abortifacient properties as well as stimulant effects on uterine muscle and menstrual flow. When applied topically, rosemary is an irritant and may increase circulation.

## USES

Used for flatulence, gout, toothache, cough, eczema, and as a poultice for poor wound healing. Also used to aid digestion, ease dyspepsia, promote menstrual flow, induce abortion, increase appetite, and relieve headaches, liver and gallbladder complaints, and blood pressure problems. Used topically as an insect repellent and to treat baldness, circulatory disturbances, joint or musculoskeletal pain, myalgia, sciatica, and neuralgia. Rosemary is also popularly used in cooking, cosmetics, and various teas.

## DOSAGE & ADMINISTRATION

*Bath:* 50 g of leaves added to 1 L hot water and added to bath water.
*Liquid extract (1:1 in 45% alcohol):* 2 to 4 ml P.O. t.i.d.
*Oral:* 4 to 6 g of leaves P.O. q.d.
*Tea:* Prepared by steeping 1 or 2 g of leaves in 5 oz boiling water for 15 minutes, then straining; 1 cup taken t.i.d.
*Topical:* 6% to 10% essential oil in semisolid or liquid preparations.

## ADVERSE REACTIONS

**CNS:** *seizures* at high doses.
**Respiratory:** asthma (from repeated occupational exposure).
**Skin:** contact dermatitis, photosensitivity.

## INTERACTIONS

**Herb-drug.** *Disulfiram:* Herbal products that contain alcohol may cause a disulfiram-like reaction. Advise patient to avoid using together.
**Herb-lifestyle.** *Sunlight:* Topical forms may cause photosensitivity. Encourage patient to take precautions and to use sunscreen.

## CAUTIONS

Pregnant and breast-feeding women should avoid this herb, as should children, patients with seizure disorders, and patients hypersensitive to rosemary products.

## NURSING CONSIDERATIONS

• Find out why patient is using the herb.
**⚕ALERT:** Undiluted oil shouldn't be ingested. Overdose may cause spasms, vomiting, gastroenteritis,

---

*Bold italic type* indicates that reaction may be life-threatening.

uterine bleeding, kidney irritation, deep coma, and possibly death.
• Rosemary is unlikely to have adverse effects when the leaves and oil are used in amounts typically found in foods. Herb is generally recognized as safe by the FDA. Maximum level of leaves is 0.41% in baked goods and 0.003% in oil.
• Repeated occupational exposure to rosemary may lead to asthma.

**Patient teaching**
• Warn patient not to ingest undiluted rosemary oil.
• Advise patient to consult with his health care provider before using an herbal preparation because a treatment with proven efficacy may be available.
• Tell patient to remind pharmacist of any herbal and dietary supplements that he's taking, when filling a new prescription.
• Advise pregnant patients, patients trying to get pregnant, and breastfeeding patients not to use rosemary in amounts greater than those found in food.
• Advise patient with seizure disorder not to ingest large amounts of rosemary.
• Inform patient that repeated occupational exposure to rosemary may lead to asthma.
• Advise parents not to give children amounts greater than those found in food.
• Advise patients to use sunscreen and limit sun exposure if rosemary is being applied topically.
• Warn patient to keep all herbal products away from children and pets.

## royal jelly

**Common trade names**
*Bee Complete, Bee Pollen Complex, Energy Elixir, Pure Energy, Royal Bee Power, Super Energy Up, Ultra Virile-Actin*

**HOW SUPPLIED**
Available as capsules, creams, lotions, milk baths, and honey.
*Capsules:* 62.5 mg, 100 mg, 125 mg, 250 mg, 500 mg

**ACTIONS & COMPONENTS**
Obtained from milky white secretion produced by worker bees of the species *Apis mellifera* for exclusive growth and development of the queen bee. Contains a complex mixture of proteins, sugar, fats, and variable amounts of minerals, vitamins, and pheromones. It's rich in B vitamins, especially pantothenic acid. About 15% of royal jelly is 10-hydroxy-trans-(2)-decanoic acid, which has weak antimicrobial activity. Royal jelly may also have antitumor activity.

**USES**
Used orally as a health tonic and for reducing cholesterol levels, promoting rejuvenation, enhancing sexual performance, improving the immune system, and treating bronchial asthma, liver disease, kidney disease, pancreatitis, insomnia, stomach ulcers, bone fractures, skin disorders, and hyperlipidemia. Applied topically as a skin tonic and hair growth stimulant.

## DOSAGE & ADMINISTRATION
*Hyperlipidemia:* 50 to 100 mg, P.O. q.d.

## ADVERSE REACTIONS
**Respiratory:** asthma.
**Skin:** rash, dermatitis, skin irritation.
**Other:** *anaphylaxis.*

## INTERACTIONS
None reported.

## CAUTIONS
Pregnant and breast-feeding women should avoid this herb, as should patients hypersensitive to related products and patients with seasonal allergies or dermatitis.

## NURSING CONSIDERATIONS
• Find out why patient is using the herb.

🔲**ALERT:** Royal jelly should be used with extreme caution by patients with asthma because allergic reactions to royal jelly have led to asthma, anaphylaxis, and death.
• One case of severe adverse GI reactions has been reported; it included abdominal pain, hemorrhagic colitis, diarrhea, GI hemorrhage, and mucosal edema of the sigmoid colon.
• Topical application may worsen existing dermatitis.
• Don't confuse royal jelly with bee pollen and honey bee venom.

## Patient teaching
• Advise patient to consult with his health care provider before using an herbal preparation because a treatment with proven efficacy may be available.

• Tell patient to remind pharmacist of any herbal and dietary supplements that he's taking, when filling new prescription.
• Tell patient that royal jelly may worsen asthma and lead to anaphylaxis. Warn patient to seek medical attention if shortness of breath develops after taking royal jelly.
• Advise women to avoid royal jelly while pregnant and breast-feeding.
• Advise patient that topical use of royal jelly may worsen existing dermatitis.

## rue

*Ruta graveolens,* herb of grace, herbygrass, rue

**Common trade names**
*Rue*

## HOW SUPPLIED
Available as dried leaves, compresses, capsules, tincture*, oil, and tea. Because of the risk of toxicity, rue is available only from specialty herb suppliers.

## ACTIONS & COMPONENTS
Obtained from above-ground plant parts of *Ruta graveolens.* Contains such essential oils as limonene, pinene, anisic acid, and phenol. Flavonoids such as rutin and quercitin may have a strengthening effect on capillaries; alkaloids arborinine, gamma-fagarine, and graveoline may have antispasmodic and abortifacient activity. Furanocoumarins such as bergapten, psoralen, and xanthotoxin have a photosensitizing effect with topical use. Chalepensin inhibits fertility, and coumarin de-

---

*Bold italic type* indicates that reaction may be life-threatening.

rivatives and alkaloids are spasmo-lytic. Rue also contains hypericin, tannin, pectin, choline, and iron.

## USES
Used internally for amenorrhea, Bell's palsy, colic, cough, epilepsy, hypertension, hysteria, multiple sclerosis, skin inflammation, oral and pharyngeal cavities, cramps, hepatitis, dyspepsia, diarrhea, in-testinal parasites, and worm infec-tions. Also used as a uterine stimu-lant for abortions. Used externally for backache, ear infection, eye soreness, gout, headache, muscle spasms, varicose veins, sprains, bruising, rheumatism, sore throat, and wounds. Applied topically as an insect repellant.

## DOSAGE & ADMINISTRATION
*Daily internal dosage:* 0.5 g to 1 g P.O. q.d.
*Tea:* 1 heaping tsp (about 3 g) to ¼ L of water, P.O.

## ADVERSE REACTIONS
**CNS:** dizziness, vertigo, tremors, depression, sleep disorders, deliri-um, melancholic mood, fatigue.
**CV:** *bradycardia.*
**EENT:** swelling of the tongue.
**GI:** vomiting, epigastric pain, ab-dominal pain.
**GU:** *severe kidney damage.*
**Hepatic:** *hepatotoxicity.*
**Skin:** contact dermatitis, clammy skin, photosensitivity, phototoxic-ity.

## INTERACTIONS
None reported.

## CAUTIONS
Pregnant and breast-feeding women shouldn't use this herb. Large doses of rue used as an abortifacient can be toxic or fatal to the mother.

## NURSING CONSIDERATIONS
• Find out why patient is using the herb.
• Discourage use of rue for any reason because of its toxic effects.
• If patient chooses to use rue, it should be under strict supervision by a health care provider with ex-tensive herbal experience.
• Pregnant women have died after using rue to induce miscarriage.
• Rue oil can cause contact derma-titis.
• Phototoxic reactions causing der-matoses have been reported from the prepared oil and from rubbing fresh leaves on the skin.
• Large doses may cause photosen-sitivity.
• Topical use may cause dermatitis.

### Patient teaching
• Advise patient to consult with his health care provider before using an herbal preparation because a treatment with proven efficacy may be available.
• Tell patient to remind pharmacist of any herbal and dietary supple-ments that he's taking, when filling a new prescription.
• Warn patient to avoid rue because of its potential toxicity and the avail-ability of safer treatments.
• Warn patient to keep all herbal products away from children and pets.

# S

## S-adenosylmethionine

methionine, Sammy

**Common trade names**
*SAM-e*

**HOW SUPPLIED**
Available as tablets.
*Enteric-coated tablets:* 200 mg

**ACTIONS & COMPONENTS**
A naturally occurring amino acid found in all living cells. Plays an integral role in methylation processes, including DNA methylation, protein methylation (critical for cell growth and repair), and phospholipid methylation, which maintains flexibility of cell membranes. Also helps produce cysteine, an amino acid needed for glutathione, the main antioxidant in the liver. Also helps limit homocysteine levels. Increased homocysteine levels may increase the risk of CV disease.

**USES**
Used to treat depression, including postpartum and menopausal, as well as osteoarthritis, fibromyalgia, fatigue, and liver disorders. Also used to prevent heart disease.

**DOSAGE & ADMINISTRATION**
*For arthritis:* 200 mg to 1,600 mg P.O. q.d. in divided doses.
*For depression:* 400 mg q.d. or 200 mg b.i.d. P.O. before breakfast and lunch. Patients sensitive to drugs or supplements may start with 200 mg q.d. Increased to 800 mg q.d.

or 400 mg b.i.d. if no improvement occurs after 2 weeks.

**ADVERSE REACTIONS**
**CNS:** headache.
**GI:** diarrhea, nausea, GI disturbances.

**INTERACTIONS**
None known.

**CAUTIONS**
Patients with bipolar depression should avoid this product because of the risk of inducing mania.

**NURSING CONSIDERATIONS**
• Find out why patient is using the product.
• Some patients try to diagnose or treat severe or life-threatening depression on their own. Determine the extent of the patient's depression and make appropriate referrals for psychiatric help, as needed.
• Although no chemical interactions have been reported in clinical studies, consider the pharmacologic properties of the product and the risk that it could interfere with therapeutic effects of conventional drugs.
• Product can be stopped without adverse effects, although depression may recur.
• Doses up to 3,600 mg have caused no adverse effects. No deaths have been reported from overdose.

**Patient teaching**
• Advise patient to consult with his health care provider before using

---

*Liquid may contain alcohol.

this product because a treatment with proven efficacy may be available.

• Tell patient to remind pharmacist of any herbal and dietary supplements that he's taking, when filling a new prescription.

• Warn patient about the danger of treating depression on his own.

• Instruct patient to have a medical evaluation before taking this product for depression or other symptoms.

• Tell patient that the effects of the herb may not be noticable for two weeks.

• Recommend that patient promptly notify health care provider about new symptoms or adverse effects.

• Warn patient to keep all herbal products away from children and pets.

## safflower

*Carthamus tinctorius,* American saffron, bastard saffron, dyer's saffron, fake saffron, false saffron, hoang-chi, koosumbha, parrot plant, zaffer

**Common trade names**
*Safflower and Safflower Oil*

### HOW SUPPLIED
Available as oil and powdered flowers.

### ACTIONS & COMPONENTS
Obtained from flowers of *Carthamus tinctorius.* Oil contains unsaturated fatty acids, including linoleic (76% to 79%), oleic (13%), palmitic (6%), and stearic (3%) acids. It also contains lignans, polysaccha-

rides, carthamone, a pigment. Linoleic acid is an omega-6 fatty acid that may help lower cholesterol.

### USES
Oil is commonly used in cooking as a source of polyunsaturated fats to help lower dietary cholesterol levels. Also used to treat wounds, amenorrhea, stomach tumors, scabies, arthritis, and chest pain. Also used to help stimulate movement of stagnant blood and to help alleviate pain when used topically and systemically.

### DOSAGE & ADMINISTRATION
*Average daily dose:* Decoction, 1 g P.O. t.i.d.

### ADVERSE REACTIONS
None reported.

### INTERACTIONS
None known.

### CAUTIONS
Pregnant or breast-feeding women shouldn't use flowers and seeds. Purified oil is probably safe to use during pregnancy.

### NURSING CONSIDERATIONS
• Find out why patient is using the herb.

• Excessive intake of omega-6 oils, such as safflower, without intake of appropriate amounts of omega-3 fatty acids can be deleterious to general health.

• Monitor patient's serum cholesterol levels, as needed.

---

*Bold italic type* indicates that reaction may be life-threatening.

**Patient teaching**
- Advise patient to consult with his health care provider before using an herbal preparation because a treatment with proven efficacy may be available.
- Tell patient to remind pharmacist of any herbal and dietary supplements that he's taking, when filling a new prescription.
- Tell patient to avoid excessive intake of omega-6 oils, such as safflower, without appropriate intake of omega-3 fatty acids.
- Warn patient to seek medical evaluation before taking any herbal or dietary supplement.
- Tell patient to notify a health care provider immediately about new or worsened symptoms.
- Recommend that women notify a health care provider about planned, suspected, or known pregnancy.
- Warn patient to keep all herbal products away from children and pets.

## saffron

*Crocus sativus,* nagakeshara, saffron crocus, Spanish saffron, zang hong hua

**Common trade names**
*Saffron*

### HOW SUPPLIED
Available as dried powder; often adulterated with American saffron.

### ACTIONS & COMPONENTS
Obtained from flower stigmas and styles of *Crocus sativus,* grown mainly in Spain and France. Contains a xanthophyll carotenoid, cro-

cetin, which increases oxygen diffusion in blood plasma and, in turn, may help prevent or treat atherosclerosis. The rarity of CV disease in parts of Spain may result from daily consumption of saffron. Saffron also contains essential oils such as cineole, safranal, and terpenes; crocin, a bitter glycoside; and vitamins $B_1$ and $B_2$.

Purified crocetin products in development are more likely than the crude herb to help increase plasma oxygen levels.

### USES
Used to stimulate digestion and to treat amenorrhea, atherosclerosis, bronchitis, sore throat, headache, vomiting, and fever. Also used as an abortifacient and a sedative.

### DOSAGE & ADMINISTRATION
Dosages not well documented.

### ADVERSE REACTIONS
None reported.

### INTERACTIONS
None reported.

### CAUTIONS
Pregnant or breast-feeding women shouldn't use this herb.

### NURSING CONSIDERATIONS
- Find out why patient is using the herb.
- ⚡ALERT: Saffron may be lethal at doses above 12 g. Overdose may cause central paralysis, dizziness, stupor, vomiting, intestinal colic, bloody diarrhea, and hemorrhaging of skin on the nose, lips, and eyelids. Treatment involves empty-

*Liquid may contain alcohol.

ing the stomach by gastric lavage and giving activated charcoal, if needed. Symptomatic treatment includes diazepam to control seizures and sodium bicarbonate to correct acidosis. In severe cases, patient may need intubation and artificial respiration.

• Saffron is generally safe for use as a spice.

**Patient teaching**

• Advise patient to consult with his health care provider before using an herbal preparation because a treatment with proven efficacy may be available.

• Tell patient to remind pharmacist of any herbal and dietary supplements that he's taking, when filling a new prescription.

• Caution patient to avoid using saffron medicinally without consulting a qualified health care pro-vider.

• Instruct patient to promptly notify a health care provider about new or worsened symptoms.

• Warn patient not to take herb before seeking medical attention because doing so may delay diagnosis of a potentially serious medical condition.

• Warn patient to keep all herbal products away from children and pets.

## sage

*Salvia officinalis,* Dalmatian sage, garden sage, meadow sage, red sage, scarlet sage, tree sage

**Common trade names**
*Alcohol-Free Sage, Sage*

**HOW SUPPLIED**
Available as dried leaves, extract*, tincture*, and essential oil. Also used in shampoos and conditioners.

**ACTIONS & COMPONENTS**
Contains volatile oils (including thujone, cineole, and camphor), tannins, diterpene bitter principles, triterpenes, steroids, flavones, and flavonoid glycosides. Herb has antibacterial, fungistatic, virustatic, astringent, antioxidative, antispasmodic, secretion-promoting, and perspiration-inhibiting properties.

**USES**
Used topically to treat itching from insect bites, herpes lesions, shingles, and psoriasis. Also used to prevent hair loss and preserve hair color. Used internally for loss of appetite, excessive perspiration, laryngitis, tonsillitis, pharyngitis, halitosis, canker sores, gum disease, fatigue, and Alzheimer's disease. Also used as a vaginal douche to treat vaginal yeast infection.

**DOSAGE & ADMINISTRATION**
*Dry herb (leaves):* 4 g to 6 g P.O. q.d.
*Essential oil:* 0.1 g to 0.3 g P.O. q.d.
*Fluidextract or tincture (1:2 and 1:5 alcohol):* 6 ml to 12 ml P.O. in divided dose, t.i.d.
*For halitosis:* A few leaves chewed, as necessary.
*For inflamed mucous membranes:* Undiluted alcohol extract, applied p.r.n.
*For inflammation of bronchial mucous membranes:* 50 g of powdered herb mixed with 80 g honey and used as an expectorant.

---

*Bold italic type* indicates that reaction may be life-threatening.

*Gargle or mouth rinse:* 2.5 g dry herb or 2 to 3 gtt essential oil in 100 ml of water, or 9 ml of alcoholic extract in 1 glass of water.

## ADVERSE REACTIONS
**CNS:** *seizures,* vertigo.
**CV:** tachycardia.

## INTERACTIONS
**Herb-drug.** *Disulfiram:* Herbal products that contain alcohol may cause a disulfiram-like reaction. Advise patient to avoid using together.

## CAUTIONS
Pregnant or breast-feeding women shouldn't use this herb. It should be used cautiously by patients with a history of epilepsy or other seizure disorders.

## NURSING CONSIDERATIONS
• Find out why patient is using the herb.
• Although no chemical interactions have been reported in clinical studies, consider the pharmacologic properties of the herbal product and the risk that it will interfere with therapeutic effects of conventional drugs
• Chemical content of the dry herbal product is likely to vary widely, depending on where the herb is grown, time of harvest, storage time, and drying method used.

### Patient teaching
• Advise patient to consult with his health care provider before using an herbal preparation because a treatment with proven efficacy may be available.

• Tell patient to remind pharmacist of any herbal and dietary supplements that he's taking, when filling a new prescription.
🗲 **ALERT:** Advise patient to avoid using large amounts of sage, especially tincture or essential oil, because large amounts of thujone may be toxic.
• Warn patient not to take herb before seeking medical attention because doing so may delay diagnosis of a potentially serious medical condition.
• Tell patient to promptly notify health care provider about new symptoms or adverse effects.
• Warn patient to keep all herbal products away from children and pets.

## St. John's wort

*Hypericum perforatum,* amber, goatweed, hardhay, herb John, hexenkraut, Johanniskraut, John's wort, klamath weed, millepertuis, Saint John's word, tipton weed, titson weed

### Common trade names
*Alterra, Hypercalm, Kira, Quanterra Emotional Balance, St. John's Wort Extracts, Tension Tamer, various combination products*

## HOW SUPPLIED
Available as tablets, pellets, capsules of standardized extract, powdered or dried herb, liquid extract*, tincture, and transdermal forms.
*Capsules (extended-release, standardized at 0.3% hypericin):* 450 mg, 900 mg, 1,000 mg

---

*Liquid may contain alcohol.

*Capsules (standardized at 0.3% hypericin):* 125 mg, 150 mg, 250 mg, 300 mg, 350 mg, 370 mg, 375 mg, 400 mg, 424 mg, 434 mg, 450 mg, 500 mg, 510 mg
*Extract:* 1:1
*Injection:* 1%
*Liquid:* 300 mg/5 ml, 250 mg/ml
*Liquid dilutions:* 3x, 6x, 30x, 12c, 30c
*Pellets:* 3x, 6x, 12x, 12c, 30c
*Tablets (standardized at 0.3% hypericin):* 100 mg, 150 mg, 300 mg, 450 mg
*Tincture:* 1:10
*Transdermal:* 900 mg/24 hr

## ACTIONS & COMPONENTS

Obtained from *Hypericum perforatum.* Contains naphthodianthrones, including hypericin and pseudohypericin; hyperoside; quercitrin; rutin; isoquercitrin; bioflavonoids, including amentoflavone; 1,3,6,7-tetrahydroxy-xanthone; hyperforin; adhyperforin; aliphatic hydrocarbons, including 2-methyloctane and undecane; dodecanol; mono- and sesquiterpenes, including alphapinene and caryophyllene; 2-methyl-3-but-3-en-2-ol, oligomeric procyanidines; catechin tannins; and caffeic acid derivatives, including chlorogenic acid. St. John's wort may have a slight inhibitory effect on MAO inhibitors and reuptake of serotonin. Hypericin has antiviral activity and also inhibits catechol O-methyltransferase and receptors for adenosine, benzodiazepines, GABA-A, GABA-B, and inositol triphosphate. Certain constituents have also shown antibacterial activity.

## USES

Used orally for mild to moderate depression, anxiety, psychovegetative disorders, sciatica, and viral infections, including herpes simplex virus types 1 and 2, hepatitis C, influenza virus, murine cytomegalovirus, and poliovirus. St. John's wort has also been used to treat bronchitis, asthma, gallbladder disease, nocturnal enuresis, gout, and rheumatism, although it hasn't proven effective in these cases. Used topically for contusions, inflammation, myalgia, burns, hemorrhoids, and vitiligo. In traditional Chinese medicine, St. John's wort has been used as a gargle for tonsillitis and as a lotion for dermatoses.

## DOSAGE & ADMINISTRATION

*Capsules or tablets for mild to moderate depression:* Initially, 900 mg P.O. q.d.; maintenance, 300 to 600 mg P.O. q.d.
*For depression:* 2 to 4 g dried herb P.O. q.d., or 0.2 to 1 mg hypericin.
*For wounds, bruising, and swelling:* Applied topically to affected area.
*Liquid extract:* 2 to 4 ml P.O. q.d.
*Tea:* 2 to 3 g of dried herb in boiling water.
*Tincture:* 2 to 4 ml P.O. q.d.

## ADVERSE REACTIONS

**CNS:** fatigue, neuropathy, restlessness, headache.
**GI:** digestive complaints, fullness sensation, constipation, diarrhea, nausea, abdominal pain, dry mouth.
**Skin:** photosensitivity reaction, pruritus.
**Other:** delayed hypersensitivity.

---

*Bold italic type* indicates that reaction may be life-threatening.

## INTERACTIONS

**Herb-drug.** *Amitriptyline, chemotherapy drugs, cyclosporine, digoxin, drugs metabolized by the cytochrome P-450 enzyme system, oral contraceptives, protease inhibitors, theophylline, and warfarin:* Decreased effectiveness, requiring possible dosage adjustment. Monitor patient closely; advise patient to avoid using together.

*Barbiturates:* Decreased sedative effects. Monitor patient closely.

*MAO inhibitors, including phenelzine and tranylcypromine:* May increase effects and cause possible toxicity and hypertensive crisis. Advise patient to avoid using together.

*Narcotics:* Increased sedative effects. Advise patient to avoid using together.

*Reserpine:* Antagonized effects of reserpine. Advise patient to avoid using together.

*Selective serotonin reuptake inhibitors, such as citalopram, fluoxetine, paroxetine, sertraline:* Increased risk of serotonin syndrome. Advise patient to avoid using together.

**Herb-herb.** *Herbs with sedative effects, such as calamus, calendula, California poppy, capsicum, catnip, celery, couch grass, elecampane, German chamomile, goldenseal, gotu kola, Jamaican dogwood, kava, lemon balm, sage, sassafras, skullcap, shepherd's purse, Siberian ginseng, stinging nettle, valerian, wild carrot, and wild lettuce:* Possible enhanced effects of either herb. Monitor patient closely, and advise him to avoid using together.

**Herb-food.** *Tyramine-containing foods such as beer, cheese, dried meats, fava beans, liver, yeast, and wine:* May cause hypertensive crisis when used together. Advise patient to separate administration times.

**Herb-lifestyle.** *Alcohol use:* Possible increased sedative effects. Advise patient to avoid using together. *Sun exposure:* Increased risk of photosensitivity reactions. Urge patient to avoid unprotected sun exposure.

## CAUTIONS

Pregnant patients and men and women planning pregnancy shouldn't take St. John's wort because of mutagenic risk to developing cells and fetus. Transplant patients maintained on cyclosporine therapy should avoid this herb because of the risk of organ rejection.

## NURSING CONSIDERATIONS

- Find out why patient is using the herb.
- St. John's wort has been effective in treating mild to moderate depression.
- Recommended duration of therapy for depression is 4 to 6 weeks; if no improvement occurs, a different therapy should be considered.
- Monitor patient for response to herbal therapy, as evidenced by improved mood and lessened depression.
- By using standardized extracts, patient can better control the dosage. Clinical studies have used formulations of standardized 0.3% hypericin as well as hyperforin-stabilized version of the extract.

*Liquid may contain alcohol.

- St. John's wort interacts with many other products; they must be considered before patient takes it with other prescription or OTC products.
- Serotonin syndrome may cause dizziness, nausea, vomiting, headache, epigastric pain, anxiety, confusion, restlessness, and irritability.
- Because St. John's wort decreases the effect of certain prescription drugs, watch for signs of drug toxicity if patient stops using the herb. Drug dosage may need to be reduced.
- St. John's wort has mutagenic effects on sperm cells and oocytes and adverse effects on reproductive cells; therefore, it shouldn't be used by pregnant patients or those planning pregnancy (including men).
- Topically, the volatile plant oil is an irritant. Monitor affected site for adverse effects and improvement.
- Monitor patient for sedative effects and GI complaints.

**Patient teaching**
- Advise patient to consult with his health care provider before using an herbal preparation because a treatment with proven efficacy may be available.
- Tell patient to remind pharmacist of any herbal and dietary supplements that he's taking, when filling a new prescription.
- Instruct patient to consult a health care provider for a thorough medical evaluation before using St. John's wort.
- Encourage patient to discuss depression and to seek regular psychiatric help, as indicated.

- If patient takes St. John's wort for mild to moderate depression, explain that several weeks may pass before effects occur. Tell patient that a new therapy may be needed if no improvement occurs in 4 to 6 weeks.
- Inform patient that St. John's wort interacts with many other prescription and OTC products and may reduce their effectiveness.
- Tell patient that St. John's wort may cause increased sensitivity to direct sunlight. Recommend protective clothing, sunscreen, and limited sun exposure.
- Inform patient that a sufficient wash-out period is needed after stopping an antidepressant before switching to St. John's wort.
- Tell patient to report adverse effects to a health care provider.
- Warn patient to keep all herbal products away from children and pets.

## santonica

*Artemisia cina*, levant, santonica, sea wormwood, wormseed

**Common trade names**
*None known*

**HOW SUPPLIED**
Available as powder, lozenges, and in combination products.

**ACTIONS & COMPONENTS**
Obtained from *Artemisia cina*. Contains sesquiterpene lactone beta-santonin, which gives herb its action against intestinal worms,

---

particularly ascarids. It also may reduce fever.

## USES
Used to treat intestinal parasites such as *Ascaris* and *Oxyuris*.

## DOSAGE & ADMINISTRATION
*For intestinal worms:* For adults, 25 mg powder P.O. For children, child's age in years multiplied by 2 gives dose amount in mg.

## ADVERSE REACTIONS
**CNS:** headache, muscle twitching, stupor.
**EENT:** visual disorders, xanthopsia.
**GI:** gastroenteritis, nausea, vomiting.
**GU:** kidney irritation.
**Other:** allergic reactions.

## INTERACTIONS
None known.

## CAUTIONS
Patients allergic to members of the Compositae family, which includes ragweed, chrysanthemums, marigolds, and daisies, should avoid this herb.

## NURSING CONSIDERATIONS
• Find out why patient is using the herb.
🖉 **ALERT:** Fatal poisonings have been reported after ingestion of less than 10 g of this herb.
• To treat intestinal worms, herb must be taken with a laxative to ensure expulsion.
• Monitor patient's response to the herb.

• Although no chemical interactions have been reported in clinical studies, consider the pharmacologic properties of the herb and its potential to interfere with therapeutic effects of conventional drugs.

## Patient teaching
• Advise patient to consult with his health care provider before using an herbal preparation because a treatment with proven efficacy may be available.
• Tell patient to remind pharmacist of any herbal and dietary supplements that he's taking, when filling a new prescription.
• Advise patient to avoid using this herb if he's allergic to members of the Compositae family, which includes ragweed, chrysanthemums, marigolds, daisies, and other herbs.
• Warn patient not to take herb before seeking medical attention because doing so may delay diagnosis of a potentially serious medical condition.
• Instruct patient to promptly notify health care provider about new symptoms or adverse effects.

## sarsaparilla

*Smilax officinalis,* anantamul, anantamula, gopakanya, Indian sarsaparilla, kapuri, khao yen, naga-jihva, sariva, sarsa, smilax

**Common trade names**
*EveCare, Renalka, Sarsaparilla Root, Styplon*

## HOW SUPPLIED
Available as dried root, capsules, and tablets.

*Liquid may contain alcohol.

## ACTIONS & COMPONENTS
Obtained from dried root of *Smilax officinalis*. Contains saponins, phytosterols, resin, shikimic acid, terpene alcohols, glycosides, tannins, and essential oils. Detoxifying effect of herb is based on its ability to bind endotoxins. Antimicrobial and antipsoriatic activity may be caused by saponins. Herb also may act against *Treponema pallidum*, the organism that causes syphilis. It also has diuretic, anti-inflammatory, and hepatoprotective effects.

## USES
Used to treat psoriasis, rheumatism, kidney problems (including kidney stones), other urinary problems, syphilis, and venereal disease. Used as a tonic to improve appetite, digestion, vitality, and virility; popular among bodybuilders. Used to improve ailments and excretion of wastes from the blood. Used with other herbs such as burdock root, sassafras, red clover, and yellow dock. Also used as a flavoring agent in medicines.

## DOSAGE & ADMINISTRATION
*Capsules or tablets:* 9 g of dried root P.O. t.i.d., in divided doses.
*Decoction:* 3 cups P.O. q.d. Prepared by placing 1 to 2 tsp root in 1 cup of water and simmering for 10 to 15 minutes.
*Tincture:* 1 to 2 ml in 1 cup of warm water P.O. t.i.d.

## ADVERSE REACTIONS
**GI:** GI irritation, nausea.
**GU:** kidney irritation.

**Respiratory:** occupational asthma from root dust.

## INTERACTIONS
None reported.

## CAUTIONS
Patients with recurrent kidney stones should avoid this herb. No one should take large doses for long periods.

## NURSING CONSIDERATIONS
• Find out why patient is using the herb.
• Monitor patient's response to herbal therapy.

**Patient teaching**
• Advise patient to consult with his health care provider before using an herbal preparation because a treatment with proven efficacy may be available.
• Tell patient to remind pharmacist of any herbal and dietary supplements that he's taking, when filling a new prescription.
• If patient takes a drug that contains digitalis or bismuth, tell him to stop taking sarsaparilla.
• Advise patient to avoid heavy meals and animal-based foods.
• Tell patient to drink sufficient fluids to help the excretion process.
• Urge patient to promptly notify a health care provider about new symptoms or adverse effects.

---

*Bold italic type* indicates that reaction may be life-threatening.

## sassafras

*Sassafras albidum, S. officinale, S. radix, S. variifolia*, ague tree, cinnamon wood, kuntze saloop, laurus sassafras, saloop, sassafrax, saxifras

**Common trade names**
*None known*

### HOW SUPPLIED
Available as dried root.

### ACTIONS & COMPONENTS
Obtained from root of *Sassafras albidum*. Volatile oil contains safrole (up to 90%); other constituents include anethole, asarone, camphor, eugenol, myristicin, and pinene apiole. Herb elicits a mild antidiuretic response. Safrole and its major metabolite, 1-hydroxysafrole, are carcinogenic and neurotoxic.

### USES
Used orally to treat eye or mucous membrane inflammation, catarrh, bronchitis, high blood pressure, kidney disorders, arthritis, cancers, and syphilis; as a tonic and blood purifier; and as a flavoring agent. Used topically as an antiseptic and to treat skin eruptions, insect bites and stings, rheumatism, gout, sprains, and swelling.

### DOSAGE & ADMINISTRATION
*Infusion:* 50 g added to 1 L of water.
*Tea:* 1 tsp added to boiling water and strained after 10 minutes.

### ADVERSE REACTIONS
**CNS:** ataxia, CNS depression, hallucinations, hot flashes, paralysis, shakes, stupor, exhaustion, spasm.
**CV:** hypertension, tachycardia, *CV collapse.*
**EENT:** dilated pupils, ptosis.
**GI:** vomiting.
**Hepatic:** *liver cancer.*
**Skin:** contact dermatitis, diaphoresis.
**Other:** carcinogenesis, *hypersensitivity,* hypothermia.
**GU:** miscarriage.

### INTERACTIONS
**Herb-drug.** *Barbiturates, sedatives:* May cause additive effects. Advise patient to avoid using together.
*Drugs metabolized by cytochrome P-450 and P-488, phenytoin:* Increased metabolism and decreased blood levels of drugs metabolized by these pathways. Advise patient to avoid using together.
**Herb-herb.** *Herbs with sedative effects, including calamus, calendula, California poppy, capsicum, catnip, celery, couch grass, elecampane, German chamomile, goldenseal, gotu kola, hops, Jamaican dogwood, kava, lemon balm, sage, shepherd's purse, Siberian ginseng, skullcap, stinging nettle, St. John's wort, valerian, wild carrot, and wild lettuce:* May enhance therapeutic and adverse effects. Advise patient to avoid using together.
*Safrole-containing herbs, including basil, camphor, cinnamon, and nutmeg:* Potential additive toxicity. Advise patient to avoid using together.

---

*Liquid may contain alcohol.

**Herb-lifestyle.** *Alcohol use:* May enhance CNS depressant effects. Advise patient to avoid using together.

## CAUTIONS
Because of its carcinogenic potential, sassafras shouldn't be used in any form.

## NURSING CONSIDERATIONS
• Find out why patient is using the herb.

🗲**ALERT:** Sassafras has been banned by the FDA as a drug or food product; it may be carcinogenic and has caused many adverse reactions and death.

• Sassafras will alter phenytoin levels.

**Patient teaching**
• Advise patient to consult with his health care provider before using an herbal preparation because a treatment with proven efficacy may be available.
• Tell patient to remind pharmacist of any herbal and dietary supplements that he's taking, when filling a new prescription.
• Warn patient not to take herb before seeking medical attention because doing so may delay diagnosis of a potentially serious medical condition.
• Advise patient that sassafras has been banned by the FDA as a potential carcinogen with numerous adverse effects.

## saw palmetto

*Serenoa repens,* American dwarf palm tree, cabbage palm, sabal, shrub palmetto

**Common trade names**
*Centrum Saw Palmetto, Herbal Sure Saw Palmetto, Permixon, PlusStrogen, Premium Blend Saw Palmetto, Proactive Saw Palmetto, Propalmex, Quanterra Prostate, Saw Palmetto Power, Standardized Saw Palmetto ExtractCap, Super Saw Palmetto*

## HOW SUPPLIED
Available as tablets, capsules, fresh and dried berries, and as extracts*.
*Extracts:* 60% to 70% grain alcohol

## ACTIONS & COMPONENTS
Obtained from berries of *Serenoa repens.* Contains fatty acids, fatty acid esters, sitosterols, and phytosterols. Exact mechanism of action isn't known, but sitosterols may inhibit conversion of testosterone to dihydrotestosterone (DHT), reducing prostate enlargement. May also inhibit androgenic activity by competing with DHT for androgen receptors, affecting testosterone metabolism. Herb also has anti-inflammatory and astringent properties and inhibits prolactin and growth factor-induced cell proliferation. Said to improve urine flow rate and post-void residual in BPH.

## USES
Used to treat symptoms of BPH and coughs and congestion from colds, bronchitis, or asthma. Also

---

*Bold italic type* indicates that reaction may be life-threatening.

used as a mild diuretic, urinary antiseptic, and astringent.

## DOSAGE & ADMINISTRATION
*Average daily dose:* 160 mg P.O. b.i.d. or 320 mg P.O. q.d. (1 to 2 g fresh berries or 320 mg of lipophilic extract).
*Decoction of berries:* 1 to 2 g of fresh berries in 1 cup of water, boiled, then simmered for 5 minutes. Taken t.i.d., possibly for longer than 3 months but less than 6 months.

## ADVERSE REACTIONS
**CNS:** headache.
**CV:** hypertension.
**GI:** nausea, abdominal pain, diarrhea.
**GU:** urine retention.
**Musculoskeletal:** back pain.

## INTERACTIONS
**Herb-drug.** *Adrenergics, hormones, hormone-like drugs:* Possible estrogen, androgen, and alpha-blocking effects. Drug dosages may need adjustment if patient takes this herb. Monitor patient closely.

## CAUTIONS
Pregnant or breast-feeding women and women of childbearing age shouldn't use this herb. Adults and children with hormone-dependent illnesses other than BPH or breast cancer should avoid this herb.

## NURSING CONSIDERATIONS
● Find out why patient is using the herb.
● Herb should be used cautiously for conditions other than BPH because data about its effectiveness in other conditions is lacking.

● Obtain a baseline prostate-specific antigen (PSA) test before patient starts taking herb because it may cause a false-negative PSA result.
● Be aware that saw palmetto may not alter prostate size.
● Laboratory values didn't change significantly in clinical trials using dosages of 160 mg to 320 mg daily.

**Patient teaching**
● Advise patient to consult with his health care provider before using an herbal preparation because a treatment with proven efficacy may be available.
● Tell patient to remind pharmacist of any herbal and dietary supplements that he's taking, when filling a new prescription.
● Warn patient not to take herb for bladder or prostate problems before seeking medical attention because doing so could delay diagnosis of a potentially serious medical condition.
● Tell patient to take herb with food to minimize GI effects.
● Caution patient to promptly notify health care provider about new or worsened adverse effects.
● Warn women to avoid herb if planning pregnancy, if pregnant, and if breast-feeding.

## scented geranium

*Pelargonium*

**Common trade names**
*None known*

## HOW SUPPLIED
Available as whole plant and essential oil.

*Liquid may contain alcohol.

## ACTIONS & COMPONENTS
Obtained from leaves of certain *Pelargonium* species. Contains *l*-citronellol, alcohols, esters, aldehydes, and ketones. Mechanism of antibacterial and antifungal effects is unknown.

## USES
Used for citronell effects as mosquito repellant and for antibacterial and antifungal effects. Also used as an analgesic, antidepressant, expectorant, astringent, diuretic, sedative, flavoring agent, and fragrance.

## DOSAGE & ADMINISTRATION
Dosages not well documented.

## ADVERSE REACTIONS
**CV:** edema.
**Skin:** dermatitis, erythema, vesiculation, cheilitis.

## INTERACTIONS
None known.

## CAUTIONS
Patients hypersensitive to members of the geranium family should avoid this herb.

## NURSING CONSIDERATIONS
• Find out why patient is using the herb.
• *Pelargoniums* are common annuals and houseplants of many different species and varieties. They shouldn't be confused with plants of the genus *Geranium*.

### Patient teaching
• Advise patient to consult with his health care provider before using an herbal preparation because a treatment with proven efficacy may be available.
• Tell patient to remind pharmacist of any herbal and dietary supplements that he's taking, when filling a new prescription.
• Inform patient that few data are available regarding medicinal use of geraniums. Tell him that scented geranium has questionable efficacy as a topical mosquito repellant and may cause dermatitis.
• Instruct patient to promptly notify a health care provider about new or worsened adverse effects.
• Warn patient to keep all herbal products away from children and pets.

## schisandra

*Schisandra chinensis,* gomishi, hoku-gomishi, kita-gomishi, omicha, schizandra, wu-wei-zu

**Common trade names**
*Bilberry/Schizandra Plus, Clarity, Immunity, Milk Thistle/Schizandra Plus, NutraPack, ParaCleanse, Schizandra Plus*

## HOW SUPPLIED
Available as dried berries, seeds, and fluidextract*.
*Capsules:* 560 mg, 600 mg
*Extract:* 1:1 in 12% to 15% grain alcohol or glycerin base

## ACTIONS & COMPONENTS
Obtained from *Schisandra chinensis*. Contains 10% organic acids, including carboxylic, malic, citric, tartaric, and nigranoic acids, as well as vitamins E and C. More

than 30 lignins have been identified in seeds and fruit (about 2% of fruit by weight), including schizandrin and related compounds and many gomisin compounds. Lignins may have pronounced liver protecting effects. Herb may have astringent and nervous system stimulant effects.

## USES
Used to treat dry cough, asthma, night sweats, chronic fatigue, nocturnal seminal emissions, chronic diarrhea, and various lung, liver, and kidney disorders. Also used to improve mental alertness and reflex responses, relieve eye fatigue, increase visual acuity, and ease depression caused by adrenergic exhaustion.

## DOSAGE & ADMINISTRATION
*Decoction:* 1 cup taken every 8 hours. Prepared by adding 5 g crushed berries to 100 ml water, boiling, and then simmering.
*Liquid extract (1:1 alcohol or glycerin base):* 1.25 to 3 ml P.O. t.i.d.
*Tea:* 2 to 3 cups P.O. q.d. Prepared by adding 2 to 4 tbs dried berries to 2 cups of water, boiling, and then simmering until liquid is reduced to 1 cup.

## ADVERSE REACTIONS
**CNS:** restlessness, insomnia, CNS depression.
**GI:** heartburn.
**Hepatic:** altered ALT levels.
**Respiratory:** dyspnea.

## INTERACTIONS
*Body-strengthening drugs:* May potentiate drug effects and raise blood pressure. Advise patient to avoid using together.

## CAUTIONS
Pregnant or breast-feeding patients should avoid this herb, as should patients who have epilepsy, peptic ulcers, fever, or high blood pressure.

## NURSING CONSIDERATIONS
- Find out why patient is using the herb.
- Patients with peptic ulcer may develop increased acidity.
- Monitor liver function tests.
- Advise patient to avoid taking schisandra before having liver function tests because herb may alter ALT test results.
- Chinese call this herb *wu-wei-zu* (five-taste fruit) because berries are sweet, sour, bitter, pungent (hot), and salty. Plant is considered balanced because of this wide range of flavors.

### Patient teaching
- Advise patient to consult with his health care provider before using an herbal preparation because a treatment with proven efficacy may be available.
- Tell patient to remind pharmacist of any herbal and dietary supplements that he's taking, when filling a new prescription.
- Tell patient to take herb with meals to minimize GI upset.
- Advise women to avoid using this herb when pregnant or breast-feeding.

---

*Liquid may contain alcohol.

• Warn patient to keep all herbal products away from children and pets.

## sea holly

*Eryngium campestre,* eryngio herba, eryngo, sea holme, sea hulver

**Common trade names**
*None known*

### HOW SUPPLIED
Available as leaves, powdered root, and extract*.

### ACTIONS & COMPONENTS
Obtained from *Eryngium campestre.* Above-ground parts contain triterpene saponins, caffeic acid esters such as chlorogenic acid and rosmaric acid, and flavonoids. Roots also contain procoumarins, pyranocoumarins, and oligosaccharides. Above-ground plant parts have a mild diuretic effect. Roots have antispasmodic and mild expectorant effects.

### USES
Above-ground parts are used to treat UTI, prostatitis, and inflamed bronchial mucous membranes. Roots are used to treat kidney and bladder stones, renal colic, kidney and urinary tract inflammation, urine retention, edema, cough, bronchitis, and skin and respiratory disorders.

### DOSAGE & ADMINISTRATION
*Decoction:* 2 to 3 cups q.d. Prepared by boiling 4 tsp ground root in 1 L water for 10 minutes, steeping 15 minutes, and then straining.
*Tea:* 3 to 4 cups q.d. Prepared by steeping 1 tsp ground root in 150 ml boiling water until cold, and then straining.
*Tincture:* 50 to 60 gtt P.O. q.d., divided into 3 or 4 doses. Prepared by soaking 20 g powdered root in 80 g of 60% alcohol for 10 days.

### ADVERSE REACTIONS
None known.

### INTERACTIONS
**Herb-drug.** *Disulfiram:* Herbal products that contain alcohol may cause a disulfiram-like reaction. Advise patient to avoid using together.

### CAUTIONS
Pregnant or breast-feeding women shouldn't use this herb.

### NURSING CONSIDERATIONS
• Find out why patient is using the herb.
• Monitor patient's response to herbal therapy.

**Patient teaching**
• Advise patient to consult with his health care provider before using an herbal preparation because a treatment with proven efficacy may be available.
• Tell patient to remind pharmacist of any herbal and dietary supplements that he's taking, when filling a new prescription.
• Remind patient that commercially available rubbing alcohol is denatured and isn't appropriate for oral use.

---

*Bold italic type* indicates that reaction may be life-threatening.

- Advise patient to promptly notify health care provider about adverse effects or changes in symptoms.

## self-heal

*Prunella vulgaris,* all-heal, blue curls, brownwort, brunella, carpenter's herb, carpenter's weed, heal-all, heart of the earth, Hercules woundwort, hock-heal, hook-heal, sicklewort, siclewort, slough-heal, woundwort

**Common trade names**
*Prunella, Self-Heal*

### HOW SUPPLIED
Available as dried herb, capsules, tea, and tincture*.

### ACTIONS & COMPONENTS
Obtained from *Prunella vulgaris.* Contains oleanolic acid, urosolic acid, rutin, hyperoside, caffeic acid, vitamins, carotenoids, tannis, essential oils, and alkaloids. Urosolic acid is cytotoxic against lymphocytic leukemia cells and human lung cancer cells. Also contains rosmarinic acid, an antioxidant, and prunellin, which may have anti-HIV activity. Some marginal cytotoxicity against human colon and mammary tumor cells has also been reported.

### USES
Used to treat wounds, stop bleeding, control diarrhea, support the liver, and aid circulation. Also used as a gargle for mouth and throat infections, as a cooling tea, and as a treatment for tuberculosis, jaundice, infectious hepatitis, bacillary dysentery, pleuritis with effusion, and cancer. Also used as an antibiotic, antihypertensive, antimutagenic, and antioxidant, especially in patients with HIV and cancer.

### DOSAGE & ADMINISTRATION
*Infusion:* 6 to 15 g of dried herb steeped for 10 minutes in 8 oz of water, P.O. t.i.d.
*Tincture:* 1 to 2 ml P.O. t.i.d.
*Topical:* Juice or poultice applied to affected area.

### ADVERSE REACTIONS
None known.

### INTERACTIONS
**Herb-drug.** *Disulfiram:* Herbal products that contain alcohol may cause a disulfiram-like reaction. Advise patient to avoid using together.

### CAUTIONS
Patients hypersensitive to any part of the herb shouldn't take self-heal. Pregnant or breast-feeding women shouldn't use this herb. Safety in children isn't known.

### NURSING CONSIDERATIONS
- Find out why patient is using the herb.
- Because entire plant is used, sensitivity reactions are possible.
- Patients may combine topical and liquid forms of prunella with other herbal products. Read product ingredients carefully.
- Although no chemical interactions have been reported in clinical studies, consider the pharmacologic properties of the herb and its po-

---

*Liquid may contain alcohol.

tential to interfere with therapeutic effects of conventional drugs.

**Patient teaching**
• Advise patient to consult with his health care provider before using an herbal preparation because a treatment with proven efficacy may be available.
• Tell patient to remind pharmacist of any herbal and dietary supplements that he's taking, when filling a new prescription.
• Advise patients with allergies to flowers, such as hayfever and ragweed, to use this herb cautiously.
• Urge patient to consult with his health care provider before taking self-heal.
• Tell patient to promptly notify his health care provider about adverse effects or changes in symptoms.

## senega

*Polygala senega,* milkwort, mountain flax, northern senega, plantula marilandica, poligala raiz, polygala virginiana, polygalae radix, polygale de virginie, rattlesnake root, senega snakeroot, senegawurzel, snake root, snakeroot yuan zhi

**Common trade names**
*Seneca, Senega.*
Combination products: Antibron, Asthma 6-N, Bronchial, Bronchiplant, Bronchiplant Light, Bronchocodin, Bronchozone, Broncofluid, Broncovial, Calmarum, Chest Mixture, Cocillana-Etyfin, Combitorax, Desbly, Dinacode, Dinacode avae Codeine,

Expectoran Codeine, Fluidin Antiasmatico, Fluidin Infantil, Hederix, Makatussin, Makatussin forte, Neo-Codion, Nyl Bronchitis, Pastillas Pectoral Kely, Patussol, Pectocalamine, Pectoral N, Phol-Tux, Polery, Pulmofasa, Pulmofasa Antihist, Quintopan, Senega and Ammonia, Sirop Pectoral Adulte, Sirop Santitussif Wyss a Base de Codeine, Sirop Wyss Contre La Toux, Stodol, Tussimont, Wampole Bronchial Cough Syrup

**HOW SUPPLIED**
Available as dried root, liquid extract*, infusion, syrup, lozenges, tea, and tincture*.

**ACTIONS & COMPONENTS**
Obtained from *Polygala senega.* Contains triterpenoid saponins (senegenin, polygalin, and polygalic acid), which exert expectorant action on the lining of the upper GI tract and stomach. Irritation of the gastic mucosa may lead to reflex stimulation of bronchial mucous gland secretion.

**USES**
Used with other expectorants for chronic bronchitis and for treating pneumonia or the second stage of acute bronchial catarrh. Currently used mainly as an expectorant by patients with bronchitis who have poor sputum output. Also used as an antidote for some poisons, as a poultice for external wounds, and as an abortifacient. Also used for general ailments.

## DOSAGE & ADMINISTRATION

*Fluidextract (1:1 in 60% alcohol):* 0.3 to 1 ml (6 to 20 gtt) P.O. t.i.d. or 1.5 to 3 g P.O. q.d.

*Infusion:* 0.5 to 1 g of herb in 1 cup of water P.O. b.i.d. or t.i.d. In severe cases, q 2 hr as long as patient is being monitored for adverse effects.

*Root:* 1.5 to 3 g P.O. q.d.

*Tincture (1:4 in 60% alcohol):* 2.5 to 5 ml (50 to 100 gtt) P.O. t.i.d. or 2.5 to 7.5 g P.O. q.d.

## ADVERSE REACTIONS

**GI:** nausea, vomiting, GI irritation, diarrhea.
**Respiratory:** increased bronchial secretion.
**Skin:** diaphoresis.

## INTERACTIONS

**Herb-drug.** *Disulfiram:* Herbal products that contain alcohol may cause a disulfiram-like reaction. Advise patient to avoid using together.

## CAUTIONS

Patients hypersensitive to senega shouldn't use this herb. Patients with GI disorders (such as peptic ulcer disease and inflammatory bowel disease) and those who are pregnant or breast-feeding also shouldn't use this herb. Pediatric effects are unknown and use isn't recommended.

## NURSING CONSIDERATIONS

• Find out why patient is using the herb.
• Prolonged use has been linked to GI irritation.

⚡**ALERT:** Monitor patient for nausea, diaphoresis, vomiting, GI complaints, and diarrhea. These problems may indicate an overdose, an adverse reaction, or sensitivity to senega. Emetic properties of the herb at high doses make further toxicity self-limiting.

• Monitor patients, especially those with diagnosed respiratory conditions, for shortness of breath or other respiratory difficulties from increased bronchial secretions.

### Patient teaching

• Advise patient to consult with his health care provider before using an herbal preparation because a treatment with proven efficacy may be available.
• Tell patient to remind pharmacist of any herbal and dietary supplements that he's taking, when filling a new prescription.
• Tell patient to read product labels carefully because senega is usually taken with other herbs or substances.
• Caution patient against prolonged use.
• Recommend that patient stop taking senega if he develops nausea, GI discomfort, vomiting, diarrhea, or increased respiratory problems.
• Tell patient that liquid forms may contain alcohol, which can interact with other drugs.

---

*Liquid may contain alcohol.

## senna

*Cassia acutifolia,* Alexandria senna, Alexandrian senna, Cassia senna, India senna, Khartoum senna, sennae folium, tinnevelly senna

**Common trade names**
*Black-Draught, Dr. Caldwell Senna Laxative, Fletcher's Castoria, Gentlax, Senexon Senna-Gen, Senokot, SenokotXTRA, Senolax, X-Prep Bowel Evacuant*

### HOW SUPPLIED
Available as granules, fluidextract, suppository, syrup, and tablets.
*Granules:* 326 mg/tsp, 1.65 g/½ tsp
*Suppositories:* 652 mg
*Syrup:* 218 mg/5 ml
*Tablets:* 187 mg, 217 mg, 600 mg

### ACTIONS & COMPONENTS
Obtained from dried leaves and pods of *Cassia acutifolia* or *C. angustifolia.* Contains 1.2% to 6% dianthrone glycosides—primarily sennosides A, $A_1$, and B with lesser amounts of C, D, E, F, and G—together with other anthraquinone derivatives that contribute to the laxative effect. Senna increases peristalsis, probably by direct effect on intestinal smooth muscle. It probably either irritates the muscles or stimulates the colonic intramural plexus. Senna is activated in the colon to rheinanthrone. Because activation takes 6 to 12 hours, a bedtime dose typically produces a morning bowel movement. It also promotes fluid accumulation in the colon and small intestine.

### USES
Used as a laxative to treat constipation or ease bowel evacuation after rectal-anal surgery or if patient has anal fissures or hemorrhoids. Also used for colon evacuation before rectal and bowel exams or surgery. It's commonly used to treat constipation caused by narcotics. Senna has been investigated as a treatment for fecal soiling, herpes simplex, and infections with *Escherichia coli* or *Candida albicans.*

### DOSAGE & ADMINISTRATION
The following are general ranges; dosage should be individualized to the smallest dose needed to produce a soft stool. Elderly, debilitated, antepartum, and postpartum patients start with smallest doses. If comfortable elimination doesn't occur by the second day, dosage can be adjusted until evacuation occurs.
*For adults, to evacuate colon for rectal and bowel examinations:* Single 75-ml dose of a standardized senna preparation (1 ml standardized to 26 mg sennoside B).
*For adults with constipation:* 0.5 to 3.0 g crude herb or 15 to 40 mg sennosides (standardized preparations) P.O., ideally h.s.
*For children:* Several OTC products are available for children older than age 6 or who weigh more than 60 lb (27 kg). See product labels.
*Infusion:* Prepared either by adding 0.5 to 2.0 g of powdered herb to 150 ml hot (not boiling) water for 10 to 15 minutes and then strainings or by steeping macerated herb in cold water for 10 to 12 hours and then straining.

---

*Bold italic type* indicates that reaction may be life-threatening.

## ADVERSE REACTIONS

**CV:** *arrhythmias,* disorders of heart function.

**EENT:** rhinoconjunctivitis.

**GI:** GI cramping or gripping, diarrhea, nausea, perianal irritation, aggravated constipation.

**GU:** yellowish-brown or red urine, nephritis, nephropathies, albuminuria, hematuria, damage to renal tubules.

**Metabolic:** loss of fluid and electrolytes, especially potassium; hyperaldosteronism.

**Musculoskeletal:** accelerated bone deterioration, muscle weakness.

**Respiratory:** asthma.

**Other:** reversible finger clubbing, IgE-mediated allergy.

## INTERACTIONS

**Herb-drug.** *Antiarrhythmics, cardiac glycosides including digoxin, lanoxin:* Overuse or abuse of senna may interfere with drug action via loss of potassium. For extended use, monitor patient's serum potassium levels and heart rate. Advise patient to avoid using together.

*Corticosteroids:* May increase risk of hypokalemia and potentiation of cardioactive steroids, and may rarely cause heart arrhythmias. For extended use, monitor patient's serum potassium levels, vital signs, and ECG.

*Estrogen:* Decreased serum estrogen levels. Advise patient to avoid using together.

*NSAIDs:* May decrease effect of senna. Advise patient to avoid using together.

*Oral drugs:* Absorption of some drugs may be decreased by rapid transit time in the colon. Monitor patient for loss of therapeutic response, especially patients previously well controlled.

*Thiazide diuretics, including furosemide, lasix:* May increase risk of hypokalemia. For extended use, monitor patient's serum potassium levels and ECG.

**Herb-herb.** *Potassium-depleting herbs such as gossypol, horsetail plant, licorice:* Increased risk of hypokalemia. For extended concurrent use, monitor patient's serum potassium levels.

*Stimulant laxative herbs such as aloe dried leaf sap, black root, blue flag rhizome, butternut bark, cascara bark, castor oil, colocynth fruit pulp, gamboge bark exudate, jalap root, manna bark exudate, podophyllum, rhubarb root, senna leaves and pods, wild cumber fruit, and yellow dock root:* Increased risk of hypokalemia. For extended use, monitor patient's serum potassium levels.

## CAUTIONS

Senna should be avoided by patients with intestinal obstruction, diarrhea, abdominal pain of unknown origin, fluid or electrolyte imbalance, and acute inflammatory intestinal diseases, such as appendicitis, colitis, Crohn's disease, and irritable bowel syndrome. Those with renal disease should use the herb cautiously.

There's no consensus in international labeling regarding use of senna by pregnant or breast-feeding women. In Britain and Germany, senna is contraindicated for these conditions. In the United States, no

---

*Liquid may contain alcohol.

label restrictions appear on standardized OTC products. Studies haven't shown that standardized senna products stimulate uterine contractions in pregnant women.

The German Commission E doesn't recommend senna for children younger than age 12; however, several OTC products available in the United States provide dose recommendations for children older than age 6 or who weigh more than 60 pounds.

## NURSING CONSIDERATIONS
- Find out why patient is using the herb.
- Although senna may be taken as a tea, dosages are difficult to determine or adjust using this unstandardized form. Many OTC products with standardized ingredients and doses are available. Adult dosages for senna can range from 20 to 60 mg of hydroxyanthracene derivatives.
- Infusions made in cold water may contain less of the compounds suspected to cause abdominal pain.
- Geriatric patients are usually advised to start with half the typical adult dose.
- Herb takes effect 6 to 8 hours after administration and isn't suitable for rapid emptying of the bowels.
- Long-term use is undesirable; however, if patient has chronic constipation, long-term use may be warranted with proper care, including potassium replacement.
- Long-term use may reduce spontaneous bowel function and lead to "cathartic colon" and laxative-dependency syndrome.

- Typical symptoms of laxative abuse include: abdominal pain, weakness, fatigue, thirst, vomiting, edema, bone pain caused by osteomalacia, fluid and electrolyte imbalance, hypoalbuminemia caused by protein-losing gastroenteropathy, and syndromes that mimic colitis.
- Evidence of overdose includes vomiting, severe GI spasms, and thin, watery stools. Large overdoses may also cause nephritis.
- Melanosis coli develops in about 5% of people who use anthranoids long-term (4 to 13 months). It resolves after discontinuation. There's no definite link between anthracene drugs and colon cancer.
- Other anthranoids, such as cassic acid, appear in breast milk in small amounts and may give milk a brownish tint. No data exist to determine whether the anthranoid level causes diarrhea in nursing infants.
- Senna preparations may contain alcohol or sugar.
- Monitor patient's serum potassium level during concurrent use of senna and cardiac glycosides, thiazide diuretics, corticosteroids, antiarrhythmics, licorice, potassium-depleting herbs, or other stimulant laxative herbs.

### Patient teaching
- Advise patient to consult with his health care provider before using an herbal preparation because a treatment with proven efficacy may be available.
- Tell patient to remind pharmacist of any herbal and dietary supple-

---

*Bold italic type* indicates that reaction may be life-threatening.

ments that he's taking, when filling a new prescription.
- Encourage patient to first try lifestyle changes—such as increasing dietary fiber, fluid intake, and exercise—to restore normal bowel function. Patient can also use a bulk laxative.
- Tell patient that senna may turn urine yellowish-brown or red.
- Recommend that pregnant or breast-feeding patients consult a health care provider before using senna.
- Inform patient that senna preparations may contain alcohol or sugar; patient should check product label if he has alcohol or sugar restrictions.
- Instruct patient not to take stimulant laxatives for longer than 1 or 2 weeks without seeking medical advice.
- Warn patient not to exceed maximum recommended dose.
- Advise patient that overuse of laxatives can lead to severe electrolyte imbalances, intestinal sluggishness, and a dependency on laxatives.
- Advise patient that rectal bleeding or failure to have a bowel movement after using a laxative may indicate a serious condition.
- Instruct patient to stop using senna if he has or develops nausea, vomiting, abdominal pain, loose stools, or diarrhea.
- Tell patient to contact a health care provider if his bowel habits change suddenly for 2 weeks or longer.
- Warn patient to keep all herbal products away from children and pets.

*Liquid may contain alcohol.

## shark cartilage

*Sphyrna lewini, Squalus acanthias* and other shark species, squalamine

**Common trade names**
*BeneFin, Cartilade*

**HOW SUPPLIED**
Available as powder and capsules. *Capsules:* 200 g, 500 g

**ACTIONS & COMPONENTS**
Obtained from shredded and dried cartilage of the hammerhead shark *(Sphyrna lewini)* and the spiny dogfish shark *(Squalus acanthias)* captured in the Pacific Ocean. Shark cartilage is purported to have anticancer properties by inhibiting angiogenesis (new blood vessel formation) in tumors. Another hypothesis for the anticancer effect involves a class of proteins normally present in cartilage and bone called tissue inhibitors of metalloproteinases (TIMPs). TIMPs block enzymes that tumors use to invade surrounding tissue. An inhibitor, or series of inhibitors, of neovascularization present in shark cartilage has been identified as guanidine extractable protein. A family of complex carbohydrates and mucopolysaccharides may be the primary anti-inflammatory components.

**USES**
Used to treat or prevent cancer and to treat osteoarthritis, rheumatoid arthritis, psoriasis, lupus, eczema, and enteritis. Also used to assist in bone and wound healing and to maintain proper bone and joint

function. Powder is also used as a retention enema. Data from ongoing studies may help define the role of shark cartilage in the treatment of lung cancer, AIDS-associated Kaposi's sarcoma, and prostate cancer.

**DOSAGE & ADMINISTRATION**

No consensus exists on the dosage for anticancer effects or other uses. *For benefit of additional cartilage protein and calcium:* 6 g powder in 1 glass of water or juice P.O. *To maintain proper bone and joint function:* 4 g powder in 1 glass of water or juice P.O.

**ADVERSE REACTIONS**

None known.

**INTERACTIONS**

None reported.

**CAUTIONS**

Shark cartilage shouldn't be used by children or by pregnant or breast-feeding women. Patients recovering from MI or CVA shouldn't use this product because inhibition of angiogenesis may interfere with revascularization of an infarcted area.

**NURSING CONSIDERATIONS**

● Find out why patient is using the product.
● No data exist regarding toxicity of shark cartilage.

**Patient teaching**

● Advise patient to consult with his health care provider before using this product because a treatment with proven efficacy may be available.

● Tell patient to remind pharmacist of any herbal and dietary supplements that he's taking, when filling a new prescription.

● Warn patient not to take shark cartilage before seeking medical attention because doing so may delay diagnosis of a potentially serious medical condition.

● Tell patient not to use shark cartilage if pregnant or breast-feeding unless advised by a knowledgeable health care provider. Effects of shark cartilage on pregnant or breast-feeding women are unknown.

● Warn patient not to take shark cartilage after a recent MI or CVA. Explain that shark cartilage may inhibit the body's ability to form new blood vessels, which may obstruct healing in the injured heart or brain area.

## shepherd's purse

*Capsella bursa pastoris,* Bursae pastoris herba, blindweed, capsella, case-weed, cocowort, lady's purse, Mother's heart, pepper-and-salt, pick-pocket, poor man's parmacettie, rattle pouches, sanguinary, shepherd's heart, shepherd's purse herb, shepherd's scrip, shepherd's sprout, shovelweed, St. James' weed, toywort, witches' pouches

**Common trade names**
*None known*

---

*Bold italic type* indicates that reaction may be life-threatening.

## HOW SUPPLIED
Available as dried herb and liquid extract*.

## ACTIONS & COMPONENTS
Obtained from *Capsella bursa pastoris*. Contains the amino acid proline, cardioactive steroids, and a peptide with hemostatic oxytocin-like activity. Also contains saponins, flavonoids, large amounts of potassium salts, oxalates, vitamin C, and sinigrin. Sinigrin can be degraded to allyl isothiocyanate, which is linked to goiter and abnormal thyroid function. Shepherd's purse increases uterine contractions by stimulating smooth muscle. Cardioactive steroids in the seeds cause positive and negative inotropic and chronotropic effects. Muscarine-like, dose-dependent hypertensive and antihypertensive effects are also reported.

## USES
Used internally to treat dysmenorrhea, mild menorrhagia, and metrorrhagia. Also used for headache, mild cardiac insufficiency, arrhythmia, hypotension, nervous heart complaints, premenstrual complaints, hematemesis, hematuria, diarrhea, and acute catarrhal cystitis. Topically, it's used as a styptic for nosebleeds and other superficial bleeding injuries.

## DOSAGE & ADMINISTRATION
*Dried above-ground parts:* 10 to 15 g P.O. q.d. May be taken as 1 to 4 g of dried herb t.i.d.
*Fluidextract (1:1 in 25% alcohol):* 5 to 8 g or 1 to 4 ml P.O. t.i.d.

*Tea:* 1 to 4 g dried herb steeped in 150 ml of boiling water for 15 minutes and then strained.
*Topical form:* 3 to 5 g of herb steeped in 180 ml of boiling water for 10 to 15 minutes and then strained. Fluid is applied to affected area.

## ADVERSE REACTIONS
**CNS:** sedation.
**CV:** palpitations, hypertension, hypotension.
**GU:** increased uterine contractions, abnormal menstruation.
**Other:** abnormal thyroid function.

## INTERACTIONS
**Herb-drug.** *Antihypertensives, antihypotensives:* Possible reduced effect. Monitor blood pressure closely.
*CV drugs:* Possible reduced effect. Monitor vital signs, and assess patient for palpitations.
*Disulfiram:* Herbal products that contain alcohol may cause a disulfiram-like reaction. Advise patient to avoid using together.
*Sedatives:* Additive effects. Monitor patient for sedation.
*Thyroid medications:* Allyl isothiocyanate may interfere with thyroid therapy. Monitor thyroid function in patients previously well controlled.
**Herb-herb.** *Herbs with sedative effects, including calamus, calendula, California poppy, capsicum, catnip, celery, cough grass, elecampane, German chamomile, goldenseal, gotu kola, hops, Jamaican dogwood, kava, lemon balm, sage, sassafras, Siberian ginseng, skullcap, stinging nettle, St. John's wort, va-*

---

*Liquid may contain alcohol.

*lerian, wild carrot, wild lettuce, and yerba maté:* Possible additive effects. Monitor patient for sedation.

## CAUTIONS
Shepherd's purse is a uterine stimulant and may induce miscarriage; it shouldn't be used by women planning pregnancy or those who are pregnant or breast-feeding. Patients with a history of kidney stones should use shepherd's purse cautiously because of its oxalate content. Shepherd's purse commonly harbors endophytic fungi such as *Albugo candida* and *Peronospora parasitica.* Because it may contain mycotoxins, patients with compromised immune systems should use the herb cautiously.

## NURSING CONSIDERATIONS
• Find out why patient is using the herb.
• The use of shepherd's purse instead of ergot for uterine bleeding is inappropriate because of inadequate activity.
• Monitor blood pressure, which may increase or decrease, and thyroid function in patients taking thyroid medication who were previously well controlled.
• Monitor patient for palpitations, especially if susceptible to arrhythmias.
• Monitor patient for changes in menstruation.

## Patient teaching
• Advise patient to consult with his health care provider before using an herbal preparation because a treatment with proven efficacy may be available.

• Tell patient to remind pharmacist of any herbal and dietary supplements that he's taking, when filling a new prescription.
• Warn patient not to use alcohol-containing forms if he takes disulfiram, metronidazole, or any other drug that interacts with alcohol.
• Inform women that shepherd's purse may cause abnormal menstruation.
• Tell patient that this herb may aggravate kidney stones, CV therapy, thyroid therapy, and antihypertensive or antihypotensive therapy. Affected patients should use shepherd's purse cautiously and only under direct supervision by a knowledgeable health care provider.
• Advise patient that herb may cause or increase sedation and the adverse effects of other herbs or drugs that cause sedation.
• Caution patient to avoid hazardous tasks until full sedative effects of herb are known.
• Urge patient to promptly notify health care provider about new symptoms or adverse effects.
• Tell patient to store herb away from light and moisture, and to keep it away from children and pets.

## skullcap

*Scutellaria lateriflora,* blue pimpernel, helmet flower, hoodwort, mad-dog weed, madweed, Quaker bonnet, skullcap, Virginian skull cap

**Common trade names**
*Skullcap, Wild American Skullcap, Wild Countryside Skullcap*

## HOW SUPPLIED
Available as dried herb, extracts, and capsules.
*Capsules:* 425 mg, 430 mg

## ACTIONS & COMPONENTS
Obtained from roots and leaves of *Scutellaria lateriflora* and *S. baicalensis.* Contains flavonoids such as apigenin, baicalein, baicalin, hispidulin, scutellarein, and scutellarin. Also contains sesquiterpenes such as cadinene, caryophyllene, catapol, limonene, and terpineol. Other compounds include wogonin and its glucuronide, which can inhibit sialidase, an enzyme linked to some cancers. Lignin and various tannins are also present. Extracts from *S. baicalensis* may modulate hemopoiesis, scavenge free radicals, and increase nitric oxide production. Extracts may have some bacteriostatic, bactericidal, anti-inflammatory, and antiviral activity.

## USES
Used as an anticonvulsant, antispasmodic, anti-inflammatory, and sedative. Also used as an adjunct to chemotherapy to enhance immune response.

## DOSAGE & ADMINISTRATION
*Dried herb:* 1 to 2 g as a tea P.O. t.i.d.
*Liquid extract (1:1 in 25% alcohol):* 2 to 4 ml P.O. t.i.d.

## ADVERSE REACTIONS
**CNS:** confusion, headache, *seizures.*
**CV:** *arrhythmias.*
**Hepatic:** *hepatotoxicity.*

## INTERACTIONS
**Herb-drug.** *Disulfiram:* Herbal products that contain alcohol may cause a disulfiram-like reaction. Advise patient to avoid using together.

## CAUTIONS
Pregnant or breast-feeding women shouldn't use this herb.

## NURSING CONSIDERATIONS
• Find out why patient is using the herb.
• Skullcap preparations may be contaminated with other substances.
• Monitor patient for adverse effects and response to herbal treatment.

## Patient teaching
• Advise patient to consult with his health care provider before using an herbal preparation because a treatment with proven efficacy may be available.
• Tell patient to remind pharmacist of any herbal and dietary supplements that he's taking, when filling a new prescription.
• Warn patient not to take herb before seeking medical attention because doing so may delay diagnosis of a potentially serious medical condition.
• Instruct patient to promptly notify health care provider about any new symptoms or adverse effects.
• Warn patient to keep all herbal products away from children and pets.

*Liquid may contain alcohol.

## skunk cabbage

*Symplocarpus foetidus,*
dracontium, meadow cabbage,
pole-cat cabbage,
polecatweed, skunkweed

**Common trade names**
*None known*

### HOW SUPPLIED
Available as powdered root, extract*, and tincture.

### ACTIONS & COMPONENTS
Obtained from seeds, rhizomes, and roots of *Symplocarpus foetidus.* Contains starch, gum sugar, fixed and volatile oils, iron, various alkaloids, phenolic compounds, glycosides, and tannins. The leaves are also said to contain *n*-hydroxytryptamine. The root contains calcium oxalate.

### USES
Used for treating chest tightness, as in asthma and bronchitis, and as an antispasmodic, diaphoretic, emetic, expectorant, and sedative.

### DOSAGE & ADMINISTRATION
*Liquid extract (1:1 in 25% alcohol):* 0.5 to 1 ml P.O. t.i.d.

### ADVERSE REACTIONS
**CNS:** headache, vertigo.
**EENT:** burning of mucous membranes or a hot sensation when taken orally; vision impairment.
**GI:** nausea, vomiting.
**GU:** renal damage.
**Skin:** irritation.

### INTERACTIONS
**Herb-drug.** *Disulfiram:* Herbal products that contain alcohol may cause a disulfiram-like reaction. Advise patient to avoid using together.

### CAUTIONS
Pregnant or breast-feeding women shouldn't use this herb.

### NURSING CONSIDERATIONS
• Find out why patient is using the herb.
• Monitor patient's response to herbal therapy.

**Patient teaching**
• Advise patient to consult with his health care provider before using an herbal preparation because a treatment with proven efficacy may be available.
• Tell patient to remind pharmacist of any herbal and dietary supplements that he's taking, when filling a new prescription.
• Warn patient not to take herb for asthma or bronchitis before seeking medical attention because doing so may delay diagnosis of a potentially serious medical condition.
• Instruct patient to seek appropriate medical attention if he's short of breath or has a persistent cough.
• Warn patient to keep all herbal products away from children and pets.

---

*Bold italic type* indicates that reaction may be life-threatening.

## slippery elm

*Ulmus rubra,* American elm, Indian elm, moose elm, red elm, sweet elm

**Common trade names**
*None known*

### HOW SUPPLIED
Available as powdered bark, liquid extract*, lozenges, and capsules.
*Capsules:* 370 mg
*Liquid extract:* 1:1 in 60% alcohol

### ACTIONS & COMPONENTS
Obtained from inner bark of *Ulmus rubra.* Contains mucilage composed of hexoses, methylpentoses, pentoses, and polyuronides. Other constituents include phytosterols, sesquiterpenes, calcium oxalate, cholesterol, and tannins that may have astringent activity.

### USES
Used externally as a demulcent to soothe and soften skin and as an emollient that coats and protects irritated tissues. Also used to treat wounds, burns, and various skin conditions. Used internally to treat diverticulitis, gastritis, gastric and duodenal ulcers, herpes, and syphilis. Also used as an abortifacient, a lubricant to ease labor, and a nutritional source in baby food.

### DOSAGE & ADMINISTRATION
*Decoction (1:8 with alcohol):* 4 to 16 ml P.O. q.d.
*For GI discomfort:* 5 ml liquid extract P.O. t.i.d.

*Topical use:* Poultice is prepared from powdered bark in boiling water. Applied to affected area.

### ADVERSE REACTIONS
**Skin:** contact dermatitis.
**Other:** allergic reaction.

### INTERACTIONS
**Herb-drug.** *Disulfiram:* Herbal products that contain alcohol may cause a disulfiram-like reaction. Advise patient to avoid using together.

### CAUTIONS
Pregnant or breast-feeding women shouldn't use this herb.

### NURSING CONSIDERATIONS
● Find out why patient is using the herb.
● Although no chemical interactions have been reported in clinical studies, consider the pharmacologic properties of the herb and its potential to interfere with therapeutic effects of conventional drugs.
● Monitor patient's response to herbal therapy.

**Patient teaching**
● Advise patient to consult with his health care provider before using an herbal preparation because a treatment with proven efficacy may be available.
● Tell patient to remind pharmacist of any herbal and dietary supplements that he's taking, when filling a new prescription.
● Warn patient not to use herb for burns or wounds before seeking medical attention because doing so

*Liquid may contain alcohol.

may delay diagnosis of a potentially serious medical condition.
- Instruct patient to promptly notify health care provider about new symptoms and adverse effects.
- Warn patient to keep all herbal products away from children and pets.

## soapwort

*Saponaria officinalis,* bouncing bet, bruisewort, crow soap, dog cloves, Fuller's herb, latherwort, old maid's pink, soap root, soapwood, sweet Betty, wild sweet William

**Common trade names**
*None known*

### HOW SUPPLIED
Available as dried leaves, root, fluidextract.

### ACTIONS & COMPONENTS
Obtained from leaves, roots, and rhizomes of *Saponaria officinalis.* Contains saponin, sapotoxin, saponarine, and other saporins. Other components include flavonoids, resin, and gum. Saponins are cytotoxic compounds that may be active against various cancers, including lymphoma, leukemia, melanoma, and breast cancer. The seeds of *S. officinalis* have ribosome inactivating activity.

### USES
Used as an expectorant for cough and other respiratory tract disorders, a gargle for tonsillitis, a diaphoretic, and a diuretic. Also used for GI complaints, liver and kidney disorders, rheumatic gout, and such skin conditions as acne, eczema, psoriasis, and poison ivy. Also used to alter metabolism. Externally, its lathering action has led to use in shampoo and bath preparations.

### DOSAGE & ADMINISTRATION
**Soapwort herb.** *Constipation:* Decoction of leaves, 2 glasses P.O. q.d.
*Daily dose:* Aqueous extract, 1 to 2 g q.d.
**Soapwort root.** *Decoction:* 10 to 180 g root added to 1 g sodium carbonate and simple syrup to make 200 g.
*Expectorant:* 9 ml (about 2 tsp) of the decoction P.O. q 2 hours.
*Tea:* 0.4 g of medium fine cut root; 1 tsp contains about 2.6 g of herb.

### ADVERSE REACTIONS
**CNS:** neurotoxicity.
**GI:** GI irritation, nausea, vomiting, diarrhea.
**GU:** *nephrotoxicity.*
**Hepatic:** *hepatotoxicity.*
**Skin:** localized irritation, mucous membrane irritations.

### INTERACTIONS
None reported.

### CAUTIONS
Internal use isn't recommended. Women who are pregnant or breastfeeding shouldn't use this herb. Patients with GI disorders should avoid using this herb because it irritates the gastric mucosa.

### NURSING CONSIDERATIONS
- Find out why patient is using the herb.

---

*Bold italic type* indicates that reaction may be life-threatening.

- Although no chemical interactions have been reported in clinical studies, consider the pharmacologic properties of the herb and its potential to interfere with therapeutic effects of conventional drugs.
- Patients who take soapwort should have liver and renal function monitored periodically.
- If patient takes herb internally, watch for adverse effects, such as vomiting and diarrhea.
- Observe patient for localized skin reactions.

**Patient teaching**
- Advise patient to consult with his health care provider before using an herbal preparation because a treatment with proven efficacy may be available.
- Tell patient to remind pharmacist of any herbal and dietary supplements that he's taking, when filling a new prescription.
- Warn patient not to take herb for extended periods before seeking medical attention because a persistent cough may indicate a potentially serious medical condition.
- Instruct patient to notify a health care provider about adverse effects, such as localized skin reactions or nausea.
- Tell patient to store herb in a tightly sealed container that protects it from light and moisture.
- Warn patient to keep all herbal products away from children and pets.

## sorrel

*Rumex acetosa,* cuckoo's meate, cuckoo sorrow, dock, garden sorrel, green sauce, green sorrel, sour dock, sourgrass, sour sauce, soursuds

**Common trade names**
*None known*

### HOW SUPPLIED
Available as a tea, liquid extract*, and coated tablets.

### ACTIONS & COMPONENTS
Obtained from leaves, berries, and roots of *Rumex acetosa*. Contains oxalates (such as oxalic acid and calcium oxalate) and anthracene derivatives, such as physcion, chryosphanol, emodin, and rhein. Other components include ascorbic acid, tartaric acid, and tannins.

### USES
Used for acute and chronic inflammation of nasal passages and respiratory tract. Also used as an adjunct to antibacterial therapy and as an antiseptic, an astringent, and a diuretic.

### DOSAGE & ADMINISTRATION
*Liquid extract (19% alcohol):* 50 gtt P.O. t.i.d.
*Tablets:* For adults, 2 coated tablets t.i.d.

### ADVERSE REACTIONS
**CNS:** headache.
**GI:** nausea, flatulence.
**GU:** renal damage.
**Hepatic:** liver damage.

*Liquid may contain alcohol.

## INTERACTIONS

**Herb-drug.** *Disulfiram:* Herbal products that contain alcohol may cause a disulfiram-like reaction. Advise patient to avoid using together.

## CAUTIONS

Pregnant or breast-feeding women shouldn't use this herb.

## NURSING CONSIDERATIONS

• Find out why patient is using the herb.

⚡**ALERT:** High oxalate salt content may lead to significant toxicity and even death if enough herb is ingested. Such oxalate poisoning can occur with consumption of large quantities of leaves as a salad.

• Closely monitor patient's response to herbal therapy.

## Patient teaching

• Advise patient to consult with his health care provider before using an herbal preparation because a treatment with proven efficacy may be available.

• Tell patient to remind pharmacist of any herbal and dietary supplements that he's taking, when filling a new prescription.

• Warn patient not to take herb for inflammatory or respiratory symptoms before seeking medical attention because doing so may delay diagnosis of a potentially serious medical condition.

• Instruct patient to promptly notify his health care provider about adverse effects or a change in symptoms.

• Warn patient to keep all herbal products away from children and pets.

## southernwood

*Artemisia abrotanum,* appleringie, boy's love, garde robe, lad's love, old man, southern wormwood

**Common trade names**
*None known*

## HOW SUPPLIED

Available as dried herb and fluid-extract.

## ACTIONS & COMPONENTS

Obtained from *Artemisia abrotanum.* Contains a volatile essential oil, mostly absinthol, as well as artemisitin, hydroxycoumarins such as umbelliferone and isofraxidin, and tannins. Recently, four flavonols possessing spasmolytic activity have been isolated. Herb has tonic, antiseptic, antimicrobial, anthelmintic, and stimulant effects.

## USES

Used internally to treat fever, infections, irregular menstruation, and worm infestations, especially roundworm and pinworm in children, and as a bitter to improve digestion. Applied externally to treat baldness and dandruff, poorly healing or gangrenous wounds, ulcers, and insect bites. Also used to repel moths, fleas, flies, and mosquitoes.

## DOSAGE & ADMINISTRATION

*Fluidextract:* ½ to 1 dram.

---

*Bold italic type* indicates that reaction may be life-threatening.

*To stimulate menstruation:* 1 oz of herb added to 1 pint boiling water, P.O. t.i.d.

*To treat worm infestations:* 1 tsp powdered herb P.O. morning and h.s.

## ADVERSE REACTIONS
**Hepatic:** liver damage.

## INTERACTIONS
**Herb-drug.** *Alkaloids, glycosides, heavy metal ions such as aluminum and zinc:* Tannic acid may form insoluble complexes. Advise patient to avoid using together.

*Antiplatelet drugs such as aspirin, heparin, low-molecular-weight heparin, warfarin:* Altered coagulation. Monitor PT and INR closely.

## CAUTIONS
Pregnant or breast-feeding women should avoid this herb, as should patients with a history of liver disease. Using herb to treat burns has caused toxicity.

## NURSING CONSIDERATIONS
• Find out why patient is using the herb.
• Southernwood shouldn't be consumed in large amounts.
• Significant amounts of tannic acid present in the plant may lead to liver damage.
• Monitor patient for signs of bleeding, especially if he takes an anticoagulant.
• Monitor patient's response to herbal therapy.
• Don't confuse southernwood with a related species, field southernwood *(Artemisia campestris)*.

## Patient teaching
• Advise patient to consult with his health care provider before using an herbal preparation because a treatment with proven efficacy may be available.
• Tell patient to remind pharmacist of any herbal and dietary supplements that he's taking, when filling a new prescription.
• Instruct patient to have a medical evaluation before taking this herb and not to consume large quantities of it.
• Tell patient to consult with his health care provider if he takes the herb for any medical condition that doesn't improve in 2 weeks.
• Tell patient to store herb in a sealed container protected from light.
• Warn patient to keep all herbal products away from children and pets.

## soy

*Glycine max, Glycine soja,* soya, soyabean, soybean

**Common trade names**
*None known*

## HOW SUPPLIED
Available as soy protein or isoflavone supplements in powder, capsules, or tablets. Also available as beans, flour, and many food items such as sprouts, tofu, tempeh, soy milk, textured and hydrolyzed vegetable protein, meat substitutes, miso, and soy sauce.

## ACTIONS & COMPONENTS

Obtained from beans (seeds) of *Glycine max.* Contains soy protein; isoflavones; saponins; phenolic acids; lecithin; phytoestrols; vitamins A, E, K, and some B; minerals such as calcium, potassium, iron, and phosphorus; and amino acids.

Isoflavones are molecularly similar to natural body estrogens (phytoestrogens). The isoflavones in soy, particularly genistein and daidzen, have antioxidant and phytoestrogenic properties. Saponins enhance immune function and bind to cholesterol to limit its absorption in the intestines. Phenolic acids have antioxidant properties. Phytoestrols and other components, including lecithin, may lower cholesterol levels.

Isoflavones may reduce the risk of hormone-dependent cancers, such as breast and prostate cancer, as well as other forms of cancer. Increased consumption of soy in Asian populations helps account for decreased rates of CV disease. Soy-based diets lead to significant decreases in total cholesterol, HDL levels, and LDL levels. The FDA officially supports the claim that soy protein may decrease blood cholesterol levels.

The mild estrogenic activity of soy isoflavones may help to alleviate menopausal symptoms in some women. However, no clinical data exist concerning the effect of soy on other symptoms of menopause, such as night sweats, insomnia, vaginal dryness, or changes in sexual desire. Soy consumption may also help regulate hormone levels in premenopausal women. Soy may also have a beneficial effect on GI function.

## USES

Used to treat cancers, CV disease, menopausal symptoms, and osteoporosis. Also used as a detoxicant, a circulatory stimulant, and a popular dietary protein supplement.

## DOSAGE & ADMINISTRATION

No consensus exists. The FDA currently recommends 25 g soy protein P.O. daily. Other sources suggest beneficial CV effects with doses of 30 to 50 g P.O. daily.

## ADVERSE REACTIONS

**Respiratory:** asthma.
**Other:** allergic reaction.

## INTERACTIONS

**Herb-drug.** *Calcium, iron, zinc:* Decreased absorption. Advise patient to avoid using together. *Estrogen, raloxifene, tamoxifen:* Possible reduced effects. Advise patient to avoid using together.

## CAUTIONS

Patients hypersensitive to soy or soy-containing products shouldn't use this product. High doses of soy protein may have harmful effects in women with breast cancer. Infants shouldn't be fed soy-based formulas because of high isoflavone content. Inhalation of soy dust led to an asthma outbreak in 26 workers exposed to soy powder when unloading the product.

---

*Bold italic type* indicates that reaction may be life-threatening.

## NURSING CONSIDERATIONS

- Find out why patient is using the herb.
- Certain constituents of soy may interfere with thyroid function, but the clinical importance of this problem is unclear.
- Soybeans and soybean products are an excellent source of protein, vitamins, and minerals.
- Monitor patient's response to herbal therapy.

### Patient teaching

- Advise patient to consult with his health care provider before using an herbal preparation because a treatment with proven efficacy may be available.
- Tell patient to remind pharmacist of any herbal and dietary supplements that he's taking, when filling a new prescription.
- If patient takes estrogen, tamoxifen, or raloxifene, tell her to inform a health care provider if she also takes soy. Soy may interfere with therapeutic effects of these drugs.
- To avoid disturbed absorption, instruct patient to separate consumption of zinc, iron, or calcium supplements by several hours from any soy products.
- Warn patient to keep all herbal products away from children and pets.

## spirulina

*Spirulina maxima, Spirulina platensis,* blue green algae, blue-green micro-algae, dihe, tecuitlatl

**Common trade names**
*Chinese Spirulina, Green Earth Food, Spirulina*

### HOW SUPPLIED

Available as a powder, flakes, capsules, and tablets.
*Capsules:* 380 mg
*Tablets:* 500 mg

### ACTIONS & COMPONENTS

Obtained from the blue-green algae *Spirulina maxima* and *S. platensis.* Contains about 65% protein and all essential amino acids. Spirulina is a concentrated source of other nutrients, including chlorophyll, beta-carotene, other carotenoids, high levels of B-complex vitamins, minerals, and essential fatty acids, including gamma linolenic acid and omega-3 fatty acid. Spirulina may enhance disease resistance, inhibit allergic reactions, and exert hepatoprotective and hypocholesteremic effects.

The protein content of spirulina is comparable to other sources, such as meat and milk. The vitamin $B_{12}$ in spirulina has no activity in humans and may even block assimilation of regular vitamin $B_{12}$.

### USES

Used as a nutritional supplement and energy booster and to treat obesity, diabetes mellitus, and oral cancers.

*Liquid may contain alcohol.

## DOSAGE & ADMINISTRATION
*Average daily dose:* 2,000 to 3,000 mg P.O. q.d. in divided doses.

## ADVERSE REACTIONS
**Metabolic:** inhibited vitamin $B_{12}$ absorption.
**Other:** allergic reaction.

## INTERACTIONS
None reported.

## CAUTIONS
Spirulina grown in contaminated water may concentrate such toxic metals as lead, mercury, and cadmium.

## NURSING CONSIDERATIONS
• Find out why patient is using the herb.
• Assess patient's knowledge of herb use.
• Monitor patient's response to herbal therapy.

## Patient teaching
• Advise patient to consult with a health care provider before using an herbal preparation because a treatment with proven efficacy may be available.
• Tell patient to remind pharmacist of any herbal and dietary supplements that he's taking, when filling a new prescription.
• Advise patient to store product in a cool, dry place, not to freeze it, and to keep it away from children and pets.

## squaw vine

*Mitchella repens,* checkerberry, deerberry, deer berry, one berry, partridgeberry, partridge berry, squawberry, squawvine, winter clover

**Common trade names**
*None known*

## HOW SUPPLIED
Available as dried herb, extract, and tincture.

## ACTIONS & COMPONENTS
Obtained from above-ground parts of *Mitchella repens.* Contains resin, dextrin, mucilage, saponin, wax, alkaloids, glycosides, and tannins. Herb has tonic, antispasmodic, diuretic, and astringent effects.

## USES
Used to treat dysmenorrhea or amenorrhea and to aid labor and childbirth. After delivery, herb is used to treat sore nipples. Also used to stimulate lactation and to treat insomnia, colitis, dysuria, diarrhea, heart failure, liver failure, and seizures.

## DOSAGE & ADMINISTRATION
*For sore nipples:* 2 oz fresh herb added to 1 pint boiling water, strained, and added to an equal amount of cream. Mixture is boiled to a soft consistency, allowed to cool, then applied to nipples after each breast-feeding session.
*Infusion:* 1 tsp of herb added to 1 cup boiling water, steeped for 10 to 15 minutes and taken t.i.d.

---

***Bold italic type*** indicates that reaction may be life-threatening.

*Strong decoction:* 2 to 4 oz fresh herb added to 1 pint boiling water, strained, cooled; then 2 to 4 oz taken P.O. b.i.d. or t.i.d.
*Tincture:* 1 to 2 ml P.O. t.i.d.

## ADVERSE REACTIONS
**Hepatic:** liver damage.

## INTERACTIONS
**Herb-drug.** *Cardiac glycosides:* May have increased effects. Advise patient to avoid using together.

## CAUTIONS
Pregnant or breast-feeding women should use herb cautiously.

## NURSING CONSIDERATIONS
● Find out why patient is using the herb.
● Human toxicity is rare and is only likely to occur after ingestion of large amounts of tannic acid.
● Monitor patient's response to herbal therapy.

**Patient teaching**
● Advise patient to consult with his health care provider before using an herbal preparation because a treatment with proven efficacy may be available.
● Tell patient to remind pharmacist of any herbal and dietary supplements that he's taking, when filling a new prescription.
● Advise patient to consult with his health care provider if taking the herb for any condition that doesn't improve within 2 weeks. Chronic symptoms may indicate a more serious problem.

● Instruct patient to promptly notify a health care provider about new symptoms or adverse effects.
● Tell patient not to exceed recommended dosage.
● Advise patient to store herb in a cool, dry place, not to freeze it, and to keep it away from children and pets.

## squill

*Urginea indica, U. maritima,* European squill, Indian squill, Mediterranean squill, red squill, sea onion, sea squill, white squill

**Common trade names**
*None known*

## HOW SUPPLIED
Available as powder or syrup.
*Syrup of squill, USP*

## ACTIONS & COMPONENTS
Obtained from bulbs of *Urginea maritima* and *U. indica.* Contains several cardioactive steroid glycosides, including scillaren A, glucoscillaren A, scillaridin A, and scilliroside and proscillaridin A that exert digitalis-like activity. Squill components also have diuretic, natriuretic (increases urinary sodium excretion), stimulant, expectorant, and emetic action. One component, silliglaucosidin, has shown anticancer activity.

## USES
Used to treat cancer, arthritis, gout, dysmenorrhea, and warts. Also used to treat mild (New York Heart Association I and II) cardiac insuf-

---

*Liquid may contain alcohol.

ficiency, arrhythmias, and reduced kidney capacity. However, squill extracts have been superseded by widespread use of digitalis glycosides. Squill is a component of some cough preparations because of its weak expectorant effect.

Red squill has been used externally in hair tonics for dandruff and seborrhea; however, it's mainly used as a rodenticide.

## DOSAGE & ADMINISTRATION
*Cardiotonic:* 0.1 to 0.5 g standardized squill powder P.O.
*Expectorant (Syrup of squill, USP):* 30 minims P.O.

## ADVERSE REACTIONS
**CNS:** fatigue, dizziness, *seizures, coma,* headache.
**CV:** *life-threatening cardiac effects, arrhythmias, bradycardia,* hypotension.
**GI:** vomiting, nausea, diarrhea, loss of appetite.

## INTERACTIONS
**Herb-drug.** *Calcium, digoxin, diuretics, extended glucocorticoid therapy, laxatives, quinidine:* Increased risk of digitalis-like toxicity. Advise patient to avoid using together.
*Methylxanthines, such as theophylline; phosphodiesterase inhibitors, including inamrinone, cilostazol, and milrinone; quinidine; sympathomimetics, including epinephrine and phenylephrine:* Increased risk of cardiac arrhythmias. Advise patient to avoid using together. Monitor ECG closely if these drugs are taken together.

## CAUTIONS
Squill should be avoided by patients with second- or third-degree AV block, hypercalcemia, hypokalemia, hypertrophic cardiomyopathy, carotid sinus syndrome, ventricular tachycardia, thoracic aortic aneurysm, or Wolff-Parkinson-White syndrome.

## NURSING CONSIDERATIONS
• Find out why patient is using the herb.
🗲 **ALERT:** All squill species can cause digitalis-like toxicity, which may cause nausea, vomiting, diarrhea, fatigue, dizziness, arrhythmias, bradycardia, hypotension, seizures, and coma.
• In patients with GI symptoms and bradyarrhythmias from presumed herbal poisoning, suspect cardiac glycoside poisoning as the cause.
• Because of the narrow therapeutic index of squill glycosides, adverse effects could occur rapidly in some patients even at therapeutic doses.
• Monitor vital signs and ECG, as indicated.
• Monitor patient's response to herbal therapy.

### Patient teaching
• Advise patient to consult with his health care provider before using an herbal preparation because a treatment with proven efficacy may be available.
• Tell patient to remind pharmacist of any herbal and dietary supplements that he's taking, when filling a new prescription.

---

*Bold italic type* indicates that reaction may be life-threatening.

• Instruct patient to consult a health care provider if taking the herb for any condition that doesn't improve within 2 weeks. Chronic symptoms may indicate a more serious medical condition.

• Warn patient to contact a health care provider if he has an irregular heartbeat, fainting, difficulty breathing, nausea, appetite loss, vomiting, diarrhea, or unusual weakness, tiredness, or drowsiness.

• Instruct patient to store herb in a cool, dry place, not to freeze it, and to keep it away from children and pets.

## stone root

*Collinsonia canadensis,* citronella, hardback, hardhack, heal-all, horseweed, knob grass, knob root, knobweed, richleaf, richweed

**Common trade names**
*Stoneroot Extract*

### HOW SUPPLIED
Available as dried root or rhizome, tea, liquid extract\*, and tincture\*.

### ACTIONS & COMPONENTS
Obtained from *Collinsonia canadensis.* Contains volatile oils, tannins, saponins, resin, mucilage, and caffeic acid derivatives.

### USES
Used for bladder inflammation, kidney stones, water retention, hyperuricuria, edema, GI disorders, headaches, and indigestion. In homeopathic medicine, stone root is used for hemorrhoids and constipation.

### DOSAGE & ADMINISTRATION
*Dried root:* 1 to 4 g in 150 ml boiling water, steeped 5 to 10 minutes, and then strained. Consumed t.i.d.
*Liquid extract (1:1 in 25% alcohol):* 1 to 4 ml P.O. t.i.d.
*Tincture (1:5 in 40% alcohol):* 2 to 8 ml P.O. t.i.d.

### ADVERSE REACTIONS
**CNS:** dizziness, numbness with ingestion of large quantities.
**GI:** irritation, abdominal pain, nausea.
**GU:** painful urination.

### INTERACTIONS
**Herb-drug.** *Diuretics, including acetazolamide, furosemide, hydrochlorothiazide:* Possible additive effects. Advise patient to use cautiously with other diuretics.
**Herb-herb.** *Other herbs with diuretic action, such as gum acacia, Chinese cucumber, ginkgo, sassafras:* Possible additive effects. Advise patient to use cautiously with other diuretics.

### CAUTIONS
Pregnant or breast-feeding women should avoid this herb.

### NURSING CONSIDERATIONS
• Find out why patient is using the herb.

• Stone root "citronella" is not the same as true citronella oil *(Cymbopogon),* which is used as an insect repellent.

• Because stone root may have diuretic effects, caution should be used when patient takes it with other herbs or drugs that have diuretic effects.

---

\*Liquid may contain alcohol.

- Although no chemical interactions have been reported in clinical studies, consider the pharmacologic properties of the herb and their potential to interfere with therapeutic effects of conventional drugs.
- Monitor intake and output, as indicated.
- Monitor patient's response to herbal therapy.

**Patient teaching**
- Advise patient to consult with his health care provider before using an herbal preparation because a treatment with proven efficacy may be available.
- Tell patient to remind pharmacist of any herbal and dietary supplements that he's taking, when filling a new prescription.
- Inform patient that stone root normally has a strong, unpleasant odor.
- Advise pregnant and breast-feeding patients not to take stone root.
- If patient takes a diuretic herb or drug, tell him to consult a health care provider before using stone root.
- Warn patient not to take herb for urinary or abdominal complaints before seeking medical attention because doing so may delay diagnosis of a potentially serious medical condition.
- Instruct patient to promptly notify health care provider about adverse effects or new symptoms.
- Warn patient to keep all herbal products away from children and pets.

## sundew

*Drosera ramentacea, D. rotundifolia,* dew plant, drosera, lustwort, red rot, ros solis, round-leafed sundew, sonnenthau, youthwort

**Common trade names**
*B&T Natural Relief - Cough*

**HOW SUPPLIED**
Available as dried herb, tea, liquid extract*, and tincture*.

**ACTIONS & COMPONENTS**
Obtained from *Drosera ramentacea, D. rotundifolia, D. intermedia, D. anglica,* and others. Contains naphthoquinone, thought to have antitussive, antimicrobial, secretolytic, and bronchospasmolytic effects. May also have immunostimulant effects.

**USES**
Used orally for bronchitis, asthma, pertussis, coughing fits, and dry cough. May be used topically for warts.

**DOSAGE & ADMINISTRATION**
*Average daily dose:* 3 g dried plant P.O.
*Liquid extract (1:1 in 25% alcohol):* 0.5 to 2 ml P.O. t.i.d.
*Tea:* 1 to 2 g in 150 ml boiling water, steeped for 5 to 10 minutes, strained, and taken t.i.d.
*Tincture (1:5 in 60% alcohol):* 0.5 to 1 ml P.O. t.i.d.

**ADVERSE REACTIONS**
None known.

---

*Bold italic type* indicates that reaction may be life-threatening.

## INTERACTIONS
**Herb-drug.** *Disulfiram:* Herbal products that contain alcohol may cause a disulfiram-like reaction. Advise patient to avoid using together.

## CAUTIONS
Pregnant or breast-feeding women shouldn't use this herb.

## NURSING CONSIDERATIONS
• Find out why patient is using the herb.
• Although few chemical interactions have been reported in clinical studies, consider the pharmacologic properties of the herb and its potential to interfere with therapeutic effects of conventional drugs.
• Monitor patient's response to herbal therapy.

**Patient teaching**
• Advise patient to consult with his health care provider before using an herbal preparation because a treatment with proven efficacy may be available.
• Warn patient not to take herb before seeking medical attention because doing so may delay diagnosis of a potentially serious medical condition.
• Advise women not to use this herb while pregnant or breast-feeding.
• Warn patient that herb has a bitter, sour, hot taste.
• Warn patient not to take herb for persistent cough or difficulty breathing before seeking medical attention because doing so may delay diagnosis of a potentially serious medical condition.

• Instruct patient to promptly notify a health care provider about adverse effects or changes in symptoms.
• Warn patient to keep all herbal products away from children and pets.

## sweet cicely

*Myrrhis odorata,* British myrrh, cow chervil, shepherd's needle, smooth cicely, sweet bracken, sweet chervil, sweet-cus, sweet-fern, sweet-humlock, sweets, the Roman plant

**Common trade names**
*None known*

## HOW SUPPLIED
Available as ground root, a tonic, or infusion. Also available as a salve.

## ACTIONS & COMPONENTS
Obtained from *Myrrhis odorata.* Volatile oils and flavonoids may act as a digestive aid, an expectorant, and a carminative.

## USES
Used orally for asthma, breathing difficulties, intestinal gas and colic, and for urinary tract, chest, and throat complaints. Also used as an expectorant, a blood purifier, and a digestive aid. Used topically to treat gout pain and acute wounds and sores.

## DOSAGE & ADMINISTRATION
*For wounds, sores, pain of gout:* Fresh herb salve applied topically, p.r.n.

## ADVERSE REACTIONS
None known.

## INTERACTIONS
None reported.

## CAUTIONS
Pregnant or breast-feeding women shouldn't use this herb.

## NURSING CONSIDERATIONS
• Find out why patient is using the herb.
• Herb is generally thought to be harmless in typical quantities.
• Although no chemical interactions have been reported in clinical studies, consider the pharmacologic properties of the herb and its potential to interfere with therapeutic effects of conventional drugs.
• Monitor patient's response to herbal therapy.

## Patient teaching
• Advise patient to consult with his health care provider before using an herbal preparation because a treatment with proven efficacy may be available.
• Tell patient to remind pharmacist of any herbal and dietary supplements that he's taking, when filling a new prescription.
• Warn patient not to take herb for breathing problems before seeking medical attention because doing so may delay diagnosis of a potentially serious medical condition.
• Discuss alternative, proven therapies with patient.
• Tell patient to promptly notify his health care provider about adverse effects or changes in symptoms.

• Warn patient to keep all herbal products away from children and pets.

## sweet flag

*Acorus calamus,* bacc, beewort, calamus, cinnamon sedge, gladdon, myrtle-flag, myrtle-grass, myrtle sedge, rat root, sweet cane, sweet grass, sweet myrtle, sweet root, sweet rush, sweet sedge, vakhand

**Common trade names**
*None known*

## HOW SUPPLIED
Available as oil, extract*, tincture*, and dried and powdered rhizome.

## ACTIONS & COMPONENTS
Obtained from *Acorus calamus* or *A. gramineus.* There are four types of sweet flag, based on their content of asarone, a carcinogen. The North American type (*A. calamus* var. *americanus*) contains none of this component, but varieties from India do. Sweet flag also contains acorin, choline, resin, starch, calcium oxalate, tannins, mucilage, and asarone. Asarone is chemically related to reserpine.

## USES
Used orally for childhood colic, digestive complaints, fever, sore throat. Also used as a sweat inducer. Used topically to treat rheumatism, angina, and gingivitis. Use of sweet flag as a flavoring agent in dental products, drinks, and medi-

---

*Bold italic type* indicates that reaction may be life-threatening.

cines has been banned in the United States.

## DOSAGE & ADMINISTRATION
*Average daily dose:* 1 to 3 g P.O. t.i.d.
*Liquid extract (1:1 in 60% alcohol):* 1 to 3 ml P.O. t.i.d.
*Tea:* One cup of tea P.O. t.i.d. Made from 1 to 3 g rhizome in 150 ml boiling water, steeped for 5 to 10 minutes, and strained.
*Tincture (1:5 in 60% alcohol):* 2 to 4 ml P.O. t.i.d.
*Wash:* 250 to 500 g added to bath water.

## ADVERSE REACTIONS
**CNS:** sedation, tremors, *seizures.*
**GU:** kidney damage.

## INTERACTIONS
**Herb-drug.** *CNS depressants, MAO inhibitors:* Possible additive adverse reactions. Monitor patient closely, if used together.
*H₂-receptor antagonists, proton pump inhibitors:* Decreased effect caused by acidifying effect of herb. Monitor patient closely, if used together.
**Herb-herb.** *Other herbs that cause sedation, including calendula, California poppy, capsicum, catnip, celery, couch grass, elecampane, German chamomile, goldenseal, gotu kola, hops, Jamaican dogwood, kava, lemon balm, sage, sassafras, shepherd's purse, Siberian ginseng, skullcap, stinging nettle, St. John's wort, valerian, wild carrot, wild lettuce, withania root, and yerba maté:* Additive effects. Advise patient to use together cautiously.

**Herb-lifestyle.** *Alcohol use:* Possible additive sedative effects. Advise patient to avoid using together.

## CAUTIONS
Pregnant or breast-feeding women shouldn't use this herb.

## NURSING CONSIDERATIONS
• Find out why patient is using the herb.
**ALERT:** Because of its potential cancer-causing properties, sweet flag is banned by the FDA for use in foods, medicine, and beverages in the United States. The cancer-causing component of sweet flag, asarone, usually isn't found in North American variety; however, sweet flag from India contains large amounts of this chemical.
• Chemical content of the supplement—and its safety—can't be assured.
• If a patient is taking sweet flag, other sedative herbs or drugs should be avoided because of possible additive effects.

### Patient teaching
• Advise patient to consult with his health care provider before using an herbal preparation because a treatment with proven efficacy may be available.
• Tell patient to remind pharmacist of any herbal and dietary supplements that he's taking, when filling a new prescription.
• Advise patient to avoid this herb in any form because of its cancer-causing potential.
• Inform patient taking sweet flag that other herbs or drugs that cause

drowsiness should be avoided because of possible additive effects.

● Caution patient to avoid hazardous tasks until full sedative effects of herb are known.

● Tell patient to avoid alcohol while taking sweet flag because of possible additive sedative effects.

● Instruct patient to promptly notify his health care provider about adverse effects or change in symptoms.

● Warn patient to keep all herbal products away from children and pets.

## sweet violet

*Viola odorata,* garden violet, sweet violet herb, violet

**Common trade names**
*Acnetonic, Herbal Pumpkin, Sweet Violet Lotion*

### HOW SUPPLIED
Available as dried or fresh root, dried flowers, and leaves.

### ACTIONS & COMPONENTS
Obtained from *Viola odorata.* Contains saponins that, in high doses, can irritate mucous membranes. In low doses, they act as expectorants. Also contains salicylic acid, methyl esters, and alkaloids. Herb has antimicrobial and bronchosecretolytic effects caused by saponin content.

### USES
Used as an expectorant in acute and chronic bronchitis, bronchial asthma, cough and cold symptoms, and late flu symptoms. Also used as a sedative or relaxant, for urinary incontinence, and for GI complaints, such as heartburn, flatulence, and digestion problems.

### DOSAGE & ADMINISTRATION
*Average daily dose of root:* 1 g.
*Decoction:* 1 tbs in boiling water in proportion to make a 5% water to volume preparation, steeped for 10 to 15 minutes, and then strained. 1 tbs taken P.O. 5 to 6 times q.d.
*Tea:* 2 tsp herb in 250 ml boiling water, steeped for 10 to 15 minutes, then strained. Taken P.O. b.i.d. to t.i.d.

### ADVERSE REACTIONS
None known.

### INTERACTIONS
None reported.

### CAUTIONS
Caution pregnant or breast-feeding women that full effects of sweet violet haven't been studied.

### NURSING CONSIDERATIONS
● Find out why patient is using the herb.

● Sweet violet is often used in combination preparations for oral and topical use.

● Although no chemical interactions have been reported in clinical studies, consider the pharmacologic properties of the herb and its potential to interfere with therapeutic effects of conventional drugs.

● Monitor patient's response to herbal therapy.

---

*Bold italic type* indicates that reaction may be life-threatening.

**Patient information**

• Advise patient to consult with his health care provider before using an herbal preparation because a treatment with proven efficacy may be available.

• Tell patient to remind pharmacist of any herbal and dietary supplements that he's taking, when filling a new prescription.

• If patient takes sweet violet for respiratory problems, tell him to seek medical attention if it fails to relieve symptoms.

• Instruct patient not to use more than recommended amounts because higher amounts can irritate the lining of the mouth, stomach, intestines, and lungs.

• Urge pregnant or breast-feeding patients to consult a health care provider before using sweet violet.

• Warn patient to keep all herbal products away from children and pets.

*Liquid may contain alcohol.

# T

## tansy

*Chrysanthemum vulgare, Tanacetum vulgare,* bitter buttons, buttons, daisy, hindheal, parsley fern, tansy flower, tansy herb

**Common trade names**
*None known*

### HOW SUPPLIED
Available as oil, extract, and combination products.

### ACTIONS & COMPONENTS
Obtained from leaves and flowers of *Tanacetum vulgare.* Contains volatile oil with thujone, a neurotoxin. Other components include sesquiterpenes and flavones. Caffeic acid may have bile-inducing effects. Thujone is probably responsible for liver toxicity. Tansy toxicity varies greatly among subtypes.

### USES
Used orally to stimulate menstrual flow, induce abortion, improve digestion, and treat migraines and GI worm infestations in children. Used topically for scabies, sunburn, toothache, sores, sprains, and insect repellent. Also used in perfumes and as a green dye source, but the toxic potential of the herb precludes its use in herbal medicine.

### DOSAGE & ADMINISTRATION
Tansy use is strongly discouraged. Deaths have been reported after ingestion of oil, powdered form, or tea. Lethal dosage is 15 to 30 g of essential oil.
*Average daily dose:* 0.1 g P.O.

### ADVERSE REACTIONS
**CNS:** *seizures*, tremors, vertigo, restlessness, loss of consciousness, tonic-clonic spasms.
**CV:** tachycardia, irregular heart rate.
**EENT:** dilated pupils.
**GI:** vomiting, gastroenteritis, abdominal pain, *liver toxicity.*
**GU:** *kidney damage,* uterine bleeding.
**Skin:** local mucous membrane irritation, contact dermatitis, severe facial flushing.
**Other:** allergic reaction.

### INTERACTIONS
**Herb-drug.** *Hypoglycemics:* Altered control of blood glucose level and increased effect of hypoglycemics. Monitor blood glucose level closely. Advise patient to avoid use.
**Herb-herb.** *Other herbs that may contain thujone, including cedar leaf oil, oak moss, oriental arborvitae, sage, tree moss, and wormwood:* Increased toxicity. Warn patient to avoid use.
**Herb-lifestyle.** *Alcohol use:* Because of the thujone component, tansy may increase and change the effects of alcohol. Advise patient to avoid use.

### CAUTIONS
Pregnant or breast-feeding women shouldn't use this herb. Tansy pro-

---

*Liquid may contain alcohol.

ducts shouldn't be used by patients allergic to ragweed, chrysanthemums, arnica, sunflowers, yarrow, marigolds, daisies, and similar plants.

**NURSING CONSIDERATIONS**
• Find out why patient is using the herb.
⚡**ALERT:** Deaths have occurred from as little as 10 gtt of oil taken orally. Take a careful history if a patient uses tansy. Be sure to note if the patient has also taken any other herbs containing thujone, a potent toxin.
• Tansy poisoning may cause a weak tachycardic pulse, severe gastritis, violent spasms, and seizures.
• Gastric lavage and emesis have been used to treat symptomatic toxicity.
• Don't confuse with tansy ragwort *(Senecio jacoboea).*

**Patient teaching**
• Advise patient to consult with his health care provider before using an herbal preparation because a treatment with proven efficacy may be available.
• Tell patient to remind pharmacist of any herbal and dietary supplements that he's taking, when filling a new prescription.
• Warn patient that tansy is toxic at very low doses and is unsafe for any medicinal use.
⚡**ALERT:** If patient takes tansy, caution him to watch for signs of toxicity, such as a rapid and weak pulse, severe abdominal pain, and seizures. Urge patient to seek emergency care immediately if adverse effects or toxic reactions develop.
• Advise patient that tansy may cause severe dermatitis.
• If patient has a history of allergy to any member of the Compositae family, such as arnica, yarrow, or sunflower, tell him not to take tansy because a cross-reaction may occur.
• Warn patient to keep all herbal products away from children and pets.

## tea tree

*Melaleuca alternifolia,*
paperbark tree

**Common trade names**
*Tea Tree Oil, Tea Tree Oil Lotion, Tea Tree Soap*

**HOW SUPPLIED**
Available as essential oil, creams, lotions, suppositories, and soaps.

**ACTIONS & COMPONENTS**
Obtained from leaves of *Melaleuca alternifolia.* Contains 2% of a pale-yellow volatile oil. Oil contains cineole and terpinen-4-ol. The latter supplies most antifungal and antibacterial activity of tea tree oil. Tea tree oils with high cineole content are lower quality and more likely to cause skin irritation. Therapeutic concentrations range from 0.25% to 0.5%, but may contain up to 10% essential oil.

**USES**
Used as a topical antiseptic that's more effective than phenol for superficial skin infections, minor

---

burns, cuts, sore throats, ingrown or infected toenails, sunburn, tinea (athlete's foot), *Candida* species (including *C. albicans*), ulcers, cold sores, pimples, and acne. Also used in aromatherapy and as a mouthwash and shampoo. In bath form, it's used to treat vaginal infections. It can also be added to vaporizers for respiratory disorders.

## DOSAGE & ADMINISTRATION
*For mouth ulcers, sore gums, or plaque:* 3 gtt oil in water P.O. b.i.d.
*For skin conditions:* Concentrated tea tree oil diluted with almond or vegetable oil and applied with a cotton ball to the affected area t.i.d.
*Respiratory vaporizer:* A few drops of oil added to water in vaporizer.
*Vaginal douche:* A few drops of oil added to water for sitz bath.

## ADVERSE REACTIONS
**CNS:** ataxia, drowsiness, weakness, confusion.
**EENT:** itching, burning.
**Hematologic:** neutrophil leukocytosis.
**Skin:** contact dermatitis, rash.

## INTERACTIONS
**Herb-drug.** *Drugs that affect histamine release:* Possible altered effects. Advise patient to avoid using together.

## CAUTIONS
Patients shouldn't apply tea tree products to dry skin, cracked or broken skin, open wounds, or areas affected by rash that's not fungal.

## NURSING CONSIDERATIONS
• Find out why patient is using the herb.
• Because of systemic toxicity, tea tree oil shouldn't be used internally.
• Essential oil should be used externally only after being diluted, especially by people with sensitive skin.
• Tea tree oil may cause burns or itching in tender areas and shouldn't be used around nose, eyes, and mouth.
• Diluted essential oil, even as low as 0.25% or 0.5%, is active against microbes.
• Vaginal douches using concentrations as strong as 40% require extreme caution and supervision by a health care provider.
• Pure (100%) essential tea tree oil is rarely used and only with close supervision by a health care provider.
• Other related *Melaleuca* species are also known as tea trees, such as *M. cajeputi, M. dissitiflora,* and *M. linariiflora,* but tea tree oil can be obtained only from *M. alternifolia.*

### Patient teaching
• Advise patient to consult with his health care provider before using an herbal preparation because a treatment with proven efficacy may be available.
• Tell patient to remind pharmacist of any herbal and dietary supplements that he's taking, when filling a new prescription.
• Tell patient to use very dilute tea tree oil (0.25% to 0.5%) as a topical anti-infective.

- Explain that a few drops are sufficient in mouthwash, shampoo, or sitz bath.
- Caution patient not to apply oil to wounds or to skin that's dry or cracked.
- If patient will be using the douche form of this product, stress the need for medical supervision.
- Warn patient to keep all herbal products away from children and pets.

## thuja

*Thuja occidentalis,* American arborvitae, arborvitae, hackmatack, northern white cedar, swamp cedar, thuja oil, tree of life, white cedar

**Common trade names**
*Fresh Thuja Leaf Oil*

**HOW SUPPLIED**
Available as oil, extract*, ointment, and homeopathic products.

**ACTIONS & COMPONENTS**
Obtained by steam distillation of leaves and twigs of *Thuja occidentalis.* Contains thujone, a neurotoxin. Also contains glycoproteins and polysaccharides, which have antiviral and immunostimulating properties. Thuja also has uterine-stimulant activity. Some thuja preparations are certified thujone-free.

**USES**
Used orally as an immune stimulant, expectorant, and diuretic. Misused as an abortifacient. Used topically as an insect repellent and a treatment for skin diseases, in-fected wounds and burns, joint pain, arthritis, rheumatism, condyloma, warts, and cancers. Also used as a fragrance in personal care items and as a flavoring. Thuja is used in food items in the United States only if it's certified thujone-free.

**DOSAGE & ADMINISTRATION**
*Extract (1:1 in 50% alcohol, 1:10 in 60% alcohol):* 1 to 2 ml P.O. t.i.d. *Tincture:* 100 parts thuja powder and 1,000 parts diluted spirit of wine mixed together.

**ADVERSE REACTIONS**
**CNS:** *seizures,* neurotoxicity.
**CV:** hypotension, tachycardia.
**GI:** nausea, vomiting, diarrhea.
**GU:** uterine stimulation and cramping, miscarriage.
**Other:** mucous membrane hemorrhaging.

**INTERACTIONS**
**Herb-herb.** *Other herbs that contain thuja, such as oak moss, oriental arborvitae, sage, tansy, tree moss, wormwood:* Increased risk of toxicity. Advise patient to avoid using together.
**Herb-lifestyle.** *Alcohol use:* Possible additive CNS effects. Advise patient to avoid using together.

**CAUTIONS**
Pregnant or breast-feeding women shouldn't use this herb. Thuja shouldn't be used by transplant patients or those with a history of seizures or immune-related diseases, such as lupus, rheumatoid arthritis, or AIDS, because it may

---

*Bold italic type* indicates that reaction may be life-threatening.

activate the immune system and accelerate the disease.

**NURSING CONSIDERATIONS**
• Find out why patient is using the herb.

⚡**ALERT:** Thuja preparations intended for oral or topical use shouldn't contain thujone, a neurotoxin. Some thuja and thuja oil preparations are said to be thujone-free. However, if you suspect thujone toxicity, call a poison control center immediately.
• For homeopathic thuja preparations, patient must not eat or drink for 15 minutes before and after taking the remedy to prevent its dilution.
• Monitor patient's response to therapy and for adverse effects.
• Don't confuse this *Thuja* species with *T. orientalis,* the Oriental arborvitae.

**Patient teaching**
• Advise patient to consult with his health care provider before using an herbal preparation because a treatment with proven efficacy may be available.
• Tell patient to remind pharmacist of any herbal and dietary supplements that he's taking, when filling a new prescription.
• Caution patient not to take thuja if he has a history of seizures.
• If patient intends to take thuja leaf oil by mouth, warn him to make sure it's certified thujone-free.
• If patient intends to take a homeopathic remedy, urge him not to eat or drink for 15 minutes before and after doing so.

• If patient takes a form that contains alcohol, caution him to avoid hazardous activities until full CNS effects of the herb are known.
• Warn patient to immediately contact a poison control center or seek emergency treatment if he becomes ill after taking thuja orally.
• Warn patient to keep all herbal products away from children and pets.

## thunder god vine

*Tripteryigium wilfordii,* huang-t'engken, lei gong teng, lei-kung t'eng, threewingnut, tsao-ho-hua, yellow vine

**Common trade names**
*None known*

**HOW SUPPLIED**
Available as an extract.

**ACTIONS & COMPONENTS**
Obtained from leaves and roots of *Tripteryigium wilfordii.* Contains tripchlorolide, tribromoline, and demethylzeylesteral constituents, which have immunosuppressive effects. Triptolide and tripdiolide may depress spermatogenesis and exert anti-inflammatory and immunosuppressive effects.

**USES**
Used for male antifertility effects. Also used to treat rheumatoid arthritis, inflammation, abscesses and boils, heavy menstrual periods, and autoimmune diseases.

*Liquid may contain alcohol.

## DOSAGE & ADMINISTRATION
*For rheumatoid arthritis:* 30 mg extract P.O. q.d.
*Male antifertility effects:* About ⅓ of the dose used for anti-inflammatory effects. Fertility usually returns 6 weeks after herb is stopped.

## ADVERSE REACTIONS
**CV:** hypotension, *shock.*
**GI:** stomach upset, vomiting, diarrhea.
**GU:** amenorrhea, infertility, *renal failure.*
**Hematologic:** decreased white blood cell and lymphocyte count.
**Skin:** rash.

## INTERACTIONS
**Herb-drug.** *Immunosuppressants:* Enhanced immunosuppressive effects. Advise patient to avoid using together.

## CAUTIONS
Patients who take immunosuppressive drugs or have CV disease, a previous transplant, or immune disorders should avoid taking this herb. Men of childbearing age and women who are pregnant or breast-feeding shouldn't use this herb.

## NURSING CONSIDERATIONS
● Find out why patient is using the herb.
🖝ALERT: Herb may cause death in patients with a history of MI, coronary artery disease, or heart failure. The one reported death involved a patient with coexisting cardiac damage. This patient experienced profuse vomiting, diarrhea, decreased serum WBCs, renal failure, hypotension, and shock before death.
● Men considering fatherhood shouldn't use this herb because of its antifertility effect.
● When herb is taken as a male antifertility agent, fertility usually returns to normal 6 weeks after stopping herb.

## Patient teaching
● Advise patient to consult with his health care provider before using an herbal preparation because a treatment with proven efficacy may be available.
● Tell patient to remind pharmacist of any herbal and dietary supplements that he's taking, when filling a new prescription.
● If patient has a history of heart disease, MI, or heart failure, tell him not to use this herb.
● Advise pregnant patients, those trying to become pregnant, and those not using adequate pregnancy prevention to avoid this herb. Tell patient to make sure she's not pregnant before use.
● Inform men considering fatherhood about herb's antifertility effects.
● Advise against using herb if patient has a disease or condition that alters the immune system or if he takes other herbs or drugs that lower the immune system.
● If patient is using herb as a male contraceptive, tell him that sperm levels and activity should return to normal 6 weeks after stopping herb.
● Warn patient to keep all herbal products away from children and pets.

---

*Bold italic type* indicates that reaction may be life-threatening.

## thyme

*Thymus serpyllum, T. vulgaris,* common thyme, French thyme, garden thyme, rubbed thyme, Spanish thyme, thymi herba

**Common trade names**
*Candistroy, Dentarone Plus Toothpaste, Fenu-Thyme, Respirtonic, Thyme Beautiful Skin Tea, Thyme Leaf & Flower, Thyme Leaf, Thyme (liquid), Ultimate Respiratory Cleanse*

### HOW SUPPLIED
Available as 100% oil, dry herb, powder, liquid extract*, and dry extract.

### ACTIONS & COMPONENTS
Obtained from above-ground parts of *Thymus serpyllum* or *T. vulgaris.* Contains thymol, flavonoids, and carvacrol, which have expectorant, antispasmodic, and antitussive effects. Thymol and carvacrol may also have antibacterial and antifungal effects. Rosmarinic acid may have antiedema and macrophage-inhibiting effects. Herb may also act as a menstrual stimulant. Common thyme (*T. vulgaris*) contains more oil than wild thyme (*T. serpyllum*) or Spanish thyme (*T. zygis*).

### USES
Used for bronchitis, pertussis, laryngitis, tonsillitis, dyspepsia, diarrhea, rheumatic diseases, and pediatric enuresis. Also used as a diuretic, an antibacterial, and an antiflatulent. Used externally to treat wounds resistant to healing and as a mouthwash and gargle for mouth and throat inflammations. Also used as a spice and flavoring agent.

### DOSAGE & ADMINISTRATION
*Average daily dose:* 1 to 2 g dried leaf or flower P.O. several times a day. Maximum, 10 g of dried leaf q.d.
*Bath:* 0.004 g thyme oil (the minimum dose) added to 1 L water, filtered, and then added to 95° to 100.4° F (35° to 38° C) bath water. Or, 500 g of herb added to 4 L boiling water, filtered, and then added to bath water as directed above.
*Fluidextract:* 1 to 2 g P.O. up to t.i.d.
*Tea:* 1 to 2 g dried leaf or flower in 150 ml boiling water, steeped for 10 minutes, strained, and taken several times q.d.
*Topical:* 5 g in 100 ml boiling water (5% infusion), steeped for 10 minutes, strained, cooled slightly, and used as gargle or applied as compress.

### ADVERSE REACTIONS
**Skin:** irritation, mild sensitivity reactions.

### INTERACTIONS
None known.

### CAUTIONS
Pregnant or breast-feeding women should avoid this herb, as should patients allergic to oregano. Patients with GI disorders, such as ulcers, and those with urinary tract inflammation should use thyme cautiously. Patients with widespread skin injuries or skin disease, high fever, infectious disease, or cardiac problems should be very cautious when

*Liquid may contain alcohol.

using any herb as an ingredient in a whole-body bath.

## NURSING CONSIDERATIONS
● Find out why patient is using the herb.
● Although no chemical interactions have been reported in clinical studies, consider the pharmacologic properties of the herb and its potential to interfere with therapeutic effects of conventional drugs.
● Monitor patient's response to herbal therapy.

### Patient teaching
● Advise patient to consult with his health care provider before using an herbal preparation because a treatment with proven efficacy may be available.
● Tell patient to remind pharmacist of any herbal and dietary supplements that he's taking, when filling a new prescription.
● Advise patients who are pregnant or breast-feeding not to use thyme in medicinal quantities.
● Tell patient who uses thyme as an expectorant that he may receive increased benefit by adding honey as a sweetener, if he has no sugar restrictions in his diet.
● If patient is allergic to oregano, explain that thyme may cause mild allergic reactions.
● Warn patient not to take herb for persistent bronchitis or cough before seeking medical attention because doing so may delay diagnosis of a potentially serious medical condition.
● Instruct patient to contact a health care provider if he develops a skin reaction.

● If patient has urinary tract inflammation, urge him to be cautious when taking thyme because it may be aggravated.
● If patient has widespread skin injuries or skin disease, high fever, infectious disease, or cardiac problems, instruct him to be very cautious when using any herb as an ingredient in a whole-body bath.
● Instruct patient to promptly notify health care provider about adverse effects or changes in symptoms.
● Warn patient to keep all herbal products away from children and pets.

## tonka bean

*Dipteryx odorata, Coumarouna odorata,* curmaru, Dutch tonka, English tonka, tonca seed, tongo bean, tonka, tonka seed, tonquin bean, torquin bean

**Common trade names**
*None known*

### HOW SUPPLIED
Beans aren't used medicinally. No longer available in the United States.

### ACTIONS & COMPONENTS
Obtained from beans of *Dipteryx odorata (Coumarouna odorata).* Contains 1% to 3% coumarin, but can be as high as 10%. Also contains a fatty oil. Coumarin may increase venous and lymphatic return, thus reducing edema and inflammation.

---

*Bold italic type* indicates that reaction may be life-threatening.

## USES
Used as a tonic and for cachexia, cramps, lymphedema, spasms, tuberculosis, ulcers, earache, and sore throat. Some people claimed the beans had aphrodisiac properties. Coumarin has been used as a flavoring for cakes, tobacco, soaps, and preserves.

## DOSAGE & ADMINISTRATION
*Usual daily dose:* 60 mg (coumarin content) P.O. q.d.

## ADVERSE REACTIONS
**CNS:** insomnia, dizziness, stupor, headache.
**CV:** *cardiac arrest* with large doses.
**GI:** nausea, vomiting, diarrhea.
**GU:** testicular atrophy.
**Hepatic:** *hepatotoxicity,* elevated liver enzymes, liver damage.
**Other:** growth retardation.

## INTERACTIONS
**Herb-drug.** *Anticoagulants, antiplatelets such as aspirin, clopidogrel bisulfate, warfarin:* Potential coagulation disturbances. Monitor PT, INR, and patient closely. Advise patient to avoid using together.
**Herb-herb.** *Angelica, anise, arnica, bogbean, boldo, capsicum, celery, chamomile, clove, danshen, fenugreek, feverfew, garlic, ginger, ginkgo, ginseng, horse chestnut, horseradish, licorice, meadowsweet, onion, passion flower, poplar, prickly ash, red clover, turmeric, wild carrot, wild lettuce, and willow:* Potential coagulation disturbances. Advise patient to avoid using together.

## CAUTIONS
Pregnant patients, breast-feeding patients, and patients with a history of liver disease shouldn't use this herb.

## NURSING CONSIDERATIONS
• Find out why patient is using the herb.
• High doses or long-term consumption of tonka bean should be avoided because of the risk of liver damage and cardiac arrest.
• Take a careful history that includes any recent foreign travel or purchase and use of foodstuffs abroad.
• Take a thorough drug history to assess the patient's use of antiplatelet drugs or anticoagulants.
• Don't confuse coumarin with such anticoagulants as warfarin, dicumarol, or bishydroxycoumarin, but do recognize the potential for additive antiplatelet or anticoagulant effects.
• Vanilla extract and possibly other flavoring extracts purchased in foreign countries may contain coumarin impurities and are unsafe for consumption.
• Monitor patient for signs of bleeding, such as easy bruising and gum bleeding.

### Patient teaching
• Advise patient to consult with his health care provider before using an herbal preparation because a treatment with proven efficacy may be available.
• Tell patient to remind pharmacist of any herbal and dietary supplements that he's taking, when filling a new prescription.

---

*Liquid may contain alcohol.

- Caution patient not to purchase or consume flavorings, preservatives, or beverages that contain tonka beans or their chemical component, coumarin, when traveling outside the United States.
- Warn patient to avoid tonka bean if he takes blood thinners of any type.
- Warn pregnant and breast-feeding patients to avoid tonka bean.
- Explain the signs of bleeding, and urge patient to promptly notify a health care provider if this or any other adverse effect develops.
- Tell patient to avoid high doses and long-term use of tonka bean.
- Instruct patient to seek emergency medical care if he develops cardiac symptoms (chest pain, shortness of breath, diaphoresis) while taking tonka bean.

## tormentil

*Potentilla erecta, Tormentillae rhizoma*, biscuits, bloodroot, cinquefoil, earthbank, English sarsaparilla, ewe daisy, flesh and blood, potentilla, septfoil, shepherd's knapperty, shepherd's knot, thormantle, tormentilla

**Common trade names**
*Immune Master*

### HOW SUPPLIED
Available as root, powder, tincture*, and fluidextract.

### ACTIONS & COMPONENTS
Obtained from *Potentilla erecta*. Contains tannins, flavonoids, resins, ellagic acid, and kinovic acid.

Tannins are probably responsible for pharmacologic actions.

### USES
Used orally to treat diarrhea, mild gastroenteritis, and fever. Used topically as a mouth rinse for mild oral inflammation and mild superficial bleeding. Fluidextract is also used to promote wound healing. Used with galangal, marshmallow root, and powdered ginger to treat diarrhea and dysentery.

### DOSAGE & ADMINISTRATION
*Tea for diarrhea:* 2 to 3 g of root in 150 ml boiling water, steeped for 10 to 15 minutes, strained, and taken b.i.d. to q.i.d. One tsp powdered root = 4 g of drug.
*Tincture:* 10 to 20 gtt (1:10) in a glass of water P.O., swished as a mouth rinse once q.d.

### ADVERSE REACTIONS
**GI:** nausea, vomiting, abdominal complaints.

### INTERACTIONS
**Herb-drug.** *Disulfiram, metronidazole:* Herbal products that contain alcohol may cause a disulfiram-like reaction. Advise patient to avoid using together.
**Herb-food.** *Milk products:* Decreased antidiarrheal effect. Advise patient to avoid using together.

### CAUTIONS
Pregnant or breast-feeding women should avoid this herb, as should alcoholic patients and those with liver disease.

---

## NURSING CONSIDERATIONS
• Find out why patient is using the herb.
• Milk products may bind the tannins in tormentil used as an antidiarrheal, thus decreasing both beneficial and adverse effects.
• Monitor patient's response to herbal therapy.

**Patient teaching**
• Advise patient to consult with his health care provider before using an herbal preparation because a treatment with proven efficacy may be available.
• Tell patient to remind pharmacist of any herbal and dietary supplements that he's taking, when filling a new prescription.
• Tell pregnant and breast-feeding patients not to use tormentil.
• Inform patient that milk products may bind the active ingredient in tormentil when used to treat diarrhea, thus reducing its effectiveness.
• Urge patient to stop using tormentil and to contact his health care provider if diarrhea gets worse or continues for longer than 2 days.
• Tell patient to promptly notify a health care provider about adverse effects or changes in symptoms.
• Warn patient to keep all herbal products away from children and pets.

## tragacanth

*Astragalus gummifer,* goat's thorn, green dragon, gum dragon, gum tragacanth, hog gum, Syrian tragacanth, tragacanth gum

**Common trade names**
*Normacol, Tragacanth Mucilage*

### HOW SUPPLIED
Available as powder.

### ACTIONS & COMPONENTS
Obtained from *Astragalus gummifer*. Contains tragacanthin and bassorin, which form a colloidal solution and a thick gel, respectively, when wet. Tragacanth promotes peristaltic movement, has adhesive properties, and may inhibit cancer cell growth.

### USES
Used for diarrhea and constipation. Also used as a stabilizer, a thickener, a suspending agent in food and pharmaceutical products, a binder, an emulsifier, and an ingredient in denture adhesives. Mucilage is used as an adjunct for burns.

### DOSAGE & ADMINISTRATION
*Average daily dose:* 1 tsp granulated herb added to 250 to 300 ml liquid, P.O.

### ADVERSE REACTIONS
**GI:** esophageal pain or blockage, *ileal obstruction*.
**Skin:** contact dermatitis.

### INTERACTIONS
None known.

## CAUTIONS
Patients allergic to quillaja bark *(Quillaja saponaria)* may be sensitive to tragacanth preparations. Pregnant or breast-feeding women should avoid this herb, as should patients with esophageal strictures or intestinal obstructions.

## NURSING CONSIDERATIONS
• Find out why patient is using the herb.
• Tragacanth is relatively safe, but should be taken P.O. with a full glass of water to avoid expansion of the compound in the esophagus and potential blockage or esophageal damage.
• Tragacanth may inhibit absorption of oral drugs, herbs, and foods. Doses of preparations that contain large amounts of tragacanth should be separated from other oral intake by 2 hours.
• Monitor patient for adverse effects, including difficulty swallowing and esophageal pain.

### Patient teaching
• Advise patient to consult with his health care provider before using an herbal preparation because a treatment with proven efficacy may be available.
• Tell patient to remind pharmacist of any herbal and dietary supplements that he's taking, when filling a new prescription.
• Instruct patient to drink a full glass of water with each dose of tragacanth to avoid expansion of the compound in the esophagus and possible blockage or damage.
• Warn patient to seek medical help immediately if he can't swallow or has significant pain, vomiting, or esophageal bleeding after taking tragacanth.
• Warn patient to keep all herbal products away from children and pets.

## tree of heaven

*Ailanthus altissima,* ailanto, a-lan-thus, Chinese sumach, heaven tree, paradise tree, vernis de Japon

**Common trade names**
*Chun Pi*

### HOW SUPPLIED
Available as trunk or root bark, tincture*, tea, or infusion.

### ACTIONS & COMPONENTS
Obtained from *Ailanthus altissima.* Quassinoid constituents such as ailanthin and quassin may have cytotoxic effects. Tannins and alkaloids may have astringent, antipyretic, and antispasmodic properties. Herb also has cardiac depressant activity and purgative action, and it may have antimalarial properties.

### USES
Used for pathologic leukorrhea, diarrhea, chronic dysentery, dysmenorrhea, cramps, asthma, tachycardia, gonorrhea, epilepsy, and tapeworm infestation.

### DOSAGE & ADMINISTRATION
*Infusion:* 1 tsp taken b.i.d. Prepared by adding 50 g bark to 75 g hot water, straining, and cooling.

---

*Bold italic type* indicates that reaction may be life-threatening.

*Tincture:* 5 to 60 gtt (about 7 to 20 grains) per dose P.O. b.i.d. to q.i.d.

**ADVERSE REACTIONS**
**CNS:** headache, limb tingling, dizziness.
**CV:** decreased cardiac function.
**GI:** nausea, diarrhea.
**Skin:** dermatitis after contact with leaves.

**INTERACTIONS**
**Herb-drug.** *Disulfiram:* Herbal products that contain alcohol may cause a disulfiram-like reaction. Advise patient to avoid using together.

**CAUTIONS**
Pregnant or breast-feeding women should avoid this herb, as should patients with compromised cardiac function, such as heart failure, coronary artery disease, or a history of MI.

**NURSING CONSIDERATIONS**
• Find out why patient is using the herb.
• Bark preparations have an offensive smell commonly described as burnt peanuts.
• Although no chemical interactions have been reported in clinical studies, consider the pharmacologic properties of the herb and its potential to interfere with therapeutic effects of conventional drugs.
• Monitor patient's response to herb.
• Monitor patient carefully for adverse GI or CNS effects.
• If patient has diarrhea, monitor intake and output as indicated.

• Don't confuse tree of heaven *(Ailanthus)* with tree of life *(Thuja occidentalis).*

**Patient teaching**
• Advise patient to consult with his health care provider before using an herbal preparation because a treatment with proven efficacy may be available.
• Tell patient to remind pharmacist of any herbal and dietary supplements that he's taking, when filling a new prescription.
• Advise patient to avoid use of herb while pregnant and breast-feeding.
• Caution parents not to give this herb to children.
• Warn patient not to take herb for diarrhea, dysmenorrhea, or other undiagnosed symptoms before seeking medical attention because doing so may delay diagnosis of a potentially serious medical condition.
• Inform patient that bark preparations smell something like burnt peanuts.
• Tell patient to store herb in a dry, well-ventilated area away from moths.
• Warn patient to keep all herbal products away from children and pets.

## true unicorn root

*Aletris farinosa,* ague grass, ague-root, aloe-root, bettie grass, bitter grass, black-root, blazing star, colic-root, crow corn, devil's bit, star grass, starwort, true unicorn stargrass, unicorn root, whitetube stargrass

**Common trade names**
*Extraction Aletridis Alcoholicum, Menopause Support*

### HOW SUPPLIED
Available as powdered or dried root, fluidextract*, and infusion.

### ACTIONS & COMPONENTS
Obtained from *Aletris farinosa.* Contains some steroidal components that may have estrogenic properties. Also contains alkaloids, oil, saponin, and resins.

### USES
Used for rheumatism, gynecologic disorders (particularly dysmenorrhea and amenorrhea), miscarriage, and symptoms caused by a prolapsed vagina. Also used as a sedative, a general tonic, a laxative, an antiflatulent, an antidiarrheal, a diuretic, and an antispasmodic.

### DOSAGE & ADMINISTRATION
*Fluidextract (1:1 in 45% alcohol):* 0.3 to 0.6 g P.O. t.i.d.
*Infusion:* 1.5 g of herb to 100 ml water; 0.3 to 0.6 g P.O. t.i.d.

### ADVERSE REACTIONS
**CNS:** vertigo.
**GI:** colic.

### INTERACTIONS
**Herb-drug.** *Antacids, histamine $H_2$-antagonists, proton pump inhibitors, sucralfate:* Possible increased gastric acidity and reduced drug effects. Monitor patient closely.
*Disulfiram, metronidazole:* Herbal products that contain alcohol may cause a disulfiram-like reaction. Advise patient to avoid using together.
*Estrogens, hormonal contraceptives:* Possible additive effect. Patient may need dosage adjustment or a change to nonhormonal birth control. Advise patient to avoid using together.
*Pitocin:* May antagonize effects. If drug and herb must be used together, monitor patient closely.

### CAUTIONS
Pregnant or breast-feeding women should avoid this herb, as should patients being treated for alcoholism or liver disease.

### NURSING CONSIDERATIONS
• Find out why patient is using the herb.
• Some patients may use true unicorn for repeated miscarriage despite repeated warnings against such use.
• Monitor patient's response to herb.

### Patient teaching
• Advise patient to consult with his health care provider before using an herbal preparation because a treatment with proven efficacy may be available.
• Tell patient to remind pharmacist of any herbal and dietary supple-

---

*Bold italic type* indicates that reaction may be life-threatening.

ments that he's taking, when filling a new prescription.

- Advise patient that true unicorn root may increase stomach acid and interfere with the action of antacids and other drugs used to limit or stop stomach acid production.
- Caution women of childbearing age and those attempting to conceive that using herb while pregnant and breast-feeding may have adverse effects.
- Warn patient not to take herb before seeking medical attention because doing so may delay diagnosis of a potentially serious medical condition.
- Instruct patient to promptly notify his health care provider about adverse effects or changes in symptoms.

## turmeric

*Amomum curcuma, Curcuma domestica, Curcuma longa, Curcuma rotunda,* Indian saffron, turmeric root

**Common trade names**
*Inflam-Aid, Lipolytics Plus, Phyto Quench Supreme, Pitta Balancing Elixir, Stone Free, Turmeric Catechu Supreme*

### HOW SUPPLIED
Available as powdered root or tincture*.

### ACTIONS & COMPONENTS
Obtained from *Curcuma longa* and other species. Root contains volatile oils and diaryl heptanoids thought to have anti-inflammatory effects.

Diaryl heptanoids may also have bile-stimulating and liver-protecting effects. Antispasmodic activity has also been noted. Other components include turmerone, atlantone, zingiberone, and more than six minor components of the oil. Two compounds, ukonon A and ukonon D, may possess anticancer activity via activation of phagocytosis and the reticuloendothelial system.

### USES
Used orally for dyspepsia, abdominal bloating, flatulence, liver and gallbladder complaints, headaches, and chest infections. Used topically for analgesia, oral mucosa inflammation, inflammatory skin conditions, and ringworm. Also used as a flavoring and coloring agent in foods.

### DOSAGE & ADMINISTRATION
*Average daily dose:* 0.5 to 1 g of powdered root P.O. several times a day between meals. Usual maximum dose is 1.5 to 3 g P.O. q.d.
*Infusion:* 2 to 3 cups taken P.O. between meals. Prepared by scalding 0.5 to 1 g powdered root in boiling water, covering and steeping for 5 minutes, and then straining. Infusion isn't the preferred method of administration because turmeric contains volatile oils that aren't water soluble.
*Tincture:* 10 to 15 gtt P.O. t.i.d. or b.i.d.

### ADVERSE REACTIONS
**GI:** indigestion.
**GU:** increased weight of sexual organs, increased sperm motility.

**Hematologic:** decreased WBC and RBC counts, depression of clotting factors.

## INTERACTIONS
**Herb-drug.** *Antiplatelet drugs including aspirin, clopidogrel bisulfate, dipyridamole:* Potential additive effects. Monitor PT, INR, and patient closely. Advise patient to use together cautiously.
**Herb-herb.** *Angelica, anise, arnica, bogbean, boldo, capsicum, celery, chamomile, clove, danshen, fenugreek, feverfew, garlic, ginger, ginkgo, ginseng, horse chestnut, horseradish, licorice, meadowsweet, onion, passion flower, poplar, prickly ash, red clover, wild carrot, wild lettuce, willow:* Potential additive antiplatelet activity. Advise patient to use together cautiously.

## CAUTIONS
Patients with bile duct obstruction, gallstones, gastric ulcers, or hyperacidity shouldn't use turmeric. Turmeric should be used cautiously in patients who take other herbs or drugs that have antiplatelet activity.

## NURSING CONSIDERATIONS
● Find out why patient is using the herb.
● Patients who take indomethacin or reserpine may have a reduced risk of drug-induced gastric or duodenal ulcers when they also take turmeric.
● Monitor patient's response to herb.

## Patient teaching
● Advise patient to consult with his health care provider before using an herbal preparation because a treatment with proven efficacy may be available.
● Tell patient to remind pharmacist of any herbal and dietary supplements that he's taking, when filling a new prescription.
● If patient takes an antiplatelet drug with turmeric, advise him to do so with caution.
● Tell patient to contact his health care provider immediately if he develops frequent nosebleeds or other evidence of excessive anticoagulation.
● Warn patient not to take herb before seeking medical attention because doing so may delay diagnosis of a potentially serious medical condition.
● Instruct patient to protect turmeric from light and to keep all herbal products away from children and pets.

---

*Bold italic type* indicates that reaction may be life-threatening.

# V

## valerian, valerian root

*Valeriana officinalis,* all-heal, amantilla, baldrian, Belgium valerian, capon's tail, garden heliotrope, Indian valerian, Mexican valerian, Pacific valerian, radix, setewale, setwall, vandal root

**Common trade names**
*Herbal Sure Valerian Root, NuVeg Valerian Root, Quanterra Sleep, Valerian Root*

### HOW SUPPLIED
Available as dried root, essential oil, tea, tincture*, extract, capsules, tablets, and combination products.
*Capsules:* 100 mg, 250 mg, 380 mg, 400 mg, 445 mg, 475 mg, 493 mg, 495 mg, 500 mg, 530 mg, 550 mg, 1,000 mg
*Tablets:* 160 mg, 550 mg

### ACTIONS & COMPONENTS
Obtained from *Valeriana officinalis.* Multiple constituents, including essential oils, seem to contribute to sedating properties of valerian. Valeric acid, the main component of the root, inhibits the enzyme system responsible for breaking down the neurotransmitter GABA, thus increasing its level in the brain. Valerian may also have mild pain relief properties and some hypotensive effects.

### USES
Used to treat menstrual cramps, restlessness and sleep disorders from nervous conditions, and other symptoms of psychological stress, such as anxiety, nervous headaches, and gastric spasms. Used topically as a bath additive for restlessness and sleep disorders.

### DOSAGE & ADMINISTRATION
*Bath additive:* 100 g of root mixed with 2 L of hot water and added to one full bath.
*For hastening sleep and improving sleep quality:* 400 to 800 mg root P.O. up to 2 hours before h.s. Some patients need 2 to 4 weeks of use for significant improvement. Maximum, 15 g q.d.
*For restlessness:* 220 mg of extract P.O. t.i.d.
*Tea:* 1 cup P.O. b.i.d. to t.i.d., and h.s.
*Tincture (1:5 in 45% to 50% alcohol):* 15 to 20 gtt in water several times q.d.

### ADVERSE REACTIONS
**CNS:** headache, morning drowsiness, uneasiness, restlessness.
**CV:** cardiac disturbances.
**GI:** GI complaints.
**Skin:** contact allergies.
**Other:** withdrawal symptoms, including increased agitation and decreased sleep.

### INTERACTIONS
**Herb-drug.** *Barbiturates, benzodiazepines:* Possible additive effects. Monitor patient closely.
**Herb-herb.** *Herbs with sedative effects, such as catnip, hops, kava, passion flower, skullcap:* May po-

*Liquid may contain alcohol.

tentiate sedative effects. Monitor patient closely.

**Herb-lifestyle.** *Alcohol use:* May potentiate sedative effects. Advise patient to avoid using together.

## CAUTIONS
Pregnant or breast-feeding women should avoid this herb. Patients with acute or major skin injuries, fever, infectious diseases, cardiac insufficiency, or hypertonia shouldn't bathe with valerian products.

## NURSING CONSIDERATIONS
• Find out why patient is using the herb.
• Valerian seems to have a more pronounced effect on those with disturbed sleep or sleep disorders.
⚡ALERT: Evidence of valerian toxicity includes difficulty walking, hypothermia, and increased muscle relaxation.
• Withdrawal symptoms, such as increased agitation and decreased sleep, can occur if valerian is abruptly stopped after prolonged use.
• Monitor CNS status and patient response to herb.

**Patient teaching**
• Advise patient to consult with his health care provider before using an herbal preparation because a treatment with proven efficacy may be available.
• Tell patient to remind pharmacist of any herbal and dietary supplements that he's taking, when filling a new prescription.
• If patient takes valerian, tell him to do so 1 to 2 hours before his desired sleep time. Explain that pa-

tient may not feel herb's effect for 2 to 4 weeks.
• Inform patient that most adverse effects occur only after long-term use.
• Instruct patient to promptly notify a health care provider about adverse effects.
• Warn patient not to take herb for insomnia before seeking medical attention because doing so may delay diagnosis of a potentially serious medical condition.
• If patient takes valerian for a long time, caution that amount should be tapered to avoid withdrawal symptoms, which may include increased agitation and decreased sleep.
• Instruct patient to avoid hazardous activities until full CNS effects of herb are known.
• Tell patient to protect herb from light and to keep tincture in a tightly closed plastic container at room temperature.
• Warn patient to keep all herbal products away from children and pets.

## vervain

*Verbena officinalis,* common vervain, eisenkraut, enchanter's plant, herb of grace, herb of the cross, holywort, Juno's tears, pigeon's grass, pigeonweed, verbena

**Common trade names**
*Quanterra Sinus, Sinupret, Verbena, Vervain*

---

*Bold italic type* indicates that reaction may be life-threatening.

## HOW SUPPLIED
Available as tablets, liquid extract*, tincture*, and combination products.
*Quanterra Sinus:* Combination containing 29 mg verbena
*Sinupret tablets:* Combination containing 36 mg verbena

## ACTIONS & COMPONENTS
Obtained from above-ground parts of *Verbena officinalis.* Contains iridoid glycosides, including verbascoside, verbenalin, and verbenin. Actions are many and varied. Small amounts of verbenin appear to stimulate sympathetic activity; larger amounts inhibit it. Verbenin may also stimulate milk secretion. Verbenalin may be a uterine stimulant and abortifacient. Verbascoside may have analgesic and antihypertensive action and may enhance the antitremor action of levodopa.

## USES
Used to treat sore throats and other oral and pharyngeal inflammation, asthma, whooping cough, and sinusitis. Also used to stimulate secretion of breast milk. Used topically to treat wounds, abscesses, arthritis pain, contusions, itching, and minor burns. Used as a gargle for cold symptoms.

## DOSAGE & ADMINISTRATION
*Liquid extract (1:1 in 25% alcohol):* 2 to 4 ml P.O. q.d.
*Tea:* 1 cup P.O. t.i.d. Prepared by adding 2 to 4 g dried herb to 150 ml boiling water.
*Tincture (1:1 in 40% alcohol):* 5 to 10 ml P.O. t.i.d.

## ADVERSE REACTIONS
**CNS:** paralysis, stupor, *seizures,* sedation.
**CV:** hypotension.
**GI:** vomiting.
**Other:** uterine stimulation.

## INTERACTIONS
**Herb-drug.** *Disulfiram:* Herbal products that contain alcohol may cause a disulfiram-like reaction. Advise patient to avoid using together.
*Hormone therapy:* Excessive amounts of vervain can interfere with hormone therapy. Monitor patient closely.
**Herb-lifestyle.** *Alcohol use:* Possible additive sedative effects. Advise patient to avoid using together.

## CAUTIONS
Pregnant or breast-feeding women should avoid this herb, as should patients using hormone therapies.

## NURSING CONSIDERATIONS
• Find out why patient is using the herb.
• Monitor patient closely for adverse CNS effects and response to herb.
• Evidence of excessive intake of the verbenalin component includes CNS paralysis, stupor, and seizures.

## Patient teaching
• Advise patient to consult with his health care provider before using an herbal preparation because a treatment with proven efficacy may be available.
• Tell patient to remind pharmacist of any herbal and dietary supple-

---

*Liquid may contain alcohol.

ments that he's taking, when filling a new prescription.

• If patient is using hormone therapy, warn him against using this herb.

• Tell patient to refrain from using alcohol and other sedatives because they may cause increased sedative effects.

• If patient takes disulfiram and an herbal product that contains alcohol, warn him about possible adverse reactions.

• Advise patient that taking excessive amounts of vervain can cause CNS depression.

• Warn patient to keep all herbal products away from children and pets.

# W

## wahoo

*Euonymus atropurpureus,* arrow wood, bitter ash, bleeding heart, burning bush, bursting heart, fish wood, fusanum, fusoria, gatten, Indian arrowroot, pigwood, spindle tree

**Common trade names**
*Wahoo, Wahoo Root*

### HOW SUPPLIED
Available as dried bark and seeds.

### ACTIONS & COMPONENTS
Obtained from stems, root bark, and berries of *Euonymus atropurpureus.* Seeds and bark contain cardioactive steroid glycosides similar to digoxin. Also contains various alkaloids, caffeine, and theobromine. Wahoo is thought to stimulate bile flow and to have laxative and diuretic effects. In larger amounts, it can affect the heart.

### USES
Bark is used orally to treat indigestion and stimulate bile production. Also used as a laxative, a diuretic, and a tonic.

### DOSAGE & ADMINISTRATION
No consensus exists.

### ADVERSE REACTIONS
**CNS:** stupor, severe tonic-clonic spasms with lockjaw, *coma.*
**CV:** *circulatory collapse.*
**GI:** upset stomach, severe bloody diarrhea.
**Respiratory:** dyspnea.
**Other:** fever.

### INTERACTIONS
**Herb-drug.** *Digoxin, other cardioactive drugs:* Increased risk of cardiac or cardiac glycoside toxicity. Advise patient to avoid using together.
*Macrolide antibiotics, tetracyclines:* May increase the risk of cardiac glycoside toxicity. Advise patient to avoid using together.
*Potassium-depleting diuretics:* Increased risk of cardiac glycoside toxicity. Advise patient to avoid using together.
*Stimulant laxatives:* Potassium depletion can increase glycoside toxicity. Advise patient to avoid using together.
**Herb-herb.** *Horsetail, licorice, stimulant laxative herbs (including aloe, cascara bark, yellow dock):* May increase the risk of cardiac toxicity from potassium depletion. Advise patient to avoid using together.

### CAUTIONS
Patients with obstructive biliary disease should avoid use because wahoo can stimulate the flow of bile.

### NURSING CONSIDERATIONS
• Find out why patient is using the herb.
⚠ ALERT: Wahoo is poisonous. Ingesting just 36 berries can be fa-

tal. Signs of toxicity include upset stomach, bloody diarrhea, fever, shortness of breath, collapse, stupor increasing to unconsciousness, severe tonic-clonic spasms with locked jaw muscles, and coma.
● Wahoo interacts with many drugs.
● Monitor patient's response to herb and patient's cardiac status closely.

**Patient teaching**
● Advise patient to consult with his health care provider before using an herbal preparation because a treatment with proven efficacy may be available.
● Tell patient to remind pharmacist of any herbal and dietary supplements that he's taking, when filling a new prescription.
● Warn patient of potential dangers of using wahoo, and discourage its use.
● Inform patient that safer, clinically proven treatments may be available for his condition.
● Warn patient not to take herb before seeking medical attention because doing so may delay diagnosis of a potentially serious medical condition.
● Warn patient to keep all herbal products away from children and pets.

## watercress

*Nasturtium officinale,* agrao, berro, brunnenkressenkraut, crescione di fonte, Indian cress, mizu-garushi, nasilord, nasturtii herba, oranda-garashi, scurvy grass, selada-air, tall nasturtium

**Common trade names**
*Watercress*

**HOW SUPPLIED**
Available as fresh or dried herb, juice, and capsules.
*Capsules:* 500 mg

**ACTIONS & COMPONENTS**
Obtained from *Nasturtium officinale.* Contains mustard oil, vitamin C, beta carotene, minerals, and vitamins $B_1$, $B_2$, E, and K. Herb has diuretic and slight antibiotic activity; both may result from mustard oil.

**USES**
Used for treating catarrh (an inflammation of the air passages usually involving the nose, throat, or lungs), chronic bronchitis, and respiratory tract mucous membrane inflammation. Also used as a poultice for skin irritation, a detoxifying agent, a diuretic, a spring tonic, and an appetite stimulant. Watercress is also widely cultivated as a salad herb.

**DOSAGE & ADMINISTRATION**
*Average daily dose:* 4 to 6 g of dried herb, 20 to 30 g fresh herb, or 60 to 150 g freshly pressed juice.
*Tea:* 150 ml boiling water poured over 2 g of drug (about 1 to 2 tsp),

---

*Bold italic type* indicates that reaction may be life-threatening.

covered for 10 to 15 minutes, and then strained. 2 to 3 cups taken P.O. q.d. before meals.

**ADVERSE REACTIONS**
**GI:** GI irritation.
**GU:** kidney damage.
**Skin:** irritation.

**INTERACTIONS**
**Herb-drug.** *Chlorzoxazone, orphenadrine citrate:* May potentiate effects. Monitor patient closely.
*Diuretics:* Possible additive effects. Monitor patient closely.
*Warfarin:* May antagonize anticoagulant effects of warfarin because of high vitamin K content. Monitor PT and INR closely.

**CAUTIONS**
Pregnant or breast-feeding women should avoid this herb, as should children younger than age 4 and patients with gastric ulcers, intestinal ulcers, or inflammatory kidney disease.

**NURSING CONSIDERATIONS**
• Find out why patient is using the herb.
• Use caution if patient also takes an anticoagulant because of high vitamin K content.
• Consuming large amounts of watercress may cause GI irritation.
• Watercress can be used topically as a poultice or compress, but watch for skin irritation.
• Monitor patient's response to herb.

**Patient teaching**
• Advise patient to consult with his health care provider before using an herbal preparation because a treatment with proven efficacy may be available.
• Tell patient to remind pharmacist of any herbal and dietary supplements that he's taking, when filling a new prescription.
• Caution patient about possible GI irritation from irritating effect of mustard oil on mucous membranes.
• If patient takes an anticoagulant, warn that herb has a vitamin K content. Instruct patient to watch for signs of bleeding, such as easy bruising and bleeding gums.
• Warn patient not to take herb before seeking medical attention because doing so may delay diagnosis of a potentially serious medical condition.
• Warn patient to keep all herbal products away from children and pets.

## wild cherry

*Prunus serotina,* black cherry, black choke, choke cherry, rum cherry bark, Virginian prune, wild black cherry

**Common trade names**
*Black Cherry, Wild Cherry*

**HOW SUPPLIED**
Available as dried bark, liquid extract*, and combination products.

**ACTIONS & COMPONENTS**
Obtained from stem bark of *Prunus serotina* or *P. virginiana.* Contains prunasin, a cyanogenic glycoside that's hydrolyzed to toxic hydrocyanic acid (HCN) and benzalde-

*Liquid may contain alcohol.

hyde. Herb has astringent, antitussive, and sedative effects. Bark collected in the fall has higher HCN content—about 0.15%—than bark collected in the spring—about 0.05%.

## USES
Widely used in cough syrups because of its sedative, expectorant, and antitussive effects. Also used for colds, bronchitis, whooping cough, other lung problems, nervous digestive disorders, and diarrhea. It's used in foods and beverages as a flavoring agent.

## DOSAGE & ADMINISTRATION
*Liquid extract (alcohol 12% to 14% by volume):* 5 to 12 gtt in water P.O. t.i.d. or b.i.d.

## ADVERSE REACTIONS
**Other:** *fatal poisoning* with ingestion of large amounts.

## INTERACTIONS
None known.

## CAUTIONS
Pregnant or breast-feeding women shouldn't use this herb because prunasin, one of its constituents, may be teratogenic.

## NURSING CONSIDERATIONS
• Find out why patient is using the herb.
⚡ALERT: Wild cherry should be avoided because of its HCN content. Deaths have occurred among children who ate fruit or leaves.
• Wild cherry is best used only in very small amounts as a component of cough syrups because of the risk of poisoning at larger doses.
• Although no chemical interactions have been reported in clinical studies, consider the pharmacologic properties of the herb and its potential to interfere with therapeutic effects of conventional drugs.
• Monitor patient's response to herbal therapy.

**Patient teaching**
• Advise patient to consult with his health care provider before using an herbal preparation because a treatment with proven efficacy may be available.
• Tell patient to remind pharmacist of any herbal and dietary supplements that he's taking, when filling a new prescription.
• Instruct patient to use wild cherry only in combination cough syrups, as directed by a health care provider or pharmacist.
• Caution patient about dangers of excessive use of wild cherry.
• Warn patient not to take herb for respiratory problems before seeking medical attention because doing so may delay diagnosis of a potentially serious medical condition.
• Warn patient to keep all herbal products away from children and pets.

---

*Bold italic type* indicates that reaction may be life-threatening.

## wild ginger

*Asarum canadense, Asarum europaeum*, asarabacca, cat's foot, false coltsfoot, hazelwort, Indian ginger, public house plant, snakeroot, wild nard

**Common trade names**
*Wild Ginger Extract*
Combination products: *Bronchaid, Immunaid*

### HOW SUPPLIED
Available as dried root, dried rhizome, and liquid extract*.
*Liquid extract:* 45% alcohol

### ACTIONS & COMPONENTS
Obtained from *Asarum canadense* or *A. europaeum*. Contains phenylpropanol, trans-isoasarone, and aristolochic acid. Mode of action unknown, but constituents of rhizome may have antibiotic, antiseptic, antispasmodic, anti-inflammatory, expectorant, and sedative properties. Phenylpropanol may be responsible for effects on bronchitis and bronchial asthma. Some products are standardized for this constituent. Trans-isoasarone may cause emetic and spasmolytic effects. Aristolochic acid may be carcinogenic and nephrotoxic.

### USES
*Asarum canadense* is used for GI spasms, gas, and chronic pulmonary conditions, such as bronchitis. Also used to produce sweating and promote menstruation. May be added to multiple-ingredient products and promoted for chronic cough, bronchitis, or immune system support.

Extract of *A. europaeum* is used in Europe for acute and chronic bronchitis, bronchial spasms, and bronchial asthma. Also used as a menstrual stimulant and antitussive and to treat angina pectoris, migraines, liver disease, jaundice, and pneumonia.

### DOSAGE & ADMINISTRATION
*Typical doses of A. canadense:* ½ oz of powdered root in 1 pint boiling water as tea; taken hot.
*Typical doses of A. europaeum:* 30 mg dry extract P.O. for adults and children older than age 13.

### ADVERSE REACTIONS
**CNS:** partial paralysis.
**EENT:** burning of tongue.
**GI:** nausea, vomiting, gastroenteritis, diarrhea.
**GU:** *acute renal failure.*
**Skin:** dermatitis.

### INTERACTIONS
*Disulfiram, metronidazole:* Herbal products that contain alcohol may cause a disulfiram-like reaction. Advise patient to avoid using together.

### CAUTIONS
Pregnant or breast-feeding women should avoid this herb, as should patients with kidney disorders or infectious or inflammatory GI conditions.

### NURSING CONSIDERATIONS
• Find out why patient is using the herb.

*Liquid may contain alcohol.

• Although no chemical interactions have been reported in clinical studies, consider the pharmacologic properties of the herb and its potential to interfere with therapeutic effects of conventional drugs.
• Monitor kidney function with long-term use.
• Monitor patient's response to herb.
• Don't confuse with bitter milkwort *(Polygala amara)* or senega *(P. senega),* also known as snake root.

**Patient teaching**
• Advise patient to consult with his health care provider before using an herbal preparation because a treatment with proven efficacy may be available.
• Tell patient to remind pharmacist of any herbal and dietary supplements that he's taking, when filling a new prescription.
• Caution patient not to use herb long-term because of possible kidney problems and carcinogenic effects of aristolochic acid in the herb.
• Warn patient to keep all herbal products away from children and pets.

## wild indigo

*Baptisia tinctoria,* American indigo, false indigo, horse-fly weed, rattlebush, rattleweed, yellow broom, yellow indigo

### Common trade names
*Wild Indigo Extract, Wild Indigo Root Caps*
Combination products: *Echinacea & Baptisia, Echinacea Throat Relief, Esberitox, Immune Boost, Re-Zist*

**HOW SUPPLIED**
Available as dried root, root powder, capsules, tablets, suppositories, drops, homeopathic injection, and liquid extracts*.

**ACTIONS & COMPONENTS**
Obtained from *Baptisia tinctoria.* Contains polysaccharides, glycoproteins, quinolizidine alkaloids, isoflavonoids, and hydroxycoumarins. Herb may have immunostimulant properties and a mild estrogenic effect.

**USES**
Used to treat infections such as typhoid and scarlet fever. Large doses used to induce bowel evacuation and vomiting. Also used for ear, nose, and throat infections and for inflamed lymph glands and fever. Used as a mouthwash to treat mouth sores and gum disease. Herb is thought to stimulate the immune system when combined with herbs, such as echinacea. In homeopathic medicine, wild indigo has been used to treat confusion and blood poisoning.

**DOSAGE & ADMINISTRATION**
*Decoction:* ½ to 1 tsp of root in a cup of water, boiled, and then simmered 10 to 15 minutes. Taken P.O. t.i.d.
*Homeopathic dose:* 5 to 10 gtt, 1 tablet, or 5 to 10 globules P.O. up to t.i.d.; for injection solution, 1 ml twice weekly S.C.
*Liquid extract or tincture (1:1 in 60% alcohol):* 1 to 2 ml P.O. t.i.d.
*Ointment:* 1:8 parts liquid extract to ointment base; applied topically to affected area.

---

*Bold italic type* indicates that reaction may be life-threatening.

## ADVERSE REACTIONS
**GI:** vomiting, diarrhea, inflammation of the GI tract, spasms.
**Skin:** irritation.

## INTERACTIONS
*Disulfiram, metronidazole:* Herbal products that contain alcohol may cause a disulfiram-like reaction. Advise patient to avoid using together.

## CAUTIONS
Pregnant or breast-feeding women should avoid this herb, as should patients with inflammatory GI conditions.

## NURSING CONSIDERATIONS
• Find out why patient is using the herb.
• Although no chemical interactions have been reported in clinical studies, consider the pharmacologic properties of the herb and its potential to interfere with therapeutic effects of conventional drugs.
• Monitor patient's response to herbal therapy.
• Don't confuse wild indigo with the root of false blue indigo *(B. australis)* or *B. alba.*

### Patient teaching
• Advise patient to consult with his health care provider before using an herbal preparation because a treatment with proven efficacy may be available.
• Tell patient to remind pharmacist of any herbal and dietary supplements that he's taking, when filling a new prescription.
• Warn patient not to take herb before seeking medical attention be-

cause doing so may delay diagnosis of a potentially serious medical condition.
• Tell patient to watch for adverse effects, including local reactions, if used topically as an ointment. Urge him to promptly notify health care provider about any change in symptoms.
• Warn patient to keep all herbal products away from children and pets.

## wild lettuce

*Lactuca canadensis, Lactuca virosa,* bitter lettuce, green endive, lactucarium, lettuce opium, poison lettuce

**Common trade names**
*Hydro, Hypericum Pro (contains multiple ingredients), Sahivah Blend, Spirit Walk, Turkhash, Vision Quest, Wild Lettuce Extract*

## HOW SUPPLIED
Available as dried or powdered herb, oil, dried sap, and extracts*.

## ACTIONS & COMPONENTS
Obtained from *Lactuca canadensis* and *L. virosa.* The milky latex can cause mydriasis. Lactucin, a component of the latex, may have sedative and CNS depressant properties. Trace amounts of morphine have been found in *Lactuca* species, but not enough to exert pharmacologic effects.

## USES
Latex is used as a sedative and a treatment for colic and cough. Seed oil is used for arteriosclerosis and

*Liquid may contain alcohol.

as a substitute for wheat germ oil. Leaf is used for insomnia, restlessness, dry irritated cough, and muscle or joint pain. Latex and leaf are used for excitability in children, priapism, painful menses, swollen genitals, and as an opium substitute in cough preparations. Leaf and dried sap are smoked recreationally as legal substitutes for marijuana and hashish. Crude extract has been injected I.V. for the same purpose. Also used as an analgesic and a GI aid.

## DOSAGE & ADMINISTRATION

*Infusion:* 1 or 2 tsp leaves to 1 cup boiling water, steeped for 10 to 15 minutes. Taken P.O. t.i.d.
*Tincture:* 1 to 2 ml P.O. t.i.d.

## ADVERSE REACTIONS

**CNS:** dizziness, somnolence, *coma.*
**CV:** tachycardia.
**EENT:** pupil dilation, tinnitus.
**Respiratory:** tachypnea.
**Skin:** contact dermatitis.
**Other:** allergic reaction.

## INTERACTIONS

**Herb-drug.** *Antihistamines, OTC cold medicines, sedatives:* May have additive sedative effects. Monitor patient closely. Advise patient to avoid using together.
*Disulfiram, metronidazole:* Herbal products that contain alcohol may cause a disulfiram-like reaction. Advise patient to avoid using together.
**Herb-herb.** *Herbs with anticoagulant or antiplatelet effects:* Increased risk of bleeding. Monitor

patient for bleeding. Monitor PT and INR, as indicated.
*Herbs with sedative effects:* May enhance adverse effects. Advise patient to avoid using together.
**Herb-lifestyle.** *Alcohol use:* Additive CNS effects. Advise patient to avoid using together.

## CAUTIONS

Pregnant or breast-feeding women should avoid this herb, as should patients hypersensitive to members of the Compositae family and patients with a history of glaucoma or BPH.

## NURSING CONSIDERATIONS

• Find out why patient is using the herb.
• Monitor patient's response to herbal therapy.
• Monitor patient for bleeding, and check PT and INR, if indicated.

## Patient teaching

• Advise patient to consult with his health care provider before using an herbal preparation because a treatment with proven efficacy may be available.
• Tell patient to remind pharmacist of any herbal and dietary supplements that he's taking, when filling a new prescription.
• Advise the patient to use caution if combining wild lettuce with other sedating drugs or with alcohol.
• Caution patient to avoid hazardous activities until CNS effects of herb are fully known.
• Warn patient not to take herb before seeking medical attention because doing so may delay diagno-

---

*Bold italic type* indicates that reaction may be life-threatening.

sis of a potentially serious medical condition.

• Tell patient to promptly notify a health care provider about adverse effects or changes in symptoms.

• Warn patient to keep all herbal products away from children and pets.

## wild yam

*Dioscorea composita, D. villosa*, Atlantic yam, barbasco, China root, colic root, devil's bones, Mexican wild yam, rheumatism root, yuma

### Common trade names
Combination products: *Bone Strengthener Formula, Born Again Wild Yam Gel, Ease Wild Yam Extract, FemPro, MexiYam, Mexican Wild Yam, Progesterone Plus, Prostan, Resolve, Super Female Formula, Ultra Diet Pep, Wild Yam & Chaste Tree, Wild Yamcon, Wild Yam/Dong Quai Formula, Wild Yam EFX, Wild Yam Extract, Wild Yam-False Unicorn Virtue, Wild Yam Root, Yamcon Pro, Yamcon Vaginal, Yam Extract Plus 30*

### HOW SUPPLIED
Available as capsules, creams, gels, and liquid extracts*.
*Cream and gel:* 3% to 10% yam extract with or without added progesterone or other herbs. Added progesterone content runs from 0.5% to 1.5%, about 24 to 72 mg per tsp, depending on the product.
*Liquid extracts:* 1:1, 1:2; 250 mg/ml
*Root powder capsules:* 400 mg, 500 mg

*Standardized extract capsules:* 200 mg, usually standardized to 10% diosgenin

### ACTIONS & COMPONENTS
Obtained from *Dioscorea composita* or *D. villosa.* Contains a glycoside, diosgenin, saponins, and tannins. Diosgenin is a steroid precursor used in the first commercial production of oral contraceptives, topical hormones, estrogens, progestogens, androgens, and other sex hormones. However, compounds in wild yam can't be used as hormones by the human body. Diosgenin may have some weak estrogenic effects, but not progesterogenic actions. Progesterogenic effects are sometimes obtained from wild yam cream by adding "natural" progesterone, which is absorbed through the skin. Diosegenin prevents estrogen-induced bile flow suppression. It may stimulate the growth of mammary tissue.

### USES
Commercial wild yam cream and oral preparations may have hormonal properties and are used to relieve menopausal symptoms, premenstrual syndrome (PMS), and other gynecologic symptoms. Wild yam doesn't, however, contain hormones or compounds such as dihydroepiandrosterone (DHEA) that are converted into hormones in the human body. Orally, wild yam is used as a "natural alternative" for estrogen replacement, postmenopausal vaginal dryness, PMS, osteoporosis, increasing energy and libido in men and women, and breast enlargement. It may also be used

for diverticulosis, gallbladder colic, painful menstruation, cramps, and rheumatoid arthritis.

Wild yam cream with progesterone added from other sources does exert physiologic effects from the absorbed progesterone. Progesterone cream may be useful in treating menopausal symptoms. However, progesterone has been shown to be an ineffective treatment for PMS even at much higher doses.

Wild yam is also used in multiple-ingredient commercial formulas promoted for menopause, osteoporosis prevention, PMS, threatened abortion, weight loss, women's general health, and men's prostate health. Diosgenin, a yam constituent, is promoted as a natural precursor to DHEA to increase athletic performance and slow the aging process.

**DOSAGE & ADMINISTRATION**
*Oral dosage:* No consensus exists. For adults, 1 to 6 g powder P.O. q.d. or 6 to 12 ml P.O. q.d. of liquid extract, in divided doses.
*Topical dosage:* No consensus exists. Yam cream without progesterone, ¼ to ½ tsp q.d. Cream with progesterone, ⅛ to ½ tsp q.d. (progesterone dose of 4 to 33 mg q.d.) depending on the product. Rubbed onto belly, breasts, inner thighs, or under the upper arms. Some manufacturers recommend using their product only 14 to 21 days per month.

**ADVERSE REACTIONS**
**CNS:** dizziness, headache, fatigue.
**GI:** nausea, vomiting, diarrhea, abdominal pain.

**GU:** abnormal menstrual flow, including amenorrhea, spotting, breakthrough bleeding.
**Other:** breast pain, infection.

**INTERACTIONS**
**Herb-drug.** *Disulfiram, metronidazole:* Herbal products that contain alcohol may cause a disulfiram-like reaction. Advise patient to avoid using together.
*Estrogen-containing drugs, progesterone:* May increase blood glucose level and adverse effects of prescribed progestins. Advise patient to avoid using together and to consult a health care provider.
*Indomethacin:* Decreased anti-inflammatory effect. If used together, monitor patient for lack of therapeutic effect.

**CAUTIONS**
The addition of progesterone and the amount added may not be obvious on package labeling. Pregnant or breast-feeding women should avoid wild yam. Progesterone-containing products shouldn't be used by patients with breast cancer, liver disease, liver cancer, or undiagnosed uterine or urinary tract bleeding.

**NURSING CONSIDERATIONS**
• Find out why patient is using the herb.
• The term *natural progesterone* means that it's identical to human progesterone. It's produced synthetically from soybeans or other plant sources.
• Topical creams that contain progesterone may increase the adverse effects of prescribed progestins.

---

*Bold italic type* indicates that reaction may be life-threatening.

- Topical progesterone alone may not reduce the risk of osteoporosis.
- Breast examinations should be performed routinely, especially with prolonged progestin use.
- Monitor patient for adverse effects.

**Patient teaching**
- Advise patient to consult with his health care provider before using an herbal preparation because a treatment with proven efficacy may be available.
- Tell patient to remind pharmacist of any herbal and dietary supplements that he's taking, when filling a new prescription.
- Instruct patient to have appropriate medical evaluation before beginning any new herbal or dietary supplement.
- Urge patient to talk to her health care provider before using products containing progesterone.
- Warn patient not to take herb before seeking medical attention because doing so may delay diagnosis of a potentially serious medical condition.
- Instruct patient to apply cream to alternate body areas daily to ensure optimum absorption.
- Tell patient to promptly notify a health care provider about adverse effects or changes in symptoms.
- Caution pregnant and breastfeeding women that effects of this herb are unknown.
- Warn patient to keep all herbal products away from children and pets.

*Liquid may contain alcohol.

# willow

*Salix alba, S. nigra,* bay willow, black American willow, black willow, brittle willow, crack willow, Daphne willow, laurel willow, purple osier, pupurweide, violet willow, white willow

**Common trade names**
*Black Willow Bark Caps, White Willow Liquid Extract, Willow Bark caps, Willowprin*
Combination products: *Allerelief, Arth Plus, Cold-Control, Coldrin, Congest Ease, Menstrual-Ease, Migracin, PMS.O.S.*

**HOW SUPPLIED**
Available as crude inner bark, capsules, and dry and liquid extracts*. Extracts are often combined with root powder in commercial products.
*Capsules:* Powdered bark, 400 mg
*Dry extract:* 1:5 strength or standardized to 15% salicin

**ACTIONS & COMPONENTS**
Obtained from *Salix alba* or *S. nigra.* Bark contains 2% to 11% salicin, which is converted by the body into salicylic acid—similar to aspirin in its analgesic, antiinflammatory, and fever-reducing properties. Also contains 10% to 20% tannins, which have astringent properties, and flavonoids.

**USES**
Used for reducing fever, treating inflamed joints, easing GI disorders, and relieving pain. Also used in combination products for colds, flu, allergies, menstrual pain, pre-

menstrual syndrome, migraines, arthritis, and general pain and inflammation.

## DOSAGE & ADMINISTRATION
*Capsules:* One 400-mg capsule of willow bark with high salicin content equals $\frac{1}{10}$ of a 300-mg aspirin tablet. One capsule of a high-potency dry willow extract may equal $\frac{1}{4}$ aspirin tablet. Amount of willow in combination products would be much less.
*Decoction:* 1 or 2 tsp of bark added to 1 cup water, boiled, and then simmered 10 to 15 minutes; taken P.O. t.i.d. Manufacturers typically recommend 600 to 3,000 mg of bark equivalent up to 6 times q.d.

## ADVERSE REACTIONS
**GI:** stomach upset, esophageal cancer.
**GU:** kidney damage.
**Hepatic:** *liver necrosis.*
**Skin:** rash.
**Other:** bleeding episodes.

## INTERACTIONS
**Herb-drug.** *Anticoagulants:* Increased bleeding risk. Monitor patient for bleeding. Also, monitor PT and INR, as indicated. Advise patient to use together cautiously.
*Disulfiram, metronidazole:* Herbal products that contain alcohol may cause a disulfiram-like reaction. Advise patient to avoid using together.
*NSAIDs, including aspirin, ibuprofen:* Possible GI bleeding and ulceration. Monitor patient closely. Advise patient to avoid using together.

**Herb-herb.** Use with other herbal products should be avoided because of the risk that the tannin component will precipitate alkaloids.

## CAUTIONS
Willow shouldn't be used by patients hypersensitive to aspirin or salicylates or by those with gastritis, peptic ulcer disease, or kidney or liver dysfunction. It shouldn't be given to feverish children or adolescents because salicylates may cause Reye's syndrome. Pregnant women shouldn't use willow because it contains salicylates similar to aspirin, which are usually contraindicated in pregnancy.

## NURSING CONSIDERATIONS
• Find out why patient is using the herb.
🖉 ALERT: Willow bark products may be marketed as *aspirin-free* but may cause some of the same adverse reactions as aspirin, such as Reye's syndrome and salicylate hypersensitivity.
• Problems in breast-fed infants with usual analgesic doses of aspirin or willow haven't been documented. However, salicylates appear in breast milk and may cause macular rashes in breast-fed infants.
• Monitor patient for adverse reactions and signs of bleeding. Routinely check PT and INR, as indicated.
• Watch for sedative effects if patient takes a form that contains alcohol.

---

*Bold italic type* indicates that reaction may be life-threatening.

## Patient teaching

- Advise patient to consult with his health care provider before using an herbal preparation because a treatment with proven efficacy may be available.
- Tell patient to remind pharmacist of any herbal and dietary supplements that he's taking, when filling a new prescription.
- Ask whether patient has had adverse reactions to aspirin.
- Advise pregnant and breast-feeding women that effects of this herb are unknown and that aspirin, which is similar to some components in willow, is usually contraindicated in pregnancy.
- Caution parents not to give willow-containing products to feverish children or adolescents.
- Tell patient that taking willow with meals may reduce stomach upset.
- Instruct patient to separate doses of willow from other oral drugs to avoid interactions.
- Urge patient to have an appropriate medical evaluation before beginning an herbal supplement.
- Warn patient not to take herb before seeking medical attention because doing so may delay diagnosis of a potentially serious medical condition.
- Tell patient to promptly notify a health care provider about adverse effects or changes in symptoms.
- Warn patient to keep all herbal products away from children and pets.

## wintergreen

*Gaultheria procumbens,* boxberry, Canada tea, checkerberry, deerberry, gaultheria oil, ground berry, hillberry, mountain tea, partridge berry, spiceberry, teaberry, wax cluster

**Common trade names**
*Koong Yick Hung Fa Oil, Olbas Oil, Wintergreen Oil*

### HOW SUPPLIED
Available as oil, cream, lotion, gel, and liniment*.

### ACTIONS & COMPONENTS
Obtained from *Gaultheria procumbens.* Contains a volatile oil and a monotropitoside, gaultherin. 96% to 98% of volatile oil is methyl salicylate, and during steam distillation of the leaves, gaultherin is enzymatically hydrolyzed to methyl salicylate. Topical counterirritant and analgesic effects result from methyl salicylate, which is percutaneously absorbed and inhibits prostaglandin synthesis.

### USES
Used as an anodyne, analgesic, antasthmatic, digestive stimulant, antiseptic, and aromatic. Used to treat neuralgia, gastralgia, pleurisy, pleurodynia, ovarialgia, orchitis, epididymitis, diaphragmitis, uratic arthritis, and dysmenorrhea. Used topically as an antiseptic and to treat musculoskeletal pain and rheumatoid arthritis. Also used as a flavoring agent in candies and foods.

---

*Liquid may contain alcohol.

## DOSAGE & ADMINISTRATION

*Gels, lotions, ointments, liniments containing 10% to 60% methyl salicylate:* For adults and children older than age 2, herb is applied t.i.d. to q.i.d. topically to affected area.

*Oil:* 1 tsp wintergreen oil = about 7,000 mg salicylate or 21.5 adult aspirin (325 mg) tablets.

*Tea:* 1 tsp dried leaves added to 1 cup boiling water, P.O. q.d.

## ADVERSE REACTIONS

**CNS:** confusion.
**CV:** *pulmonary edema and collapse.*
**EENT:** tinnitus.
**GI:** GI distress, nausea, vomiting.
**GU:** *renal failure.*
**Hepatic:** *liver failure.*
**Metabolic:** metabolic acidosis.
**Musculoskeletal:** *rhabdomyolysis.*
**Respiratory:** hyperventilation, respiratory alkalosis.
**Skin:** contact dermatitis, diaphoresis.

## INTERACTIONS

**Herb-drug.** *Anticoagulants, antiplatelet drugs:* Increased bleeding risk. Monitor PT, INR, and patient closely.

*Antidiabetics, salicylates:* Large doses of topical or oral wintergreen may increase hypoglycemia. Monitor blood glucose level and patient closely.

**Herb-lifestyle.** *Alcohol use:* Use of oral wintergreen with alcohol may increase the risk for GI irritation. Advise patient to avoid using together.

## CAUTIONS

Women who are or wish to become pregnant or who are breast-feeding should avoid wintergreen, as should patients with severe asthma, nasal polyps, peptic or duodenal ulcers, or allergies to salicylates. Because methyl salicylate may play a role in Reye's syndrome, wintergreen shouldn't be used in infants, children, or adolescents during or after flulike symptoms.

## NURSING CONSIDERATIONS

• Find out why patient is using the herb.

⚡**ALERT:** Ingestion of more than small amounts of methyl salicylate is hazardous. Although the average lethal dose of methyl salicylate is estimated to be 10 ml for children and 30 ml for adults, as little as 4 ml has caused death in infants and 5 ml in children. Because of this toxicity, no drug product may contain more than 5% methyl salicylate or it will be regarded as misbranded. The FDA requires child-resistant containers for liquid forms that contain more than 5% methyl salicylate.

• The highest concentration of methyl salicylate used in candy flavoring is 0.04%.

• Monitor blood glucose level in patients who take large doses of wintergreen.

• Assess patient's response to herb.

## Patient teaching

• Advise patient to consult with his health care provider before using an herbal preparation because a treatment with proven efficacy may be available.

---

*Bold italic type* indicates that reaction may be life-threatening.

• Tell patient to remind pharmacist of any herbal and dietary supplements that he's taking, when filling a new prescription.

• Advise patient to inform health care provider before using wintergreen.

• Caution patient not to use a heating pad with topical wintergreen and not to apply topical wintergreen after strenuous exercise, especially on a hot, humid day. These situations increase transdermal absorption of wintergreen.

• Warn parents not to use wintergreen in infants, children, or adolescents during or after flulike symptoms.

• Instruct diabetic patient to closely monitor blood glucose level and to report changes to a health care provider. Review the signs and symptoms of hypoglycemia.

• If patient is taking wintergreen oil orally, stress the importance of proper dosing, because amounts from 4 to 10 ml of the oil have been fatal.

• Explain the sign and symptoms of salicylism, including tinnitus, nausea, vomiting, sweating, and hyperventilation. Tell patient to seek medical attention immediately if symptoms occur.

• Caution patient not to consume alcohol while taking this herb.

• Warn patient to keep all herbal products away from children and pets.

## witch hazel

*Hamamelis virginiana,* hamamelis water, hazel nut, snapping hazel, spotted alder, striped alder, tobacco wood, winter bloom

**Common trade names**
*Grandpa Soap Witch Hazel, Superhazel Medicate, Superhazel Medicated Pads, Thayer's Herbal Astringent, Tucks Medicated Pads, Witch Hazel Aftershave, Witch Hazel & Aloe Face Pads, Witch Hazel Beauty Gel/Lotion, Witch Hazel Leaf Low Alcohol, Witch Hazel Protective Gel*

### HOW SUPPLIED
Available as poultices, medicated pads and toilettes, soap, shampoo, aftershave, ointment and gel, decoction, suppositories, liquid*, liquid extract*, and gargle.
*Extracts:* Semisolid and liquid preparations corresponding to 5% to 10% drug
*Liquid extract:* 1:1 with 45% alcohol
*Ointment or gel:* 5 g witch hazel extract in 100-g ointment base
*Poultices:* 20% to 30% in a semisolid preparation
*Suppositories:* 0.1 to 1 g

### ACTIONS & COMPONENTS
Obtained from dried or fresh bark, leaves, and roots of *Hamamelis virginiana.* Contains flavonoids such as kaempferol and quercetin, tannins (up to 8%), and a volatile oil (about 0.5%). Oil contains small amounts of safrole and eugenol, sesquiterpenes, resin, wax, and

*Liquid may contain alcohol.

choline. Witch hazel's astringent and hemostatic properties result from high levels of tannins in leaf, bark, and extract. Extracts may cause vasoconstriction, decrease vascular permeability, tighten distended vessels, restore vessel tone, and stop bleeding immediately. Hamamelis water, or witch hazel water, doesn't contain tannins, so its astringent properties may result from other constituents or from alcohol content.

## USES

Used orally for diarrhea, mucous colitis, hematemesis, and hemoptysis. Primarily used topically for itching, insect bites, minor burns, local inflammation of skin and mucous membranes, varicose veins, hemorrhoids, and bruises. Witch hazel may enhance solar protection factor (SPF) when combined with other skin protective agents.

## DOSAGE & ADMINISTRATION

*Compress:* 5 to 10 g leaf or bark simmered in 250 ml of water.
*Hamamelis liquid extract (1:1 in 45% alcohol):* 2 to 4 ml P.O. t.i.d.
*Hamamelis water in 14% to 15% alcohol:* For anorectal disorders, applied up to 6 times q.d. or after each bowel movement. For minor cuts, burns, and wounds, affected area is soaked b.i.d. to q.i.d. for 15 to 30 minutes, or a compress is applied, soaked in the solution, and reapplied every few minutes for 20 to 30 minutes, 4 to 6 times q.d.
*Ointment:* 5 g witch hazel extract in 100 g ointment base. Applied topically.

*Suppository:* 1 suppository P.R. taken once q.d. to t.i.d.
*Tea:* 150 ml boiling water poured over 2 to 3 g drug and strained after 10 minutes. Taken P.O. t.i.d.

## ADVERSE REACTIONS

**GI:** nausea, vomiting, constipation, fecal impaction.
**Hepatic:** *liver damage.*
**Other:** contact allergy.

## INTERACTIONS

**Herb-drug.** *Disulfiram:* Herbal products that contain alcohol may cause a disulfiram-like reaction. Advise patient to avoid using together.

## CAUTIONS

Pregnant or breast-feeding women shouldn't use this herb. Although extracts of witch hazel are available commercially, internal use isn't recommended because of tannin and safrole content.

## NURSING CONSIDERATIONS

• Find out why patient is using the herb.
• Witch hazel water (hamamelis water) isn't intended for internal use.
• In doses of 1 g, witch hazel has caused nausea, vomiting, or constipation, possibly leading to fecal impaction.
• Long-term use may cause liver damage, possibly from tannin content.
• Monitor patient for adverse effects.

### Patient teaching

• Advise patient to consult with his health care provider before using

---

an herbal preparation because a treatment with proven efficacy may be available.

• Tell patient to remind pharmacist of any herbal and dietary supplements that he's taking, when filling a new prescription.

• Advise pregnant or breast-feeding patient to avoid oral use of this herb.

• Warn patient against taking more than 1 g of witch hazel to reduce the risk of nausea, vomiting, or constipation, possibly leading to fecal impaction.

• Inform patient that long-term oral use may lead to hepatic damage, possibly because of herb's tannin content.

• Warn patient not to take herb before seeking medical attention because doing so may delay diagnosis of a potentially serious medical condition.

• Tell patient to promptly notify a health care provider about adverse effects or changes in symptoms.

• Warn patient to keep all herbal products away from children and pets.

## wormwood

*Artemisia absinthium,* absinth, absinthe, absinthii herba, absinthium, ajenjo, armoise, green ginger, herbe d'absinthe, wermut, wermutkraut, wurmkraut

### Common trade names
*Wormwood Capsules, Wormwood Combo, Wormwood Organo Capsules, Wormwood Tincture*

### HOW SUPPLIED
Available as fresh or dried herb, powder, extract, and tincture*.

### ACTIONS & COMPONENTS
Obtained from fresh or dried shoots and leaves of *Artemisia absinthium.* Contains bitter principles absinthine, anabsinthin, artabsin, and others; a volatile oil containing up to 12% thujone; and flavones. Bitter principles may stimulate receptors in the taste buds of the tongue, triggering increased stomach acid secretion. Flavones may have spasmolytic activity. Thujone acts as an anthelmintic, causing expulsion of roundworms. It also acts on the same receptor in the brain as tetrahydrocannabinol, the active principle of marijuana. Interaction with these receptors may contribute to appetite stimulation and to the CNS toxicity seen with higher doses.

### USES
Used orally for anthelmintic and diaphoretic effects and to treat appetite loss, dyspepsia, bloating, and biliary dyskinesia. Used topically for wounds, skin ulcers, and insect bites. Also used as a flavoring agent for foods and aromatic alcoholic beverages such as vermouth. Extracts have been investigated for antimalarial, antimicrobial, and antifungal properties. The FDA has classified wormwood as an unsafe herb, although thujone-free derivatives have been approved for use in foods.

---

*Liquid may contain alcohol.

**DOSAGE & ADMINISTRATION**
Total oral daily dose shouldn't exceed 3 g of the herb as an aqueous extract.
*Decoction:* 1 handful of herb added to 1 L of boiling water for 5 minutes.
*Infusion:* 150 ml boiling water poured over ½ tsp of herb and strained after 10 minutes.
*Liquid extract:* 1 or 2 ml P.O. t.i.d.
*Tea:* 1 g of herb in 1 cup of water, P.O. 30 minutes before each meal.
*Tincture:* 10 to 30 gtt in sufficient water, P.O. t.i.d.

**ADVERSE REACTIONS**
**CNS:** headache, dizziness, restlessness, vertigo, trembling of the limbs, numbness of extremities, loss of intellect, paralysis, *seizures,* delirium, unconsciousness.
**GI:** vomiting, stomach and intestinal cramping, thirst.
**GU:** renal dysfunction.
**Skin:** topical eruptions.

**INTERACTIONS**
**Herb-drug.** *Acid-inhibitors, such as antacids, H₂-antagonists, proton pump inhibitors, or sucralfate:* Increased stomach acidity, decreased drug action. If used together, monitor patient's response closely.
*Anticoagulants, antiplatelet drugs:* May increase bleeding risk. Monitor PT, INR, and patient closely.
*Anticonvulsants:* May decrease effectiveness. Advise patient to avoid using together.
*Disulfiram, metronidazole:* Herbal products that contain alcohol may cause a disulfiram-like reaction.

Advise patient to avoid using together.
*Hypoglycemics:* May potentiate hypoglycemic effect. Monitor blood glucose level closely.
**Herb-herb.** *Thujone-containing herbs, such as oak moss, oriental arborvitae, sage, tansy, thuja, yarrow:* May increase risk of CNS toxicity. Advise patient to avoid using together.
**Herb-lifestyle.** *Alcohol use:* May cause CNS toxicity, especially with large doses or continuous use of wormwood. Advise patient to avoid using together.

**CAUTIONS**
Because of thujone content, consumption of large doses or continuous use of wormwood isn't recommended. Pregnant or breastfeeding women should avoid this herb, as should children, patients allergic to members of the Compositae family (such as sunflower seeds, chamomile, pistachios, hazelnuts, ragweed, chrysanthemums, marigolds, daisies), and patients with seizure disorders, bile duct obstruction, gallbladder inflammation, gallstones, liver disease, renal dysfunction, or gastric or duodenal ulcers.

**NURSING CONSIDERATIONS**
• Find out why patient is using the herb.
⚠ALERT: Many tinctures contain significant levels of alcohol, up to 20%, and may not be suitable for children, alcoholic patients, patients with liver disease, or patients who take disulfiram or metronidazole.

---

*Bold italic type* indicates that reaction may be life-threatening.

- The FDA has classified wormwood as an unsafe herb, although thujone-free derivatives have been approved for use in foods.
- Wormwood is aromatic and has a very bitter taste.
- Monitor INR and PT closely if patient takes an anticoagulant.
- Monitor blood glucose level and check for signs of hypoglycemia.
- If patient has a seizure disorder, watch for lack of anticonvulsant effectiveness and lack of seizure control.
- Monitor patient for adverse effects, such as absinthism, a CNS disorder characterized by vertigo, restlessness, and delirium.

**Patient teaching**
- Advise patient to consult with his health care provider before using an herbal preparation because a treatment with proven efficacy may be available.
- Tell patient to remind pharmacist of any herbal and dietary supplements that he's taking, when filling a new prescription.
- Advise patient to inform health care provider before using wormwood.
- Tell patient not to use wormwood in large doses or for continuous periods of time.
- Caution pregnant and breast-feeding women to avoid herb.
- Warn patient not to drink alcohol with this herb.
- Tell patient to promptly notify a health care provider about adverse effects or changes in symptoms.
- Instruct patient to store wormwood in a sealed container, protected from light.

- Warn patient to keep all herbal products away from children and pets.

## woundwort

*Anthyllis vulneraria,* kidney vetch, ladies' fingers, lamb's toes, staunchwort

**Common trade names**
*None known*

**HOW SUPPLIED**
Available as dried flowers and extract*.

**ACTIONS & COMPONENTS**
Obtained from *Anthyllis vulneraria.* Contains tannins, saponins, flavonoids, isoflavonoids, and lectins. Tannins provide astringent, hemostatic, anti-inflammatory, and antibacterial properties. Tannins may also exert vasoconstriction, decrease vascular permeability, tighten distended vessels, restore vessel tone, and stop bleeding immediately. Alcohol extract may have antiherpetic properties. Flavonoids in other herbs have been found to exert spasmolytic properties, which may account for woundwort's effect in controlling vomiting.

**USES**
Used internally for oral-pharyngeal disorders and both externally and internally for ulcers and wounds. Also used for cramps, dizziness, fever, gout, and menstrual disorders. Combined with other herbs to purify blood and to treat coughs and vomiting.

*Liquid may contain alcohol.

## DOSAGE & ADMINISTRATION

*Extract or poultice:* Applied externally.
*Tea:* 9 ml flowers to 250 ml of water.

## ADVERSE REACTIONS

**GI:** digestive complaints, nausea, vomiting, constipation, impaction.
**Hepatic:** *liver toxicity.*

## INTERACTIONS

None known.

## CAUTIONS

Because of tannin content, excessive ingestion of woundwort isn't recommended. Woundwort shouldn't be taken by children and patients who are pregnant, planning to become pregnant, or breast-feeding.

## NURSING CONSIDERATIONS

● Find out why patient is using the herb.
● Although no chemical interactions have been reported in clinical studies, consider the pharmacologic properties of the herb and its potential to interfere with therapeutic effects of conventional drugs.
● Monitor patient for GI symptoms, including nausea, vomiting, and constipation.
● Monitor patient's response to herb.
● Don't confuse woundwort with other herbs, such as *Stachys palustris,* marsh woundwort, or *S. sylvatica,* hedge woundwort. Other plants called woundwort include *Prunella vulgaris* and *Achillea millefolium.*

## Patient teaching

● Advise patient to consult with his health care provider before using an herbal preparation because a treatment with proven efficacy may be available.
● Tell patient to remind pharmacist of any herbal and dietary supplements that he's taking, when filling a new prescription.
● Tell patient to consult with health care provider before using woundwort.
● Inform patient that if woundwort is taken orally in large amounts, the tannin content may lead to nausea, vomiting, constipation, and possible fecal impaction.
● Warn patient not to take herb before seeking medical attention because doing so may delay diagnosis of a potentially serious medical condition.
● Inform patient that long-term use of herbs containing tannins may lead to liver toxicity.
● Warn patient to keep all herbal products away from children and pets.

---

*Bold italic type* indicates that reaction may be life-threatening.

Y

## yarrow

*Achillea millefolium,* achilee, Achillea, acuilee, band man's plaything, bauchweh, birangasifa, bloodwort, carpenter's weed, civan percemi, devil's plaything, erba da cartentieri, erba da falegname, gemeine schafgarbe, green arrow, herbe aux charpentiers, katzenkrat, milefolio, milfoil, millefolii flos, millefolii herba, millefolium, millefuille, noble yarrow, nose bleed, old man's pepper, roga mari, sanguinary, soldier's woundwort, staunchweed, tausendaugbram, thousand-leaf, woundwort

**Common trade names**
*Alcohol-Free Yarrow Flowers, Tincture of Yarrow, Yarrow Capsules, Yarrow Dock Tea, Yarrow Extract, Yarrow Flower*

### HOW SUPPLIED
Available as dried flower or herb, liquid extract*, tincture*, tea, or capsules.
*Capsules:* 340 mg, 350 mg
*Liquid:* 1:1, 250 mg/ml

### ACTIONS & COMPONENTS
Obtained from dried flowers and dried or fresh above-ground parts of *Achillea millefolium*. Contains a volatile oil (0.2% to 1.0%) composed of sesquiterpene lactones, terpinen-4-ol, polyenes, alkamids, flavonoids, tannins, thujone, and betaines. The sesquiterpene lactones found in the volatile oil are azulenes and chamazulenes. Azulenes may have antispasmodic and anti-inflammatory effects; tannins may have astringent effects. Terpinen-4-ol may have diuretic effects. Alcohol extracts and chamazulene may be active against *Staphylococcus aureus, Bacillus subtilis, Candida albicans, Mycobacterium smegmatis, Escherichia coli, Shigella sonnei*, and *Shigella flexneri*. These properties would explain the benefit of yarrow in controlling diarrhea and dysentery. Bitter principles found in yarrow may stimulate receptors in taste buds of the tongue, triggering increased stomach acid secretion.

Thujone, found in small amounts in yarrow, may contribute to appetite stimulation. The antipyretic and hypotensive effects of yarrow may be caused by alkaloids. Yarrow's volatile oil may exert CNS depressant effects.

### USES
Used orally for inducing sweating and for fever, common cold, hypertension, amenorrhea, dysentery, diarrhea, loss of appetite, mild or spasmodic GI tract discomfort, and specifically for thrombotic conditions with hypertension, including cerebral and coronary thromboses. Used topically for antibacterial and astringent properties in wound healing. Also used to treat bleeding hemorrhoids, menstrual complaints, and as a bath to remove perspiration. In the United States,

*Liquid may contain alcohol.

yarrow is only approved for use in alcoholic beverages, and the finished product must be thujone-free.

## DOSAGE & ADMINISTRATION
Total oral daily dose shouldn't exceed 4.5 g of yarrow herb, 3 g of yarrow flower, or 3 tsp of pressed juice from fresh plants.
*Liquid extract (1:1 in 25% alcohol):* 2 to 4 ml P.O. t.i.d.
*Partial bath:* 100 g of herb in 20 L water.
*Tea:* 2 g of herb added to boiling water; covered, steeped for 10 to 15 minutes, and then strained. 1 cup freshly made tea, taken t.i.d. to q.i.d.
*Tincture (1:5 in 45% alcohol):* 2 to 4 ml P.O. t.i.d.

## ADVERSE REACTIONS
**CNS:** sedation, CNS toxicities, headache, dizziness.
**GI:** vomiting, stomach and intestinal cramping.
**GU:** diuresis, renal dysfunction.
**Metabolic:** hypoglycemia.
**Skin:** contact dermatitis.

## INTERACTIONS
**Herb-drug.** *Acid-inhibiting drugs, such as antacids, H₂-antagonists, proton pump inhibitors, sucralfate:*

*Acid-inhibiting drugs, such as antacids, $H_2$-antagonists, proton pump inhibitors, sucralfate:* Increased stomach acid may decrease effectiveness. Advise patient to avoid using together.
*Anticoagulants:* May decrease effectiveness. Monitor PT, INR, and patient closely.
*Antidiabetics:* May potentiate hypoglycemic effect. Monitor blood glucose level closely.

*Antihypertensives, hypotensives:* Possible reduced effects. Monitor blood pressure closely.
*Barbiturates, benzodiazepines:* May increase sedative effects. Advise patient to avoid using together.
*Disulfiram, metronidazole:* Herbal products that contain alcohol may cause a disulfiram-like reaction. Advise patient to avoid using together.
*Sedative-hypnotics:* May increase sedative effects. Advise patient to avoid using together.
**Herb-herb.** *Sedative herbs:* May increase sedative effects. Advise patient to avoid using together.
*Thujone-containing herbs, such as oak moss, oriental arborvitae, sage, tansy, thuja, wormwood:* May increase the risk of CNS toxicity. Advise patient to avoid using together.
**Herb-lifestyle.** *Alcohol use:* May increase CNS toxicity. Advise patient to avoid using together.

## CAUTIONS
Pregnant or breast-feeding women should avoid this herb, as should patients allergic to members of the Compositae family, such as wormwood, honey, sunflower seeds, chamomile, pistachios, hazelnuts, ragweed, chrysanthemums, marigolds, and daisies.

## NURSING CONSIDERATIONS
● Find out why patient is using the herb.
● Closely monitor INR and PT in patients who take anticoagulants with this herb.

---

*Bold italic type* indicates that reaction may be life-threatening.

- Closely monitor patient's serum electrolytes, blood pressure, and blood glucose level.

**Patient teaching**

- Advise patient to consult with his health care provider before using an herbal preparation because a treatment with proven efficacy may be available.
- Tell patient to remind pharmacist of any herbal and dietary supplements that he's taking, when filling a new prescription.
- Advise patient to consult with his health care provider before using yarrow.
- Caution patient not to drink alcohol with this herb.
- Tell patient that taking yarrow with sedatives or other CNS depressant drugs may cause increased sedation or lethargy.
- Tell patient to avoid hazardous activities until full CNS effects of herb are known.
- Advise patient to protect yarrow from light and moisture and not to store essential oil in a synthetic container.
- Warn patient to keep all herbal products away from children and pets.

## yellow root

*Xanthorrhiza simplicissima,*
parsley-leaved yellow root,
shrub yellow root, yellow wort

**Common trade names**
*Yellowroot Liquid Extract*

**HOW SUPPLIED**
Available as a tincture*.

**ACTIONS & COMPONENTS**
Obtained from roots of *Xanthorrhiza simplicissima.* Contains several alkaloids: berberine, jatrorhizine, and mognoflorine. Berberine is the most abundant. Two isoquinoline alkaloids, iriodenine and palmitin, also have been identified. Most pharmacologic activity is from berberine, which may have antihypertensive, antitumor, antibacterial, antifungal, and antiprotozoal effects.

**USES**
Used to treat diabetes, hypertension, and infections. Recent studies documenting antineoplastic effects may lead to expanded interest in berberine-containing plants, such as yellow root, in treating cancer.

**DOSAGE & ADMINISTRATION**
Not well documented.

**ADVERSE REACTIONS**
**CNS:** tremors, sedation.
**CV:** reflex tachycardia.
**GI:** GI irritation, vomiting.
**Other:** *arsenic poisoning.*

**INTERACTIONS**
**Herb-drug.** *Heparin:* Reduced effectiveness. Monitor PT, INR, and patient closely if used together. *Paclitaxel:* Reduced effectiveness. Advise patient to avoid using together.

**CAUTIONS**
Pregnant or breast-feeding women shouldn't use this herb. Patients with cardiac conditions or diabetes should use it cautiously.

*Liquid may contain alcohol.

## NURSING CONSIDERATIONS

• Find out why patient is using the herb.
• Monitor patient's response to herbal therapy.
• Don't confuse yellow root with goldenseal, which is also known as yellow root and also contains berberine.

### Patient teaching

• Advise patient to consult with his health care provider before using an herbal preparation because a treatment with proven efficacy may be available.
• Tell patient to remind pharmacist of any herbal and dietary supplements that he's taking, when filling a new prescription.
• Explain the berberine content of this herb and its effects on blood pressure and blood clotting.
• Warn patient not to take herb before seeking medical attention because doing so may delay diagnosis of a potentially serious medical condition.
• Caution patient not to confuse yellow root with other herbs with similar names.
• Tell patient to promptly notify a health care provider about adverse effects or changes in symptoms.
• Warn patient to keep all herbal products away from children and pets.

## yerba maté

*Ilex paraguariensis,*
Bartholomew's tea, campeche, gaucho, ilex, jaguar, Jesuit's tea, la hoja, la mulata, mate, oro verde, Paraguay tea, payadito

**Common trade names**
*None known*

### HOW SUPPLIED

Available as dried leaves and as liquid extract*.
*Extract:* 1:1 in 25% alcohol

### ACTIONS & COMPONENTS

Obtained from *Ilex paraguariensis.* Leaves contain several methylxanthines, chiefly caffeine (0.2% to 2.0%) theobromine (0.1% to 0.2%), and theophylline (0.05%). Leaves also contain flavonoids kaempferol and quercetin, as well as terpenoids, ursolic acid, beta-amyrin, ilexides A and B, and tannins (4% to 16%). Carotene, vitamins A and D, riboflavin, ascorbic acid, and nicotinic acid are present as well. Hepatotoxic pyrrolizadine alkaloids have also been reported. Most pharmacologic effects, including diuresis, appetite suppression, smooth muscle relaxation, and CNS, respiratory, skeletal, and cardiac muscle stimulation, are caused by the methylxanthines, especially caffeine.

### USES

Used as a CNS stimulant for drowsiness or fatigue and as a mild analgesic for headaches caused by fatigue. It's also been used as a diuretic and appetite suppressant.

---

*Bold italic type* indicates that reaction may be life-threatening.

## DOSAGE & ADMINISTRATION

Average effective daily dose of caffeine in adults is 100 to 200 mg, about 1 to 2 cups of coffee.

*Infusion:* 1 tsp or 2 to 4 g dried leaves steeped in 1 cup hot water for 5 to 10 minutes and then strained. 3 cups taken P.O. q.d.

*Tincture (1:1 in 25% alcohol):* 2 to 4 ml P.O. t.i.d.

## ADVERSE REACTIONS

**CNS:** sleeplessness, restlessness, irritability, anxiety, tremor, headache and sleep disturbances.
**CV:** palpitations.
**EENT:** *esophageal cancer.*
**GU:** *bladder cancers.*
**Hepatic:** *liver toxicity.*

## INTERACTIONS

**Herb-drug.** *Other CNS stimulants:* Additive stimulatory and diuretic effects. Advise patient to avoid using together.
**Herb-food.** *Caffeine:* Additive stimulatory and diuretic effects. Advise patient to avoid using together.

## CAUTIONS

Pregnant or breast-feeding women should avoid this herb, as should patients with CV disease (such as hypertension), ischemic heart disease, or chronic liver disease.

## NURSING CONSIDERATIONS

• Find out why patient is using the herb.
• Watch for evidence of excessive stimulation, such as hypertension, restlessness, and sleeplessness.

• Headache and sleep disturbances are signs of withdrawal from yerba maté.
• Consumption of products containing caffeine may cause additive effects.
• Monitor patient's response to herb.

**Patient teaching**

• Advise patient to consult with his health care provider before using an herbal preparation because a treatment with proven efficacy may be available.
• Tell patient to remind pharmacist of any herbal and dietary supplements that he's taking, when filling a new prescription.
• Inform patient that this herb is a source of caffeine and theophylline, and combining with other caffeine-containing beverages or other stimulants could lead to excessive stimulation.
• Caution patient about possible liver toxicity and possible increased cancer risk.
• If evidence of excessive stimulation arises, suggest that patient decrease or eliminate consumption of herb.
• Urge patient to promptly notify a health care provider about adverse effects or changes in symptoms.
• Tell patient that he may have withdrawal symptoms, such as headache and sleep disturbances, when he stops taking yerba maté.
• Warn patient to keep all herbal products away from children and pets.

## yerba santa

*Eriodictyon californicum,* bear's weed, consumptive's weed, gum bush, gum plant, holy weed, mountain balm, sacred herb, tarweed

**Common trade names**
*Feminease, Respirtone*

**HOW SUPPLIED**
Available as fresh or dried herb, powdered herb, liquid, and ointment.

**ACTIONS & COMPONENTS**
Obtained from *Eriodictyon californicum.* Contains at least 12 flavonoids, including eriodictyonine (6%), eriodictyol (0.5%), and eriodictine, as well as four flavones: cirsimaritin, chrysoeriol, hispidulin, and chrysin. Eriodictyol is a mild expectorant. Resins in the plant have a pleasant taste and aroma, explaining why it's used to mask bitter taste of certain drugs or as a flavoring in foods and beverages. Several flavones and flavonoids inhibit formation of active metabolites of the carcinogen benzopyrene, thus showing chemopreventive potential. Herb is also a mild diuretic.

**USES**
Used orally to treat coughs, colds, asthma, and bronchitis. Used topically to treat bruises, sprains, skin wounds, poison ivy, and insect bites.

**DOSAGE & ADMINISTRATION**
*Fresh leaves:* Chewed p.r.n.

*Tea:* 1 tsp dried or fresh leaves added to 1 cup hot water, taken P.O. 30 minutes before h.s.

**ADVERSE REACTIONS**
**GI:** sticky residue on teeth after chewing fresh leaves.

**INTERACTIONS**
None reported.

**CAUTIONS**
Pregnant or breast-feeding women shouldn't use this herb.

**NURSING CONSIDERATIONS**
• Find out why patient is using the herb.
• Although no chemical interactions have been reported in clinical studies, consider the pharmacologic properties of the herb and its potential to interfere with therapeutic effects of conventional drugs.
• Monitor patient's response to herbal therapy.

**Patient teaching**
• Advise patient to consult with his health care provider before using an herbal preparation because a treatment with proven efficacy may be available.
• Tell patient to remind pharmacist of any herbal and dietary supplements that he's taking, when filling a new prescription.
• Advise patient that chewing the fresh leaves will leave a sticky residue on his teeth.
• Warn patient not to take herb for a chronic cough or cold before seeking medical attention because doing so may delay diagnosis of a

---

*Bold italic type* indicates that reaction may be life-threatening.

potentially serious medical condition.

• Instruct patient to promptly notify a health care provider about adverse effects or changes in symptoms.

• Warn patient to keep all herbal products away from children and pets.

## yew

*Taxus baccata, T. brevifolia, T. canadenis, T. cuspidata, T. cuspididata, T. floridana,* American yew, chinwood, English yew, globe-berry, Japanese yew, Oregon yew, Pacific or Western yew

**Common trade names**
*Vital Yew, Yew Tea*

### HOW SUPPLIED
Available as a tincture*, capsules, and a salve of yew bark.

### ACTIONS & COMPONENTS
Obtained from bark and branch tips of *Taxus brevifolia*. Contains a mixture of about 19 taxane-type diterpene esters referred to as taxines. Most prominent of these are paclitaxel and taxine A and B. Other constituents include taxicatin, milossine, and ephedrine. Paclitaxel inhibits cell division by binding to the β-tubulin subunit of microtubules, which prevents the disassembly of microtubules. Cells are thus arrested in mitosis.

### USES
Used for promoting menstruation, eliminating tapeworms, and treating tonsillitis. Taxol is the trade name for the drug paclitaxel, which is isolated from the bark of *T. brevifolia*. Taxotere is the trade name of docetaxel, a more potent analogue of paclitaxel. Paclitaxel is FDA-approved for treating metastatic, ovarian, and breast cancers. Pending results of clinical trials, it may be approved for other cancers, such as melanoma and lung and esophageal cancers.

### DOSAGE & ADMINISTRATION
*For cancers:* Optimal doses and administration protocols are still being determined in ongoing clinical trials.
*Infusion:* Bark or needles are added to 1 cup hot water. Taken P.O. once q.d.
*Tinctures:* Doses of yew bark tinctures vary widely.

### ADVERSE REACTIONS
**CNS:** dizziness, *unconsciousness.*
**CV:** *bradycardia,* tachycardia, hypotension, *heart failure.*
**EENT:** mydriasis, dry mouth, reddened lips.
**GI:** abdominal cramps, nausea, vomiting.
**GU:** miscarriage.
**Respiratory:** dyspnea, *respiratory failure.*
**Skin:** rash, pallor, cyanosis.

### INTERACTIONS
**Herb-drug.** *Other chemotherapeutic drugs:* Potentiation of myelosuppression and interactions with other chemotherapeutic drugs. Advise patient to use together only with extreme caution and only un-

---

*Liquid may contain alcohol.

der direct supervision of a health care provider.

## CAUTIONS
Women who are pregnant or breast-feeding shouldn't use this herb. Because of the potential toxicity of multiple constituents, herbal formulations of the yew tree should be used only with extreme caution, if at all.

## NURSING CONSIDERATIONS
• Find out why patient is using the herb.

⚠ALERT: Most parts of the yew plant are highly poisonous. Ingestion of 50 to 100 g of yew needles or berries has been fatal and is especially dangerous in children. Treatment includes digoxin-specific fragment antigen-binding antibodies and gastric lavage followed by administration of charcoal. Supportive measures to treat cardiac effects and other symptoms may also be indicated.

• Keep emergency equipment readily available.

• Monitor vital signs and ECG if large amounts of the herb are ingested.

• Because of the potential extreme toxicity of this herb, only prescription forms of paclitaxel should be used, and then only under the careful guidance of an oncologist.

• Some common hypersensitivity reactions to paclitaxel have been reduced by giving the drug as a slow infusion over 6 to 24 hours.

• Monitor patient's level of consciousness, and report changes immediately to a health care provider.

## Patient teaching
• Advise patient to consult with his health care provider before using an herbal preparation because a treatment with proven efficacy may be available.

• Tell patient to remind pharmacist of any herbal and dietary supplements that he's taking, when filling a new prescription.

• If patient chooses to use this herb for a cancerous condition, warn him to use it only on the recommendation of an oncologist.

• Advise patient of the need for regular follow-up care with an oncologist if taking this herb for cancer.

• Urge patient to report adverse effects promptly to a health care provider.

• Tell patient to seek emergency medical care if he develops adverse effects or a toxic response.

• Warn patient of the danger of taking this toxic herb without medical supervision.

• Warn patient to keep all herbal products away from children and pets.

## yohimbe

*Corynanthe yohimbi,*
*Pausinystalia yohimbe,*
aphrodien, corynine, yohimbehe, yohimbine

### Common trade names
*Aphrodyne, Dayto Himbin, Potensan, Yobinol, Yocon, Yohimbine HCL, Yohimbehe, Yohimbe Power MAX for Women, Yohimmex*

---

## HOW SUPPLIED
Available as tablets and tinctures*.
*Tablets:* Yohimbine hydrochloro-
thiazide (HCL) 3 mg, 5.4 mg
*Tinctures:* Standardized to yohim-
bine

## ACTIONS & COMPONENTS
Obtained from bark of *Pausinystalia yohimbe.* Contains tannins
and 2.7% to 5.9% indole alkaloids,
especially yohimbine. Other alkaloids include ajamalicin, dihydro-
yohimbine, corynanthein, and others. Effects of yohimbine are medi-
ated mostly via selective blockade
of alpha$_2$ receptors, primarily in
CNS. At higher levels, yohimbine
acts as an agonist at alpha$_1$, serotonin, and dopamine receptors.
Yohimbine may also inhibit MAO
and slow L-type calcium channels
in heart and blood vessels.

Yohimbe increases penile cav-
ernous blood flow in men with
erectile dysfunction. It also increases autonomic nerve activity
from the brain to genital tissues
and increases reflex excitability in
the sacral region of the spinal cord.

## USES
Primarily used as an aphrodisiac
and to treat organic and psychogenic erectile dysfunction in men.
Also used at higher doses to treat
orthostatic hypotension.

## DOSAGE & ADMINISTRATION
*For erectile dysfunction:* 5.4 mg
P.O. t.i.d. Doses of 20 to 30 mg
have been shown to significantly
increase blood pressure. Yohimbe
bark alcoholic extracts are usually
standardized to contain a certain
amount of yohimbine.

## ADVERSE REACTIONS
**CNS:** nervousness, anxiety, irritability, increased motor activity,
headache, anorexia, dizziness, insomnia, manic or psychotic episodes, paralysis.
**CV:** tachycardia, hypotension, hypertension.
**GI:** abdominal discomfort, diarrhea, nausea.
**GU:** *acute renal failure.*

## INTERACTIONS
**Herb-drug.** *Antihypertensives, including adrenergics and clonidine:*
May precipitate clonidine withdrawal hypertensive crisis. Advise
patient to avoid using together.
*Anxiolytics:* May block action of
these drugs. Advise patient to
avoid using together.
*CNS-stimulating drugs:* Enhanced
effects. Advise patient to avoid using together.
*Naltrexone:* Increased sensitivity
to yohimbe, potentiating adverse
reactions. Advise patient to avoid
using together.
*Selective serotonin reuptake in-
hibitors and tricyclic antidepressants:* May cause serum serotonin
levels to increase dangerously. Advise patient to avoid using together.
**Herb-food.** *Caffeine:* Enhanced effect. Advise patient to avoid using
together.
*Tyramine-containing foods:* Because of its reported weak MAO-
inhibiting activity, yohimbe may
interact with tyramine-containing
foods. Advise patient to avoid using together.

*Liquid may contain alcohol.

**Herb-lifestyle.** *Alcohol use:* May have additive effects. Advise patient to avoid using together.

## CAUTIONS
Yohimbe shouldn't be used by children, geriatric patients, pregnant women, breast-feeding women, and people with psychiatric disorders, liver disease, kidney disease, hyperthyroidism, angina pectoris, or CV disease, especially hypertension.

## NURSING CONSIDERATIONS
• Find out why patient is using the herb.
• Herb is used mainly by men to help with impotence, but some women may also take it for an aphrodisiac effect.
• Be alert for possible CNS and blood pressure changes.
• Herb can significantly increase blood pressure in patients with orthostatic hypotension caused by autonomic failure or multisystem atrophy.
• Follow patient's vital signs and ECG closely.
• Monitor patient for adverse effects or changes in condition.

**Patient teaching**
• Advise patient to consult with his health care provider before using an herbal preparation because a treatment with proven efficacy may be available.
• Tell patient to remind pharmacist of any herbal and dietary supplements that he's taking, when filling a new prescription.

• Inform patient that herb is considered by many to have a high risk-to-benefit ratio.
• Instruct patient not to take caffeine products while also taking this herb.
• Warn patient not to take herb for erectile dysfunction before seeking medical attention because doing so may delay diagnosis of a potentially serious medical condition.
• Instruct patient to report adverse effects promptly to a health care provider.
• Warn patient to keep all herbal products away from children and pets.

---

*Bold italic type* indicates that reaction may be life-threatening.

# Supplemental vitamins and minerals

| Name and recommended daily allowances | Actions | Special considerations |
|---|---|---|
| **Vitamin A (retinol)** *Women:* 800 mcg retinol equivalents (RE), or 4,000 IU *Pregnant women:* Supplement with beta-carotene to form necessary retinol. *Men:* 1,000 mcg RE, or 5,000 IU | • Promotes growth, differentiates and maintains epithelial tissue • Fights infection • Aids in bone and teeth formation • Promotes wound healing • Maintains good vision (rod and cone function; adaptation to light changes) | • Best food sources include liver, fish liver oil, tuna, mackerel, eggs, cheese, fortified milk, and fruits and vegetables containing beta-carotene that can be converted to retinol in the body. • Best if taken with B complex; vitamins C, D, and E; and calcium, phosphorus, and zinc. • Mineral oil may decrease GI absorption of vitamin A. • Supplementation of over 6,000 IU daily of retinol without beta-carotene is associated with birth defects. • Should be taken during or shortly after a meal. • Vitamin A and accutane enhance the toxicity of each. • Patients taking colestipol may need more vitamin A. |
| **Beta-carotene** Forms vitamin A when retinol isn't in the diet. The amount of beta-carotene needed to meet the vitamin A requirement is roughly double that of retinol: 6 mcg beta-carotene = 1 mcg RE = 3.33 IU. Safe supplementation range is 5-25,000 IU. | • Same as retinol • Taken with other antioxidants, may help prevent cancer • Enhances immune system | • Best food sources include dark green and yellow fruits and vegetables, such as carrots, cantaloupe, sweet potato, papaya, apricots, and squash. • Best if taken with a meal, because fat facilitates absorption. • Should be taken with a network of other antioxidants: vitamins E and C, selenium, zinc. • Hypercarotenemia causes yellowing of the palms, nasolabial folds, and soles of the feet, but not of the sclerae, which distinguishes it from jaundice. |
| **Vitamin $B_1$ (thiamine)** *Women:* 1-1.1 mg | • Aids digestion, especially carbohydrates • Improves mental attitude and maintains | • Best food sources include brewer's yeast, whole brown rice, soybeans, tofu, whole *(continued)* |

| Name and recommended daily allowances | Actions | Special considerations |
|---|---|---|
| **Vitamin B₁** *(continued)* *Pregnant women:* 1.5 mg *Men:* 1-1.5 mg | a healthy nervous system • Stimulates good muscle tone and appetite | wheat, oatmeal, wheat germ, milk, and most vegetables. • Best if taken with B complex, vitamin C, and manganese. • Increased physical activity combined with carbohydrate loading may promote depletion. • Allicin, a factor in onions and garlic, promotes the absorption of vitamin B₁. • No known toxic ranges with oral supplementation because B vitamins are water soluble. • Chronic alcoholism inhibits absorption of vitamin B₁ from the intestinal lumen. • Long-term use of loop diuretics depletes vitamin B₁. |
| **Vitamin B₂ (riboflavin)** *Women:* 1.2-1.3 mg *Pregnant women:* 1.6 mg *Men:* 1.2-1.5 mg | • Needed for carbohydrate, protein, and fat metabolism • Aids in RBC formation • Promotes healthy vision, nails | • Best food sources include milk, brewer's yeast, liver, cheese, fish, eggs, leafy green vegetables, broccoli, beef, and pork. • Riboflavin needs gastric acids to be released from foods. • Best if taken with B complex, folic acid, and vitamin C. • Urine will become discolored with high doses of riboflavin, which can affect urinalysis results. |
| **Vitamin B₃ (niacin, nicotinic acid)** *Women:* 15 mg *Pregnant women:* 17 mg *Men:* 19-20 mg | • Improves circulation and reduces cholesterol level • Needed for carbohydrate, fat, and protein metabolism • Needed for healthy skin, nervous system, and digestive tract | • Best food sources include eggs, organ meats, fortified grains, peanuts, peanut butter, brewer's yeast, cottage cheese, broccoli, peas, and mushrooms. • Best if taken with B complex, vitamin C, magnesium, and potassium. • Hepatotoxicity is more likely with high-dose, sustained- |

| Name and recommended daily allowances | Actions | Special considerations |
|---|---|---|
| **Vitamin B$_3$** *(continued)* | | release niacin therapy. Such therapy shouldn't be used without a doctor's supervision. |
| **Vitamin B$_5$ (pantothenic acid)** *Women:* 4-7 mg *Pregnant women:* 4-7 mg *Men:* 4-7 mg | • Aids in stress resistance • Assists in release of energy from carbohydrates, fat, and protein metabolism • Needed for healthy skin, nervous system, and digestive tract | • Best food sources include meats, whole grain cereals, chicken, milk, corn, avocado, nuts, and eggs. • Best if taken with B complex and vitamin C. |
| **Vitamin B$_6$ (pyridoxamine)** | • Needed for carbohydrate, fat, and protein metabolism • Aids in antibody and RBC formation • Helps maintain balance of sodium and phosphorus • Acts as a natural diuretic • Essential for neurotransmitter synthesis • Maintains immune function | • Best food sources include brewer's yeast, liver, bananas, soybeans, cabbage, brown rice, avocado, peanuts, and walnuts. • Best if taken with B complex, vitamin C, magnesium, and potassium. • Oral contraceptives, theophylline, isoniazid, cycloserine, penicillamine, and hydralazine interfere with vitamin B$_6$ metabolism or action. • Caution must be used when prescribing large daily doses for premenstrual syndrome, and nausea and vomiting of pregnancy because of potential risk of neurotoxicity. |
| **Vitamin B$_9$ (folic acid)** *Women:* 150-180 mcg *Pregnant women:* 400 mcg *Men:* 150-200 mcg | • Helps prevent birth defects and improve lactation • Important in RBC formation • Needed for growth and division of body cells • May relieve depression and certain headaches | • Best food sources include green leafy vegetables, beans, liver, egg yolk, brewer's yeast, whole wheat, peanuts, beef liver, and soybean flour. • Best if taken with B complex, vitamin B$_{12}$, vitamin C, and biotin. |

*(continued)*

| Name and recommended daily allowances | Actions | Special considerations |
|---|---|---|
| **Vitamin B$_9$** *(continued)* | • Protects against osteoporosis<br>• Indicated with vitamin B$_{12}$ for macrocytic anemia | • Vitamin C helps reduce the amount of folic acid lost to excretion.<br>• Estrogens, alcohol, some chemotherapy drugs, sulfasalazine, barbiturates, and anticonvulsants interfere with folate absorption.<br>• High-dose folic acid supplementation should be used with extreme caution in those with epilepsy. It may increase seizure activity.<br>• Because folic acid supplementation can mask vitamin B$_{12}$ deficiency, which can lead to irreversible neurologic damage, folic acid supplementation should always include vitamin B$_{12}$. |
| **Vitamin B$_{12}$ (cyanocobalamin)** *Women:* 2.0 mcg *Pregnant women:* 2.2 mcg *Men:* 2.0 mcg | • Needed for all blood cell formation and a healthy nervous system<br>• Helps to improve the appetite and increase energy<br>• Needed for carbohydrate, fat, and protein metabolism<br>• Together with folic acid and vitamin B$_6$, vitamin B$_{12}$ has been shown to reduce high plasma levels of homocysteine, which is an independent risk factor for CV disease | • Best food sources include liver, kidney, milk, eggs, fish, cheese, and yogurt.<br>• Best if taken with B complex, folic acid, vitamin C, potassium, and calcium.<br>• Vegetarians are at a higher risk for low B$_{12}$ levels than nonvegetarians.<br>• People need adequate gastric intrinsic factor to convert oral vitamin B$_{12}$ to its active form.<br>• Parenteral cyanocobalamin given for B$_{12}$ deficiency caused by malabsorption should be given I.M. or by deep S.C. route but never I.V. |
| **B complex** | • Helps nervous system function and maintains a healthy digestive tract | • Best food sources include brewer's yeast, liver, wheat germ, whole grains, nuts, and beans. |

| Name and recommended daily allowances | Actions | Special considerations |
|---|---|---|
| **B complex** *(continued)* | • Needed for carbohydrate, fat, and protein metabolism<br>• Maintains the health of eyes, skin, hair, and liver | • Best if taken with vitamin C, vitamin E, calcium, and phosphorus.<br>• A balanced B complex helps to ensure proper absorption of all the B vitamins. |
| **Vitamin C** *Women:* 60 mg *Pregnant women:* 70 mg *Men:* 60 mg | • Helps heal wounds and burns and helps prevent hemorrhaging<br>• Reduces serum cholesterol level<br>• Aids in preventing many bacterial and viral infections<br>• Fights toxins caused by smoke pollution<br>• Maintains healthy blood vessels<br>• Useful in treating allergies<br>• Aids in iron absorption<br>• Protects against cancer | • Best food sources include citrus fruits, berries, tomatoes, broccoli, green and red pepper, dark leafy greens, kiwi, papaya, strawberries, Brussels sprouts, and potatoes.<br>• More effective with all other vitamins, minerals, calcium, and magnesium.<br>• Interferes with blood tests for vitamin $B_{12}$.<br>• High doses of more than 2,000 mg daily can cause diarrhea, gas, or stomach upset.<br>• Buffered vitamin C is available if regular vitamin C upsets the stomach.<br>• Cooking vegetables decreases their vitamin C content. |
| **Vitamin D** *Women:* 200 IU *Pregnant women:* 400 IU *Men:* 200 IU *Adults ages 51-70:* 400 IU | • Needed for absorption and utilization of calcium and phosphorus, to form strong bones and teeth<br>• Helps maintain normal heart action and stable nervous system<br>• Helps to control blood glucose level<br>• Reduces cartilage damage in people with osteoarthritis and may decrease the severity of rheumatoid arthritis | • Best food sources include fortified milk, fish liver oil, sardines, tuna, salmon, and mackerel.<br>• Sunlight is the most common natural source: a fair-skinned person needs 20 to 30 minutes daily; a dark-skinned person needs about 3 hours daily.<br>• More than 1,000 IU of vitamin D daily can cause illness. Symptoms include excessive thirst, vomiting, diarrhea, muscle problems, and itching skin.<br>• Drug interactions that may cause mineral imbalances include: digoxin, verapamil, and thiazide diuretics. |

*(continued)*

| Name and recommended daily allowances | Actions | Special considerations |
| --- | --- | --- |
| **Vitamin E**<br>*Women:* 12 IU<br>*Pregnant women:* 15 IU<br>*Men:* 15 IU<br>The recommended dose for disease prevention and treatment for adults is 400-800 IU/day. | • Potent antioxidant that, along with vitamin C, helps prevent the breakdown of cells by free radicals<br>• Protects lungs against air pollution<br>• Alleviates fatigue and protects RBCs<br>• Prevents blood clots<br>• Helps wounds heal faster | • Best food sources include wheat germ, soybeans, nuts, leafy greens, sunflower, walnut, and safflower oils, sweet potato, whole wheat, and liver.<br>• Best if taken with B complex, vitamin C, magnesium, and selenium.<br>• Natural vitamin E (d-alpha-tocopherol) is the preferred form because it's absorbed best and most actively.<br>• Chronic alcoholism depletes vitamin E stores in the liver.<br>• May prolong bleeding time and enhance antiplatelet drugs.<br>• High doses may interfere with vitamin K activity.<br>• Cholestyramine and colestipol may decrease absorption of vitamin E.<br>• Selenium enhances antioxidant activity of vitamin E.<br>• Improves vitamin A effectiveness.<br>• Considered generally nontoxic. In doses of more than 1,200 IU daily, it can cause nausea, gas, diarrhea, and heart palpitations. |
| **Vitamin H (biotin)**<br>*Women:* 30-100 mcg<br>*Pregnant women:* 30-100 mcg<br>*Men:* 30-100 mcg<br>Because biotin is synthesized in the intestinal microflora, deficiency is rare. | • Needed for carbohydrate, fat, and protein metabolism<br>• Helps fatty acid and amino acid synthesis<br>• Improves blood glucose control in diabetic patients by enhancing insulin sensitivity<br>• Needed for healthy hair, skin, and nails | • Best food sources include liver, almonds, peanuts, pecans, walnuts, cooked eggs, cauliflower, brewer's yeast, oat bran, and unpolished rice.<br>• Works best when taken with B complex and vitamin C.<br>• Isn't absorbed if taken with raw egg whites.<br>• Requirements may rise if a person takes sulfa drugs or estrogen, or drinks alcohol. |

| Name and recommended daily allowances | Actions | Special considerations |
|---|---|---|
| **Vitamin H** *(continued)* | | • Deficiency may result from prolonged use of anticonvulsant drugs or antibiotics.<br>• Biotin is nontoxic; no adverse effects have been noted, even at high doses.<br>• Food processing can destroy biotin. |
| **Vitamin K (phytomenadione)** *Women:* 65 mcg *Pregnant women:* 65 mcg *Men:* 80 mcg | • Needed for prothrombin formation and blood coagulation; for normal liver functioning; and for the bones to use calcium<br>• May prevent kidney stones | • Best food sources include dark green leafy vegetables, especially kale, spinach, turnip greens, broccoli, and cabbage; beef liver; egg yolk; and safflower oil.<br>• Natural vitamin K taken orally is generally nontoxic.<br>• Large doses of the synthetic form of vitamin K, which are usually given to prevent bleeding in certain conditions, may cause anemia and liver damage.<br>• Vitamin K can interfere with the action of anticoagulants such as warfarin.<br>• X-rays and radiation can raise vitamin K requirements.<br>• Extended use of antibiotics may result in vitamin K deficiency.<br>• Aspirin, cholestyramine, and mineral oil laxatives may decrease vitamin K levels.<br>• Freezing foods may destroy vitamin K, but heating doesn't affect it. |
| **Calcium** *Women:* 800-1,200 mg *Pregnant women:* 1,200 mg *Men:* 800-1,200 mg | • Needed in developing and maintaining bones and teeth, in maintaining heartbeat and proper blood pressure, and in | • Best food sources include milk, yogurt, cottage cheese, cheese, broccoli, dark leafy greens, canned salmon, mackerel, sardines, fortified orange juice, soymilk, soybean nuts, |

*(continued)*

| Name and recommended daily allowances | Actions | Special considerations |
|---|---|---|
| **Calcium** *(continued)* | transmitting nerve impulses<br>• Reduces pregnancy risks, such as high blood pressure and preeclampsia<br>• Helps maintain proper cholesterol levels | hard or mineral water, almonds, and brazil nuts.<br>• Supplements should be taken in small doses throughout the day.<br>• High-protein diets cause calcium excretion.<br>• Increased urinary calcium loss is also caused by sodium, phosphorus, sugar, saturated fats, caffeine, alcohol, and aluminum-containing antacids.<br>• Excess calcium can interfere with the absorption of iron, zinc, magnesium, iodine, manganese, and copper.<br>• Doses of 5,000 mg daily are toxic.<br>• Doses above 2,000 mg daily may increase the risk of kidney stones and soft-tissue calcification.<br>• Several types of calcium supplements exist; check dosage for the type of calcium ingested. |
| **Magnesium**<br>*Women:* 280-300 mg<br>*Pregnant women:* 320 mg<br>*Men:* 270-400 mg | • Needed in protein synthesis and amino acid activation<br>• May correct heart arrhythmias<br>• Needed for nerve transmission and muscle contraction and relaxation<br>• Needed to develop teeth and bones<br>• Needed for many metabolic reactions; acting as an enzyme cofactor, it produces energy, synthesizes lipids and proteins, regulates calcium | • Best food sources include tofu, legumes, whole grains, green leafy vegetables, brazil nuts, almonds, cashews, pumpkin and squash seeds, pine nuts, oatmeal, bananas, and baked potatoes with skin.<br>• Vitamin $B_6$ assists in the body's accumulation of magnesium and works with magnesium in many enzyme systems.<br>• Magnesium and calcium don't inhibit each other's absorption, but increased magnesium intake may result in excess calcium excretion.<br>• Magnesium should be taken with a full glass of water with each dose to avoid diarrhea. |

| Name and recommended daily allowances | Actions | Special considerations |
|---|---|---|
| **Magnesium** *(continued)* | flow, forms urea, and relaxes muscles | • Some foods, drinks, and drugs can cause magnesium loss. These include sodium, sugar, caffeine, alcohol, fiber, riboflavin in high doses, insulin, diuretics, and digoxin.<br>• Magnesium supplements shouldn't be taken by those with severe heart or kidney disease without talking to a health care provider. |
| **Potassium** *Women:* 3,500 mg/day *Pregnant women:* 3,500 mg/day *Men:* 3,500 mg/day | • Treats symptoms of hypokalemia, which include weakness, lack of energy, stomach disturbances, irregular heartbeat, and abnormal ECG<br>• Controls or prevents hypertension<br>• Reduces the mortality associated with acute MI (used in combination with glucose and insulin)<br>• Treats muscle weakness<br>• Protects against stroke | • Best food sources include fresh, unprocessed food such as meats, fish, vegetables, especially potatoes; fruits, especially avocados; and citrus juices, milk, and cereals.<br>• Potassium supplements, other than those in a multivitamin, shouldn't be taken unless recommended by a health care provider.<br>• Patients with renal insufficiency should use with caution. Those with severe renal impairment should avoid use of potassium.<br>• Care should be taken when prescribing potassium supplements to geriatric patients because of decreased renal functions.<br>• Potassium-depleting drugs include thiazides, furosemide, bumetanide, and ethacrynic acid.<br>• Other drugs interacting with potassium include potassium-sparing diuretics, NSAIDs, ACE inhibitors, beta blockers, heparin, digoxin, and trimethoprim. |

*(continued)*

| Name and recommended daily allowances | Actions | Special considerations |
|---|---|---|
| **Iron**<br>*Women:* 15 mg<br>*Pregnant women:* 30 mg<br>*Men:* 10 mg | • Improves the symptoms of iron-deficient anemia<br>• Helps deliver oxygen from the lungs to all parts of the body | • Best food sources include liver, lean red meat, poultry, fish, dried beans, fruits, and vegetables.<br>• Iron supplements should be kept in childproof bottles and away from children.<br>• Children between the ages of 12 and 24 months are at highest risk of iron poisoning from accidental ingestion.<br>• Vitamin C enhances absorption of iron.<br>• Antacids can reduce the absorption of iron.<br>• Iron reduces absorption of the antibiotics ciprofloxacin, norfloxacin, ofloxacin, and tetracycline.<br>• Supplemental oral iron may cause GI disturbances, such as nausea, diarrhea, constipation, heartburn, and upper gastric discomfort. |
| **Selenium**<br>*Women:* 50 mcg<br>*Pregnant women:* 65 mcg<br>*Men:* 70 mcg | • Acts as antioxidant to boost the immune system and prevent age-related diseases, such as cancer<br>• Helps with reproductive health and needed for proper fetal development<br>• Prevents MI and stroke by lowering low-density lipoprotein (LDL) cholesterol level<br>• Required for antioxidant protection of the eye lens; helps prevent cataract formation<br>• Promotes proper liver and metabolic function | • Best food sources include brewer's yeast, wheat germ, liver, butter, fish, shellfish, sunflower seeds, and brazil nuts.<br>• The amount of selenium in foodstuffs corresponds directly to selenium levels in the soil.<br>• Food-source selenium is destroyed during processing.<br>• Selenium should be taken with vitamin E, because the two act synergistically.<br>• Vitamin C may increase risk of selenium toxicity.<br>• Although rare, extended high intake, exceeding 1,000 mcg daily, may lead to toxicity.<br>• Chemotherapy drugs may increase selenium requirements. |

| Name and recommended daily allowances | Actions | Special considerations |
|---|---|---|
| **Zinc**<br>*Women:* 12 mg<br>*Pregnant women:* 15 mg<br>*Men:* 15 mg | • Needed for more than 200 enzymatic reactions in the body<br>• Needed for proper growth and development, especially in early life<br>• Needed to maintain proper vision, taste, and smell<br>• Improves wound healing<br>• Improves immune system function | • Best food sources include oysters, shrimp, crab, and other shellfish; red meat; lima beans, pinto beans, soybeans; whole grains, miso, tofu, brewer's yeast, cooked greens, and pumpkin seeds.<br>• Zinc sulfate can cause GI irritation.<br>• Zinc toxicity is rare, usually occurring only after a dose of 2,000 mg or more has been ingested.<br>• High doses of zinc interfere with the assimilation of other trace minerals, such as copper and iron.<br>• High doses of calcium may interfere with zinc absorption.<br>• Because of the many interactions between zinc and other nutrients, people should take a balanced multiple vitamin with mineral, containing zinc, copper, iron, and folate to help prevent deficiencies of these nutrients. |
| **Manganese**<br>Estimated safe and adequate daily dietary intakes:<br>*Adults:* 2.0-5.0 mg | • Aids in forming connective tissue, fats, and cholesterol, bones, blood clotting factors, and proteins<br>• Needed for normal brain function<br>• Is a component of manganese superoxide dismutase (MnSOD), an antioxidant that protects the body from toxic substances | • Best food sources include pecans, almonds, wheat germ, whole grains, leafy vegetables, liver, kidney, legumes, and dried fruits.<br>• There's no RDA for manganese.<br>• Manganese deficiency hasn't been documented.<br>• Manganese is the least toxic of the trace elements. Toxicity is more common in those exposed to manganese dust |

*(continued)*

| Name and recommended daily allowances | Actions | Special considerations |
|---|---|---|
| **Manganese** *(continued)* | | found in steel mills and mines and certain chemical industries.<br>• Excess manganese may produce iron-deficiency anemia. |
| **Copper**<br>Estimated safe and adequate daily dietary intakes:<br>*Adults:* 1.5-3.0 mg | • Needed for hemo-globin formation<br>• Involved in many reactions to produce and release energy<br>• Needed to develop and maintain skeletal structures<br>• Plays a role in proper functioning of the immune system | • Best food sources include seafood, organ meats, nuts, legumes, chocolate, fruits and vegetables, black pepper, black-strap molasses, and water that flows through copper piping.<br>• Copper supplements should be kept away from children. A dose as little as 3.5 g may be lethal.<br>• Excess copper can interfere with absorption of zinc.<br>• Copper absorption may be affected by calcium, iron, manganese, zinc, vitamin $B_6$, high levels of vitamin C, and antacids in high amounts.<br>• Copper deficiency may be aggravated by alcohol, eggs, and fructose.<br>• Copper deficiency is rare.<br>• Low copper levels may reduce thyroid function. |

# Herb-drug interactions

| Herb | Drug | Possible effects |
|------|------|------------------|
| Aloe | Cardiac glycosides, antiarrhythmics | Ingestion of aloe juice may lead to hypokalemia, which may potentiate cardiac glycosides and antiarrhythmics. |
| | Thiazide diuretics, licorice, and other potassium-wasting drugs | Additive effect of potassium wasting with thiazide diuretics, and other potassium-wasting drugs. |
| | Orally administered drugs | Potential for decreased absorption of drugs because of more rapid GI transit time. |
| Bilberry | Antiplatelets, anticoagulants | Decreases platelet aggregation. |
| | Insulin, hypoglycemics | May increase serum insulin levels, causing hypoglycemia; additive effect with diabetes drugs. |
| Capsicum | Antiplatelets, anticoagulants | Decreases platelet aggregation and increases fibrinolytic activity, prolonging bleeding time. |
| | NSAIDs | Stimulates GI secretions to help protect against NSAID-induced GI irritation. |
| | ACE inhibitors | May cause cough. |
| | Theophylline | Increases absorption of theophylline, possibly leading to higher serum levels or toxicity. |
| | MAO inhibitors | Decreased effects resulting from the increased catecholamine secretion by capsicum. |
| | CNS depressants such as opioids, benzodiazepines, barbiturates | Increased sedative effect. |
| | $H_2$ blockers, proton pump inhibitors | Potential for decreased effectiveness because of increased acid secretion by capsicum. |
| Chamomile | Drugs requiring GI absorption | May delay drug absorption. |

*(continued)*

| Herb | Drug | Possible effects |
|------|------|------------------|
| Chamomile *(continued)* | Anticoagulants | Warfarin constituents may enhance anticoagulant therapy and prolong bleeding time. |
| | Iron | Tannic acid content may reduce iron absorption. |
| Echinacea | Immunosuppressants | Echinacea may counteract immuno-suppressant drugs. |
| | Hepatotoxics | Hepatotoxicity may increase with drugs known to elevate liver enzyme levels. |
| | Warfarin | Increased bleeding time without an increased INR. |
| Evening primrose | Anticonvulsants | Lowered seizure threshold. |
| Feverfew | Antiplatelets, anticoagulants | May decrease platelet aggregation and increase fibrinolytic activity. |
| | Methysergide | May potentiate methysergide. |
| Garlic | Antiplatelets, anticoagulants | Enhances platelet inhibition, leading to increased anticoagulation. |
| | Insulin, other drugs causing hypoglycemia | May increase serum insulin levels, causing hypoglycemia, an additive effect with antidiabetics. |
| | Antihypertensives | Potential for additive hypotension. |
| | Antihyperlipidemics | May have additive lipid-lowering properties. |
| Ginger | Chemotherapy | Ginger may reduce nausea associated with chemotherapy. |
| | $H_2$ blockers, proton pump inhibitors | Potential for decreased effectiveness because of increased acid secretion by ginger. |
| | Antiplatelets, anticoagulants | Inhibits platelet aggregation by antagonizing thromboxane synthetase and enhancing prostacyclin, leading to prolonged bleeding time. |
| | Calcium channel blockers | May increase calcium uptake by myocardium, leading to altered drug effects. |

| Herb | Drug | Possible effects |
|------|------|------------------|
| Ginger *(continued)* | Antihypertensives | May antagonize antihypertensive effect. |
| Ginkgo | Antiplatelets, anticoagulants | May enhance platelet inhibition, leading to increased anticoagulation. |
| | Anticonvulsants | May decrease effectiveness of anticonvulsants. |
| | Drugs known to lower seizure threshold | Potential further reduction of seizure threshold. |
| Ginseng | Stimulants | May potentiate stimulant effects. |
| | Warfarin | Antagonism of warfarin, resulting in a decreased INR. |
| | Antibiotics | Siberian ginseng may enhance effects of some antibiotics. |
| | Anticoagulants, antiplatelets | Decreased platelet adhesiveness. |
| | Digoxin | Ginseng may falsely elevate digoxin levels. |
| | MAO inhibitors | Potentiates action of MAO inhibitors. |
| | Hormones, anabolic steroids | May potentiate effects of hormone and anabolic steroid therapies. Estrogenic effects of ginseng may cause vaginal bleeding and breast nodules. |
| | Alcohol | Increases alcohol clearance, possibly by increasing activity of alcohol dehydrogenase. |
| | Furosemide | May decrease diuretic effect with furosemide. |
| | Antipsychotics | Because of CNS stimulant activity, avoid use with antipsychotics. |
| Goldenseal | Heparin | May counteract anticoagulant effect of heparin. |
| | Diuretics | Additive diuretic effect. |
| | $H_2$ blockers, proton pump inhibitors | Potential for decreased effectiveness because of increased acid secretion by goldenseal. |

*(continued)*

| Herb | Drug | Possible effects |
|------|------|------------------|
| Goldenseal *(continued)* | General anesthetics | May potentiate hypotensive action of general anesthetics. |
| | CNS depressants, such as opioids, barbiturates, benzodiazepines | Increased sedative effect. |
| Grapeseed | Warfarin | Increased effects and INR caused by tocopherol content of grapeseed. |
| Green tea | Warfarin | Antagonism resulting from vitamin content of green tea. |
| Hawthorn berry | Digoxin | Additive positive inotropic effect, with potential for digitalis toxicity. |
| Kava | CNS stimulants or depressants | May hinder therapy with CNS stimulants. |
| | Benzodiazepines | Use with benzodiazepines has resulted in comalike states. |
| | Alcohol | Potentiates depressant effect of alcohol and other CNS depressants. |
| | Levodopa | Decreased effectiveness caused by dopamine antagonism by kava. |
| Licorice | Digoxin | Licorice causes hypokalemia, which predisposes to digitalis toxicity. |
| | Oral contraceptives | Increased fluid retention and potential for increased blood pressure resulting from fluid overload. |
| | Corticosteroids | Additive and enhanced effects of the corticosteroids. |
| | Spironolactone | Decreases the effects of spironolactone. |
| Ma huang | MAO inhibitors | Potentiates MAO inhibitors. |
| | CNS stimulants, caffeine, theophylline | Additive CNS stimulation. |
| | Digoxin | Increased risk of arrhythmias. |
| | Hypoglycemics | Decreased hypoglycemic effect because of hyperglycemia caused by ma huang. |

| Herb | Drug | Possible effects |
|------|------|------------------|
| Melatonin | CNS depressants (such as opioids, barbiturates, benzodiazepines) | Increased sedative effect. |
| Milk thistle | Drugs causing diarrhea | Increases bile secretion and often causes loose stools. May increase effect of other drugs commonly causing diarrhea. Liver membrane-stabilization and antioxidant effects leading to protection from liver damage from various hepatotoxic drugs such as acetaminophen, phenytoin, ethanol, phenothiazines, butyrophenones. |
| Nettle | Anticonvulsants | May increase sedative adverse effects; may increase risk of seizure. |
| | Narcotics, anxiolytics, hypnotics | May increase sedative adverse effects. |
| | Warfarin | Antagonism resulting from vitamin K content of aerial parts of nettle. |
| | Iron | Tannic acid content may reduce iron absorption. |
| Passion flower | CNS depressants (such as opioids, barbiturates, benzodiazepines) | Increased sedative effect. |
| St. John's wort | SSRIs, MAO inhibitors, nefazodone, trazodone | Additive effects with SSRIs, MAO inhibitors, and other antidepressants, potentially leading to serotonin syndrome, especially when combined with SSRIs. |
| | Indinavir; HIV protease inhibitors (PIs); nonnucleoside reverse transcriptase inhibitors (NNRTIs) | Induces cytochrome P450 metabolic pathway, which may decrease therapeutic effects of drugs using this pathway for metabolism. Use of St. John's wort and PIs or NNRTIs should be avoided because of the potential for subtherapeutic antiretroviral levels and insufficient virologic response that could lead to resistance or class cross-resistance. |

*(continued)*

| Herb | Drug | Possible effects |
|------|------|------------------|
| St. John's wort *(continued)* | Narcotics, alcohol | Enhances the sedative effect of narcotics and alcohol. |
| | Photosensitizing drugs | Increases photosensitivity. |
| | Sympathomimetic amines (such as pseudoephedrine) | Additive effects. |
| | Digoxin | May reduce serum digoxin concentrations, decreasing therapeutic effects. |
| | Reserpine | Antagonizes effects of reserpine. |
| | Oral contraceptives | Increases breakthrough bleeding when taken with oral contraceptives; also decreases contraceptive's effectiveness. |
| | Theophylline | May decrease serum theophylline levels, making the drug less effective. |
| | Anesthetics | May prolong effect of anesthesia drugs. |
| | Cyclosporine | Decreased cyclosporine levels below therapeutic levels, threatening transplanted organ rejection. |
| | Iron | Tannic acid content may reduce iron absorption. |
| | Warfarin | Potential to alter INR. Reduces effectiveness of anticoagulant, requiring increased dosage of drug. |
| Valerian | Sedative hypnotics, CNS depressants | Enhances effects of sedative hypnotic drugs. |
| | Alcohol | Claims no risk for increased sedation with alcohol, although debated. |
| | Iron | Tannic acid content may reduce iron absorption. |

# A listing of herbs by common uses

**Abdominal disorders**
- artichoke

**Abdominal pain**
- bitter orange
- Chinese cucumber
- Chinese rhubarb
- ground ivy
- khella

**Abortifacients**
- black hellebore
- feverfew
- pennyroyal
- pomegranate
- rosemary
- rue
- saffron
- senega
- slippery elm
- tansy
- thuja

**Abscesses**
- burdock
- castor bean
- Chinese cucumber
- echinacea
- kava-kava
- thunder god vine
- vervain

**Acne**
- acidophilus
- arnica
- asparagus
- burdock
- cat's claw
- chaste tree
- jojoba
- marigold
- pansy
- soapwort
- tea tree

**Aging**
- melatonin
- morinda
- royal jelly
- wild yam

**Agitation**
- passion flower

**AIDS**
- cat's claw
- dehydroepiandrosterone

**Allergy symptoms**
- bearberry
- bee pollen
- chaparral
- devil's claw
- fenugreek
- ginkgo
- grape seed
- methylsulfonylmethane
- nettle
- willow

**Altitude sickness**
- ginkgo

**Alzheimer's disease**
- dehydroepiandrosterone
- galanthamine
- sage

***Amanita* mushroom poisoning**
- milk thistle

**Amenorrhea**
- black hellebore
- blessed thistle
- chaste tree
- Chinese rhubarb
- false unicorn root
- mayapple
- motherwort

**Amenorrhea** *(continued)*
- parsley
- rue
- safflower
- saffron
- squaw vine
- tree unicorn root
- yarrow

**Amoebiasis**
- pill-bearing spurge

**Amyloidosis**
- autumn crocus

**Amyotrophic lateral sclerosis**
- octacosanol

**Analgesia**
- aconite
- allspice
- arnica
- bethroot
- borage
- butterbur
- capsicum
- celandine
- devil's claw
- horse chestnut
- indigo
- lemongrass
- meadowsweet
- nettle
- parsley
- passion flower
- peach
- poplar
- red poppy
- safflower
- scented geranium
- turmeric
- wild lettuce
- willow
- wintergreen
- yerba maté

**Anemia**
- bee pollen
- dong quai
- onion
- ragwort

**Angina pectoris**
- celandine
- Chinese cucumber
- comfrey
- hawthorn
- khella
- night-blooming cereus
- onion
- sweet flag
- wild ginger

**Ankylosing spondylitis**
- morinda

**Anogenital inflammation**
- oak bark

**Anorectal disorders**
- aloe
- benzoin
- bitter orange
- buckthorn
- Irish moss
- senna

**Antibiotic-induced diarrhea**
- acidophilus

**Anticoagulant effects**
- blessed thistle
- clove oil
- horse chestnut

**Antihistaminic effects**
- agrimony

**Antimicrobial effects**
- acidophilus
- aloe
- anise

- barberry
- basil
- blessed thistle
- blue cohosh
- chamomile
- chaulmoogra oil
- dill
- eyebright
- galangal
- garlic
- green tea
- hops
- methylsulfonylmethane
- olive
- scented geranium
- self-heal
- sorrel
- thyme
- wormwood
- yarrow

**Antimutagenic effects**
- cat's claw
- self-heal

**Antioxidant effects**
- grape seed
- self-heal

**Antiseptic effects**
- agrimony
- allspice
- anise
- basil
- bay
- bearberry
- buchu
- celandine
- clove oil
- feverfew
- lavender
- parsley
- pennyroyal
- poplar
- sassafras
- saw palmetto

- sorrel
- tea tree
- wintergreen

**Antispasmodic effects**
- American hellebore
- anise
- black haw
- bloodroot
- blue cohosh
- boldo
- butterbur
- cardamom
- celery
- clary
- cowslip
- dill
- fennel
- galangal
- ginger
- goldenrod
- hops
- jambolan
- lady's slipper
- lemongrass
- lovage
- madder
- parsley
- passion flower
- peppermint
- skunk cabbage
- tree unicorn root

**Antitumorigenic effects**
- acidophilus
- agrimony
- ginger
- gotu kola

**Anxiety**
- betony
- black cohosh
- black hellebore
- blue cohosh
- chamomile
- clary

**Anxiety** *(continued)*
- hops
- Jamaican dogwood
- jambolan
- kava-kava
- kelpware
- lemon balm
- mugwort
- rauwolfia
- St. John's wort
- valerian

**Aphrodisiac effects**
- burdock
- damiana
- guarana
- hops
- jambolan
- kava-kava
- tonka bean
- yohimbe

**Apocrine chromhidrosis**
- capsicum

**Appendicitis**
- Chinese cucumber

**Appetite stimulation**
- bitter orange
- blessed thistle
- bogbean
- boldo
- caraway
- centaury
- cinnamon
- condurango
- coriander
- daisy
- dandelion
- devil's claw
- elecampane
- false unicorn root
- fenugreek
- galangal
- gentian

- hops
- hyssop
- Iceland moss
- juniper
- milk thistle
- nutmeg
- onion
- oregano
- Oregon grape
- peppermint
- rosemary
- sage
- sarsaparilla
- watercress
- wormwood
- yarrow

**Appetite suppression**
- cola
- ephedra
- guarana
- khat
- yerba maté

**Aromatherapy**
- clary
- coriander
- marjoram
- tea tree

**Arrhythmias**
- broom
- chicory
- khella
- motherwort
- shepherd's purse
- squill
- tree of heaven

**Arthritis**
- autumn crocus
- bearberry
- black pepper
- bogbean
- burdock
- capsicum

- celery
- chaparral
- chaulmoogra oil
- couch grass
- evening primrose oil
- feverfew
- fumitory
- ginger
- guggul
- kelpware
- male fern
- mayapple
- meadowsweet
- methylsulfonylmethane
- morinda
- nettle
- nutmeg
- oregano
- pau d'arco
- rose hip
- safflower
- sassafras
- shark cartilage
- squill
- thuja
- thunder god vine
- vervain
- willow
- wintergreen

**Ascites**
- pipsissewa

**Asthma**
- anise
- betony
- black haw
- black pepper
- bloodroot
- blue cohosh
- catnip
- celandine
- chickweed
- coltsfoot
- cowslip
- cranberry

- elderberry
- elecampane
- ephedra
- evening primrose oil
- feverfew
- ginkgo
- hyssop
- jambolan
- jimsonweed
- khella
- lobelia
- mullein
- nettle
- onion
- pill-bearing spurge
- royal jelly
- saw palmetto
- schisandra
- skunk cabbage
- St. John's wort
- sundew
- sweet cicely
- sweet violet
- tree of heaven
- vervain
- wild ginger
- wintergreen
- yerba santa

**Astringent effects**
- agrimony
- bayberry
- bethroot
- birch
- black catechu
- borage
- clary
- daffodil
- eyebright
- green tea
- ground ivy
- horse chestnut
- lady's mantle
- lungwort
- meadowsweet
- night-blooming cereus

**Astringent effects** (continued)
- pipsissewa
- rose hip
- saw palmetto
- scented geranium
- sorrel
- yarrow

**Atherosclerosis**
- Asian ginseng
- butcher's broom
- devil's claw
- fumitory
- garlic
- green tea
- guggul
- hawthorn
- kelpware
- mistletoe
- onion
- saffron
- wild lettuce

**Athlete's foot**
- tea tree

**Autoimmune diseases**
- methylsulfonylmethane
- thunder god vine

**Autonomic dysfunction**
- jimsonweed

**Autonomic neuroses**
- mugwort

**Backache**
- butterbur
- rue

**Bacterial vaginosis**
- acidophilus

**Bacteriostatic effects**
- dill

**Bedsores**
- balsam of Peru
- benzoin
- karaya gum

**Bedwetting**
- damiana
- pumpkin
- St. John's wort
- thyme

**Bee sting**
- ragwort

**Behcet's disease**
- autumn crocus

**Belching**
- blue flag

**Bell's palsy**
- rue

**Benzodiazepine withdrawal**
- melatonin

**Bile secretion stimulation**
- butterbur
- cat's foot
- dandelion
- elecampane
- goldenseal
- horehound
- mugwort
- oregano
- wahoo

**Biliary disorders**
- autumn crocus
- wormwood

**Bilious fever**
- black root

**Bladder disorders**
- American cranesbill
- asparagus
- betony
- blackthorn
- borage
- buchu
- capsicum
- celery
- coriander
- devil's claw
- flax
- fumitory
- horsetail
- kava-kava
- parsley piert
- pau d'arco
- pipsissewa
- pumpkin
- Queen Anne's lace
- sea holly
- shepherd's purse
- stone root

**Bleeding**
- Asian ginseng
- bee pollen
- bethroot
- blessed thistle
- broom
- bugleweed
- goldenseal
- lady's mantle
- mistletoe
- night-blooming cereus
- peach
- self-heal
- shepherd's purse
- tormentil

**Blepharitis**
- eyebright

**Blind entrainment**
- melatonin

**Blisters**
- peach

**Bloating**
- anise
- bitter orange
- caraway
- cinnamon
- daisy
- oregano
- turmeric
- wormwood

**Blood disorders**
- chickweed
- safflower

**Blood glucose regulation**
- fenugreek
- fumitory
- goat's rue
- olive
- pipsissewa
- raspberry

**Blood poisoning**
- wild indigo

**Blood pressure regulation**
- aconite
- American hellebore
- balsam of Peru
- betony
- blue cohosh
- broom
- capsicum
- celery
- coenzyme Q10
- cucumber
- dong quai
- elecampane
- gotu kola
- hawthorn
- lemon balm
- mistletoe
- morinda

**Blood pressure regulation**
*(continued)*
- olive
- onion
- peach
- prickly ash
- rauwolfia
- rosemary
- rue
- sassafras
- self-heal
- shepherd's purse
- Siberian ginseng
- yarrow
- yellow root
- yohimbe

**Blood purification**
- blackthorn
- blue flag
- burdock
- fumitory
- indigo
- kelpware
- mistletoe
- nettle
- sarsaparilla
- sassafras
- sweet cicely
- woundwort

**Body composition**
- dehydroepiandrosterone

**Boils**
- black catechu
- blessed thistle
- castor bean
- peach
- thunder god vine

**Bowel preparation**
- aloe
- senna

**Bradycardia**
- hawthorn

**Brain damage**
- bee pollen

**Breast cancer**
- yew

**Breast disorders**
- bugleweed
- celandine
- chaste tree
- Chinese cucumber

**Breast enlargement**
- wild yam

**Breathing difficulty**
- sweet cicely

**Bronchitis**
- anise
- balsam of Peru
- benzoin
- betony
- black pepper
- bloodroot
- broom
- catnip
- celery
- chickweed
- clove oil
- coltsfoot
- couch grass
- elderberry
- elecampane
- fennel
- galangal
- horehound
- jambolan
- jimsonweed
- juniper
- kelpware
- lungwort
- mallow

- meadowsweet
- mullein
- onion
- peach
- pill-bearing spurge
- saffron
- sassafras
- saw palmetto
- sea holly
- senega
- skunk cabbage
- St. John's wort
- sundew
- sweet violet
- thyme
- watercress
- wild cherry
- wild ginger
- yerba santa

## Bronchospasm
- butterbur
- ephedra
- wild ginger

## Bruises
- arnica
- balsam of Peru
- blue flag
- chaulmoogra oil
- comfrey
- daisy
- grape seed
- hyssop
- mullein
- onion
- passion flower
- peach
- ragwort
- rue
- St. John's wort
- vervain
- witch hazel
- yerba santa

## Burns
- aloe
- balsam of Peru
- bloodroot
- chamomile
- daffodil
- echinacea
- figwort
- ginger
- gotu kola
- horsetail
- hyssop
- kelpware
- lavender
- marigold
- marshmallow
- mullein
- olive
- onion
- peach
- ragwort
- slippery elm
- St. John's wort
- tea tree
- thuja
- tragacanth
- vervain
- witch hazel

## Bursitis
- nettle

## Cachexia
- tonka bean

## Calculosis
- American cranesbill
- celery

## Cancer
- Asian ginseng
- asparagus
- autumn crocus
- black hellebore
- bloodroot
- buckthorn

**Cancer** *(continued)*
- burdock
- carline thistle
- celandine
- chaparral
- comfrey
- condurango
- dehydroepiandrosterone
- echinacea
- garlic
- ginger
- ginkgo
- grape seed
- green tea
- indigo
- marigold
- mayapple
- melatonin
- methylsulfonylmethane
- mistletoe
- morinda
- pau d'arco
- peach
- Queen Anne's lace
- red clover
- safflower
- sassafras
- self-heal
- shark cartilage
- Siberian ginseng
- soy
- spirulina
- squill
- thuja
- yellow root
- yew

**Canker sores**
- acidophilus
- raspberry
- rhatany
- sage

**Capillary insufficiency**
- bilberry
- bloodroot

**Carbuncles**
- castor bean
- ground ivy

**Cardiac depressant effects**
- aconite
- American hellebore

**Cardiac surgery**
- coenzyme Q10

**Cardiotonic effects**
- agrimony
- balsam of Peru
- borage
- ephedra
- figwort
- hawthorn

**Cardiovascular disorders**
- arnica
- broom
- coenzyme Q10
- cowslip
- garlic
- grape seed
- hawthorn
- khella
- lily-of-the-valley
- motherwort
- night-blooming cereus
- oleander
- pipsissewa
- raspberry
- S-adenosylmethionine
- shepherd's purse
- soy
- squill

**Catarrh**
- acacia gum
- agrimony
- betony
- boneset
- burdock
- lemon balm

- pill-bearing spurge
- pipsissewa
- plantain
- sassafras
- senega
- shepherd's purse
- watercress

## Cathartic effects
- aloe
- bloodroot
- blue flag
- broom
- mayapple
- Oregon grape

## Celiac disease
- carob

## Cerebral hemorrhage
- bee pollen

## Cerebral insufficiency
- ginkgo

## Cerebral thrombosis
- yarrow

## Cervical cancer
- bee pollen

## Cervical ripening
- evening primrose oil

## Chemotherapy adverse effects
- chondroitin
- coenzyme Q10

## Chest complaints
- coriander
- safflower
- skunk cabbage
- sweet cicely
- turmeric

## Chilblains
- rhatany

## Chills
- ephedra

## Chinese rhubarb
- clove oil
- coriander
- elderberry
- male fern
- mallow
- marigold
- meadowsweet
- prickly ash
- rosemary
- tansy

## Cholecystitis
- celandine

## Cholera
- barberry
- birch
- black pepper

## Chronic fatigue syndrome
- dehydroepiandrosterone
- evening primrose oil
- morinda
- schisandra

## Circulation
- arnica
- barberry
- bayberry
- broom
- butcher's broom
- capsicum
- condurango
- coriander
- ginkgo
- hyssop
- monascus
- mugwort
- prickly ash

## Circulation *(continued)*
- rose hip
- rosemary
- self-heal
- soy

## Cirrhosis
- autumn crocus
- cat's claw
- milk thistle

## Cluster headaches
- melatonin

## Coagulant effects
- agrimony

## Cochlear deafness
- ginkgo

## Coffee substitutes
- asparagus
- blue cohosh
- dandelion

## Colic
- black pepper
- blessed thistle
- blue cohosh
- butterbur
- calumba
- catnip
- coriander
- ginger
- hyssop
- juniper
- marjoram
- mugwort
- nutmeg
- parsley
- Queen Anne's lace
- rauwolfia
- rue
- sea holly
- sweet cicely
- sweet flag

- wild lettuce

## Colitis
- Asian ginseng
- bee pollen
- carob
- cat's claw
- ginkgo
- peppermint
- squaw vine
- witch hazel

## Colostomy care
- karaya gum

## Common cold
- anise
- balsam of Peru
- bay
- bayberry
- blackthorn
- boneset
- burdock
- catnip
- chickweed
- cinnamon
- clove oil
- coltsfoot
- couch grass
- echinacea
- ephedra
- galangal
- garlic
- hyssop
- Iceland moss
- kava-kava
- linden
- marjoram
- meadowsweet
- onion
- pau d'arco
- pennyroyal
- peppermint
- rose hip
- saw palmetto
- sweet violet

- vervain
- wild cherry
- willow
- yarrow
- yerba santa

## Concentration problems
- Asian ginseng
- Siberian ginseng

## Condylomata acuminata
- mayapple
- thuja

## Confusion
- wild indigo

## Conjunctivitis
- cornflower
- eyebright
- marjoram

## Constipation
- agar
- aloe
- asparagus
- barberry
- bee pollen
- black hellebore
- black pepper
- black root
- blessed thistle
- bloodroot
- blue cohosh
- boldo
- buchu
- buckthorn
- burdock
- butcher's broom
- cascara sagrada
- celandine
- chickweed
- chicory
- Chinese cucumber
- Chinese rhubarb
- cornflower
- couch grass
- damiana
- dandelion
- elderberry
- figwort
- flax
- glucomannan
- jambolan
- karaya gum
- kelp
- kelpware
- mallow
- marshmallow
- mayapple
- mugwort
- olive
- pansy
- pareira
- peach
- pineapple
- plantain
- rose hip
- senna
- stone root
- tragacanth
- tree unicorn root
- wahoo

## Contact dermatitis
- bearberry

## Contraception
- asparagus
- cat's claw
- gossypol
- gotu kola
- melatonin
- thunder god vine

## Cor pulmonale
- lily-of-the-valley

## Corns
- agrimony

**Coronary thrombosis**
- yarrow

**Cosmetic products**
- cacao tree
- coriander
- cucumber
- hyssop
- Irish moss
- jojoba
- juniper
- karaya gum
- lemon
- marigold
- nutmeg
- pennyroyal
- rosemary
- soapwort

**Cough**
- acacia gum
- aconite
- anise
- balsam of Peru
- bayberry
- betel palm
- betony
- borage
- burdock
- butterbur
- catnip
- chickweed
- Chinese cucumber
- clove oil
- coltsfoot
- coriander
- cornflower
- couch grass
- elderberry
- elecampane
- ephedra
- eyebright
- fennel
- galangal
- garlic
- horehound
- horse chestnut
- horseradish
- Iceland moss
- Irish moss
- jimsonweed
- linden
- lungwort
- mallow
- marshmallow
- meadowsweet
- mullein
- onion
- oregano
- peach
- pokeweed
- Queen Anne's lace
- ragwort
- red clover
- red poppy
- rosemary
- rue
- saw palmetto
- schisandra
- sea holly
- soapwort
- sundew
- sweet violet
- wild cherry
- wild ginger
- wild lettuce
- woundwort
- yerba santa

**Cramps**
- blue cohosh

**Crohn's disease**
- American cranesbill
- cat's claw
- peppermint

**Croup**
- benzoin
- bloodroot
- mullein

## Cutaneous ulcers
- balsam of Peru
- benzoin
- bethroot
- black catechu
- blessed thistle
- echinacea
- fenugreek
- figwort
- gotu kola
- horse chestnut
- jambolan
- karaya gum
- papaya
- prickly ash
- Queen Anne's lace
- rhatany
- southernwood
- tea tree
- tonka bean
- wormwood

## Cystitis
- American cranesbill
- betony
- buchu
- chamomile
- fumitory
- kava-kava
- methylsulfonylmethane
- night-blooming cereus
- parsley
- shepherd's purse

## Cytomegalovirus infection
- St. John's wort

## Dandruff
- birch
- burdock
- southernwood
- squill

## Deafness
- ginkgo

## Decongestant effects
- betony
- bloodroot
- ephedra
- ground ivy
- horseradish
- linden
- parsley
- saw palmetto

## Dehydration
- onion

## Delirium
- black pepper
- Chinese rhubarb

## Dementia
- dehydroepiandrosterone
- galanthamine
- ginkgo
- sage

## Dental health
- acacia gum
- allspice
- bay
- chaparral
- green tea

## Dental impressions
- agar

## Dental pain
- allspice
- arnica
- asparagus
- bloodroot

## Depression
- Asian ginseng
- clary
- damiana
- dehydroepiandrosterone
- ginger
- ginkgo

**Depression** *(continued)*
- jambolan
- khat
- marjoram
- melatonin
- mugwort
- S-adenosylmethionine
- scented geranium
- schisandra
- St. John's wort

**Dermatitis herpetiformis**
- autumn crocus

**Detoxification**
- soy
- watercress

**Diabetes**
- agrimony
- artichoke
- Asian ginseng
- bitter melon
- cat's claw
- dandelion
- elecampane
- glucomannan
- jambolan
- morinda
- olive
- onion
- rose hip
- Siberian ginseng
- spirulina
- yellow root

**Diabetic neuropathy**
- capsicum
- evening primrose oil

**Diabetic retinopathy**
- ginkgo

**Diaphoretic effects**
- angelica
- birch

- blackthorn
- blessed thistle
- blue cohosh
- borage
- burdock
- carline thistle
- catnip
- jaborandi
- linden
- skunk cabbage
- soapwort
- sweet flag
- wild ginger
- wormwood
- yarrow

**Diaphragmitis**
- wintergreen

**Diarrhea**
- acacia gum
- acidophilus
- agrimony
- American cranesbill
- avens
- barberry
- bayberry
- bethroot
- betony
- bilberry
- birch
- bistort
- black catechu
- black haw
- black pepper
- blessed thistle
- calumba
- carob
- catnip
- chamomile
- Chinese rhubarb
- cinnamon
- comfrey
- coriander
- flax
- green tea

- ground ivy
- horse chestnut
- Irish moss
- jaborandi
- jambolan
- lady's mantle
- lungwort
- marshmallow
- meadowsweet
- monascus
- mugwort
- nutmeg
- oak bark
- pau d'arco
- plantain
- quince
- raspberry
- rhatany
- rose hip
- rue
- schisandra
- self-heal
- shepherd's purse
- squaw vine
- thyme
- tormentil
- tragacanth
- tree of heaven
- tree unicorn root
- wild cherry
- witch hazel
- yarrow

**Dietary stimulation**
- evening primrose oil

**Digestive stimulation**
- bloodroot

**Diphtheria**
- betel palm

**Diuresis**
- agrimony
- American hellebore
- angelica

- artichoke
- asparagus
- basil
- bearberry
- black haw
- blackthorn
- blue flag
- boldo
- broom
- buchu
- butcher's broom
- carline thistle
- catnip
- cat's foot
- chicory
- coffee
- condurango
- cornflower
- couch grass
- cowslip
- dandelion
- elderberry
- elecampane
- false unicorn root
- figwort
- goat's rue
- goldenrod
- green tea
- hops
- horsetail
- jambolan
- lemon
- lovage
- madder
- marigold
- meadowsweet
- mullein
- nettle
- onion
- oregano
- papaya
- pareira
- parsley
- parsley piert
- pipsissewa
- pumpkin

**Diuresis** *(continued)*
- rose hip
- saw palmetto
- scented geranium
- soapwort
- sorrel
- thuja
- thyme
- tree unicorn root
- wahoo
- watercress
- yerba maté

**Diverticulitis**
- flax
- slippery elm

**Diverticulosis**
- cat's claw
- wild yam

**Dizziness**
- cowslip
- marjoram
- woundwort

**Doxorubicin adverse effects**
- chondroitin
- coenzyme Q10

**Dropsy**
- pipsissewa

**Drug additives**
- acacia gum
- agar
- Irish moss
- licorice
- sarsaparilla
- tragacanth

**Drug extravasation**
- chondroitin

**Dyes**
- agrimony

- indigo
- tansy

**Dysentery**
- American cranesbill
- birch
- bitter orange
- calumba
- cat's foot
- coriander
- ground ivy
- guarana
- jambolan
- peach
- Queen Anne's lace
- quince
- self-heal
- tormentil
- tree of heaven
- yarrow

**Dysmenorrhea**
- black cohosh
- black haw
- black pepper
- butterbur
- caraway
- catnip
- chaparral
- daisy
- dong quai
- false unicorn root
- feverfew
- guarana
- Jamaican dogwood
- lady's mantle
- marigold
- night-blooming cereus
- parsley
- passion flower
- peach
- peppermint
- ragwort
- shepherd's purse
- squaw vine
- squill

- tree of heaven
- tree unicorn root
- valerian
- wild lettuce
- wild yam
- willow
- wintergreen

**Dyspepsia**
- acidophilus
- allspice
- artichoke
- avens
- bee pollen
- bitter orange
- black pepper
- blackthorn
- blessed thistle
- bogbean
- boldo
- capsicum
- cardamom
- carline thistle
- carob
- catnip
- centaury
- chaparral
- chicory
- condurango
- coriander
- damiana
- dandelion
- dill
- elecampane
- feverfew
- galangal
- ginger
- goldenseal
- guarana
- horehound
- hyssop
- Iceland moss
- juniper
- kelpware
- milk thistle
- monascus

- mugwort
- nutmeg
- onion
- oregano
- parsley
- peach
- peppermint
- pineapple
- rosemary
- rue
- stone root
- sweet violet
- thyme
- turmeric
- wahoo
- wormwood

**Dysuria**
- parsley piert
- rauwolfia
- squaw vine

**Ear cancer**
- bloodroot

**Ear infection**
- betel palm
- castor bean
- kava-kava
- rue
- wild indigo

**Ear wax softening**
- olive

**Earache**
- male fern
- mullein
- peach

**Eclampsia**
- black hellebore
- rauwolfia

**Eczema**
- balsam of Peru

**Eczema** *(continued)*
- borage
- burdock
- celandine
- chaulmoogra oil
- chickweed
- cornflower
- echinacea
- evening primrose oil
- figwort
- fumitory
- marigold
- nettle
- pansy
- peach
- red clover
- rosemary
- shark cartilage
- soapwort

**Edema**
- broom
- Chinese rhubarb
- ephedra
- grape seed
- horse chestnut
- horseradish
- horsetail
- lovage
- night-blooming cereus
- papaya
- parsley piert
- peach
- pineapple
- Queen Anne's lace
- rose hip
- sea holly
- stone root

**Emetic effects**
- black root
- bloodroot
- blue flag
- bogbean
- broom
- false unicorn root

- indigo
- lobelia
- pokeweed
- skunk cabbage
- wild indigo

**Emphysema**
- coltsfoot
- kelpware

**Encephalitis**
- black hellebore

**Endometriosis**
- evening primrose oil

**Energy enhancement**
- bee pollen
- creatine monohydrate
- damiana
- spirulina
- wild yam

**Enuresis**
- damiana
- pumpkin
- St. John's wort
- thyme

**Epididymitis**
- wintergreen

**Epilepsy**
- black hellebore
- blue cohosh
- dehydroepiandrosterone
- elderberry
- mistletoe
- mugwort
- rue
- tree of heaven

**Erectile dysfunction**
- dehydroepiandrosterone
- yohimbe

**Erysipelas**
- mullein

**Esophageal cancer**
- yew

**Euphoric effects**
- broom
- corkwood
- damiana
- jimsonweed
- khat

**Exanthema**
- pansy

**Excitability**
- wild lettuce

**Expectoration**
- bethroot
- betony
- blackthorn
- blessed thistle
- bloodroot
- blue cohosh
- cornflower
- cowslip
- eucalyptus
- fennel
- goldenseal
- horehound
- horse chestnut
- hyssop
- licorice
- lungwort
- nettle
- oregano
- parsley
- scented geranium
- senega
- skunk cabbage
- soapwort
- squill
- sweet cicely
- sweet violet

- thuja
- wild cherry

**Extrasystoles**
- khella

**Eye disorders**
- bilberry
- corkwood
- cornflower
- eyebright
- flax
- ginkgo
- jaborandi
- marigold
- quince
- ragwort
- rue
- sassafras
- schisandra

**Facial dressing**
- betel palm

**Familial Mediterranean fever**
- autumn crocus

**Fatigue**
- Asian ginseng
- bee pollen
- cola
- dehydroepiandrosterone
- evening primrose oil
- jambolan
- khat
- morinda
- onion
- S-adenosylmethionine
- sage
- schisandra
- Siberian ginseng
- yerba maté

**Fever**
- aconite
- American hellebore

## Fever *(continued)*
- avens
- balsam of Peru
- barberry
- bayberry
- blessed thistle
- bloodroot
- boneset
- burdock
- catnip
- Chinese cucumber
- cinnamon
- coriander
- cornflower
- couch grass
- cranberry
- daisy
- elderberry
- ephedra
- eucalyptus
- galangal
- garlic
- goat's rue
- horse chestnut
- hyssop
- Iceland moss
- indigo
- linden
- marigold
- onion
- pau d'arco
- prickly ash
- saffron
- southernwood
- sweet flag
- tormentil
- wild indigo
- willow
- woundwort
- yarrow

## Fever blisters or cold sores
- acidophilus
- tea tree

## Fibrocystic breast disease
- chaste tree

## Fibromyalgia
- S-adenosylmethionine

## Fish-spine wounds
- onion

## Fistulas
- gotu kola

## Flatulence
- allspice
- anise
- black pepper
- blessed thistle
- calumba
- capsicum
- caraway
- cardamom
- celery
- chamomile
- cinnamon
- coriander
- dandelion
- fennel
- galangal
- ginger
- hyssop
- jambolan
- juniper
- lemon
- lemon balm
- lovage
- marjoram
- motherwort
- nutmeg
- onion
- parsley
- peppermint
- Queen Anne's lace
- rauwolfia
- rosemary
- sweet cicely
- sweet violet

- thyme
- tree unicorn root
- turmeric
- wild ginger

**Flavoring agents**
- agrimony
- allspice
- anise
- bitter orange
- black pepper
- blessed thistle
- caraway
- carob
- coriander
- dill
- galangal
- guarana
- horseradish
- hyssop
- Iceland moss
- juniper
- lemon
- mullein
- onion
- pennyroyal
- pipsissewa
- sarsaparilla
- sassafras
- scented geranium
- sweet flag
- thuja
- thyme
- tonka bean
- turmeric
- wild cherry
- wintergreen
- wormwood

**Fluid retention**
- burdock

**Food and beverage products**
- acacia gum
- asparagus
- bitter orange

- cacao tree
- caraway
- carob
- chicory
- coffee
- coriander
- dandelion
- guarana
- hops
- hyssop
- juniper
- karaya gum
- lemon
- lemongrass
- licorice
- madder
- papaya
- pokeweed
- red poppy
- rosemary
- safflower
- slippery elm
- thuja
- tragacanth
- watercress
- yarrow

**Fractures**
- butcher's broom
- royal jelly
- shark cartilage

**Fragrances**
- clary
- coriander
- cucumber
- hyssop
- juniper
- lemon
- lemongrass
- marigold
- marjoram
- pennyroyal
- scented geranium
- tansy
- thuja

## Frostbite
- balsam of Peru
- horsetail
- hyssop
- mullein
- poplar

## Fungal infection
- acidophilus
- bitter orange
- bloodroot
- cornflower
- elderberry
- garlic
- olive
- pau d'arco
- sage
- tea tree

## Furuncles
- marigold
- onion

## Gallbladder disorders
- agrimony
- American cranesbill
- artichoke
- black root
- blessed thistle
- boldo
- broom
- carline thistle
- celandine
- cornflower
- dandelion
- fumitory
- galangal
- hyssop
- milk thistle
- onion
- pennyroyal
- peppermint
- pipsissewa
- rose hip
- rosemary
- St. John's wort

- turmeric
- wild yam

## Gastric secretion stimulation
- bogbean
- gentian
- mugwort

## Gastrointestinal disorders
- acacia gum
- acidophilus
- agrimony
- allspice
- American cranesbill
- angelica
- anise
- artichoke
- avens
- barberry
- bee pollen
- betel palm
- bistort
- bitter melon
- bitter orange
- black catechu
- black pepper
- blackthorn
- blessed thistle
- blue flag
- buchu
- burdock
- calumba
- capsicum
- caraway
- cardamom
- carline thistle
- catnip
- cat's claw
- centaury
- chaparral
- chicory
- cinnamon
- comfrey
- condurango
- coriander
- daisy

- dandelion
- devil's claw
- dill
- elecampane
- fennel
- fenugreek
- feverfew
- flax
- fumitory
- galangal
- ginger
- green tea
- ground ivy
- hops
- hyssop
- Irish moss
- jambolan
- juniper
- kava-kava
- lavender
- lemon balm
- lemongrass
- marjoram
- marshmallow
- meadowsweet
- methylsulfonylmethane
- monascus
- morinda
- mugwort
- nutmeg
- oregano
- Oregon grape
- papaya
- parsley
- pennyroyal
- peppermint
- pulsatilla
- Queen Anne's lace
- quince
- raspberry
- rose hip
- rosemary
- rue
- saffron
- shark cartilage
- slippery elm

- soapwort
- stone root
- sweet cicely
- sweet flag
- sweet violet
- tansy
- tormentil
- wild cherry
- wild ginger
- wild lettuce
- willow
- wintergreen
- yarrow

**Genitourinary disorders**
- boldo
- kava-kava
- kelpware
- pulsatilla
- wild lettuce

**Gingivitis**
- avens
- rhatany
- sage
- sweet flag
- wild indigo

**Glaucoma**
- jaborandi

**Goiter**
- kelp
- kelpware

**Gonorrhea**
- autumn crocus
- black pepper
- cat's claw
- pipsissewa
- quince
- tree of heaven

**Gout**
- autumn crocus
- betony

**Gout** *(continued)*
- bogbean
- boldo
- broom
- buchu
- burdock
- celandine
- celery
- chickweed
- Chinese rhubarb
- cowslip
- daisy
- elderberry
- fenugreek
- horsetail
- mistletoe
- pennyroyal
- Queen Anne's lace
- ragwort
- rose hip
- rosemary
- rue
- soapwort
- squill
- St. John's wort
- sweet cicely
- woundwort

**Guillain-Barré syndrome**
- capsicum

**Gynecologic wounds**
- gotu kola

**Hair dryness**
- olive

**Hair growth**
- asparagus
- burdock
- jojoba
- parsley
- rosemary
- royal jelly
- sage

- southernwood

**Halitosis**
- avens
- basil
- chaparral
- coriander
- parsley
- peach
- sage

**Hallucinogenic effects**
- corkwood
- damiana
- jimsonweed
- nutmeg
- peyote
- wild lettuce

**Hand soak**
- mugwort

**Hay fever**
- nettle

**Headache**
- black pepper
- blue flag
- butterbur
- castor bean
- catnip
- Chinese rhubarb
- clary
- cola
- cowslip
- daisy
- damiana
- dehydroepiandrosterone
- dong quai
- elderberry
- ephedra
- feverfew
- ginkgo
- green tea
- guarana
- Jamaican dogwood

- kava-kava
- lady's slipper
- lemon balm
- marjoram
- meadowsweet
- melatonin
- morinda
- passion flower
- peach
- peppermint
- pulsatilla
- ragwort
- rosemary
- rue
- saffron
- shepherd's purse
- stone root
- tansy
- turmeric
- valerian
- wild ginger
- willow
- yerba maté

**Heart failure**
- coenzyme Q10
- motherwort
- squaw vine
- squill

**Heartburn**
- betony
- blessed thistle
- blue flag
- devil's claw
- juniper
- meadowsweet
- Oregon grape
- sweet violet

**Helminthic infection**
- false unicorn root
- morinda
- onion
- wormwood

**Hematemesis**
- shepherd's purse
- witch hazel

**Hematoma**
- bethroot

**Hematuria**
- shepherd's purse

**Hemoglobin $A_{1C}$ reduction**
- fenugreek

**Hemophilia**
- broom

**Hemoptysis**
- night-blooming cereus
- witch hazel

**Hemorrhoids**
- aloe
- balsam of Peru
- bethroot
- bilberry
- buckthorn
- butcher's broom
- cat's claw
- celandine
- coriander
- figwort
- ground ivy
- horse chestnut
- lungwort
- mullein
- pomegranate
- poplar
- rhatany
- senna
- St. John's wort
- stone root
- witch hazel
- yarrow

## Hepatitis
- dong quai
- rue
- self-heal
- St. John's wort

## Herpesvirus infection
- capsicum
- goldenseal
- motherwort
- octacosanol
- peach
- pokeweed
- sage
- senna
- slippery elm
- St. John's wort

## Hiccups
- blue cohosh
- Queen Anne's lace

## HIV infection
- cat's claw
- dehydroepiandrosterone

## Hives
- acidophilus
- catnip
- nettle

## Hoarseness
- eyebright
- mallow

## Hot flushes
- black cohosh

## Hyperactivity
- evening primrose oil

## Hypercholesterolemia
- acacia gum
- acidophilus
- artichoke
- celandine

- evening primrose oil
- fenugreek
- garlic
- ginger
- glucomannan
- guggul
- monascus
- oats
- olive
- onion
- plantain
- royal jelly
- safflower

## Hyperglycemia
- goat's rue
- pipsissewa

## Hyperlipidemia
- artichoke
- glucomannan
- green tea
- royal jelly

## Hypersensitivity reactions
- bearberry

## Hypertension
- aconite
- American hellebore
- basil
- betony
- blue cohosh
- broom
- capsicum
- celery
- coenzyme Q10
- cucumber
- dong quai
- elecampane
- gotu kola
- lemon balm
- mistletoe
- morinda
- olive
- onion

- peach
- rauwolfia
- rue
- sassafras
- self-heal
- yarrow
- yellow root

**Hyperthyroidism**
- bugleweed
- motherwort

**Hypertonia**
- khella

**Hypertriglyceridemia**
- garlic
- guggul
- monascus

**Hyperuricuria**
- stone root

**Hypnotic effects**
- cowslip
- lady's slipper
- passion flower

**Hypochondriasis**
- mugwort

**Hypoglycemia**
- fumitory

**Hypotension**
- balsam of Peru
- broom
- cucumber
- mistletoe
- prickly ash
- shepherd's purse
- Siberian ginseng
- yohimbe

**Hysteria**
- blue cohosh

- celery
- mistletoe
- passion flower
- rue

**Ifosfamide extravasation**
- chondroitin

**Ileitis**
- peppermint

**Ileostomy care**
- karaya gum

**Immune system enhancement**
- black hellebore
- cat's claw
- echinacea
- figwort
- marigold
- melatonin
- methylsulfonylmethane
- morinda
- rose hip
- royal jelly
- skullcap
- thuja
- wild ginger
- wild indigo

**Impetigo**
- pansy

**Impotence**
- ginger
- ginkgo

**Incontinence**
- caraway
- sweet violet

**Infection**
- acidophilus
- asparagus
- balsam of Peru
- birch

**Infection** (continued)
- bloodroot
- blue cohosh
- burdock
- chaparral
- cinnamon
- clove oil
- couch grass
- cranberry
- echinacea
- eucalyptus
- fumitory
- galangal
- garlic
- Iceland moss
- indigo
- kava-kava
- linden
- male fern
- marigold
- olive
- onion
- pau d'arco
- pulsatilla
- senna
- slippery elm
- southernwood
- St. John's wort
- wild indigo
- yellow root

**Infertility**
- chaste tree
- Siberian ginseng

**Inflammation**
- agrimony
- American cranesbill
- arnica
- balsam of Peru
- betel palm
- bilberry
- blackthorn
- blue cohosh
- blue flag
- boldo

- boneset
- borage
- buchu
- butcher's broom
- castor bean
- chamomile
- chaulmoogra oil
- Chinese rhubarb
- clary
- coffee
- comfrey
- couch grass
- daisy
- devil's claw
- fenugreek
- flax
- gentian
- ginger
- goldenrod
- ground ivy
- indigo
- jambolan
- lemon
- marigold
- marshmallow
- meadowsweet
- methylsulfonylmethane
- nettle
- oak bark
- octacosanol
- onion
- pansy
- papaya
- pau d'arco
- peach
- pineapple
- plantain
- prickly ash
- pulsatilla
- rue
- sassafras
- skullcap
- sorrel
- St. John's wort
- thunder god vine
- turmeric

- willow
- witch hazel

**Inflammatory bowel disease**
- acidophilus
- cat's claw
- evening primrose oil

**Influenza**
- boneset
- chickweed
- ephedra
- jimsonweed
- lungwort
- pau d'arco
- peppermint
- pokeweed
- rose hip
- St. John's wort
- sweet violet
- willow

**Injuries**
- arnica
- cat's claw
- papaya
- quince

**Insect bites and stings**
- kelpware
- ragwort
- sage
- sassafras
- southernwood
- witch hazel
- wormwood
- yerba santa

**Insect repellents**
- basil
- elderberry
- lemongrass
- pennyroyal
- rosemary
- rue
- scented geranium

- southernwood
- tansy
- thuja

**Insecticides**
- false unicorn root
- feverfew

**Insulin regulation**
- fenugreek

**Intermittent claudication**
- ginkgo

**Intervertebral disc herniation**
- papaya

**Iodine sources**
- kelp
- kelpware

**Irrigation**
- asparagus
- carline thistle
- nettle

**Irritability**
- mugwort

**Irritable bowel syndrome**
- acidophilus
- flax
- marshmallow
- meadowsweet
- peppermint
- plantain

**Ischemic heart disease**
- coenzyme Q10

**Jaundice**
- broom
- celandine
- Chinese rhubarb
- ground ivy
- pineapple

**Jaundice** *(continued)*
- self-heal
- wild ginger

**Jet lag**
- melatonin

**Joint symptoms**
- comfrey
- daffodil
- daisy
- juniper
- Queen Anne's lace
- quince
- ragwort
- rosemary
- thuja
- wild lettuce
- willow

**Kaposi's sarcoma**
- shark cartilage

**Keloids**
- papaya

**Keratoses**
- mayapple

**Kidney disorders**
- American cranesbill
- angelica
- blackthorn
- borage
- buchu
- celery
- devil's claw
- dill
- elecampane
- horsetail
- lungwort
- pareira
- parsley
- peach
- pipsissewa
- royal jelly

- sarsaparilla
- sassafras
- schisandra
- soapwort
- squill

**Kidney stones**
- asparagus
- betony
- birch
- broom
- burdock
- butterbur
- Chinese rhubarb
- couch grass
- cranberry
- goldenrod
- horseradish
- juniper
- lovage
- madder
- nettle
- parsley piert
- pipsissewa
- Queen Anne's lace
- rose hip
- sarsaparilla
- sea holly
- stone root

**Labor**
- blue cohosh

**Lactation**
- blessed thistle
- caraway
- chaste tree
- goat's rue
- parsley
- raspberry
- squaw vine
- vervain

**Lactose intolerance**
- acidophilus

## Larvicidal effects
- nutmeg

## Laryngeal papilloma
- mayapple

## Laryngeal spasm
- pill-bearing spurge

## Laryngitis
- benzoin
- bloodroot
- coltsfoot
- mallow
- nettle
- pokeweed
- poplar
- sage
- thyme

## Leg pain and edema
- horse chestnut

## Leg ulcers
- balsam of Peru
- bethroot
- rhatany

## Leprosy
- chaulmoogra oil
- gotu kola
- kava-kava

## Leukorrhea
- buchu
- tree of heaven

## Lice
- anise

## Liniments
- aconite

## Lip conditions
- benzoin
- marigold

## Liver disorders
- American cranesbill
- autumn crocus
- black root
- blessed thistle
- boldo
- celandine
- cornflower
- daisy
- dandelion
- devil's claw
- dong quai
- elderberry
- fumitory
- galangal
- ginger
- gotu kola
- hyssop
- milk thistle
- morinda
- parsley
- peach
- pennyroyal
- peppermint
- pineapple
- rauwolfia
- rosemary
- royal jelly
- rue
- S-adenosylmethionine
- schisandra
- soapwort
- squaw vine
- St. John's wort
- turmeric
- wild ginger

## Liver protectant effects
- artichoke
- bilberry
- indigo
- milk thistle
- self-heal

## Locked jaw
- peach

## Lung cancer
- mayapple
- shark cartilage
- yew

## Lung disorders
- Chinese cucumber
- peach
- pennyroyal
- schisandra
- senega
- wild cherry
- wild ginger

## Lupus
- shark cartilage

## Lymphadenopathy
- pokeweed
- wild indigo

## Lymphedema
- figwort
- horse chestnut
- tonka bean

## Macular degeneration
- bilberry
- ginkgo

## Malaria
- guarana

## Mania
- galanthamine

## Mastectomy pain
- capsicum

## Mastitis
- Chinese cucumber
- evening primrose oil

## Measles
- coriander

## Melanoma
- yew

## Memory enhancement
- blessed thistle
- blue cohosh

## Meningitis
- black hellebore

## Menopausal symptoms
- black cohosh
- borage
- chaste tree
- clary
- devil's claw
- dong quai
- red clover
- soy
- wild yam

## Menorrhagia
- broom
- bugleweed
- chaste tree
- horsetail
- lungwort
- night-blooming cereus
- raspberry
- shepherd's purse
- thunder god vine

## Menstrual disorders
- bethroot
- blessed thistle
- blue cohosh
- broom
- bugleweed
- caraway
- catnip
- cat's claw
- celery
- chaste tree
- Chinese rhubarb
- cornflower
- devil's claw

- dong quai
- elecampane
- false unicorn root
- feverfew
- ground ivy
- guarana
- horsetail
- kava-kava
- lady's mantle
- lovage
- lungwort
- mugwort
- night-blooming cereus
- onion
- oregano
- pareira
- parsley
- peach
- raspberry
- rosemary
- safflower
- saffron
- shepherd's purse
- southernwood
- squaw vine
- tansy
- thunder god vine
- tree unicorn root
- wild ginger
- woundwort
- yarrow
- yew

**Mental alertness**
- schisandra

**Mental disorders**
- Asian ginseng
- black hellebore
- clary
- damiana
- dehydroepiandrosterone
- galanthamine
- ginger
- ginkgo
- hops

- jambolan
- mugwort
- St. John's wort

**Mental fatigue**
- clary
- cola

**Metabolic enhancement**
- capsicum
- pansy
- soapwort

**Metrorrhagia**
- shepherd's purse

**Migraine**
- butterbur
- castor bean
- catnip
- clary
- cola
- daisy
- dehydroepiandrosterone
- dong quai
- feverfew
- Jamaican dogwood
- lemon balm
- passion flower
- peppermint
- pulsatilla
- tansy
- wild ginger
- willow

**Miscarriage**
- tree unicorn root
- wild yam

**Moles**
- Chinese cucumber

**Mood disturbances**
- hops

**Morning sickness**
- cola
- false unicorn root
- ginger

**Motility-enhancing effects**
- cardamom

**Motion sickness**
- chamomile
- galangal
- ginger
- marjoram

**Mucolytic agents**
- lovage
- onion

**Multiple sclerosis**
- autumn crocus
- rue

**Mumps**
- cat's foot

**Muscle pain**
- allspice
- eucalyptus
- fenugreek
- horseradish
- juniper
- male fern
- marjoram
- methylsulfonylmethane
- peppermint
- prickly ash
- rosemary
- St. John's wort
- wild lettuce
- wintergreen

**Muscle spasms**
- bay
- blue cohosh
- rue
- tonka bean

**Muscle strains**
- daffodil

**Mushroom poisoning**
- milk thistle

**Myocardial infarction**
- garlic

**Myocardial protectant effects**
- coenzyme Q10

**Myxedema**
- kelpware

**Nail disorders**
- horsetail
- tea tree

**Nasal cancer**
- bloodroot

**Nasal infection**
- wild indigo

**Nasal inflammation**
- boneset
- sorrel

**Nasal polyps**
- bloodroot

**Nausea and vomiting**
- artichoke
- black hellebore
- black pepper
- blue flag
- caraway
- carob
- cola
- false unicorn root
- galangal
- ginger
- lemon balm
- mugwort
- rauwolfia

- saffron
- woundwort

**Neck stiffness**
- lemon balm

**Nephritis**
- aconite

**Nervousness**
- betony
- bugleweed
- celery
- cowslip
- hops
- lady's slipper
- lemon balm
- lemongrass
- linden
- passion flower
- peach
- rauwolfia

**Neuralgia**
- aconite
- angelica
- betony
- black pepper
- capsicum
- cowslip
- daisy
- devil's claw
- dong quai
- elderberry
- hops
- Jamaican dogwood
- lemon balm
- male fern
- passion flower
- peppermint
- pulsatilla
- rosemary
- wintergreen

**Neurasthenia**
- mugwort

**Neurodermatitis**
- borage
- evening primrose oil

**Neurogenic bladder**
- capsicum

**Neuromuscular blockade reversal**
- galanthamine

**Neuromuscular disorders**
- galanthamine

**Nicotine addiction**
- oats

**Nicotine poisoning**
- devil's claw

**Night sweats**
- schisandra

**Nipple disorders**
- balsam of Peru
- benzoin
- marigold
- quince
- squaw vine

**Nocturnal seminal emissions**
- schisandra

**Nosebleed**
- bugleweed
- shepherd's purse

**Nutritional supplements**
- carob
- soy
- spirulina

**Obesity**
- carob
- evening primrose oil
- glucomannan

**Obesity** *(continued)*
- kelp
- kelpware
- khat
- mugwort
- spirulina

**Obstetric patients**
- barberry
- bee pollen
- black hellebore
- blue cohosh
- broom
- carob
- cola
- evening primrose oil
- false unicorn root
- ginger
- mistletoe
- olive
- parsley
- raspberry
- rauwolfia
- slippery elm
- squaw vine

**Oophoralgia**
- wintergreen

**Opium addiction**
- oats

**Oral cancer**
- spirulina

**Oral inflammation**
- agrimony
- American cranesbill
- arnica
- balsam of Peru
- bilberry
- blackthorn
- boneset
- clove oil
- coltsfoot
- jambolan

- oak bark
- peppermint
- plantain
- rhatany
- thyme
- tormentil
- turmeric
- vervain

**Oral pain**
- acidophilus

**Oral rinses and gargles**
- American cranesbill
- arnica
- bayberry
- bistort
- bitter orange
- black catechu
- blackthorn
- caraway
- carline thistle
- chaparral
- feverfew
- pomegranate
- poplar
- ragwort
- raspberry
- self-heal
- soapwort
- St. John's wort
- tea tree
- thyme
- tormentil
- vervain
- wild indigo

**Orchitis**
- wintergreen

**Osteoarthritis**
- bogbean
- capsicum
- glucosamine sulfate
- nettle
- S-adenosylmethionine

- shark cartilage

**Osteogenesis imperfecta**
- rose hip

**Osteoporosis**
- dehydroepiandrosterone
- soy
- wild yam

**Otitis**
- betel palm
- castor bean
- kava-kava

**Ovarian cancer**
- indigo
- mayapple
- yew

**Ovulation inhibition**
- blue cohosh

**Palmoplantar pustulosis**
- autumn crocus

**Palpitations**
- hawthorn
- lemon balm

**Pancreatic cancer**
- ginkgo

**Pancreatic disorders**
- jambolan
- papaya
- royal jelly

**Paralytic disorders**
- black pepper

**Parasitic infection**
- betel palm
- black hellebore
- blue cohosh
- chaparral

- false unicorn root
- feverfew
- male fern
- morinda
- mugwort
- onion
- papaya
- pau d'arco
- peach
- pomegranate
- pumpkin
- rue
- santonica
- southernwood
- tansy
- tree of heaven
- wormwood
- yew

**Parkinson's disease**
- octacosanol

**Peptic ulcers**
- capsicum
- cat's claw
- comfrey
- ginger
- Irish moss
- khat
- licorice
- lungwort
- marigold
- meadowsweet
- Oregon grape
- papaya
- pau d'arco
- royal jelly
- slippery elm

**Performance enhancement**
- bee pollen
- borage
- creatine monohydrate
- damiana
- guarana

## Performance enhancement
*(continued)*
- octacosanol
- wild yam

## Periodontal health
- acacia gum
- allspice
- avens
- broom
- chaparral
- sage
- sweet flag
- wild indigo

## Peripheral arterial disease
- ginkgo

## Personal defense products
- capsicum

## Pertussis
- black pepper
- cowslip
- horehound
- khella
- red clover
- sundew
- thyme
- vervain
- wild cherry

## Phantom limb pain
- capsicum

## Pharyngeal inflammation
- agrimony
- arnica
- balsam of Peru
- bilberry
- blackthorn
- bloodroot
- boneset
- clove oil
- coltsfoot
- jambolan

- oak bark
- peppermint
- plantain
- rhatany
- thyme
- vervain

## Phlebitis
- borage
- horse chestnut

## Plague
- goat's rue

## Pleurisy
- wintergreen

## Pleuritis with effusion
- self-heal

## Pleurodynia
- wintergreen

## Pneumonia
- peach
- pennyroyal
- senega
- wild ginger

## Poison ivy
- soapwort
- yerba santa

## Poisoning
- devil's claw
- milk thistle
- senega

## Polio
- pokeweed
- St. John's wort

## Polydipsia
- jambolan

**Postherpetic neuralgia**
- capsicum

**Postpartum complications**
- coriander
- bethroot
- broom
- goldenseal

**Pregnancy symptoms**
- blue cohosh
- carob
- cola
- false unicorn root
- ginger
- olive

**Premenstrual symptoms**
- black cohosh
- bugleweed
- chaste tree
- clary
- couch grass
- dong quai
- evening primrose oil
- ginkgo
- morinda
- nettle
- shepherd's purse
- wild yam
- willow

**Prenatal health**
- bee pollen

**Pressure ulcers**
- balsam of Peru
- benzoin
- karaya gum

**Priapism**
- wild lettuce

**Prostaglandin synthesis inhibition**
- galangal

**Prostate cancer**
- shark cartilage

**Prostate disorders**
- autumn crocus
- bee pollen
- buchu
- cat's claw
- evening primrose oil
- horse chestnut
- motherwort
- nettle
- poplar
- pumpkin
- saw palmetto
- sea holly
- wild yam

**Pruritus**
- balsam of Peru
- capsicum
- motherwort
- pansy
- peppermint
- pokeweed
- sage
- vervain
- witch hazel

**Pseudogout**
- autumn crocus

**Psoriasis**
- anise
- autumn crocus
- burdock
- capsicum
- chaulmoogra oil
- chickweed
- feverfew
- figwort
- fumitory
- gotu kola
- jojoba
- khella
- lavender

**Psoriasis** (continued)
- olive
- Oregon grape
- red clover
- sage
- sarsaparilla
- shark cartilage
- soapwort

**Pulmonary embolism**
- arnica

**Purgative effects**
- allspice
- blackthorn
- mayapple

**Quinsy**
- cat's foot

**Radiation sickness**
- bee pollen

**Raynaud's disease**
- evening primrose oil

**Rectal prolapse**
- bitter orange

**Reflex sympathetic dystrophy**
- capsicum

**Relaxation**
- broom
- chamomile
- lavender
- sweet violet

**Renal colic**
- sea holly

**Reptile bites**
- broom
- cat's foot
- goat's rue
- pareira

- rauwolfia

**Respiratory tract disorders**
- angelica
- blackthorn
- blue flag
- chickweed
- coltsfoot
- elecampane
- ephedra
- fenugreek
- ground ivy
- hyssop
- mallow
- mullein
- oregano
- pansy
- raspberry
- red poppy
- sea holly
- soapwort
- tea tree
- watercress

**Respiratory tract infection**
- echinacea
- eyebright
- fennel
- Irish moss
- kava-kava
- peach
- pennyroyal
- poplar
- rose hip
- senega
- wild ginger

**Restlessness**
- chamomile
- hops
- kava-kava
- mugwort
- pulsatilla
- valerian
- wild lettuce

**Retention enema**
- shark cartilage

**Rheumatic diseases**
- aconite
- angelica
- arnica
- asparagus
- autumn crocus
- birch
- blessed thistle
- bloodroot
- blue cohosh
- bogbean
- boldo
- boneset
- borage
- broom
- capsicum
- cat's claw
- celery
- chaparral
- chaulmoogra oil
- chickweed
- daisy
- elderberry
- eucalyptus
- evening primrose oil
- feverfew
- fumitory
- galangal
- horsetail
- juniper
- kava-kava
- kelpware
- lemon balm
- mayapple
- meadowsweet
- mullein
- nettle
- night-blooming cereus
- nutmeg
- parsley
- pau d'arco
- pokeweed
- poplar

- prickly ash
- ragwort
- rue
- sarsaparilla
- shark cartilage
- St. John's wort
- sweet flag
- thuja
- thunder god vine
- thyme
- tree unicorn root
- wild yam
- wintergreen

**Rhinitis**
- dong quai
- grape seed
- marjoram
- nettle

**Ringworm**
- turmeric

**Rodenticide**
- squill

**Rubefacients**
- pipsissewa

**Scabies**
- anise
- balsam of Peru
- birch
- black pepper
- celandine
- ground ivy
- safflower
- tansy

**Scarlatina**
- black pepper

**Scarlet fever**
- wild indigo

**Schizophrenia**
- ginkgo

**Sciatica**
- aconite
- broom
- male fern
- nettle
- ragwort
- rose hip
- rosemary
- St. John's wort

**Scleroderma**
- autumn crocus

**Scrofulosus**
- celandine
- oregano

**Scurvy**
- peach
- rose hip

**Seborrhea**
- pansy
- squill

**Secretion reduction**
- balsam of Peru
- cowslip

**Sedation**
- agrimony
- American hellebore
- betony
- borage
- celery
- chamomile
- chicory
- cowslip
- feverfew
- hawthorn
- kava-kava
- lady's slipper
- lavender

- lemon balm
- lovage
- morinda
- mugwort
- mullein
- oregano
- papaya
- passion flower
- red poppy
- saffron
- scented geranium
- skullcap
- skunk cabbage
- sweet violet
- tree unicorn root
- wild cherry
- wild lettuce

**Seizure disorders**
- black hellebore
- blue cohosh
- dehydroepiandrosterone
- elderberry
- kava-kava
- mistletoe
- mugwort
- passion flower
- skullcap
- squaw vine
- tree of heaven

**Sexual function**
- celery
- damiana
- dehydroepiandrosterone
- ginger
- ginkgo
- royal jelly
- wild yam
- yohimbe

**Shift-work disorder**
- melatonin

**Shingles**
- capsicum

- motherwort
- peach
- sage

**Shortness of breath**
- night-blooming cereus

**Sinusitis**
- betony
- vervain

**Sjögren's syndrome**
- evening primrose oil

**Skin conditions**
- agrimony
- aloe
- anise
- arnica
- autumn crocus
- balsam of Peru
- bearberry
- benzoin
- birch
- black catechu
- blackthorn
- blessed thistle
- bloodroot
- bogbean
- borage
- burdock
- capsicum
- carline thistle
- castor bean
- celandine
- chamomile
- chaulmoogra oil
- chickweed
- Chinese rhubarb
- echinacea
- fenugreek
- feverfew
- figwort
- flax
- fumitory
- green tea

- hyssop
- jambolan
- jojoba
- kava-kava
- kelpware
- lavender
- mallow
- marigold
- mullein
- nettle
- oak bark
- oats
- octacosanol
- oleander
- olive
- onion
- Oregon grape
- pansy
- passion flower
- peach
- pennyroyal
- peppermint
- plantain
- poplar
- pulsatilla
- ragwort
- red clover
- royal jelly
- rue
- sage
- sassafras
- sea holly
- slippery elm
- soapwort
- St. John's wort
- sweet cicely
- tea tree
- thuja
- turmeric
- vervain
- watercress
- witch hazel
- wormwood
- yerba santa

**Skin masks**
- acacia gum

**Sleep disturbances**
- black cohosh
- black pepper
- bugleweed
- catnip
- dill
- hops
- Jamaican dogwood
- lemon balm
- marjoram
- melatonin
- mugwort
- nutmeg
- passion flower
- rauwolfia
- red poppy
- royal jelly
- squaw vine
- valerian
- wild lettuce

**Smoking cessation**
- black pepper
- lobelia

**Snakebite**
- broom
- goat's rue
- pareira
- rauwolfia

**Sore throat**
- acacia gum
- agrimony
- avens
- bayberry
- benzoin
- bistort
- bitter orange
- black catechu
- bloodroot
- blue cohosh
- borage

- burdock
- galangal
- garlic
- horehound
- hyssop
- linden
- mallow
- marigold
- marshmallow
- mullein
- onion
- peach
- pomegranate
- rue
- saffron
- sage
- sweet cicely
- sweet flag
- tea tree
- vervain
- wild indigo

**Spermicidal effects**
- gossypol

**Spleen disorders**
- broom
- dandelion
- milk thistle
- monascus
- parsley

**Sprains**
- arnica
- chaulmoogra oil
- comfrey
- daisy
- meadowsweet
- ragwort
- rue
- tansy
- yerba santa

**Sprue**
- carob

**Stenocardia**
- night-blooming cereus

**Stimulant effects**
- acacia gum
- arnica
- bay
- betel palm
- birch
- buchu
- coffee
- cola
- corkwood
- galangal
- green tea
- guarana
- yerba maté

**Stingray wounds**
- onion

**Stomach cancer**
- celandine
- condurango
- indigo
- safflower

**Stomatitis**
- chamomile
- rhatany

**Stress**
- kava-kava
- valerian

**Stretch marks in pregnancy**
- olive

**Stroke**
- garlic

**Styes**
- eyebright

**Styptics**
- lady's mantle

- shepherd's purse

**Sunburn**
- cucumber
- jojoba
- poplar
- tansy
- tea tree

**Sunscreens**
- buckthorn
- cascara sagrada
- jojoba
- melatonin
- witch hazel

**Surgical patients**
- aloe
- buckthorn
- coenzyme Q10
- gotu kola

**Sweating**
- black cohosh
- sage
- schisandra

**Swelling**
- catnip
- comfrey
- horse chestnut
- pineapple
- ragwort

**Syphilis**
- condurango
- sarsaparilla
- sassafras
- slippery elm

**Tachycardia**
- khella
- motherwort
- tree of heaven

**Teething pain**
- mallow

**Tendinitis**
- meadowsweet
- nettle

**Tension**
- clary
- hops
- lady's slipper
- rauwolfia

**Testicular cancer**
- mayapple

**Thirst suppression**
- cola
- guarana

**Thrombophlebitis**
- arnica

**Thrombosis**
- yarrow

**Thrush**
- quince

**Thyroid function**
- blue flag
- bugleweed
- kelp
- kelpware
- motherwort

**Tinea lesions**
- mayapple
- tea tree
- turmeric

**Tinnitus**
- ginkgo
- melatonin

**Tongue cancer**
- carline thistle

**Tongue inflammation**
- boneset

**Tonics**
- bloodroot
- boneset
- buchu
- buckthorn
- calumba
- horse chestnut
- Irish moss
- motherwort
- mugwort
- nettle
- pareira
- royal jelly
- sarsaparilla
- sassafras
- tonka bean
- tree unicorn root
- wahoo
- watercress

**Tonsillitis**
- burdock
- figwort
- mallow
- pokeweed
- sage
- soapwort
- St. John's wort
- thyme
- yew

**Toothache**
- allspice
- asparagus
- Chinese rhubarb
- coriander
- elderberry
- male fern
- marigold
- meadowsweet

- prickly ash
- rosemary
- tansy

**Tourette syndrome**
- dehydroepiandrosterone

**Tremors**
- cowslip

**Tuberculosis**
- agrimony
- black pepper
- chaparral
- chaulmoogra oil
- chickweed
- kava-kava
- lungwort
- mullein
- pipsissewa
- self-heal
- tonka bean

**Typhoid**
- wild indigo

**Ulcerative colitis**
- avens

**Urethritis**
- buchu

**Uric acid metabolism disorders**
- rose hip

**Urinary retention**
- sea holly

**Urinary tract disorders**
- angelica
- buchu
- burdock
- butterbur
- dill
- elecampane
- goldenrod

- hyssop
- lovage
- lungwort
- night-blooming cereus
- oregano
- parsley piert
- ragwort
- rose hip
- sarsaparilla
- sea holly
- sweet cicely

**Urinary tract infection**
- acidophilus
- asparagus
- birch
- blue cohosh
- couch grass
- cranberry
- echinacea
- horseradish
- juniper
- parsley piert
- sea holly

**Urinary tract irrigation**
- nettle

**Uterine contractions**
- barberry
- blue cohosh
- broom
- mistletoe
- parsley
- rauwolfia

**Uterine fibroids**
- chaste tree

**Uterine inflammation**
- blue cohosh
- kava-kava

**Uterine prolapse**
- bitter orange

**Uterine tonic during pregnancy**
- false unicorn root

**Vaginal disorders**
- acidophilus
- buchu
- cornflower
- kava-kava
- mallow

**Vaginal infection**
- pau d'arco
- sage
- tea tree

**Vaginal prolapse**
- tree unicorn root

**Varicose veins**
- bethroot
- horse chestnut
- marigold
- rue
- witch hazel

**Vascular disorders**
- bilberry
- bloodroot
- borage
- broom
- butcher's broom
- gotu kola
- grape seed
- horse chestnut
- witch hazel

**Vasodilation**
- barberry

**Venereal disease**
- autumn crocus
- black pepper
- buchu
- cat's claw
- chaparral
- condurango
- ephedra
- kava-kava
- pipsissewa
- quince
- sarsaparilla
- sassafras
- slippery elm
- tree of heaven

**Venous insufficiency**
- bilberry
- butcher's broom
- gotu kola
- grape seed
- horse chestnut

**Vertigo**
- black pepper
- ginkgo

**Vincristine extravasation**
- chondroitin

**Vindesine extravasation**
- chondroitin

**Vitiligo**
- capsicum
- St. John's wort

**Vulvar pruritus**
- pansy

**Vulvar vestibulitis**
- capsicum

**Warts**
- agrimony
- bloodroot
- mayapple
- onion
- pansy
- peach
- squill
- sundew
- thuja

**Water retention**
- stone root

**Weakness**
- bee pollen

**Weight loss**
- bee pollen
- capsicum
- glucomannan
- guarana
- guggul
- Irish moss
- wild yam

**Well-being**
- dehydroepiandrosterone

**Whooping cough**
- black pepper
- cowslip
- horehound
- khella
- red clover
- sundew
- thyme
- vervain
- wild cherry

**Worm infestation**
- betel palm
- black hellebore
- blue cohosh
- male fern
- mugwort
- peach
- pomegranate
- pumpkin
- rue
- southernwood
- tansy
- tree of heaven
- yew

**Wound debridement**
- bloodroot

- feverfew
- pineapple

**Wound healing**
- acacia gum
- aloe
- balsam of Peru
- bistort
- blessed thistle
- burdock
- chamomile
- chaparral
- Chinese rhubarb
- comfrey
- daisy
- echinacea
- fenugreek
- figwort
- goldenseal
- gotu kola
- green tea
- ground ivy
- horsetail
- juniper
- kava-kava
- lungwort
- marigold
- peach
- poplar
- prickly ash
- quince
- raspberry
- rauwolfia
- rosemary
- rue
- safflower
- self-heal
- senega
- shark cartilage
- slippery elm
- southernwood
- sweet cicely
- thuja
- thyme
- tormentil
- vervain

**Wound healing** *(continued)*
- wormwood
- woundwort
- yarrow

**Wound irrigation**
- carline thistle

# Monitoring patients using herbs

Altered laboratory values and changes in a patient's condition can help target your assessments and better meet the needs of your patient who uses herbs.

| Herb | What to monitor | Explanation |
|---|---|---|
| Aloe | • Serum electrolyte levels<br>• Weight patterns<br>• BUN and creatinine levels<br>• Heart rate<br>• Blood pressure<br>• Urinalysis | Aloe possesses cathartic properties that inhibit water and electrolyte reabsorption, which may lead to potassium depletion, weight loss, and diarrhea. Long-term use may lead to nephritis, albuminuria, hematuria, and cardiac disturbances. |
| Bilberry | • Weight patterns<br>• CBC<br>• Blood glucose level<br>• Triglyceride level<br>• Liver function tests | Bilberry contains flavonoids and chromium, which are thought to have blood glucose- and triglyceride-lowering effects. Continued intoxication may lead to wasting, anemia, and jaundice. |
| Capsicum | • Liver function tests<br>• BUN and creatinine levels | Oral administration of capsicum can lead to gastroenteritis and hepatic or renal damage. |
| Cat's claw | • Blood pressure<br>• Lipid panel<br>• Serum electrolyte levels | Cat's claw can potentially cause hypotension through inhibition of the sympathetic nervous system and its diuretic properties. May also lower cholesterol level. |
| Chamomile (German, Roman) | • Menstrual changes<br>• Pregnancy | Chamomile has been reported to cause changes in menstrual cycle and is a known teratogen in animals. |
| Echinacea | • Temperature | When echinacea is used parenterally, dose-dependent, |

*(continued)*

| Herb | What to monitor | Explanation |
|------|-----------------|-------------|
| Echinacea *(continued)* | | short-term fever, nausea, and vomiting can occur. |
| Ephedra | • Blood pressure<br>• Heart rate<br>• BUN and creatinine levels<br>• Weight patterns | Ephedra's active ingredient, ephedrine, stimulates the CNS in a similar manner to that of amphetamine. Adverse effects include hypertension, tachycardia, and kidney damage. |
| Evening primrose | • Pregnancy<br>• CBC<br>• Lipid profile | Evening primrose elevates plasma lipid levels and reduces platelet aggregation. It may increase the risk of pregnancy complications, including rupture of membranes, oxytocin augmentation, arrest of descent, and vacuum extraction. |
| Fennel | • Liver function tests<br>• Blood pressure<br>• Serum calcium level<br>• Blood glucose level | Fennel contains trans-anethole and estrogole. Trans-anethole has estrogenic activity, whereas estrogole is a procarcinogen with the potential to cause liver damage. Adverse effects include photodermatitis and allergic reactions, particularly in those sensitive to carrots, celery, and mugwort. |
| Feverfew | • CBC<br>• Pregnancy<br>• Sleep patterns | Feverfew may inhibit blood platelet aggregation and decrease neutrophil and platelet secretory activity. It can cause uterine contractions in full-term, pregnant women. Adverse effects include mouth ulceration, tongue irritation and inflammation, abdominal pain, indigestion, diarrhea, flatulence, nausea, and vomiting. Post-feverfew syndrome includes nervousness, headache, insomnia, joint pain, stiffness, and fatigue. |

| Herb | What to monitor | Explanation |
|---|---|---|
| Flaxseed | • Lipid panel<br>• Blood pressure<br>• Serum calcium level<br>• Blood glucose level<br>• Liver function tests | Flaxseed possesses weak estrogenic and antiestrogenic activity. May cause a reduction in platelet aggregation and serum cholesterol level. Oral administration with inadequate fluid intake can cause intestinal blockage. |
| Garlic | • Blood pressure<br>• Lipid panel<br>• Blood glucose level<br>• CBC<br>• PT and PTT | Garlic is associated with hypotension, leukocytosis, inhibition of platelet aggregation, and decreased blood glucose and cholesterol levels. Postoperative bleeding and prolonged bleeding time can occur. |
| Ginger | • Blood glucose level<br>• Blood pressure<br>• Heart rate<br>• Respiratory rate<br>• Lipid panel<br>• ECG | Ginger contains gingerols, which have positive inotropic properties. Adverse effects include platelet inhibition, hypoglycemia, hypotension, hypertension, and stimulation of respiratory centers. Overdoses cause CNS depression and arrhythmias. |
| Ginkgo | • Respiratory rate<br>• Heart rate<br>• PT and PTT | Consumption of ginkgo seed may cause difficulty breathing, weak pulse, seizures, loss of consciousness, and shock. Ginkgo leaf is associated with infertility, as well as GI upset, headache, dizziness, palpitations, restlessness, lack of muscle tone, weakness, bleeding, subdural hematoma, subarachnoid hemorrhage, and a bleeding iris. |
| Ginseng (American, Panax, Siberian) | • BUN and creatinine levels<br>• Blood pressure<br>• Serum electrolyte levels | Ginseng contains ginsenosides and eleutherosides that can affect blood pressure, CNS activity, platelet aggregation,<br>*(continued)* |

| Herb | What to monitor | Explanation |
|------|-----------------|-------------|
| Ginseng *(continued)* | • Liver function tests<br>• Serum calcium level<br>• Blood glucose level<br>• Heart rate<br>• Sleep patterns<br>• Menstrual changes<br>• Weight patterns<br>• PT, PTT, and INR | and coagulation. A reduction in glucose and hemoglobin $A_{1C}$ levels has also been reported. Adverse effects include drowsiness, mastalgia, vaginal bleeding, tachycardia, mania, cerebral arteritis, Stevens-Johnson syndrome, cholestatic hepatitis, amenorrhea, decreased appetite, diarrhea, edema, hyperpyrexia, pruritus, hypotension, palpitations, headache, vertigo, euphoria, and neonatal death. |
| Goldenseal | • Respiratory rate<br>• Heart rate<br>• Blood pressure<br>• Liver function tests<br>• Mood patterns | Goldenseal contains berberine and hydrastine. Berberine improves bile secretion and bilirubin level, increases coronary blood flow, and stimulates or inhibits cardiac activity. Hydrastine causes hypotension, hypertension, increased cardiac output, exaggerated reflexes, seizures, paralysis, and death from respiratory failure. Other adverse effects include digestive disorders, constipation, excitatory states, hallucinations, delirium, GI upset, nervousness, depression, dyspnea, and bradycardia. |
| Kava | • Weight patterns<br>• Lipid panel<br>• CBC<br>• Blood pressure<br>• Liver function tests<br>• Urinalysis<br>• Mood changes | Kava contains arylethylene pyrone constituents that have CNS activity. It also has anti-anxiety effects. Long-term use may lead to weight loss, increased HDL cholesterol levels, hematuria, increased RBCs, decreased platelet count, decreased lymphocyte levels, reduced protein levels, and pulmonary hypertension. |

| Herb | What to monitor | Explanation |
|------|-----------------|-------------|
| Milk thistle | • Liver function tests | Milk thistle contains flavono-lignans, which have liver-protective and antioxidant effects. |
| Nettle | • Blood glucose level<br>• Blood pressure<br>• Weight patterns<br>• BUN and creatinine levels<br>• Serum electrolyte levels<br>• Heart rate<br>• PT and INR | Nettle contains significant amounts of vitamin C, vitamin K, potassium, and calcium. Nettle may cause hypergly-cemia, decreased blood pressure, decreased heart rate, weight loss, and diuretic effects. |
| Passion flower | • Liver function tests<br>• Amylase level<br>• Lipase level | Passion flower may contain cyanogenic glycosides, which can cause liver and pancreas toxicity. |
| St. John's wort | • Vision<br>• Menstrual changes | Changes in menstrual bleeding and a reduction in fertility may be caused by St. John's wort. Other adverse effects include GI upset, fatigue, dry mouth, dizziness, headache, delayed hypersensitivity, phototoxicity, and neuropathy. St. John's wort may also increase the risk of cataracts. |
| SAM-e | • Blood pressure<br>• Heart rate<br>• BUN and creatinine levels | SAM-e contains homocysteine, which requires folate, cyano-oobalamin, and pyridoxine for metabolism. Increased levels of homocysteine are associated with CV and renal disease. |
| Saw palmetto | • Liver function tests | Saw palmetto inhibits conversion of testosterone to dihydro-testosterone and may cause inhibition of growth factors. Adverse effects include cholestatic hepatitis, erectile or ejaculatory dysfunction, and altered libido.<br>*(continued)* |

| Herb | What to monitor | Explanation |
|------|-----------------|-------------|
| Valerian | • Blood pressure<br>• Heart rate<br>• Sleep patterns<br>• Liver function tests | Valerian contains valerenic acid, which increases gamma-butyric acid and decreases CNS activity. Adverse effects include cardiac disturbances, insomnia, chest tightness, and hepatotoxicity. |

# Selected references

Blumenthal, M., et al, eds. The Complete German Commission E Monographs: Therapeutic Guide to Herbal Medicines. Translated by Klein, S. Boston: Integrated Medicine Communications, 1998.

Boullata, J.I., and Nace, A.M. "Safety Issues with Herbal Medicine," Pharmacotherapy 20:257-69, 2000.

Brinker, F. Herb Contraindications and Drug Interactions, 2nd ed. Sandy, Ore: Eclectic Medical Publications, 1998.

Castleman, M. The Healing Herbs. The Ultimate Guide to the Curative Power of Nature's Medicines. Emmaus, Pa: Rodale Press, 1991.

Chevallier, A. The Encyclopedia of Medicinal Plants. New York: DK Publishing, 1996.

Culpeper, N.: Culpeper's Complete Herbal: A Book of Natural Remedies for Ancient Ills. London: Foulsham & Co Ltd, 1995.

DerMarderosian, A., et al, eds. Facts and Comparisons: The Review of Natural Products. St. Louis: Wolters Kluwer, 1999.

Duke, J.A. Handbook of Medicinal Herbs. Boca Raton, Fla: CRC Press, 1985.

Duke, J.A. The Green Pharmacy. Emmaus, Pa: Rodale Press, 1997.

Dukes, M.N.G., ed. Meyler's Side Effects of Drugs: An Encyclopedia of Adverse Reactions and Interactions, 13th ed. Amsterdam: Elsevier, 1996.

Fetrow, C.W., and Avila, J.R. The Complete Guide to Herbal Medicines. Springhouse, Pa: Springhouse Corporation, 2000.

Fleming, T., Gruenwald, J., Brendler, T., and Jaenicke, C., eds. PDR for Herbal Medicines, 2nd ed. Montvale, NJ: Medical Economics Co, 2000.

Foster, S., and Tyler, V.E. Tyler's Honest Herbal. A Sensible Guide to the Use of Herbs and Related Remedies, 4th ed. Binghamton, NY: Haworth Herbal Press, 1999.

Fugh-Berman, A. "Herb-Drug Interactions," Lancet 355:134-38, 2000.

Grieve, M., and Leyel, C.F. A Modern Herbal. New York: Dover Publications, 1978.

Harbone, J.B., and Baxter, H. Dictionary of Plant Toxins. Chichester, NJ: John Wiley & Sons, 1996.

Hoffman, D. The Complete Illustrated Holistic Herbal. A Safe and Practical Guide to Making and Using Herbal Remedies. Rockport, Mass: Element Books, 1996.

Hoffmann, D. The New Holistic Herbal. New York: Barnes & Noble Books, 1995.

Hoffmann, D., ed. The Herbal Handbook: A User's Guide to Medical Herbalism (revised edition). Rochester, Vt: Healing Arts Press, 1998.

Jellin, J.M., ed. Natural Medicines Comprehensive Database, 2nd ed. Compiled by the Editors of Pharmacist's Letter and Physician's Letter. Stockton, Calif: Therapeutic Research Faculty, 2000.

Klepser, T.B., and Klepser, M.E. "Unsafe and Potentially Safe Herbal Therapies," Am J Health-Syst Pharm 56:125-37, 1999.

Leung, A.Y., and Foster, S. Encyclopedia of Common Natural Ingredients Used in Food, Drugs, and Cosmetics, 2nd ed. New York: John Wiley & Sons, 1996.

Mabey, R. The New Age Herbalist: How to Use Herbs for Healing, Nutrition, Body Care, and Relaxation. New York: Simon & Schuster, 1988.

Macdonald, H.G. A Dictionary of Natural Products. Medford, NJ: Plexus Publishing, 1997.

McGuffin, M., et al., eds. American Herbal Products Association's Botanical Safety Handbook. Boca Raton, Fla: CRC Press, 1997.

Miller, L.G. "Herbal Medicinals: Selected Clinical Considerations Focusing on Known or Potential Drug-Herb Interactions," Arch Intern Med 158:2200-11, 1998.

Miller, L.G., and Murray, W.J., eds. Herbal Medicinals: A Clinician's Guide. Binghamton, NY: Pharmaceutical Products Press, 1998.

Mowrey, D.B. Herbal Tonic Therapies. New Canaan, Conn: Keats Publishing, 1993.

Murray, M. The Healing Power of Herbs, 2nd ed. Rocklin, Calif: Prima Publishing, 1995.

Murray, M., and Pizzorno, J. Encyclopedia of Natural Medicine, 2nd ed. Rocklin, Calif: Prima Publishing, 1998.

Newall,C.A., et al. Herbal Medicines: A Guide for Health Care Professionals. London: Pharmaceutical Press, 1996.

Nutriceutica. Database on CD-ROM. San Clemente, Calif: JAG Group, 1999.

Parfitt, K., ed. Martindale's Complete Drug Reference, 32nd ed. Micromedex Healthcare Series, vol. 103, Pharmaceutical Press, 2000.

Peirce, A. The American Pharmaceutical Association. Practical Guide to Natural Medicines. New York: Stonesong Press, 1999.

Peirce, A., and Gans, J.A. The American Pharmaceutical Association Practical Guide to Natural Medicines. New York: William Morrow and Co, 1999.

Reynolds, J., ed. Martindale: The Extra Pharmacopoeia, 32nd ed. London: Royal Pharmaceutical Society of Great Britain, 1996.

Ritchason, J. The Little Herb Encyclopedia, 3rd ed. Pleasant Grove, Utah: Woodland Health Books, 1995.

Robbers, J.E., and Tyler, V.E. Tyler's Herbs of Choice: The Therapeutic Use of Phytomedicinals. Binghamton, NY: Haworth Herbal Press, 1999.

Robbers, J.E., et al. Pharmacognosy and Pharmacobiotechnology. Baltimore, Philadelphia: Williams & Wilkins, 1996.

Schulz, V., et al. Rational Phytotherapy: A Physician's Guide to Herbal Medicine, 3rd ed. Translated by Telger, T.C. Berlin: Springer, 1998.

Squier, T.B.B. Herbal Folk Medicine. New York: Henry Holt and Company, 1997.

Tyler, V.E. Herbs of Choice: The Therapeutic Use of Phytomedicinals, 2nd ed. Binghamton, NY: Pharmaceutical Press, 1999.

Tyler, V.E. Rational Phytotherapy. Berlin: Springer, 1998.

Wichtl, M.W. Herbal Drugs and Phytopharmaceuticals: A Handbook for Practice on a Scientific Basis, 2nd ed. Edited by Bisset, N.G. Stuttgart: Medpharm Scientific Publishers, 1994.

Wren, R.C., Wren, R.W., Williamson, E.M., and Evans, F.J. Potter's New Cyclopaedia of Botanical Drugs and Preparations. Saffron Waldron, Essex, England: C.W. Daniel Company Ltd, 1988.

# Herbal resource list

**Alternative Medicine**
www.alternativemedicine.com
Burton Goldberg
1650 Tiburon Blvd., Suite 2
Tiburon, CA 94920
Phone (800) 515-4325

**American Botanical Council**
www.herbalgram.org
P.O. Box 144345
Austin, TX 78714-4345
Phone (512) 926-4900

**American Herbal Pharmacopoeia**
www.herbal-ahp.org
Box 5159
Santa Cruz, CA 95063
Phone (831) 461-6317

**American Holistic Health Association**
www.ahha.org
P.O. Box 17400
Anaheim, CA 92817-7400
Phone (714) 779-6152

**Association of Natural Medicine
Pharmacists**
www.anmp.org
P.O. Box 150727
San Rafael, CA 94915-0727
Phone (415) 453-3534

**Botanical Society of America**
www.botany.org
Office of Publications
1735 Neil Avenue
Columbus, OH 43210-1293
Phone (614) 292-3519

**Centers for Disease Control and
Prevention**
www.cdc.gov
1600 Clifton Road
Atlanta, GA 30333
Phone (404) 639-3311

**Healthy Alternatives**
www.health-alt.com
4532 W. Kennedy Blvd. #312
Tampa, FL 33609-3042

**Herb Research Foundation**
www.herbs.org
1007 Pearl Street, Suite 200
Boulder, CO 80302
Phone (800) 748-2617 or (303) 449-
2265

**Office of Dietary Supplements**
http://ods.od.nih.gov
National Institutes of Health
Building 31, Room 1B29
31 Center Drive, MSC 2086
Bethesda, MD 20892-2086
Phone (301) 435-2920

**MedHerb.com**
www.medherb.com
Editor: Paul Bergner
P.O. Box 20512
Boulder, CO 80308

**National Center for Homeopathy**
www.homeopathic.org
801 N. Fairfax Street, Suite 306
Alexandria, VA 22314
Phone (877) 624-0613 or (703) 548-
7790

**Rosenthal Center for Complementary
and Alternative Medicine**
http://cpmcnet.columbia.edu/dept/rosen-
thal
Columbia University, College of
Physicians and Surgeons
630 W. 168th Street
P.O. Box 75
New York, NY 10032
Phone (212) 543-9542

**The Special Nutritionals Adverse Event Monitoring System**
http://vm.cfsan.fda.gov/~dms/aems.html
United States Food and Drug
   Administration
Center for Food Safety and Applied
   Nutrition
200 C Street, SW
Washington, DC 20204
Phone (888) SAFEFOOD (723-3366)

**United States Department of Agriculture**
www.usda.gov/welcome.html
14th and Independence Avenue, SW
Washington, DC 20250
Phone (202) 720-2791

**abortifacient** A substance capable of inducing a miscarriage.

**adaptogen** A substance used to strengthen the body and increase resistance to disease.

**alkaloid** A substance found in plants that acts like a drug in the body. Examples include caffeine, morphine, nicotine, quinine, and strychnine. The term also applies to synthetic substances whose structures resemble that of plant alkaloids.

**antioxidant** A substance such as vitamin E that works alone or in a group to destroy disease-causing substances called free radicals.

**astringent** A substance that causes tissues to contract. It's usually used locally, as on the skin.

**Ayurvedic medicine** The ancient traditional Indian system of medicine based on Hindu philosophy. This system shares some fundamental concepts with traditional Chinese medicine: the interconnectedness of body, mind, and spirit; the belief that the cosmos is composed of five basic elements (earth, air, fire, water, and space); and the belief in a human energy field that must be kept in balance to maintain health. Ayurvedic medicine also emphasizes the importance of a person's metabolic body type *(dosha)* in determining his health, personality, and susceptibility to disease.

**binder** A substance added to a drug or herbal product to hold together the product's ingredients.

**bioflavonoid** One of a group of naturally occurring plant compounds needed to strengthen tiny blood vessels called capillaries. Some researchers believe bioflavonoids may help protect against cancer and infection.

**biomedicine** A system of medicine based on the principles of the natural sciences.

**bitter** A preparation often used to promote appetite or digestion.

**carminative** A preparation used to relieve intestinal gas.

**catarrh** Inflammation of the air passages of the nose, throat, and lungs.

**Chinese medicine, traditional** A sophisticated, complex health care system based on the belief that good health depends largely on a person's lifestyle, thoughts, and emotions. It has expanded over the centuries to embrace many theories, methods, and approaches. The cornerstone of traditional Chinese medicine, which evolved from Taoism, Confucianism, and Buddhism, is the concept of *qi,* defined as a vital life force, or energy, that flows through the body along channels called meridians.

**cholagogue** A preparation that stimulates the flow of bile from the gallbladder.

**choleretic** A preparation that stimulates the production of bile.

**Commission E** A government committee in Germany that evaluates and reviews the safety and effectiveness of herbal products.

**decoction** A drug or other substance prepared by boiling.

**Doctrine of Signatures** In herbal medicine, the archaic method of determining which plants should be used for which ailments, based on the plant's resemblance to the ailment—for example, heart-shaped leaves for heart conditions and plants with red flowers for bleeding disorders.

**dram** A unit of weight equivalent to 1/8 ounce or 60 grains.

**elixir** A mixture of a drug or herb, alcohol, water, and sugar.

**emmenagogue** A preparation that stimulates menstrual flow.

**essential oil** A naturally occurring pure oil obtained from distillation of a plant.

**extract** A concentrate prepared by extracting—that is, removing all or nearly all of the solvent and adjusting the residual amount to a prescribed standard. Most extracts are solutions of essential constituents of a plant or other complex material placed in alcohol.

**free radical** A molecule containing an odd number of electrons. Some researchers believe free radicals may play a role in cancer development by interacting with DNA (the cell's genetic material) and impairing normal cell function.

**glycerite** A solution or mixture of a medicinal substance in glycerin. Usually sweet to the taste and warm on the tongue, glycerites are an alternative to alcohol extracts and better suited to some people.

**glycoside** An active component in plants that yields sugars when it decomposes.

**herbal medicine** The use of plants for healing purposes, dating back to the ancient cultures of Egypt, China, and India, and possibly even prehistoric times. Today, more than a quarter of conventional drugs are derived from herbs and about 80% of the world's population uses herbal remedies.

**homeopathy** A method of healing in which minute amounts of a substance that causes symptoms in a healthy person are given to a sick person to cure the same symptoms. Homeopathic remedies are thought to stimulate the body's ability to heal itself.

**infusion** A method of making an herbal tea in which a dried herb is steeped in hot water for 3 to 5 minutes before drinking.

**inhalation treatment** A type of herbal treatment used mainly to open congested sinuses and lung passages, help discharge mucus, and ease breathing. In one inhalation method, 2 to 5 drops of an herbal oil are placed in a sink filled with very hot water; the steam is then inhaled for 5 minutes. In another method, dried or fresh herbs (or an aromatic oil) are added to a large pot of hot water, which is then brought to a boil, allowed to simmer for 5 minutes, and removed from the heat to cool. Then the person drapes a towel over his head to form a tent, leans over the pot, and inhales the steam for 5 minutes.

**naturopathy** An alternative system of medical practice that combines a mainstream understanding of human physiology and disease with alternative remedies, such as herbal and nutritional therapies, acupuncture, hydrotherapy, and counseling. Naturopathic practitioners favor natural treatments aimed at stimulating the body's own healing ability over drugs and surgery.

**pharmacognosy**  The study of the natural sources of drugs, such as plants, animals, and minerals and their products.

**phytomedicine**  Herbal medicine.

**phytotherapy**  Treatment by use of plants.

**poultice**  A moist paste made from crushed herbs that's applied directly to the affected area or wrapped in cloth and then applied.

**purgative**  A substance that causes bowel evacuation.

**rhizome**  A plant's underground stem, commonly thickened by deposits of reserve food material, that produces shoots above and roots below. Unlike a true root, a rhizome typically has buds, nodes, and (usually) scalelike leaves.

**spirit**  A volatile liquid, especially one that has been distilled; a volatile substance dissolved in alcohol.

**stomachic**  A preparation that improves appetite and digestion.

**tincture**  A liquid preparation that contains a drug or herb and alcohol (alcoholic solution) or a drug or herb, alcohol, and water (hydroalcoholic solution).

**tonic**  A drug or herb that restores, invigorates, refreshes, or stimulates.

**tuberous root**  A thick, fleshy storage root that lacks buds or scale leaves.

**volatile oil**  An oil that evaporates quickly. (In contrast, a fixed oil, such as castor oil or olive oil, doesn't easily evaporate.) Volatile oils occur in aromatic plants, giving them odor and other characteristics. Examples include peppermint, spearmint, and juniper. Also called distilled oil or essential oil.

# Index

# B

# R